The International Review of Child Neurology

Brain Tumors in Children
Principles of Diagnosis and Treatment

Second Edition

The International Review of Child Neurology

The International Review of Child Neurology

Brain Tumors in Children

Principles of Diagnosis and Treatment

Second Edition

Michael E. Cohen, M.D.

Chairman, Department of Neurology
Professor of Neurology and Pediatrics
State University of New York at Buffalo
School of Medicine and Biomedical Sciences
Buffalo, New York

Patricia K. Duffner, M.D.

Professor of Neurology and Pediatrics
State University of New York at Buffalo
School of Medicine and Biomedical Sciences
Buffalo, New York

Raven Press New York

Raven Press, Ltd., 1185 Avenue of the Americas, New York, New York 10036

Made in the United States of America

Library of Congress Cataloging-in-Publication Data

Cohen, Michael E., 1937–
Brain tumors in children : principles of diagnosis and treatment / Michael E. Cohen, Patricia Kressel Duffner. — 2nd ed.
p. cm. — (The International Review of Child Neurology)
Includes bibliographical references and index.
ISBN 0-7817-0064-7
1. Brain—Tumors. 2. Tumors in children I. Duffner, Patricia Kressel. II. Title. III. Series.
[DNLM: 1. Brain Neoplasms—in infancy and childhood. WL 358 C678b 1994]
RC280.B7C55 1994
618.92´99481—dc20
DNLM/DLC
for Library of Congress

93-34357
CIP

The material contained in this volume was submitted as previously unpublished material, except in the instances in which credit has been given to the source from which some of the illustrative material was derived.

Great care has been taken to maintain the accuracy of the information contained in the volume. However, neither Raven Press nor the editors can be held responsible for errors or for any consequences arising from the use of the information contained herein.

9 8 7 6 5 4 3 2

This is a facsimile of the original edition. All material contained in the original is included in this edition.

". . . if I had my choice between a moon-walk
and the life of a single child with leukemia—
I would never glance upward!"

James T. Grace Jr., M.D.
Director, Roswell Park
Cancer Institute
1967–1970

"Praise is well, compliment is well, but affection—that is the last and final and most precious reward that any man can find."

Mark Twain

To Joan and my daughters Shari, Pamela,
and Nancy for their forbearance,
encouragement, and love.

MEC

To my husband John for his insightful help
in the preparation of this manuscript,
his constant support, and his love.

PKD

Contents

Diagnosis and Management of Common Intracranial Tumors of Childhood

Complications

Contributors

Jeffrey C. Allen, M.D. *Associate Professor of Neurology and Pediatrics, Departments of Neurology and Pediatrics, New York University Medical Center, New York, New York*

Martin L. Brecher, M.D. *Associate Professor of Pediatrics, State University of New York at Buffalo, School of Medicine and Biomedical Sciences, Chairman, Department of Pediatrics, Roswell Park Cancer Institute and Chief, Division of Hematology-Oncology, Children's Hospital of Buffalo, Buffalo, New York*

Michael E. Cohen, M.D. *Chairman, Department of Neurology and Professor of Neurology and Pediatrics, State University of New York at Buffalo, School of Medicine and Biomedical Sciences, and the Children's Hospital of Buffalo, Buffalo, New York*

Patricia K. Duffner, M.D. *Professor of Neurology and Pediatrics, State University of New York at Buffalo, School of Medicine and Biomedical Sciences, Department of Neurology, Children's Hospital of Buffalo, Buffalo, New York*

Michael S. B. Edwards, M.D. *Professor, Department of Neurosurgery, University of California at San Francisco, San Francisco, California*

Steven J. Greenberg, M.D. *Assistant Professor of Neurology, State University of New York at Buffalo, School of Medicine and Biomedical Sciences, Chief, Neuro-Oncology, Roswell Park Cancer Institute, Buffalo, New York*

Roberta Hayes, Ph.D. *Assistant Professor of Neurosurgery, Department of Neurosurgery, New York University Medical Center, New York, New York*

Reid R. Heffner, Jr., M.D. *Professor of Pathology, State University of New York at Buffalo, School of Medicine and Biomedical Sciences, Buffalo, New York*

Larry E. Kun, M.D. *Professor and Chairman, Department of Radiation Oncology, University of Tennessee Medical School, St. Jude Children's Research Hospital, Memphis, Tennessee*

Daniel J. Lacey, M.D. *Associate Professor of Neurology, Wayne State University, Dayton, Ohio*

Alan Leviton, M.D. *Associate Professor of Neurology, Harvard Medical School, Director, Neuroepidemiology Unit, Children's Hospital Medical Center, Boston, Massachusetts*

Adam N. Mamelak, M.D. *Clinical Instructor, Department of Neurosurgery, University of California at San Francisco, San Francisco, California*

Foreword

The International Child Neurology Association (ICNA) is pleased to present the second edition of *Brain Tumors in Children: Principles of Diagnosis and Treatment* as one of its continuing series in the International Review of Child Neurology.

ICNA was founded in 1973 for the purpose of improving the quality of care of children with neurological disorders.

Because of modern imaging techniques and new, increasingly successful modalities of treatment, brain tumors in children require, more than ever, collaboration between child neurologists, neurosurgeons, and oncologists. This book will forward knowledge in the area to all involved in the management of these children.

Peter G. Procopis

Foreword

Children with brain tumors are among the most difficult and challenging patients seen by health-care professionals, due to both the frequent inadequacies of current therapy and the failure of many hospitals to provide multidisciplinary pediatric care. However, the years since publication of the first edition of this book have seen major advances in the approach to children with brain tumors. Drs. Cohen and Duffner, major leaders and participants in these developments, have a vantage point few other physicians share, and this second edition of *Brain Tumors in Children* eloquently addresses the therapeutic successes and limitations as well as the evolving concept of true multidisciplinary care seen in the therapy of children with these tumors.

The care of a child with a newly diagnosed brain tumor requires expertise distinct from the domain of most clinicians. The opening chapters of this book clearly define the roles of experts in pediatric neurology, pediatric neurosurgery, pediatric neuropathology, pediatric neuroradiology, pediatric oncology, and pediatric radiation therapy in treating children with benign or malignant brain tumors. A greater awareness of this need among these experts has led to the development of multidisciplinary clinics and programs where all participants work as a team. Unfortunately, far too few children and negligible numbers of teenagers are ever referred to these centers, reflecting the lack of awareness by community institutions of the advantages to the child to have specialists in pediatric care. This new edition by Drs. Cohen and Duffner, with chapters written by experts in virtually all these specialties, will hopefully provide strong rationale for universal referral to center-based care.

The largest section of *Brain Tumors in Children* reviews the presentation, therapeutic approaches, and prognosis for children with a spectrum of central nervous system tumors. Progress in the treatment of children with medulloblastoma, ependymoma, and optic pathway tumors is well summarized, reflecting the benefits of multimodality therapy. Lest this book be considered overly optimistic, the virtual lack of progress in the treatment of children with diffuse pontine gliomas is also detailed. Perhaps the most exciting tale is the history and development of chemotherapy for the treatment of young children with brain tumors. Dr. Duffner's vantage point as the head of a multigroup (POG) effort in this area allows presentation of this exciting approach in a crisp and comprehensive format.

Unfortunately, survival is not the only consideration for children with brain tumors. The damage produced by the chosen therapeutic approach frequently is substantial, and survivors may need lifelong attention to endocrinologic, intellectual, and growth insults. Drs. Cohen and Duffner are particularly well-versed in this area, with many of the seminal observations in this field resulting from their own investigations.

Brain Tumors in Children, a welcome addition to pediatric neuro-oncology, illustrates the remarkable changes in the field since the first edition. Furthermore, the hope for further increases in survival with less long-term consequences for these children, building on current approaches but incorporating newer laboratory phenotypic and genotypic studies of pediatric brain tumors, is ever present in this text. One can only imagine what Drs. Cohen and Duffner will describe in their third edition.

Henry S. Friedman, M.D.
Professor, Department of Pediatrics
Duke Comprehensive Cancer Center
Durham, North Carolina

Preface

Since the first edition of this book was written, interest in the treatment of childhood brain tumors has burgeoned. Increasingly, groups of pediatric oncologists, radiation therapists, neurosurgeons, and neurologists devote either all or a large part of their professional lives to the treatment of children with cancer of the nervous system. Although a cure remains elusive, survival of children with certain types of brain tumors has been prolonged. For malignant tumors, more aggressive radiation and chemotherapy treatment regimens have been designed. Radiosurgery and brachytherapy provide high-dose, focused radiation to the tumor bed in patients with locally confined disease. In addition, hyperfractionated radiation, i.e., radiation delivered at least twice a day, is given in an effort to decrease radiation side effects while delivering high-dose radiation. Chemotherapy has also undergone changes. With the development of hematopoietic growth factors such as colony stimulating factors (i.e., GCSF and GMCSF) and interleukins, both the dose and frequency of administration of chemotherapy can be increased dramatically without compromising bone marrow function. In a similar vein, in some centers, autologous bone marrow rescue not only is being used for patients with recurrent disease but also is now a primary treatment modality in patients with a poor prognosis.

Paradoxically, although aggressive radiation and chemotherapy regimens characterize current treatment for the more malignant tumors, there has been a recent trend to withhold radiation for the more slowly growing and potentially benign tumors. These changes in the approach to children with brain tumors reflect concerns over treatment-induced neurotoxicity. Although there was a limited literature on late effects in the mid 1980s, since then a wealth of studies has been published on the intellectual abilities, endocrine function, and risks of oncogenesis and development of leukoencephalopathy in aggressively treated children with brain tumors. In those children in whom long-term survival is anticipated or in infants in whom radiation-induced neurotoxicity is severe, treatment has been modified accordingly. For example, whereas in the first edition of this book many authors advocated routine postoperative radiation for children with low-grade astrocytomas, these recommendations are now in question. Children with low-grade astrocytomas who have had a gross total resection are currently treated with supportive therapy alone rather than either postoperative radiation or chemotherapy. With regard to those children whose tumors have been subtotally resected, a randomized study is underway testing whether postoperative radiation offers an advantage over surgery alone. As with supratentorial tumors, there has been increasing acceptance that children with optic gliomas as well as pilocytic astrocytomas of the chiasm and hypothalamus may not require treatment until there is evidence of progressive disease. This approach has been possible due to the advent of noninvasive neuroimaging, which allows close monitoring of patients while eliminating the need to rush to judgment.

The approach to infants with malignant brain tumors has also radically changed since the first edition. In 1984, a pilot study was initiated to test whether prolonged postoperative chemotherapy could delay the need for radiation in infants with malignant brain tumors. Since then a group-wide Pediatric Oncology Group study has been completed, as have several smaller single-institution studies, which have proven the validity of this approach. Future trials will test whether radiation can be eliminated entirely in those young children who have no evidence of tumor following completion of chemotherapy. These encouraging results with chemotherapy as the primary postoperative treatment modality in infants with brain tumors have been extrapolated to older children. Studies in which the dose of radiation to the neuraxis is reduced in patients with chemosensitive tumors such as medulloblastomas and germinomas are now underway to determine whether survivals equivalent to standard radiation therapy can be achieved while simultaneously limiting radiation-induced neurotoxicity.

Increasingly, knowledge gained in the laboratory has been transferred to the clinical arena. Molecular biologic techniques are being used by the pathologist to define biologic behavior. Techniques such as flow cytometry, monoclonal technology, and immunocytochemistry are used to identify neoplastic potential. Many of these techniques are currently being used to target neoplastic cells with specific toxins and/or chemotherapeutic agents. Knowledge of oncogenes, tumor suppressor genes, antisense technology, and gene transfer techniques, as well as a host of other molecular biologic advances, should become part of the therapeutic armamentarium in the not too distant future. This, coupled with increasing knowledge of how to prevent chemotherapy resistance, augers well for the future. The decades of the 1970s and 1980s were characterized by advances in neuroimaging; the major breakthrough of the 1990s will belong to the cellular and molecular biologist.

Michael E. Cohen
Patricia K. Duffner

Acknowledgments

We gratefully acknowledge the perseverance, patience, and good humor of our administrative assistant, Linda A. Amaro. We thank Lucy Wargo, head librarian, and Brian Smistek and Timothy Palaszewski of the Audiovisual Department at the Children's Hospital of Buffalo.

Introduction

In the early part of the century most authors who wrote about childhood brain tumors were concerned with classification. Koos and Miller (16) alluded to this conundrum by quoting Bailey and Gustafson : "Classification must be considered as providing merely arbitrary pockets in which we can place tumors in order that they may be easily considered—no two gliomas are identical." Although this statement continues to be prophetic, the pathologist at the turn of the twenty-first century is increasingly reaching for newer techniques of molecular biology, immunocytochemistry, and flow cytometry to aid in establishing a diagnosis.

Earlier nosologies were based on the classification of Bailey and Cushing (2) published in 1926. Kernohan and coworkers (15) in 1949 introduced a grading classification from 1 to 4 for neuroectodermal tumors. The WHO classification simplifies this approach, calling grade 1 an astrocytoma, grades 2 and 3 malignant astrocytomas, and grade 4 glioblastoma multiforme. All medulloblastomas are considered to be malignant and are not graded but subclassified depending on unusual histologic features. Although we have classified pineal parenchymal tumors and germ-cell tumors together in the chapter on pineal region tumors, the WHO classifies tumors of this region separately (25). Primitive neuroectodermal tumors, like medulloblastomas, are classified under the rubric of embryonal tumors (14) (Table I-1).

The earlier edition of this book had suggested that the classification by Rorke (23) separating neuroectodermal tumors into five different categories might replace the traditional classification schemes. This has not proven to be the case, as most authorities have not been able to agree on the central tenet of Rorke's paper that primitive tumors arise from subependymal zones at all levels of the nervous system and differentiate along similar lines regardless of the site within the nervous system. This classification has been criticized precisely because of its failure to take into consideration the biologic variability within similar histologic groupings, variability in response to treatment, and propensity to occur in various sites within the neuraxis.

The incidence of brain tumors in children over the last several decades has been stable or slightly increasing (4). Intracranial tumors continue to represent the second most common neoplasm of childhood, exceeded only by leukemia. Throughout the world, the incidence of central nervous system neoplasia for children under 15 years of age is somewhere between 2 and 3 per 100,000. Thus, in the United States population of approximately 60 million black and white children under 15 years of age approximately 1200 to

Brain Tumors in Children: Principles of Diagnosis and Treatment, 2/e, edited by M.E. Cohen and P.K. Duffner, Raven Press, Ltd., New York, 1994.

TABLE I-1. *Brain tumor classification (adapted from WHO)*

Tumors of neuroepithelial tissue	Tumors of the meninges
Astrocytic tumors	*Tumors of meningothelial cells*
Astrocytoma	Meningioma
Variants: Fibrillary	Variants: Meningothelial
Protoplasmic	Fibrous (fibroblastic)
Gemistocytic	Transitional (mixed)
Anaplastic (malignant) astrocytoma	Psammamatous
Glioblastoma	Angiomatous
Variants: Giant cell gioblastoma	Microcystic
Gliosarcoma	Secretory
Pilocytic astrocytoma	Clear cell
Pleomorphic xanthoastrocytoma	Chordoid
Subependymal giant cell astrocytoma	Lymhoplasmacyte-rich
(Tuberous sclerosis)	Metaplastic
Oligodendroglial tumors	Atypical meningioma
Oligodendroglioma	Papillary meningioma
Anaplastic (malignant) oligodendroglioma	Anaplastic (malignant) meningioma
Ependymal tumors	*Germ cell tumors*
Ependymoma	Germinoma
Variants: Cellular	Embryonal carcinoma
Papillary	Yolk sac tumor (endodermal sinus tumor)
Clear cell	Choriocarcinoma
Anaplastic (malignant) ependymoma	Teratoma
Myxopapillary ependymoma	Immature
Subependymoma	Mature
Mixed gliomas	Teratoma with malignant transformation
Oligoastrocytoma	Mixed germ cell tumors
Anaplastic (malignant) oligoastrocytoma	
Others	
Choroid plexus tumors	
Choroid plexus papilloma	
Choroid plexus carcinoma	
Neuroepithelial tumors of uncertain origin	
Astroblastoma	
Polar spongioblastoma	
Gliomatosis cerebri	
Neuronal and mixed neuronal-glial tumors	
Gangliocytoma	
Dysplastic gangliocytoma of cerebellum	
(Lhermitte-Duclos)	
Desmoplastic infantile ganglioglioma	
Dysembryoplastic neuroepithelial tumor	
Ganglioglioma	
Anaplastic (malignant) ganglioglioma	
Central neurocytoma	
Paraganglioma of the filum terminale	
Olfactory neuroblastoma	
(Esthesioneuroblastoma)	
Variant: Olfactory neuroepithelioma	
Pineal parenchymal tumors	
Pineocytoma	
Pineoblastoma	
Mixed/transitional pineal tumors	
Embryonal tumors	
Medulloepithelioma	
Neuroblastoma	
Variant: Ganglioneuroblastoma	
Ependymoblastoma	
Primitive neuroectodermal tumors (PNET)	
Medulloblastoma	
Variants: Desmoplastic medulloblastoma	
Medullomyoblastoma	
Melanocytic medulloblastoma	

From Kleihues P, Burger PC, Scheithauer BW. *Histological typing of tumours of the central nervous system.* 2nd ed. New York: Springer-Verlag; 1993.

1500 cases of CNS neoplasms are diagnosed each year. Individual subtypes are correspondingly small. Unlike adults, metastases to the central nervous system from systemic cancers are uncommon and represent a small percentage of the total number of cancers found in the central nervous system of children under 15 years of age.

As has been pointed out in several reviews (4,13), mortality rates of children with cancer has declined from 2 per 100,000 per year to less than 0.9 per 100,000 per year, suggesting that 60% of children with CNS cancer may survive into adulthood. Approximately 50% of all central nervous system tumors in the United States are managed by physicians identified with the two major children's cancer consortiums in the United States, i.e., the Pediatric Oncology Group and the Children's Cancer Study Group (3). Improvement, as documented in previous work published in the early 1980s, has been correlated to some extent with where children receive their care. It is now well recognized that patients treated at comprehensive cancer centers fare better than those who are treated in their local community (6). These settings provide state-of-the-art pediatric facilities not available at medical centers remote from comprehensive cancer treatment sites.

Of all the Surveillance, Epidemiology, End Result (SEER) registries compiled by the National Cancer Institute, the one in Connecticut continues to be the best known. This registry, like all the SEER registries, has the advantage of mandatory reporting and yearly follow-up until death. Of 488 CNS tumors occurring in children in the state of Connecticut over a 39-year period, 467 were intracranial and 21 were spinal in location. Of this group, 28% were astrocytomas of all types and locations, 25% were medulloblastomas, 9% were ependymomas, 9% were craniopharyngiomas, and 9% were glioblastoma multiforme. Eleven other tumor types made up the remaining 20% (11). Unfortunately, this study does not strictly adhere to WHO categorization of brain tumors, thereby confusing the interpretation.

We had the opportunity to report the results of the incidence of brain tumors found in all of the SEER registries reported from 1979 to 1983. Eight hundred thirty-seven children with brain tumors were identified during this period. Of these, 25% were low-grade supratentorial astrocytomas, 23% were medulloblastomas, 12% cerebellar astrocytomas, 11% high-grade supratentorial astrocytomas, 9% brainstem gliomas, and 8% ependymomas. The ratio of males to females was 1.1 to 1. Survival rates of children with high-grade astrocytomas in the SEER study were surprisingly good when compared with the results reported for adults with similar tumors. Overall, 5-year survival for the six tumor types reported was approximately 57%. The best survival rates occurred in patients with cerebellar astrocytomas and the worst in those with brain stem gliomas (Fig. I-1) (18). As confirmed by multiple series, survival rates differed significantly with age. Children less than 2 years of age had significantly lower 5-year survival rates than older children (9). As pointed out in Chapter 20, it is unclear whether young children fare

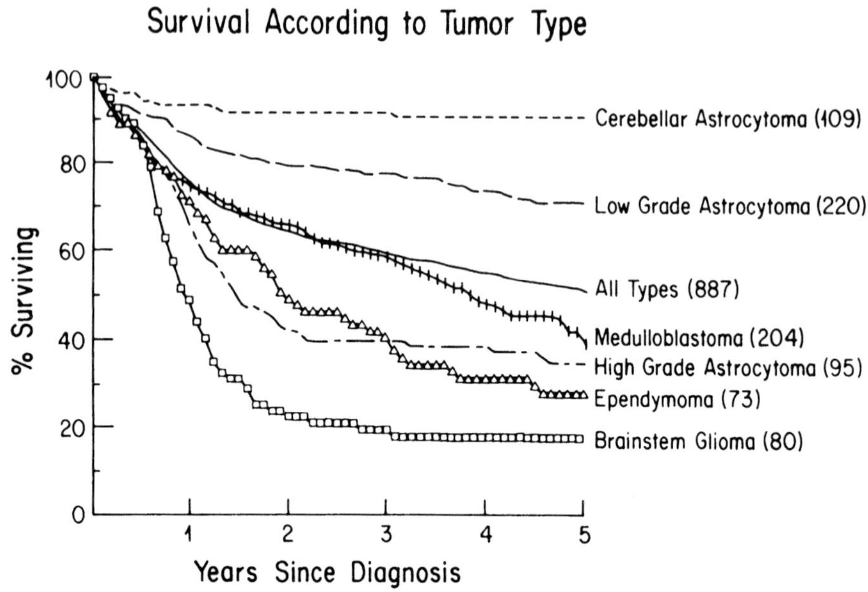

FIG. I-1. Survival rates of children according to tumor type.

worse because of high operative mortality, decreasing dosage of radiation, or the occurrence of a more malignant tumor biology.

Although the posterior fossa accounts for one-tenth of the intracranial volume, this anatomic site accounts for approximately 50 to 55% of tumors seen in childhood. During the first year of life the incidence between infratentorial and supratentorial tumors tends to be nearly equal. The incidence of infratentorial tumors is approximately 60% in the first decade of life and 40 to 45% in the second decade of life. Thereafter, the posterior fossa accounts for 25 to 30% of all intracranial tumors. In the Connecticut series, 62% were infratentorial in location; 47% were found in the cerebellum and 15% in the brain-stem. Medulloblastomas were slightly more common than cerebellar astrocytomas. Twenty-four percent were hemispheric, and 14% were located in the parasellar and chiasmatic regions (11).

For the most part, over a 30-year period the incidence of specific types of childhood brain tumors has not changed to any appreciable degree. The largest histologic grouping of CNS neoplasm is the astrocytoma, if one considers as one group astrocytomas occurring in all locations and of all grades. This cell type in most series makes up 40 to 50% of all tumors seen. Next in frequency is the medulloblastoma. Other histologic types account for the remainder of tumors. As can be seen in Table I-2, incidence figures for each tumor subtype have not varied significantly from series to series or from year to year (6,7,10,31). It is noteworthy that in those series from Western

TABLE I-2. *Incidence of childhood brain tumors in five large series*

	Craig et al., 1949		Matson, 1969		Koos and Miller, 1971		Farwell et al., 1977		Yates et al., 1979		Ertel, 1980		Duffner and Cohen et al., 1986	
	%	No.	%	No.	%	No.	%	No.	%	No.	%	No.	%	No.
Astrocytic[a]	41.3	158	49.5	372	36.7	257	42	198	45.9	316	45.2	192	57	504
Gangliogliomas	—	—	0.8	6	—	—	—	—	1.6	11	1.4	6	—	—
Oligodendrogliomas	—	—	0	0	1.4	10	1	6	0.7	5	—	—	—	—
Ependymomas	16.4	63	8.8	66	8.7	61	9	44	12.8	88	13.7	58	8	73
Medulloblastomas	22.4	86	18.5	139	17.1	120	25	117	16.3	112	10.6	45	23	204
Pineal area tumors	2.5	10	0.3	2	2.7	19	1	1	1.3	9	1.6	7	—	—
Teratomas (typical)	—	—	1.5	11	0.1	1	2	8	1.3	9	1.0	4	—	—
Craniopharyngiomas	6.8	23	9.1	68	8.8	58	9	42	6.0	41	9.8	42	—	—
Others	11.5	44	11.6	87	24.9	174	11	51	16.4	113	16.7	71	12	106
Total	384		751		700		467		704		425		887	

[a] The astrocytoma group includes all astrocytomas, glioblastoma multiforme, optic gliomas, spongioblastomas, and brain stem gliomas.

countries, teratomas and pineal area tumors represent a substantially smaller number of the total than those reported from Japan (see Chapter 16). These neoplasms, of all those considered, appear to have the greatest regional variability.

The etiology of most brain tumors remains obscure. Certain congenital rest tumors, such as dermoids and teratomas, presumably arise from errors in embryogenesis. It has been suggested that embryonic cells that persist either as a failure of migration or as a failure in differentiation may retain the ability to proliferate. This concept has been used to explain the neoplastic potential of meningiomas, medulloblastomas, craniopharyngiomas, and to a lesser extent that of hamartomas. Meningiomas are considered to arise from leptomeningeal rests, and medulloblastomas are thought to arise from retained elements of either the fetal granular layer of the cerebellum or the posterior medullary velum. The craniopharyngioma is thought to arise from retained elements of the primitive stomodeum and nasal pharyngeal duct. Although theoretically attractive, proof of this form of oncogenesis has not been forthcoming.

Several well-defined hereditary and familial syndromes are associated with CNS neoplasia. Again, the etiology remains obscure, but the genetic nature of the association is unchallenged. Neurofibromatosis, tuberous sclerosis, von Hippel-Lindau disease, and retinoblastoma are all autosomal dominant illnesses associated in varying degrees with tumors of the CNS. A less clear-cut association with brain tumors exists with Turcot's syndrome, nevoid basal cell syndrome, Wiskott-Aldrich syndrome, and ataxia telangiectasia (28). The neoplasms associated with these illnesses will be mentioned later in the volume only in relationship to the specific tumor discussed.

Of all the inherited syndromes, neurofibromatosis may provide the most information regarding oncogenesis. In the last several years NF1 has been associated with deletion of a gene on the long arm of chromosome 17 and NF2 with chromosome 22 (12). The propensity of this illness to present with a diversity and multiplicity of intracranial tumors and the ability of neurofibromas to produce local hypertrophy of bone, skin, and muscle suggests the presence of a substance capable of initiating and promoting unrestrained tissue growth. However, there is also a suggestion that a process exists that, although capable of initiating and promoting tissue growth, is also associated with factors that act to contain unrestricted growth as most neurofibromas are benign and are a limited threat to life. Despite this caveat, the patient with neurofibromatosis is at risk for the development of intracranial tumors. When intracranial tumors do arise there is some suggestion, again by no means conclusive, that these tumors may act in a more benign fashion from that of a similar tumor occurring in a patient without neurofibromatosis.

A host of implied but not proven environmental factors have been implicated in the pathogenesis of brain tumors. MacMahon (17), for instance, has suggested that cancer mortality was 40% higher in children exposed prenatally to x rays than in those not so exposed. The study of Modan et al. (20) on the increased incidence of meningiomas in patients receiving radiation for tinea capitis has become a classic (see Chapter 23).

It is well accepted that immunosuppressed patients are more apt to develop neoplasia. This has been identified in patients with ataxia telangiectasia and in those patients with the Wiskott-Aldrich syndrome. Similarly, the risk of intracranial reticulum cell sarcomas and lymphomas in immunosuppressed patients receiving renal transplants is well documented (27). The risk for the development of lymphoma after transplantation persists for as long as 5 years, and is greatest in those individuals over 40 years of age, or less than 20 years of age, at the time of transplantation. Although viral, chemical, and physical agents are known to produce CNS neoplasms in experimental animals, the relationship of environmental agents to the development of tumors in humans has not been established. Chapter 2, on epidemiology, has been expanded to explore some of these concepts.

Regardless of histologic type or grade, tumors of the CNS produce symptoms in many different ways. Symptoms may arise from either direct effects of tumors on neural tissue, secondary effects associated with interference of anatomic pathways, or an indirect effect resulting from increased intracranial pressure. Thus, not only does the biology and location of the tumor affect the choice of treatment, but treatment is also influenced by the manner in which the tumor is clinically expressed (26). Currently, cerebellar astrocytomas, subependymal giant cell tumors, craniopharyngiomas, and the occasional extra-axial neuroma may be treated with surgery alone. Medulloblastomas, ependymomas, brain stem gliomas, glioblastomas, anaplastic astrocytomas, germinomas, mixed gliomas, and primitive neuroectodermal tumors are best treated with combinations of surgery, radiation, and possibly chemotherapy (18).

Although surgery, in most cases, cannot be expected to be associated with a cure, if radiation or chemotherapy is to be effective, the tumor to be treated should be as small as possible. Presumably, radiation and chemotherapy exert their effect by a log kill hypothesis. That is, a given fraction of cells will be destroyed by a given dose of the agent to be employed. Thus, although the fraction of cells destroyed may be the same, quantitative destruction of the tumor depends on the number of tumor cells present. Whenever aggressive therapy is anticipated, surgical debulking should be considered. Chapter 4 will further explore these concepts.

Ionizing radiation produces cell damage by either indirect or direct effects on the cell nucleus. The transfer of energy induced by radiation results in damage to the DNA and RNA of cells. The end result of these events is inevitably cell death or sublethal damage to the cell. Depending on subsequent events, sublethal damage results in either death to the cell or subsequent repair. Cell viability after radiation follows an exponential curve. The fraction of cells destroyed is independent of the number of cells radiated, but, as in chemotherapy, the absolute number varies with the initial number of cells present. In general, although all cells are sensitive to radiation, sensitivity is related directly to mitotic activity in those cells entering a proliferating phase. Because most brain tumors are not undergoing active reproduction, relatively large doses of radiation are necessary to destroy these tumors (19,22,29). The radiation dosages for most tumors of the central nervous system range from 4500 to 5500 cGy given in doses of 180 per fraction over a 5- to 6-week period. The timing, dosage, and extent of radiation are in a constant state of reexamination. Controversies involving dosage, volume, and schedules of dosage are discussed in Chapter 5, on radiotherapy, as well as in the chapters devoted to the treatment of individual tumors.

As with surgery and radiation, chemotherapy is an increasingly accepted adjunct to treatment. Chemotherapy adds a dimension to the treatment of disease apart from the surgical or radiation fields. Although short-term complications from chemotherapy may be as great as or more hazardous than radiotherapy, long-term effects do not appear to be as onerous (1). Because most brain tumors have a low mitotic index, chemotherapeutic agents should be effective at any stage in the life of the cell. Cell-cycle-specific agents exert their effect only during proliferation. Other agents, cell-cycle-nonspecific drugs, act during all stages in the life of the cell. In addition to cell-cycle considerations, pharmacological effects that influence penetration into the nervous system must be considered. Chemotherapeutic agents that might be effective when given systemically may have limited effects on intracranial neoplasms because of their inability to gain access to the CNS (21,24). Properties that influence transport of a drug into the CNS include low molecular weight, high lipid solubility, nonionizing at a physiologic pH, and lack of plasma protein binding.

Complicating the concept of chemotherapy is the area of "brain adjacent tumor" (Fig. I-2). Malignant cells migrating from the center of a necrotic tumor (where the blood–brain barrier is altered) into the periphery of normal brain adjacent to the tumor may be the most viable, have the greatest capacity for proliferation, and, because of the intact blood–brain barrier, be the most inaccessible to treatment. Thus, location of tumor, rate of growth, mitotic index, and rate of entrance of drugs into the nervous system all influence the choice of agents and the route of administration.

Drug protocols are based on the efficacy of the known agents to be employed, the synergisms or additive effects of one agent with the other, and the ability of a particular drug to enter the CNS. The route of administration, the dosage intervals, and the length of duration of chemotherapy are by and large developed either by cancer consortiums or by a single oncologist. Unfortunately, no clear-cut rules guide the development of chemotherapeu-

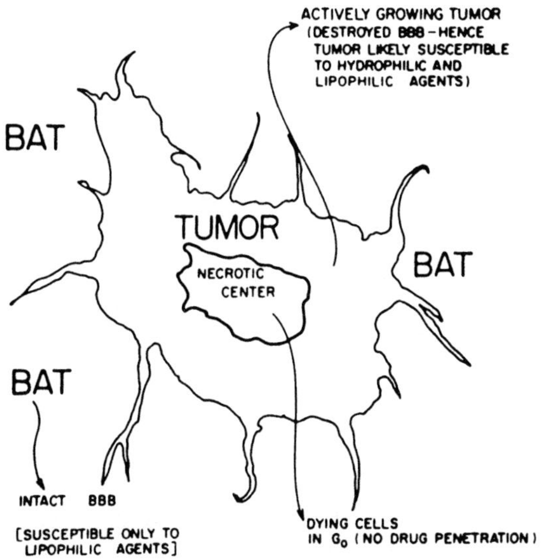

FIG. I-2. The relationship of a brain tumor to the blood–brain barrier.

tic protocols. The choice and use of chemotherapeutic agents will be explored in the chapter on principles of chemotherapy.

A chapter has been added to this edition which explores the increasing sophistication of pathologists in identifying the nature, extent, and proliferative capacity of brain tumors (Chapter 3). In addition, new information on the clinical and basic concepts of immunotherapy and molecular biology are explored in Chapters 7 and 8.

In considering approaches to treatment, the quality of life after treatment with either surgery, radiation and/or chemotherapy must constantly be assessed. Intellectual deficits caused by high-dose radiation were long suspected and are now proven. Leukoencephalopathy, endocrinopathies, and vasculopathies, among others, are increasingly being associated with high-dose radiation (5,8) and chemotherapy. The long-term pathologic and clinical effects of the current approaches to treatment are discussed in Chapters 22 and 23.

Over the 9 years since this book was first published, great changes have come about in the treatment of children with brain tumors. For the most part, these changes have resulted in prolonged survival rather than cures. An increasing understanding of the biology of cancer, application of molecular genetic techniques, the use of new radiation techniques, and changing methodology designed to alter chemotherapy resistance should, by the turn of the century, impact dramatically on survival rates of children with brain tumors.

REFERENCES

1. Allen JC. The effects of cancer therapy on the nervous system. *J Pediatr* 1978;93:903–909.
2. Bailey P, Cushing H. In: *A classification of the tumors of the glioma group on a histogenetic basis with a correlated study of prognosis.* Philadelphia: JB Lippincott; 1926.
3. Boyett JM, Vietti TJ. Role of clinical trials and cooperative group studies in cancers in children. *Cancer* 1985;56:1984–1986.
4. Cancer Statistics Review, 1973–1986, Division of Cancer Control and Prevention Surveillance Program, National Cancer Institute, Bethesda, MD, 1989.
5. Cohen ME, Duffner PK. Long-term consequences of CNS treatment for childhood cancer. I: Pathologic consequences and potential for oncogenesis. *Pediatr Neurol* 1991;7:157–163.
6. Cohen ME, Duffner PK, Tebbe CK. Brain tumors in children: diagnosis and management. In: Tebbe CK, ed. *Major topics in pediatric and adolescent oncology.* Boston: CK Hall; 1982: 240–289.
7. Craig WM, Keith HM, Kernohan JW. Tumors of the brain occurring in childhood. *Acta Psychiatr Neurol Scand* 1949;24:375–390.
8. Duffner PK, Cohen ME. Long-term consequences of CNS treatment for childhood cancer. II: Clinical consequences. *Pediatr Neurol* 1991;7:237–242.
9. Duffner PK, Cohen ME, Myers MH, Heise HW. Survival of children with brain tumors: SEER Program, 1973–1980. *Neurology* 1986;36:597–601.
10. Ertel IJ. Brain tumors in children. *Cancer* 1980;30:306–321.
11. Farwell JR, Dohrman GJ, Flannery JT. Central nervous system tumors in children. *Cancer* 1977;40:3123–3132.
12. Goldgar DE, Green P, Parry DM, Mulvihill JJ. Multipoint linkage analysis in neurofibromatosis type I: an international collaboration. *Am J Hum Genet* 1989;44:6–12.
13. Janisch W, Haas JF. Epidemiologic investigations on brain tumors in the GDR: possibilities and limits. *Arch Geschwulstforsch 1984;54:243–247.*
14. Kleihues P, Burger PC, Scheithauer BW. *Histological typing of tumours of the central nervous system.* 2nd ed. New York: Springer-Verlag; 1993.
15. Kernohan JW, Mabon RF, Svien HJ, Adson AW. Symposium on a new and simplified concept of gliomas (a simplified classification of gliomas). *Proc Mayo Clin* 1949;24:71–75.
16. Koos W Th, Miller M. *Intracranial tumors of infants and children.* St Louis: CV Mosby; 1971:11.
17. MacMahon B. Prenatal x-ray exposure and childhood cancer. *J Natl Cancer Inst* 1962;28: 1173–1191.
18. Matson DD. *Neurosurgery of infancy and childhood.* Springfield, IL: Charles C Thomas; 1969:406.
19. Mincer F, Meltzer J, Botstein C. Pinealoma: a report of twelve irradiated cases. *Cancer* 1976;37:2713–2718.
20. Modan B, Baidatz H, Mart R, Steinitz R, Levin JG. Radiation induced head and neck tumors. *Lancet* 1974;1:277–279.
21. Norrell H, Wilson C. Brain tumor chemotherapy with methotrexate given intrathecally. *JAMA* 1967;201:15–17.
22. Perez CA. Basic concepts and clinical implications of radiation therapy. In: Sutow WW, Vietti TJ, Fernbach DJ, eds. *Clinical pediatric oncology.* St Louis: CV Mosby; 1977: 139–181.
23. Rorke LB. The cerebellar medulloblastoma and its relationship to primitive neuroectodermal tumors. *J Exp Neuropathol Exp Neurol* 1983;42:1–15.
24. Rosenblum M, Reynolds AF, Smith KA. CCNU in the treatment of malignant brain tumors. *J Neurosurg* 1973;39:306–314.
25. Rubinstein LJ. In: *Tumors of the central nervous system.* Washington DC: Armed Forces Institute of Pathology; 1972:104–126.
26. Russell DS, Rubinstein LJ. *Pathology of tumors of the nervous system.* 4th ed. London: Edward Arnold; 1989.
27. Schneck SA, Penn I. De-novo brain tumors in renal transplant recipients. *Lancet* 1971;1: 983–986.
28. Shoenberg BS. Epidemiology of primary nervous system neoplasms. In: *Advances in neurology.* New York: Raven Press; 1978:475–495.

29. Sheline G. Radiation therapy of CNS tumors. *Cancer* [*Suppl*] 1975;35:957–964.
30. Wilson CB. Brain tumors. *Semin Oncol* 1975;2:5–7.
31. Yates AJ, Decker LE, Sachs LA. Brain tumors in childhood. *Childs Brain* 1979;5:31–39.
32. Young JL, Miller RW. Incidence of malignant tumors in US children. *J Pediatr* 1975;86: 254–258.
33. Zulch KJ. *Histological typing of tumors of the central nervous system*. Geneva: World Health Organization, 1979.

1

Principles of Diagnosis

CLINICAL FEATURES

Increased Intracranial Pressure

Signs and symptoms of brain tumors vary depending on location, the neurologic system with which the tumor interferes, and the age and development of the child. There are no pathognomonic features. Signs and symptomatology of a general nature without focal signature may reflect increased intracranial pressure. Pressure may result from a mass growing within a fixed volume or obstruction of spinal fluid pathways occurring within the limited volume of a relatively rigid cranial vault. Symptoms attributed to slowly developing intracranial pressure include irritability, lethargy, vomiting, anorexia, headache, and changes in behavior. Many of the tumors to be described are accompanied by unexplained changes in personality and behavior. It is well known that focal signs and symptoms may not be associated with focal disease. The abducens nerve, because of its long, free intracranial course and its proximity to bony structures, may become compromised with generalized increased intracranial pressure. Thus, the complaint of diplopia and the subsequent finding of an abducens paresis may not be lateralizing. Similarly, focal headache, ataxia, and changes in behavior may all reflect a generalized intracranial process.

The finding of papilledema should always suggest increased intracranial pressure and prompt a diligent search for its cause. In the small child, enlargement of the head or separation of cranial sutures suggests a space-occupying lesion. Visual loss and optic atrophy are a late manifestation of papilledema and may be uncommon in young children because of their expansible heads. When present, visual loss or optic atrophy implies either longstanding unrecognized pressure effects or focal pathology directly affecting the visual pathways. The earliest sign of papilledema is an increase in the cecal scotoma (blind spot) or loss of color vision (dyschromatopsia).

Because of early obstruction of the cerebrospinal fluid pathways, papilledema is more apt to be seen in tumors of the cerebellum. Early in their course, midline cerebellar tumors obstruct the outflow tract of the fourth ventricle, giving rise to obstructive hydrocephalus. Conversely, pontine tu-

---

Brain Tumors in Children: Principles of Diagnosis and Treatment, 2/e, edited by M.E. Cohen and P.K. Duffner, Raven Press, Ltd., New York, 1994.

mors, which are primarily found on the basal surface of the brain stem, are more likely to occlude the fourth ventricle late in their course. Cerebral hemispheric tumors tend to produce papilledema by mass effect rather than by obstruction of the ventricular pathways.

Other than a mild headache, chronic increased intracranial pressure usually produces few symptoms until the pressure rises high enough to impede cerebral circulation. Acute changes in intracranial pressure, unlike chronic pressure, have the potential for producing dynamic changes within the head. Intracranial mass lesions may produce pressure gradients between intracranial compartments and thus give rise to three herniation syndromes, i.e., uncal, transtentorial, and falcial herniation (16). MacEwen (14) was the first to comment on the pupillary signs associated with herniation of the medial aspect of the temporal lobe through the incisura of the tentorium. Uncal herniation occurs when a lateralized mass in the frontal or temporal lobe causes a shift of structures through the tentorial notch into the midbrain. The resultant effects consist of early meiosis followed by dilatation of the pupil secondary to compromise of the third cranial nerve as it is entrapped by the herniating uncus on the free edge of the tentorium. Compromise of the posterior circulation may produce visual symptoms. Compression of the cerebral peduncle by a herniating mass may give rise to contralateral hemiparesis. If the opposite peduncle becomes entrapped against the free edge of the contralateral tentorium (Kernohan's notch), ipsilateral rather than contralateral paresis may ensue (13). This whole syndrome may be followed by brain stem ischemia. The uncal syndrome may be followed rapidly by the bilateral brainstem features associated with a central herniation syndrome (16).

The central syndrome occurs more insidiously and is seen in patients with bilateral progressive involvement of the hemispheres or diencephalon. The first signs of the syndrome may be agitation, anxiety, or delirium followed by torpor, obtundation, and coma. Subsequently, a characteristic set of oculomotor, oculocephalic, oculovestibular, and respiratory responses occur. The pattern of responses depends on whether there is physiologic compromise at a diencephalic, mesencephalic, or medullary stage. Death is inevitable when the medullary stage is reached (16).

Cingulate herniation occurs when an expanding hemisphere results in shift of the cingulate gyrus under the falx cerebri. The major danger from this syndrome is vascular compromise of the anterior cerebral artery and the tissues that it serves. For a more comprehensive discussion of all three syndromes, a review of Plum and Posner (16) is suggested.

Posterior fossa lesions may lead to coma because of upward rather than downward shifts. Herniation of the superior vermis of the cerebellum through the tentorium may compromise midbrain diencephalic structures. Downward displacement may result in compression of the medulla. Both phenomena may interfere with the reticular formation, giving rise to alteration in levels of consciousness. With downward herniation, the cerebellar tonsils may project below the foramen magnum. This is associated with medullary compromise with subsequent respiratory and circulatory collapse. Early signs of tonsillar herniation may be head tilt and stiff neck. These signs presumably arise as a result of irritation of cervical roots by the herniating mass. Compromise of the fourth ventricle or aqueduct early in the course of a posterior fossa lesion leads to obstructive hydrocephalus and signs of increased intracranial pressure. Because most tumors are slowly evolving over weeks to months, accommodation to pressure shifts generally occurs. Herniation syndromes, when present, are usually mild and do not produce the dramatic consequences seen with more acute problems.

Nonlocalizing Signs and Symptoms

Symptoms characteristic of a brain tumor, but not specifically localizing, are vomiting, headache, and behavioral changes. These symptoms, either alone or in combination, are generally present. Because of the limited specificity associated with these symptoms, complaining children may be ignored for variable periods of time. Even then, when symptoms are brought to the attention of the unwary physician, appropriate investigation may not be initiated. Vomiting may occur with any tumor and is thought to be either secondary to generalized increased intracranial pressure or to result from direct irritation of the vagal nuclei or vomiting centers in the floor of the fourth ventricle. The vomiting may be cyclic in nature and thus passed off as a migraine equivalent or considered a functional complaint. Contrary to popular notion, vomiting associated with intracranial neoplasms does not tend to be projectile in nature. Vomiting may occur daily, usually in the early morning, and then be followed by a period of resolution. Initial symptoms may be attributed to a flu-like illness, but exacerbation of the vomiting, weeks to months later, reveals the true etiology. Abatement of the early signs of vomiting has been attributed to splitting of the intracranial sutures to accommodate the increased intracranial pressure.

Headache, although common, is an unreliable sign of tumor. Bailey et al. (1), in their book published in 1939, commented on the rarity of headache as a symptom in children and stated that when it occurs, it should suggest organic disease. Our experience has been quite the contrary. Head pain is perhaps the most common nonspecific complaint the child neurologist is asked to evaluate. This symptom, which cuts across all age groups, by itself does not herald organic disease. Most brain tumors will be clinically apparent within 4 to 6 months after the onset of head pain. Hence, clinical suspicion of a CNS neoplasm should be the greatest in a child with recent onset of headache (2,12). Location of the headache, although helpful, is certainly not pathognomonic. A headache associated with cerebellar tumors may be frontal or occipital. A focal headache, unlike a generalized headache, more likely implies organic disease and, in the absence of intracranial pressure, suggests pathology either underlying the point of head pain or a referral pattern of pain from a distant source.

Headache associated with brain tumors, as with vomiting, is more likely to occur in the early morning shortly after waking. The pain is usually mild, may occur daily, but is not protracted. The history of an increase in headache with coughing, sneezing, straining at stools, or other Valsalva type maneuvers, is a reliable but often unsolicited symptom of increased intracranial pressure. Unfortunately, this symptom is more apt to be seen in the adult or adolescent than in the young child. Because the brain parenchyma does not contain pain-bearing structures, complaints emanate from either irritation of pain fibers in the dura matter or in arterial blood vessels.

Changes in affect, energy level, motivation, or behavior are signs of abnormality more often seen in children than in adults. An early sign of CNS malfunction may be the tendency of a child to become indifferent to playmates or not want to continue previous activity. Most worrisome is the youngster who, previously a bundle of energy, becomes listless or uninterested. A change in behavior from one of unbridled energy to a more docile disposition may be the harbinger of unrecognized increased intracranial pressure. Changes in mentation, agitation, and even delirium are nonspecific signs that may herald the onset of intracranial disease. Anorexia, bulimia, weight loss or gain, somnolence, failure to thrive, sexual precocity, and/or symptoms of an autonomic nature may be nonspecific or suggest hypothalamic or pituitary dysfunction.

Signs and Symptoms of a Localizing Nature

Focal seizures, rarely an early sign of an intracranial mass, occur in less than 15% of patients with an intracranial lesion. This, in part, reflects the lower incidence of hemispheric lesions in children than in adults. Similarly, epilepsy is rarely the sine qua non of an intracranial mass. The vast majority of children with epilepsy of all types rarely have evidence of CNS neoplasia. In a study in which a CT scan was performed after an initial seizure, fewer than 1% of the patients had tumors (22). Similarly, Page et al. (15), in their review of gliomas heralded by epilepsy, stressed the rarity of this association. Nonetheless, they emphasized that alteration in behavior and school performance, changes in frequency and type of seizure, changes in the neurologic examination, and/or alterations in EEG patterns should warrant an investigation for occult neoplasm.

Visual complaints, either loss of vision or diplopia, may reflect either direct involvement of the visual axis or an indirect etiology. Complaints of visual loss are quite insidious, as most children are not aware of progressive loss of vision. This complaint may be brought to the attention of an unsuspecting parent following the failure of a school eye examination. Rarely, unless history is specifically elicited, will hemianopsias be identified. Secondary optic atrophy may occur as a result of longstanding papilledema.

Gaze paralysis is seen with brain stem lesions and is rarely found in lesions of the cerebral cortex. Nystagmus generally implies involvement of the vestibular complex and the brain stem. However, searching or pendular nystagmus may suggest visual difficulties. An erroneous diagnosis of congenital nystagmus has been associated with chiasmatic gliomas. Head tilt may occur in an effort to compensate for diplopia, or owing to cervical root irritation may reflect incipient cerebellar herniation.

Signs generally associated with supratentorial mass lesions reflect the area of the brain involved. Hemiparesis, hemisensory loss, and hemivisual defects suggest lateralized abnormalities in one of the cerebral hemispheres. Hemiparesis, rarely overt, is generally recognized by failure to use one side of the body, decreased arm swing, and a slight limp. Before 1 year of age, the history of the young child lateralizing hand use to one side suggests damage in the opposite hemisphere. Similarly, the change of handedness from one side to the other implies lateralized disease. Increasing awkwardness, failure to participate in sports, or reluctance to attend gym may suggest early motor involvement of a hemisphere. Sensory loss, when present, may be associated with parietal lobe dysfunction. Numbness, tingling, and loss of either protopathic or epicritic sensations is an uncommon complaint and rarely elicited.

Ataxia, long tract signs, and cranial neuropathies, usually without signs of pressure, suggest brain stem pathology. Classical brain stem syndromes, although described, are rarely encountered. Gait disturbances may suggest either a brain stem or cerebellar process. The child may have a history of incoordination, complaints of stiffness of gait, and increasing difficulty with hopping or running. Slightly bent posture with tightness of the hamstrings and a tendency to toe walk suggests bilateral corticospinal involvement. Examination reveals increased tone, hyperactive reflexes, and extensor plantar responses. Neuropathies involving specific cranial nerve nuclei or their axons localize the process to a specific area of the brain stem. Hypernasal speech, nasopharyngeal regurgitation, and dysarthria suggest either pseudobulbar or bulbar involvement.

Perhaps more than any other region of the brain, tumors of the cerebellum present in a specific way. Scanning speech, hypotonia, pendular reflexes, and appendicular or axial ataxia localize signs to either the cerebellar hemisphere or midline of the cerebellum. Slow, coarse nystagmus may be seen directed toward the hemisphere of involvement. Marked difficulty in walking or crawling, with limited problems in coordination when lying in bed, and little or no nystagmus, are the hallmarks of lesions in the cerebellar vermis. Truncal titubation, also a sign of vermis disease, is more apt to be seen with an infectious or metabolic etiology than with neoplasms.

Little can be added to Cushing's (4) characterization of the clinical course of a child with a cerebellar medulloblastoma. He graphically portrayed most of the clinical features seen with this tumor.

> A pre-adolescent child previously in good health begins to complain of headaches, or of sub-occipital discomfort and to have occasional attacks of vomiting without preliminary nausea, usually on first arising in the morning. Attendance at school meanwhile may continue but the teacher soon notices that the child is listless, inattentive, and the character of his work noticeably falls off. Ere long it is apparent that there is some unwanted clumsiness in movement and awkwardness in gait. The mother may find that the child quickly outgrows its caps and she thinks the head enlarges unduly fast. In course of time it is noticed, at home or in school, that the child's sight is impaired; or a beginning squint of one eye may be detected, even in the absence of any complaint of double vision. The family doctor, who has previously suspected some gastrointestinal disorder, may then have the eye grounds examined and to the surprise and shock of everyone a choked disc is found. Three or four months, on the average, have elapsed, and at about this stage of the malady many cases first come under hospital care.
>
> Should the condition not be recognized so soon, the symptoms relentlessly progress. The clumsiness increases until the gait gradually becomes so ataxic that walking without support is difficult, vomiting grows more frequent, the child begins to lose weight; the muscles become wasted and atonic; there may be a slight facial palsy; the internal squint may become bilateral and finally "fainting spells" occur, characterized by extensor rigidities that may be precipitated by slight change in position. Before this the child will have become bedridden. The whole story if uninterrupted by operation may cover a period averaging from eight to nine months.

This description described the usual course of a child with a cerebellar tumor from beginning to end. Initial manifestations are nonlocalizing features of changes in schoolwork, vomiting, enlarging head, and diplopia. This is followed by signs suggesting a midline cerebellar syndrome. Terminally, tonsillar herniation results with the development of "cerebellar fits" or more probably decerebrate rigidity. This written account of the course of a cerebellar tumor is still the most vivid one in the literature.

Thus, the overview of a child with a brain tumor is one of a youngster who, previously in good health, begins to evidence some minor behavior changes. This may lead to alterations in playtime activity, school behavior, and interpersonal relations. After this, nonspecific signs of increased intracranial pressure may develop. These signs are followed by more specific lateralizing signs, relative to an abnormality of either the posterior fossa, the brain stem, or the cerebral hemispheres. Because of the rarity of brain tumors, i.e., 2.4 per 100,000, the average pediatrician or family practitioner is apt to see few such problems in a lifetime of practice. Therefore, the physician must be ever wary and vigilant. Today, as never before, early diagnosis and prompt treatment offer the potential for cure and a good quality of life.

DIAGNOSTIC STUDIES

In the late 1920s and 1930s, electroencephalography (EEG), because of its ability to record the electrical rhythms of the brain, was heralded as a major diagnostic tool. Clinicians and physiologists alike believed that the EEG would provide an understanding of the neurophysiology of the nervous system, and this in turn would have a great diagnostic impact. Unfortunately, EEGs have not fulfilled their earlier promise of being an electrophysiologic tool capable of identifying functional and localized defects of the central nervous system. At best, EEG provides information concerning paroxysmal disorders and suggests focal or generalized abnormalities of cerebral rhythms. At worst, EEG may provide confusing and uninterpretable information. No specific patterns or electrical abnormalities allow differentiation of tumors from metabolic or vascular pathology. The findings of nonlocalizing polymorphic delta, depression of alpha rhythms, absence of sigma waves during sleep, and diffuse theta delta bursts may be compatible with intracranial neoplasms. The nonspecificity of these findings in the individual patient requires additional confirmation and further evaluation. Perhaps this is as it should be, since the EEG suggests functional rather than anatomical disturbances. With the advent of sophisticated computer technology, the assessment of electrical disturbances of the brain may provide better understanding of the functional results of tumor removal and treatment on normal brain. Evoked potentials, topographic analysis, and brain electrical activity mapping techniques have yet to reach their full potential (9,11,19).

Unlike EEG, air encephalography, introduced in the late 1920s and used through the latter part of the 1970s, provided a major diagnostic tool in assessing intracranial pathology. Air was introduced through either the lumbar theca or the lateral ventricles. Air encephalography was not nearly as complex in concept or design as the electroencephalogram, and replacement of the cerebrospinal fluid by air provided considerably more anatomic information. This technique, invasive by design, was potentially hazardous. Despite these misgivings, until the advent of computed tomography (CT), air contrast studies remained the most reliable method of assessing abnormalities of the posterior fossa or midline structures of the brain.

Arteriography, although no longer used extensively, continues to play an important role in diagnosis. This modality defines the vascular supply of the tumor and its primary feeding vessels. New vessel formation and the vascularity of the tumor provides information regarding the malignant nature of the tumor and, in addition, preoperatively assists the surgeon in formulating operative strategies. On occasion, angiography may identify an AV malformation that has been incorrectly interpreted as a neoplastic lesion by other methods (21).

Radionucleide scans have likewise been largely replaced by CT scan or MRI. Even more obsolete is the use of lumbar puncture. The risk of lumbar puncture coupled with the limited diagnostic yield has eliminated the use of this test in brain tumor diagnosis.

A major diagnostic advance in the last 15 years has been the development of CT. Every several years the quality and resolution of the CT scan has increased. Today, scans that provide thin slices of the brain in a short period of time, and with limited radiation, are available. A CT scan with judicious use of contrast enhancement provides the ability to localize and accurately describe the nature and extent of a mass (Fig. 1-1). Calcification, even when not readily seen on plain films, may easily be identified with CT scan (8). The nature of the calcification, whether punctate, diffuse, solid, or outlining a cystic cavity, can readily be ascertained. In addition, the extent of cerebral edema; dilatation and obstruction of the ventricular system; and collection and location of extracerebral fluid are readily identified. The accuracy of CT scanning in assessing central nervous system neoplasms has been reported as high as 96%. Despite this, small parasellar and brain-stem lesions may escape detection. Introduction of a water-soluble contrast agent such as metrizamide into the CSF enhances the accuracy in defining the region of the brainstem, optic canal, chiasm, sella, parasellar area, and subarachnoid space surrounding these structures (3).

Magnetic resonance imaging is rapidly replacing CT as the diagnostic agent of choice. This method not only provides superior resolution (Figs. 1-1 and

A

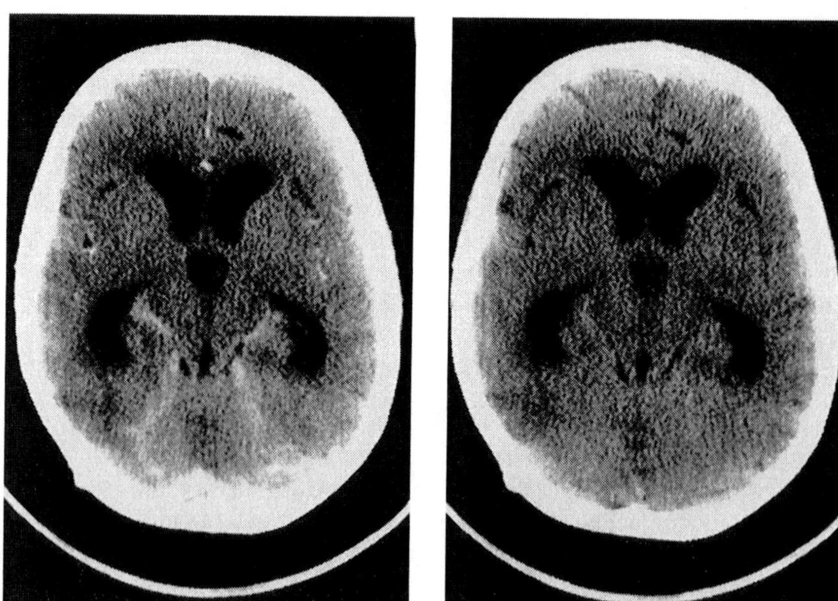

FIG. 1-1. CT scan **(A)** with and **(B)** without contrast. Note the enlarged ventricles.

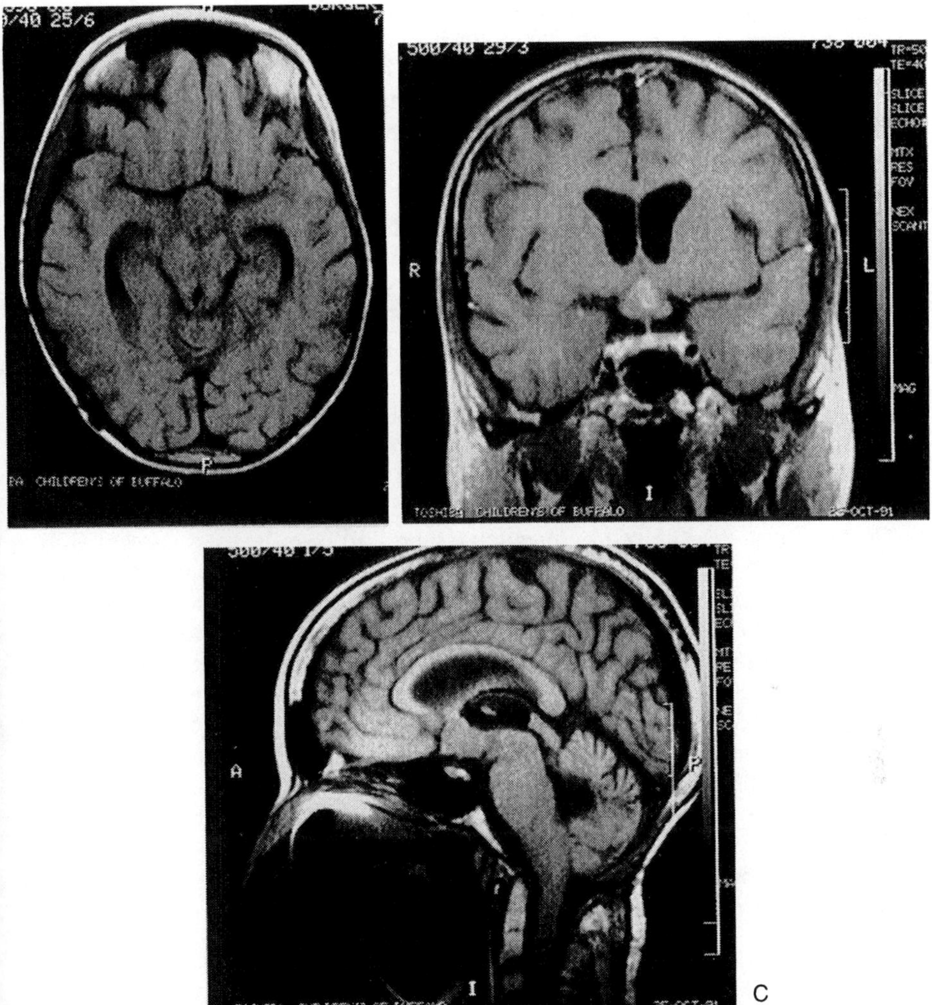

B

C

FIG. 1-2. T1-weighted MR in the **(A)** axial, **(B)** coronal, and **(C)** sagittal planes demonstrating a suprasellar mass.

1-2), but also eliminates the potential radiation danger associated with CT. The energy source for this technique, rather than ionizing radiation, is high-frequency radio waves. Low-frequency radio waves have recently been implicated as being associated with development of brain tumors, but the effects of high-frequency radio waves on human tissue have yet to be determined.

MRI provides exquisite anatomical definition and, because of the multiple paradigms of imaging, allows discrimination between healthy and diseased tissue. MRI rests on the ability to perturb the magnetic field of protons within its microenvironment. Spinning nuclei of water molecules behave like gyroscopes when their long axis is tipped away from the vertical. This motion is called precession. Radio frequency applied to a tissue sample in a rotating magnetic field can match the natural precessional frequency of molecules and influence the spin behavior of the specific nuclei in question. Upon radio excitation, nuclei reveal their location by emitting a signal of precise frequency. The term *magnetic resonance* is derived from the ability of the radio frequency of the applied electromagnetic coil to match the natural precessional frequency of the nuclei of the tissue sample in question. Computer technology then provides a pictorial reconstruction of the emitted signals, thus offering the ability to produce a graphic display of tissue in a way not available by CT. The signal that is produced depends on four factors: (a) the number of protons within the field, (b) the speed at which the tissue is moving, (c) the T1 and (d) the T2 relaxation time. T1 is described as the time needed for protons within a tissue to return to their original state of magnetization or spin; T2 refers to the time required for the coherent alignment of protons induced by magnetic energy to lose their coherence. Both T1 and T2 parameters are time-dependent. The timing of the energy administration and subsequent energy change varies between diseased and normal tissue. TR describes the repetition time between successive administrations of radio frequency energy; TE, or the echo time, describes the delay in radio frequency energy. The TR and TE are chosen to maximize the effect of differences in the T1 and T2 relaxation times, thus providing different signal energies from diseased and nondiseased tissue (4,17).

MRI can provide data from a single point, line, plane, or three-dimensional volume. Further, MRI tracers such as gadolinium can be given parenterally in much the same way as radionucleides while having the advantage of eliminating the radiation associated with the latter technique (5,7). Hydrogen molecules are currently the major source of MRI. This is fortunate, as 75% of the body is made up of water. Images of other molecules, such as phosphorus, are potentially more exciting. Phosphorus is a major constituent of high-energy molecules throughout the body. MRI may allow tracking of high-energy phosphorus molecules throughout the body and thus should provide the ability to wed function of the nervous system to structure. Magnetic resonance spectroscopy provides the ability to image signals from protons or other nuclei, allowing assessment of metabolism. For instance, phosphorus (P31 spectroscopy) allows the quantification of phosphorus-containing compounds (20). This methodology provides information concerning the distribution and utilization of high energy phosphate. This knowledge has the potential of providing information concerning the metabolic activity of the tissue under consideration.

In addition to MRI spectroscopy, MR angiography has provided a means of demonstrating, in a noninvasive way, the blood vessel supply of the nervous system (10). Blood vessels are usually seen as black in conventional MRI images owing to the effect of motion on the magnetic resonance signal. The loss of signal occurs as a result of blood flowing rapidly in and out of the imaging area. Flowing blood does not remain long enough for the radio frequency energy emitted by magnetic resonance to be detected by the scanner. Differences between moving blood and stationery tissue can then be used to form an image that shows only flowing blood, thus providing an indirect picture of the vascular supply to the area in question (Fig. 1-3). This technique provides an angiogram without the need for an intra-arterial injection of contrast material. The appearance produced is similar to conventional angiograms and can be viewed in the three-dimensional plane. The technique, although impressive, has limited resolution when compared to standard angiography and is not capable of demonstrating slow flow. Computerized graphics are now being developed that allow a specific vessel to be identified out of an entire system of vessels, thus providing the potential of demonstrating the vessels and blood supply to the area in question (10).

The last decade has not only seen a tremendous growth in MRI technology but also has witnessed the use of positron emission tomography in the field of oncology. Positron emission tomography, or PET scanning, relies on the ability of radionucleides to emit positively charged particles or positrons. Positrons travel for a few millimeters within a tissue and upon collision with electrons emit energy in the form of two gamma rays. When the gamma rays exit at 180° to each other, oppositely placed detectors can simultaneously record this event and translate it into pictorial reconstruction. Detectors are arranged circumferentially around the head to capture a large number of coincident events, and then standard computed tomography algorithms are used to generate an image. PET scanning is limited by the rate of decay of isotopes used and resolution of the image obtained. PET scanning provides

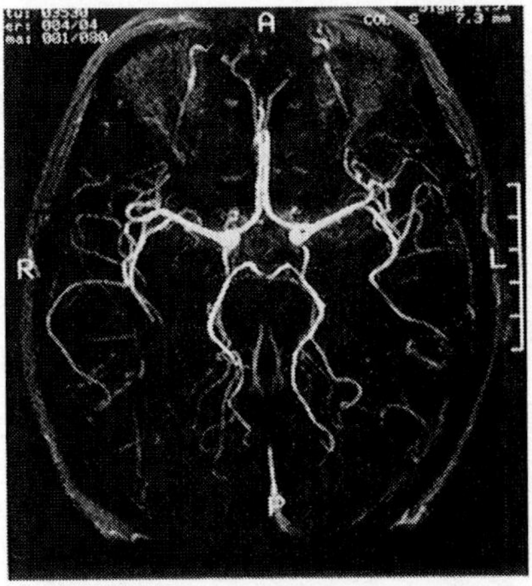

FIG. 1-3. MR angiography showing the circle of Willis in the axial plane. Note the superb detail of the intracranial vasculature.

estimates of regional cerebral metabolic rates and blood flow measurements or other metabolic parameters within a region of interest. The half lives of the presently used radionucleides range from 2 to 110 minutes. Fluorine-18 has a half life of 110 minutes; oxygen-15 has a half life of 2 minutes. Using these and other isotopes, PET has provided the ability to assess the biology of CNS neoplasms of the in vivo state. While CT and magnetic resonance imaging can eloquently define the anatomic location and extent of an intracranial lesion, they are limited by their inability to provide information regarding the functional status of the tissue in question. By looking at different rates of metabolism, PET scanning, more than any other imaging technique, is providing the ability to distinguish viable tumor from necrotic tissue. This is particularly useful in the postradiation period, when the need to distinguish necrosis from recurrent tumor is often greatest. For the most part, necrotic tumor will have decreased metabolism, and a viable tumor will have increased metabolism. Of potential use, but not firmly established, is the ability of PET to assess metabolic and physiologic changes in neoplasms following treatment and perhaps even to monitor drug delivery during treatment. This ability to acquire quantitative data portends for the future a more efficient and rational approach to understanding the current techniques used for treatment (Figs. 1-4 and 1-5) (18). Single photon emission computed tomography (SPECT), when compared to PET, is a less sensitive, cheaper technology that, for the most part, uses radioactive tracers to assess cerebral blood flow within a region of interest.

As can be readily appreciated, changing technology has significantly enhanced the ability to confirm and follow the course of intracranial neoplasms.

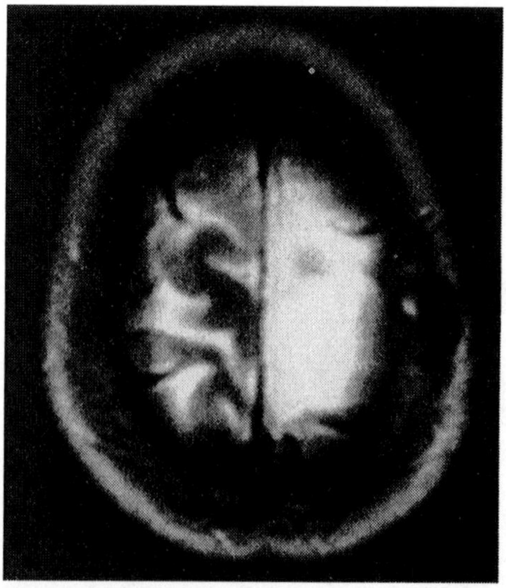

FIG. 1-4. T2-weighted MRI in axial plane demonstrating an extensive low-grade left parietal tumor.

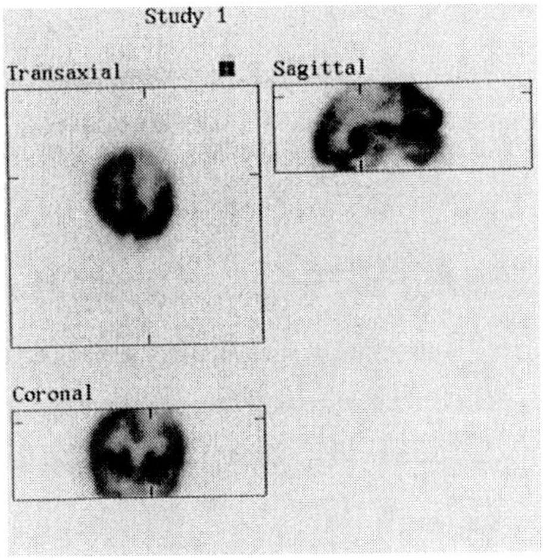

FIG. 1-5. Positron emission tomography of the patient in Fig. 1-4. Note the decreased uptake of (^{18}F) fluxodeoxyglucose in the left parietal area. Images are projected in the axial, sagittal, and coronal planes.

Fifty years ago diagnosis of a mass lesion was considered a neurologic tour de force. Even 10 years ago, MRI, magnetic resonance spectroscopy, and PET scans were not routinely available. With the advent of increasingly refined technology, the challenge for the future, as never before, is turning to treatment and cure rather than diagnosis.

REFERENCES

1. Bailey P, Buchanan DN, Bucy PC. In: *Intracranial tumors of infancy and childhood*. Chicago and London: University of Chicago Press; 1939.
2. Barlow CF. Headaches and brain tumor. *Am J Dis Child* 1982;136:99–100.
3. Bilaniuk L, Zimmerman RA, Littman P, et al. Computed tomography of brain stem gliomas in children. *Radiology* 1980;134:89–95.
4. Brody AS. New perspectives in CT and MR imaging. In: Cohen ME, Duffner PK, eds. Brain tumors in children. *neurol clin* 1991;9:273–286.
5. Cohen BH, Bury E, Packer RJ, Sutton LN, Bilaniuk LT, Zimmerman RA. Gadolinium-enhanced magnetic resonance imaging in childhood brain tumors. *Neurology* 1989;39:1178–1183.
6. Cushing H. Experiences with the cerebellar medulloblastoma: a critical review. *Acta Pathol Microbiol Scand* 1930;7:1–86.
7. Dickman CA, Rekate HL, Bird CR, Drayer BP, Media M. Unenhanced and gadolinium DTPA-enhanced MR imaging in postoperative evaluation in pediatric brain tumors. *J Neurosurg* 1989;71:49–53.
8. Duffner PK, Klein DM, Cohen ME. Calcification in brainstem gliomas. *Neurology* 1978;28:832–834.
9. Duffy FH, Burchfiel JL, Lombroso CT. Brain electrical activity mapping (BEAM): a method for extending the clinical utility of EEG and evoked potential data. *Ann Neurol* 1979;5:309–321.
10. Haacke EM, Masaryk TJ. The salient features of MR angiography. *Radiology* 1989;173:611–612.
11. Hirose G, Lombroso CT, Eisenberg H. Thalamic tumors in childhood. *Arch Neurol* 1975;32:740–744.

12. Honig PJ, Charney EB. Children with brain tumor headaches. *Am J Dis Child* 1982;136: 121–124.
13. Kernohan JW, Woltman HW. Incisura of the crus due to contralateral brain tumor. *Arch Neurol Psychiatr* 1929;21:274–287.
14. MacEwen W. The pupil in its semeiological aspects. *Am J Med Sci* 1887;94:103–146.
15. Page LK, Lombroso CT, Matson DD. Childhood epilepsy with late detection of cerebral glioma. *J Neurosurg* 1969;31:253–261.
16. Plum F, Posner JB. In: *The diagnosis of stupor and coma*. 3rd ed. Philadelphia: FA Davis; 1980.
17. Pykett IL. NMR imaging in medicine. *Sci Am* 1982;246:54–64.
18. Rozental JM, Levine RL, Nickles RJ, Dobkin JA. Glucose uptake by gliomas after treatments: a positron emission tomography study. *Arch Neurol* 1989;46:1302–1307.
19. Starr A, Achar J. Auditory brain stem responses in neurologic disease. *Arch Neurol* 1975; 32:761–768.
20. Sutton LN, Lenkinski RE, Cohen BH, Packer RJ, Zimmerman RA. Localized ^{31}p magnetic resonance spectroscopy of large pediatric brain tumors. *J Neurosurg* 1990;72:65–70.
21. Taveras JM, Wood EH. In: *Diagnostic neuroradiology*. Baltimore: Williams & Wilkins; 1964.
22. Yang PJ, Berger PE, Cohen ME, Duffner PK. Computed tomography and childhood seizure disorders. *Neurology* 1979;29:1084–1088.

2

Principles of Epidemiology

Alan Leviton

Unlike other chapters in this book, which emphasize diagnosis, classification, care, and therapy, this chapter has the underlying theme of prevention. The theme is often very subtle. Your reading of this chapter will be enhanced, however, if you keep this theme in mind.

This chapter has four parts. The first section deals mainly with epidemiologic concepts, especially as they apply to the study of brain tumors in children. The second section compares aggregate data from diverse sources, seeking differences among populations that differ in geographic location, race, sex, and age. Some investigators present data as if all brain tumors were equivalent. The main justification for this approach is the assumption that all brain tumors share some risk factors. Indeed, some oncogenic exposures are not specific. Tobacco smoke does, indeed, increase the occurrence of a number of neoplasms (25,35,60). Additional support for common antecedents is the observation that children with phakomatoses are at increased risk of multiple types of tumors throughout the brain (118).

As much of this book attests, however, brain tumors do not constitute a homogeneous entity. The third section of this chapter presents descriptive data for brain tumor subtypes, providing support for the heterogeneity of childhood brain tumors.

The fourth section includes analytic epidemiologic studies, which are almost invariably of the case-control design. Each of these has evaluated hypotheses about characteristics and exposures alleged to increase brain tumor risk.

EPIDEMIOLOGIC ISSUES

Definition

Although many of the definitions of epidemiology differ, they all emphasize two characteristics. First, epidemiology is an "observational" discipline. Although some epidemiologists conduct clinical trials, most epidemiologists collect and analyze data in order to identify sources of risk.

Brain Tumors in Children: Principles of Diagnosis and Treatment, 2/e, edited by M.E. Cohen and P.K. Duffner, Raven Press, Ltd., New York, 1994.

The second characteristic of most definitions of epidemiology is that human populations are studied. Thus, epidemiologists assume responsibility for providing what some call "external validity." For example, exposing laboratory animals to oncogenic viruses increases the risk of their developing a brain tumor (111). To date, however, epidemiologic studies have not provided convincing evidence that viruses "cause" brain tumors in children.

Types of Studies

Some people believe that only prospective epidemiologic studies can provide accurate information about exposure. Because of the infrequency of brain tumor occurrence in children, prospective studies would be prohibitively expensive. For example, for every 100,000 children under the age of 16 years, 2 or 3 children will manifest a brain tumor each year (16,20,21,22,55,121). The largest prospective study of children carried out in the United States was the Collaborative Perinatal Project, which followed approximately 40,000 children from delivery to age 7 years (86). The huge cost of such a study would be expected to identify between 5 and 10 children with brain tumors. This fact should make it clear that larger prospective epidemiologic studies of childhood brain tumors are not practical.

Unlike the prospective study that identifies children by their exposure and then follows them to see who does and who does not develop a brain tumor, the retrospective (or case-control, case-referent, or post hoc) study identifies children by whether or not they have a brain tumor. Thus, instead of following one-half million children, as might be necessary for a prospective study, a case-control study might be based on only 50 children with a specific brain tumor and a similar number of controls. The other major advantage of a retrospective study (besides its relatively low cost) is that it provides investigators an opportunity to explore multiple hypotheses. The major disadvantage to a retrospective study is that the quality of information about exposures tends not to be as good as that found in a prospective study (5). This is especially true in studies relying on parental recall of past exposures (125).

Epidemiologic Concepts

Causality

The occurrence of brain tumors in populations is not a random phenomenon. It can be described and also predicted. Two models of causation deserve comment. In the deterministic model, all children exposed to the agent in question (at a sufficiently high concentration for a sufficiently long time) should develop a brain tumor. At sublethal doses, deterministic models seem to be inappropriate in human populations. A much better description of what happens in the real world is provided by the probabilistic model. This model acknowledges that risk is rarely 100%, and that it is usually at a much lower order of magnitude. Indeed, an exposure that contributes to the risk of brain tumors in children is likely to increase the risk by only a modest amount. For example, if consumption of cured meats (with their high nitrosamine content or potential) by a woman during her pregnancy increases her child's risk of brain tumor, the risk is probably close to one per 20,000 children each year compared to a risk of one per 40,000 children each year among those whose mothers avoided cured meats (94).

Students of causal inference have suggested several criteria for evaluating cause–effect hypotheses (39,54,81). All appear to agree on five criteria.

The first criterion is biological plausibility. For example, any substance that is implicated in contributing to the occurrence of a brain tumor in a child should cross the blood–brain barrier, influence processes that can regulate intracranial cellular growth, or in some way impede DNA repair mechanisms (93). Much of what we consider biologically plausible is in keeping with "conventional wisdom."

The second criterion is the strength of the association between the exposure and the occurrence of the tumor. People are more likely to consider an exposure etiologically important if it increases the risk five-fold rather than just two-fold. This reflects the epidemiologic axiom that the higher the risk increase attributed to an exposure, the less likely is confounding (see section on biases) to account for the observed relationship.

The third criterion is consistency. Obviously, the more reproducible is the association between an exposure and the risk of childhood brain tumor, the more likely we are to acknowledge the exposure's contribution to the occurrence of the brain tumor.

The fourth criterion is temporal order. The exposure should occur in a child's life at a time in keeping with our knowledge of the interval between tumor initiation and/or promotion and the clinical presentation of that tumor.

The final criterion is what has been called a biologic gradient by some, and the dose-response relationship by others (124). For example, if radiation in utero does indeed contribute to the risk of a brain tumor, those children exposed to the greatest radiation dose should be at highest risk of brain tumor formation.

Multifactorial Model

Years ago, it was realized that not everybody exposed to the *Mycobacterium tuberculosis* bacillus developed symptoms of tuberculosis. Since then, people have come to realize that many factors influence the development of a disease process. Available evidence supports both the linear and log–linear models, which sum the contribution of each identified risk factor (56).

Interaction

Sometimes two exposures will produce a greater effect than each alone (123). The classic example of this is the exposure to tobacco smoke and particulate matter in people who develop respiratory disease. Sometimes this magnification of an adverse effect attributed to an exposure may reflect endogenous factors. Fava bean consumption by people with G-6 PD deficiency, barbiturate consumption by people with porphyria, and phenylalanine consumption by people with PKU, all serve as models of the interaction of an exposure and a unique susceptibility. This concept of interaction may prove helpful in the study of genetic tendencies to brain tumor formation, such as neurofibromatosis.

Generation and Testing of Hypotheses

Historically, epidemiologists have used two strategies to generate hypotheses about disease etiology. First, they have borrowed from laboratory studies. Reports that viruses appear to cause brain tumors in laboratory animals (111) have prompted epidemiologists to see if viral infections in humans might increase the risk of childhood brain tumors. The second strategy, which for lack of a better term may be called analogy, entails borrowing a hypothesis from a similar human disease; for example, chromosomal aberrations and congenital anomalies in children with brain tumors (14).

By and large, epidemiologists tend to be rather conservative. This has meant that a single finding should never be viewed as proving a relationship between an exposure and a disease. The first finding of such a relationship is viewed as an example of hypothesis generation. In order for that hypothesis to gain acceptance, the finding linking the exposure and the illness must be replicated. The search for replication of previously described findings is called hypothesis testing. Although the distinction may be viewed as academic, in this day of media hyperbole, such a distinction deserves more attention. For example, consider the situation in which a national news publication claims that exposure to "x" causes brain tumors in children. This might prompt some parents of children with brain tumors to blame themselves for causing their child's tumor. In addition, parents whose children do not have a brain tumor will tend to modify their behavior in order to do what they perceive is best for their children. If the exposure had other advantages, people might adversely affect their child's welfare by responding to an unproved hypothesis. Some lots of polio vaccine had been contaminated with SV-40 virus, which has oncogenic properties (88). It now appears that people inoculated with that vaccine are not at increased risk of brain tumors (82). Nevertheless, one can see the possibility of increasing the risk of polio in a vain attempt to decrease the risk of brain tumor.

Koch's Postulates

Some safeguards are needed to avoid inappropriately blaming a beneficial or innocuous exposure. Koch's postulates have been modified for viral infections, especially as causes of malignancies (130). The following are required to claim that a virus causes a childhood brain tumor.

1. The incidence of the brain tumor is higher in children infected with the putative agent than in children not so infected. Because prospective studies are unlikely to be available for brain tumor epidemiology, this criterion can be replaced with the case-control equivalent: exposure to the putative agent is more common in cases than in controls.
2. The putative agent has neoplastic potential in laboratory animals or cell cultures.
3. Inoculating laboratory animals with material from a brain tumor removed from a child results in cellular proliferation similar to that of the brain tumor.
4. Elimination of the putative agent eliminates or reduces the occurrence of the brain tumors.
5. The putative agent persists in the infected host without causing cell death (latency), or expression of viral genetic information is found in tumor cells.
6. Evidence of infection precedes manifestations of the brain tumor. Thus, the mean age of infection with the putative agent is lower than the mean age of the first manifestation of the tumor.
7. Other characteristics suggested by some students of viral oncogenesis include: immunologic specificity and a spectrum of histologic anomalies (e.g., dysplasia) antedating the occurrence of neoplasia.

To date, no viral infection has met these criteria for causation of CNS neoplasia in children.

Biases

Sackett (103) has prepared a catalog of 35 biases for epidemiologists to avoid. Some of the more important ones are discussed below.

Case Identification

Because the natural history of brain tumors includes continual growth of the tumor, rather than any appreciable probability of spontaneous regression, almost every child with a brain tumor sooner or later will come to medical attention. Thus, detection biases tend to be infrequent. Selection bias can be a problem, however, when the catchment area of a hospital is different for childhood brain tumors than it is for children with other diseases who might serve as controls. Because case identification may be a function of the completeness of a diagnostic evaluation, patients whose brain tumors have been examined histologically are more likely to have a brain tumor diagnosis on their death certificate than are people whose brain tumor evaluation was not as complete. This phenomenon was offered as an explanation for the over-representation of brain tumor diagnoses on death certificates of employees of the Eastman Kodak Company (58).

Control Identification

The ideal control for an epidemiologic study of brain tumors should be representative of all people who do not have a brain tumor. This desire to generalize the findings of any study prompts an investigator to select controls from the community in some random fashion. The potential problem here, however, is that the families of children with brain tumors might ruminate more than families of controls about experiences and exposures that could conceivably contribute to the occurrence of a brain tumor (125). To avoid this bias of selective recall, some investigators select hospitalized patients as controls. This reflects the belief that, compared to parents of healthy children, parents of seriously ill children will think more about things that might have influenced their child's health.

If community controls provide the promise of generalizability, and hospital controls provide the advantage of minimizing selective recalls, it would seem prudent to compare cases to each set of controls. Unfortunately, however, the findings may be perplexing. In their provocative hypothesis-generating study, Gold and her associates (48) found that barbiturate consumption was higher in the mothers of children with brain tumors than in the mothers of children with other malignancies, but they found a much less apparent difference between the mothers of children with brain tumors and the mothers of "normal" controls.

Confounding

Distortion of disease-exposure associations is often referred to as confounding (57). Confounding can be minimized in the design of a study by matching controls to cases. The preferred alternative is to "remove" confounding effects in the analysis. Not only is matching inefficient but also "over-matching" can impede the identification of risk factors (31). For example, in my own study of childhood brain tumors, controls were matched to cases by telephone prefix (i.e., the first three digits of the number). Although this minimizes the distortion of risk assessments that might be linked to factors that are difficult to quantify, such as socioeconomic status, it might have limited the opportunity to identify such putative risk factors of brain tumors as exposures to animals, toxins, and infections to which children are prone.

Exposure Classification

Separate from the concept of selective recall is the more diffuse problem of "misclassification of exposure" (e.g., classifying as not exposed those who really were exposed) (43). This is especially disturbing if misclassification is different in cases and controls. Even when equally distributed among cases and controls, misclassification results in reduced validity of information collected, and thus minimizes the confidence that can be attached to any exposure–outcome association. For example, memory of food consumption is distorted by recall of more recent patterns (17). This prompts me to advise caution in interpreting the finding that mothers of children who developed brain tumors (before age 24 years) were more likely than mothers of controls to acknowledge consumption of breakfast and luncheon meats before and during pregnancy (94).

Another problem that plagues epidemiologists is whether or not the correct exposures are being measured. This is akin to the inebriated person looking for his key under the street light (where the light is) and not at the place in the dark where the key was dropped. For example, should we measure stress by the number and magnitude of the major upheavals in our lives, or should we also deal with the daily problems that may contribute more on a day-to-day basis to perceived stress than do major "life events?" Perhaps we should measure support from others and the coping ability of the individuals, rather than the problems and upheavals (10).

People who use questionnaires to collect data have been concerned about reliability and validity (44). Reliability is a measure of the agreement between answers to one question obtained on one occasion with answers to that same question obtained on another occasion. Validity is a measure of how close the answer provided on a questionnaire compares with some external measure of truth.

Problems may occur by having surrogates rather than the subjects themselves provide information (53,78). A similar but related issue concerns the quality of the data provided by two people when they are interviewed together, compared with individual interviews. For example, one parent might not acknowledge alcohol or marijuana exposure when interviewed in the company of his/her spouse, but might acknowledge such exposure when interviewed alone.

Classification of Outcome

The brain is not a homogeneous organ. The cerebellum differs from the cerebrum in structure, function, and rate of development. Indeed, even within the cerebellum and the cerebrum, differences exist in structure, function, and rates of development.

I am uncertain to what extent brain tumors need to be subdivided in order to achieve biologic homogeneity. One strategy is to consider a subtype of a brain tumor homogeneous if examples of it differ minimally in histology, and if the variation in survival is minimized (104). An epidemiologic axiom is that the more homogeneous an outcome is, the greater the probability its risk factors will be identified. Thus, I am reluctant to group all brain tumors together even for hypothesis generation. Cytogenetic analysis of each child's tumor might be required if investigators are to be convinced their case group is homogeneous (6,12,26,62,64,66,109).

THE DESCRIPTIVE EPIDEMIOLOGY OF CHILDHOOD BRAIN TUMORS

For children under the age of 15 years, cancer continues to be the second leading cause of death, with brain and central nervous system tumors the most common fatal group of solid tumors in this age group (20). Yet not all brain tumors that result in death are histologically malignant. Aggressive efforts to reduce mortality have been successful, but sometimes at a high cost of function lost (29,67).

Geographic Differences

The total annual incidence of brain tumors in children is approximately 22 per million in the United States (16). This is among the highest national rates. The highest rates are from West Sweden (75), with other high rates reported from New Zealand, Israel, and Canada (21) (Table 2-1). The lowest rates of brain tumor are reported by population-based registries in India, Malaysia, Africa, and Latin America. Although differences in socioeconomic status seem to correlate with this gradient, the possibility exists that these are not true differences, but only differences in enumeration. For example, where medical care is most limited, biopsy material may not be available for all tumors. This leads to the inference that the countries most likely to devote resources to medical care are those most likely to provide the most detail about brain tumors. Unless the tumor is examined postmortem, a histologic diagnosis will never be made.

The variation among "developed" countries, however, is less likely to reflect biased ascertainment. The childhood brain tumor incidence in all Scandinavian countries (except Iceland) is approximately 60% higher than the rate in Japan. This is just the kind of difference that epidemiologists seek, because it offers an opportunity to account for the Scandinavian excess, or what might protect Japanese children.

TABLE 2-1. *Observed/expected[a] and sex ratios for the incidence of all childhood brain tumors reported from registries throughout the world*

	Observed/expected	Male/female
India (Bombay only)	0.34	1.3
Africa (blacks only)	0.50	1.6
Latin America	0.58	1.1
Singapore (Chinese)	0.59	1.0
Jamaica	0.72	2.1
Japan	0.81	1.1
Europe		
Eastern	0.94	1.1
Western	0.95	1.0
United Kingdom	1.00	1.2
United States	1.10	1.1
Canada	1.12	1.3
Israel	1.16	1.1
New Zealand (non-Maori)	1.23	1.2
Scandinavia	1.36	1.1

[a]Expected numbers calculated from age- and sex-specific rates for registries identified in previous publications.

From Breslow NE, Langholz B. Childhood cancer incidence: geographical and temporal variations. *Int J Cancer* 1983;32:703–716.

Ascertainment bias is the term applied to searching with greater scrutiny among some samples than among others. Perhaps the best example (during the pre-MRI era) of ascertainment bias in the study of childhood brain tumors is the variation among institutions to biopsy presumed neoplasms of the brain stem (85). Perhaps that is why brain-stem glioma tumors accounted for 6% of all childhood intracranial tumors in the Childhood Brain Tumor Consortium (CBTC) (where brain-stem biopsies appear to have been unusual) (113) and 14% in Cape Town (where brainstem biopsies were performed proportionately more frequently) (91).

Racial Patterns

The incidence of all major brain tumor types is slightly less among blacks than among whites in the United States (21,22) (Table 2-2). Based on data from population-based registries in Detroit and the San Francisco Bay Area between 1969 and 1980, the incidence of brain tumors increased 34% among blacks and only 18% among whites. These racial differences may reflect blacks' recently improved access to care (and thereby increased ascertainment) or true changes. Access to care (and histologic identification) might explain the much lower rates than expected among blacks in Africa and Jamaica (Table 2-1).

Children identified as Hispanic had lower rates of brain tumors in the New Mexico and Puerto Rico population-based registries than did other children (21). Lower than expected incidence rates of childhood brain tumors have

TABLE 2-2. *Age-adjusted incidence rates (per million per year) of selected brain tumors among children less than 15 years of age, based on data from population-based registries in the United States 1969–71 (TNCS) and 1973–80 (SEER)*

	Among All Children		Among Blacks		Among Whites	
Tumor type	Black	White	Girls	Boys	Girls	Boys
Glioma	13.6	14.0	13.3	12.3	14.0	14.1
Medulloblastoma	4.8	5.3	4.9	4.8	4.0	6.5
Other	2.7	3.5	3.3	2.1	3.6	3.4
Total	21.2	22.8	23.1	19.2	21.6	24.0

From Bunin G. Racial patterns of childhood brain cancer by histologic type. *J Natl Cancer Inst* 1987;78:875–880.

also been reported from Cuba, Cali, Columbia, and Saõ Paulo, Brazil. The lower than expected incidences of leukemias and lymphomas among children in most of these registries again raise the issue of underascertainment versus truly lower risks of neoplasms.

Japanese children in Hawaii tend to have brain tumors at a rate that approximates the incidence among Japanese children in Japan, but that is almost double the rate among Hawaiian children in Hawaii. The Hawaiian–Japanese difference in Hawaii is unlikely to reflect distortions in enumeration, but might reflect random phenomenon often most apparent in small samples.

Temporal Trends

Connecticut has "the longest continuously operating population-based cancer registry in the United States" (121). On the basis of data from this registry, it appears that the incidence of brain tumors increased in all childhood age groups during the interval 1935–59, with essentially stable rates since 1960 (Table 2-3). Other United States surveys and registries have shown no increase between 1970 and 1982 (55).

Increases in brain tumor incidence over time have been reported from

TABLE 2-3. *Average annual incidence rates (per million) for* malignant *central nervous system neuroplasms, Connecticut, 1935–79*

		Age 0–4	Age 5–9	Age 10–14	Age 15–19
Girls	1935–49	11.6	10.8	6.9	5.5
	1950–64	37.2	25.9	14.2	9.2
	1965–79	18.2	26.1	18.5	14.1
Boys	1935–49	11.9	21.9	6.6	11.8
	1950–64	29.9	26.5	19.8	17.6
	1965–79	39.9	25.0	22.6	18.7

From von Hoff J, Schymura MJ, Curnen MG. Trends in the incidence of childhood and adolescent cancer in the province of Perugia (Italy). *Zentralbl Bakteriol Mikrobiol Hyg* 1984;179:300–307.

Finland and Sweden (38,112). These registries, however, are rarely congruent in their findings.

Do these temporal trends reflect diagnostic changes or a true increased incidence before 1960? Before the 1960s, pneumoencephalography and angiography were available only in university medical centers. This limited availability of diagnostic capabilities could account for a low rate of tumor identification. Indeed, the apparent increased incidence does coincide with the increased availability of diagnostic methods (59). Some components of the prominent increases in the number of brain tumors in adults, however, cannot be attributed to the increasing availability of computed tomography and magnetic resonance imaging (32).

Sex

As in the past, the sex ratio (males/females) tends to be slightly greater than 1 in almost all samples (21,75,95) (Table 2-1). Among blacks in the United States, however, the sex ratio was less than 1 (22). Blacks in Jamaica and Africa have, however, a sex ratio of brain tumor incidence clearly larger than 1 (21,63). Recent studies from Germany (65) (for children less than 1 year of age), Nigeria (63), and Italy (122) have found that boys are twice as likely as girls to develop a brain tumor. These may be aberrations that are more likely to be published than are negative findings (9,23,33,36).

Primitive neuroectodermal tumors (PNET) (including medulloblastoma) have shown an elevated sex ratio even in those predominantly white populations that have a sex ratio of close to 1 for all other childhood brain tumors (22,75,113). The male preponderance is also seen among germinomas and choroid plexus papillomas (113).

Age

Data from the Connecticut tumor registries suggest that the risk of brain tumors in children decreases with increasing age (121) (Table 2-3). Among whites living in the catchment areas of cancer registries representing 10% of the United States population, however, this was much less apparent (21).

In the large CBTC representing 3,291 children who had a tissue diagnosis of a brain or spinal tumor made at one of 10 North American neurosurgical centers, 7% of all brain tumors were obtained from infants less than 1 year of age (113). Each year of age continued to represent 7 to 8% of all childhood central nervous system tumors until age 8 years, when it began to decline prominently. Fully 80% of all childhood brain tumors occur within the first 10 years of life.

An intrauterine origin for some brain tumors must be acknowledged in light of the clinical presentation of tumors in newborns (89). Some students of intrauterine neurooncogenesis have moved from limiting congenital tumors to those found in early infancy (97) to the possibility that the majority of children whose brain tumor becomes evident before age 2 years "may have been born with the tumor" (113).

Most acknowledged congenital tumors are teratomas (70). Other congenital tumors are what some view as "embryonal tumors" (including PNET) (71,102). What remains to be seen is what proportion of teratomas (including craniopharyngiomas) and PNET first evident later in childhood can be attributed to intrauterine events and exposures.

The proportion of all children with a brain tumor represented by infants less than 1 year old has varied between 1.4% (69) and 9.3% (113), but has really not increased over the years [e.g., Starr (108) reported 5.9%, whereas Koos and Miller (73) reported 2.7% (see also 18,47,68)]. This suggests that preconception and intrauterine oncogenic exposures (including those at work) are not becoming more prevalent.

THE DESCRIPTIVE EPIDEMIOLOGY OF SPECIFICS TYPES OF CHILDHOOD BRAIN TUMORS

In the previous section, data came mainly from population-based registries. This allowed an assessment of the number of children at risk. In this section the denominator is often not all children, but rather all children who had a brain tumor and who were cared for at one hospital or in one community. This allows us to see what proportion of all tumors belong to one histologic type. Wherever applicable, the data from population-based studies are presented (21,34,41). A plea has been made to supplement population-based registry data with uniform reporting of information about diagnostic procedures, staging, neuropathology, and long-term treatment effects (27).

Astrocytoma

In most series, astrocytoma is the most common histologic diagnosis (Table 2-4). In the only large series from a population-based registry, over half of the astrocytomas were located in the cerebellum, especially between the ages of 1 and 5 years (34). The vast majority of these are pilocytic astrocytomas (113), as are those in the brain stem (114). The other locations in order of decreasing frequency were cerebrum (20%), brain stem (19%), and optic chiasm (2%). The proportion located in the cerebrum is highest after age 5 years. Fibrillary and anaplastic subtypes predominate (113). The mean age at astrocytoma diagnosis in one series was 9 years (34). Cerebellar astrocytomas tend to be diagnosed at younger ages (mean = 8.4 years) than cerebral astrocytomas (mean = 10.6 years).

In adolescents, astrocytomas constitute approximately one-fourth of all intracranial tumors, with glioblastoma accounting for an additional 12% (41). Thus, in adolescents, approximately 40% of brain tumors may be of astro-

TABLE 2-4. *The percent distribution of the preponderant tumor types among case series reported 1984–91*

Citation	Location	Years	*N*	Astro-cytoma[a]	Medullo-blastoma/ PNET	Ependy-moma	Cranio-pharyn-gioma
All children							
CBTC, 1988 (113)	North America	1930–79	3291	40	20	11	7
Tomita et al., 1985 (115)	Chicago	1952–84	608	41	20	7	7
Peacock et al., 1987 (91)	Cape Town	1979–85	145	40	18	11	9
Lashley, 1991 (76)	Barbados	1978–88	29	55	17	—	7
Izuora et al., 1989 (63)	Enugu, Nigeria	1978–85	21	14	14	—	38
Less than 12 months							
Jooma et al., 1984 (68)	London	1953–81	80	36	20	18	1
Tomita et al., 1985 (115)	Chicago	1952–84	57	33	23	5	4
13–24 months							
Tomita et al., 1985 (15)	Chicago	1952–84	43	49	28	7	2
13–19 years							
Farwell et al., 1984 (41)	Connecticut	1935–75	133	40	11	5	8

[a] Includes glioblastoma.

cytic origin. On the basis of population-based registry data for the United States, the annual incidence of all astrocytic tumors in the entire childhood age group varies minimally with age, with an annual incidence of approximately 17 per million children (21). The heterogeneity of astrocytomas is suggested not only by differences in histology (e.g., fibrillary, pilocytic, etc.), but also by differences in secular trends and survival patterns (45,129).

Medulloblastoma/PNET

Although some argue for an all-inclusive designation of primitive neuroectodermal tumor (PNET), which would include medulloblastoma (101), this has not yet taken hold (79,98,116). In a number of series, PNET/medulloblastoma accounts for 20 to 25% of all childhood brain tumors. In whites, the sex ratio of medulloblastoma is 1.7 (21). In blacks, however, the sex ratio approximates 1 (22).

Ependymoma

Ependymoma is the third most common histologic type of brain tumor in children, accounting for approximately 15% of all childhood brain tumors. The majority of these tumors appear to originate in the posterior fossa (52,92,113,119). As with other specific tumor groups, boys are overrepresented (52,113).

Choroid Plexus Papilloma

In one large series of 608 childhood brain tumors, 10 of 17 choroid plexus papillomas were found in children under the age of 1 year (93). Choroid plexus papilloma represents between 10% (115) and 13% (68) of all tumors identified before children's first birthday.

Oligodendroglioma

Rarely seen in young children, oligodendroglioma tumors accounted for 1% of all childhood brain tumors in the large CBTC (113). These tumors did account for 6% of all brain tumors in adolescence in the Connecticut Tumor Registry (40).

Craniopharyngioma

In most large series, less than 10% of brain tumors in children are craniopharyngiomas (Table 2-4). Although some are obviously congenital (61,68,115), most occur later in childhood.

In the United States and Finland, approximately 38% of all craniopharyngiomas are evident before the end of adolescence (8,106). In Nigeria, however, 71% of all craniopharyngiomas diagnosed in the University College Hospital in Ibadan were in children (2). In Enugu, Nigeria, 38% of the childhood brain tumors were craniopharyngiomas (63). Why Nigeria should have such a disproportionately high rate of craniopharyngiomas remains to be determined.

THE ANALYTIC EPIDEMIOLOGY OF CHILDHOOD BRAIN TUMORS

This section is mainly a review of recent case-control (also known as case-referent) studies of the antecedents of childhood brain tumors. The findings are considered in light of a few general epidemiologic principles, and also in light of findings reported in decades past.

Because some children are born with tumors and others develop their tumors within the first years of life, it seems highly likely that events before birth contribute to the onset of early-occurring tumors. This concept has been labeled "perinatal carcinogenesis" (96).

An often unstated assumption is that what contributes to tumors in very young children also contributes to the occurrence of tumors in older children. Unfortunately, no recent case-referent study has evaluated a histologically defined tumor group in very young children only.

Familial/Genetic Factors

A number of well-recognized neurocutaneous syndromes are associated with childhood brain tumors. These include neurofibromatosis, tuberous sclerosis, Sturge-Weber syndrome, von Hippel-Lindau disease, and the multiple basal cell nevus syndrome (15,46,100,118).

The three hallmarks of familial tumors are (a) an increased risk of tumors in the families of patients with a tumor, (b) multiple tumors in some individuals, and (c) a tendency for the tumor to become manifest at an earlier age than in children without a tendency to familial tumors (72). Although this is not always confirmed (38), the families of children with brain tumor are more likely to have a history of tumors than are families of children who do not have a brain tumor (1,19,74). Children who have a brain tumor are more likely than children with another type of tumor to have a second tumor (42,117). Among children who have a brain tumor, those who have a family history of tumor are more likely to present at an earlier age than children without any familial tumor diathesis (110). All of this is consistent with the hypothesis that even among children who lack a neurocutaneous syndrome, the risk of brain tumor is increased if other (first-degree) relatives have a tumor, especially a brain tumor.

Although other familial disorders, including a propensity to stroke and seizures, had been associated with increased risk of a brain tumor in children (49), these have not been supported by recent findings (46,74). Only one study to date has reported that children with gliomas are more likely to have a relative who is mentally retarded than are controls (74).

Teratogenesis/Oncogenesis

The form of neurofibromatosis associated with brain tumors in children is now called NF-1 (84). The gene for NF-1 is on chromosome 17 (51) with the gene located on band 17q11.2 (77). What is especially intriguing is that some of the children who do not have the NF-1 gene have brain tumors with deletions or nonreciprocal translocations involving chromosome 17 (12,13,26,64,106). Support has not yet been provided that components of the short arm of chromosome 17 have tumor-suppressor capability.

The possibility that brain tumors are congenital malformations is not new. In 1924 Bailey and Cushing (7) suggested that groups of medulloblasts, which did not differentiate as they should have, persisted into early childhood and gave rise to what had been called medulloblastoma and is now called PNET. The failure of these cells to differentiate was, in essence, a congenital malformation. This concept was recently raised by those caring for a boy who, in addition to his medulloblastoma evident at age 5 months, had oomphalocele, malrotation of the intestine, and extrophy of the bladder (87). This prompted the authors to postulate that a disturbance to development during the second and third months of gestation led not only to the brain tumor but also to the anomalies of the abdomen.

Parental Preconception Exposures

Spatial–temporal clustering of childhood brain tumors was associated with parental employment in a company that manufactured electronic components and accessories (128). The parents were exposed to a large number of chemical compounds, and no single chemical or group of chemicals could be implicated.

Fathers' employment in the aerospace industry was associated with an increased risk of brain tumor before age 10 years in Washington state (90), but not with childhood brain tumors in New York state (83). Paternal exposure to pesticides or employment in the agriculture industry prior to conception was associated with brain tumor in the offspring in two studies (126,127). Increased risk of childhood brain tumor was also associated with paternal employment during the preconception period in the construction, metal, and food and tobacco industries (127). A study conducted in New York state failed to show any link between the risk of childhood brain tumor and paternal occupational exposures to hydrocarbons or electromagnetic fields, or employment in the pulp and paper manufacturing industries (83). The problems studying parental occupational exposure are indicated by the recent finding that a child's risk of brain tumor was associated with paternal exposure to ionizing radiation based on industrial codes, but not when ionizing radiation exposure was classified by occupational titles (83).

Maternal Characteristics

Characteristics of the mother are a topic of interest to epidemiologists because they might convey information about the propensity to chromosomal anomalies, congenital malformations, early fetal quality control mechanisms, and the general quality of the intrauterine environment provided by the mother. In one study of childhood astrocytoma, maternal history of miscarriage or stillbirth was associated with reduced risk of childhood astrocytoma (74), whereas in another study prior fetal death appeared to convey information about increased risk (37). Similarly, older maternal age was associated with an increased risk in some studies (37,70) but not in others (24,102). In light of these findings, it appears that maternal characteristics are not prominently associated with increased risk of childhood brain tumor.

Gestational Exposures

Use of an electric blanket by the mother during her pregnancy was associated with an increased risk of a brain tumor in her child (105). This provocative finding has yet to be confirmed.

Maternal consumption of cured meats during pregnancy was more common among the mothers of children with an astrocytoma than among mothers of controls (74). This finding can be viewed as support for the hypothesis that prenatal and early childhood exposure to N-nitroso compounds, which are oncogenic in rodents, contributes to the development of intracranial tumors in children (94).

Consumption of antinausea medications during early pregnancy has also been associated with an increased risk of childhood astrocytoma (74). What is not clear from this study is whether the need for antinausea medication or the medication itself contributes to the increased risk. For example, women who are nauseated in early pregnancy are more likely to have prominently elevated levels of chorionic gonadotrophin than are women much less disturbed by nausea (107). Thus, the nausea might be a marker of prominent hormonal changes. This is especially important in light of evidence that hormonal disturbances influence the growth of experimental brain tumors (4).

The association between maternal consumption of marijuana and the child's risk of astrocytoma is of borderline statistical significance only (74). The risk of childhood brain tumors does not appear to be associated with parental cigarette smoking (50,74) or maternal alcohol consumption (74).

Birth Characteristics

Preterm birth is not associated with an increased risk of brain tumor (94,104). Firstborn children appeared to be at increased risk of brain tumors in one study (46), but not in another (37). Increased birth weight has consistently been associated with an increased risk of childhood brain tumor, especially astrocytoma (28,37,46,80). In one explanation, augmented rates of cell division and growth are accompanied by a heightened sensitivity to carcinogenic agents in utero (49). A variation on this theme postulates that phenomena that increase fetal weight also increase fetal response to transplacental carcinogens (11,30).

Postnatal Exposures

Postnatal exposure to electric blankets does not appear to be associated with childhood brain tumors (105).

In years past, tinea capitis had been treated with radiotherapy. Such radiotherapy during childhood was associated with a prominently increased risk of brain tumors during the next 30 years (99). Unfortunately, the report describing this increased risk did not direct attention to tumors limited to the childhood years. Tinea capitis is no longer treated with radiotherapy.

EPILOGUE

Even a cursory reading of this chapter provides the impression that epidemiology has not yet shed much light on the characteristics and exposures that influence the risk of brain tumors in children. Rather than reciting a litany of possible explanations, I'd prefer to emphasize the problem of tumor heterogeneity.

Classifying all tumors as a homogeneous entity is clearly inappropriate. The recognition that all tumors that look alike are not alike should prompt a desire for the most homogeneous groupings of tumors. An epidemiologic axiom holds that nonrandom misclassification reduces the probability of identifying an association between an exposure and an outcome. In light of this axiom, the risk profile of PNET with a deletion of part of the short arm of chromosome 17 can be expected to differ from the risk profile of PNET that do not have any chromosomal abnormality. Epidemiologists need the assistance of tumor biologists if the field of epidemiology is to make a contribution to our understanding of what "causes" childhood brain tumors.

REFERENCES

1. Acqui M, Ferrante L, Vagnozzi R, Mastronardi L, Fortuna A. Occasionally occurring familial brain tumors (OFBT): reports of cases and review of the literature. *J Neurosurg Sci* 1989;33:263–269.
2. Adeloye A, Nottidge VA, Udi J. Craniopharyngioma in Nigerian children. *Childs Nerv Syst* 1988;4:128–134.
3. Asai A, Hoffman HJ, Hendrick RB, Humphreys RP, Becker LE. Primary intracranial neoplasms in the first year of life. *Childs Nerv Syst* 1989;5:230–233.
4. Avtsyn AP, Yablanowskaya LY. Effects of disturbances in the hormonal status on experimental brain tumors. *Acta Unio Contra Cancrum* 1964;20:1519–1522.
5. Baddeley A. The limitations of human memory: implications for the design of retrospective surveys. In: Moss L, Goldstein H, eds. *The recall method in social surveys*, Windsor, Berks, UK: NFER Publishing; 1979:13–27.
6. Badiali M, Pession A, Basso G, et al. N-myc and c-myc oncogenes amplification in medulloblastomas: evidence of particularly aggressive behavior of a tumor with c-myc amplification. *Tumori* 1991;77:118–121.
7. Bailey, P, Cushing H. Medulloblastoma cerebelli: a common type of midcerebellar glioma of childhood. *Arch Neurol Psychiatr* 1924;14:192–224.
8. Baskins DS, Wilson CB. Surgical management of craniopharyngiomas: a review of 74 cases. *J Neurosurg* 1986;65:22–27.
9. Berg CB, Berlin JA. Publication bias and dissemination of clinical research. *J Natl Cancer Inst* 1989;81:107–115.
10. Berkman LF. Social networks, support, and health: taking the next step forward. *Am J Epidemiol* 1986;123:559–562.
11. Berstein LM. Newborn macrosomy and cancer. In: Klein G, Weinhouse S, eds. *Advances in cancer research*. San Diego: Academic Press; 1988:231–278.
12. Bertheas MF, Frappaz D, Elian J, Brizard C, Brunon J, Freycon F. Anomalies chromosomiques des tumeurs cerebrales. *Pediatrie* 1991;46:65–69.
13. Biegel JA, Rorke LB, Packer RJ, et al. Isochromosome 17q in primitive neuroectodermal tumors of the central nervous system. *Genes Chromo Cancer* 1989;1:139–147.
14. Birch JM. Anecephaly in stillborn siblings of children with germ cell tumors. *Lancet* 1980; 1:1257.

15. Blatt J, Jaffe R, Deutsch M, Adkins JC. Neurofibromatosis and childhood tumors. *Cancer* 1986;57:1225–1229.
16. Bleyer WA. The impact of childhood cancer on the United States and the world. *CA* 1990; 40:355–367.
17. Block G, Thompson FE, Hartman AM, Larkin FA, Guire KE. Comparison of two dietary questionnaires validated against multiple dietary records collected during a 1-year period. *J Am Diet Assoc* 1992;92:686–693.
18. Bodian M, Lawson D. The intracranial neoplastic diseases of childhood. *Br J Surg* 1953; 40:368–392.
19. Bondy ML, Lustbader ED, Buffler PA, Schull WJ, Hardy RJ, Strong LC. Genetic epidemiology of childhood brain tumors. *Genet Epidemiol* 1991;8:253–267.
20. Boring CC, Squires TS, Tong T. Cancer statistics 1991. *CA* 1991;41:19–36.
21. Breslow NE, Langholz B. Childhood cancer incidence: geographical and temporal variations. *Int J Cancer* 1983;32:703–716.
22. Bunin G. Racial patterns of childhood brain cancer by histologic type. *J Natl Cancer Inst* 1987;78:875–880.
23. Chalmers TC, Frank CS, Reitman D. Minimizing the three stages of publication bias. *JAMA* 1990;263:1392–1395.
24. Choi NW, Schuman LM, Gullen WH. Epidemiology of primary central nervous system neoplasms. II: Case-control study. *Am J Epidemiol* 1970;91:467–485.
25. Clayson DB. An overview of current and anticipated methods for cancer prevention. *Cancer Lett* 1990;50:3–9.
26. Cogen PH, Daneshvar L, Metzger AK, Edwards MS. Deletion mapping of the medulloblastoma locus on chromosome 17p. *Genomics* 1990;8:279–285.
27. Cohen ME, Duffner PK, Kun LE, D'Souza B. The argument for a combined cancer consortium research data base. *Cancer* 1985;56:1897–1901.
28. Coughlin SS, Nass CC, Pickle LW, Trock B, Bunin G. Regression methods for estimating attributable risk in population-based case-control studies: a comparison of additive and multiplicative models. *Am J Epidemiol* 1991;133:305–313.
29. Craft AW, Pearson AD. Three decades of chemotherapy for childhood cancer: from cure "at any cost" to cure "at least cost." *Cancer Surv* 1989;8:605–629.
30. Daling JR, Starzyk P, Olshan AF, Weiss NS. Birthweight and the incidence of childhood cancer. *J Natl Cancer Inst* 1984;72:1039–1041.
31. Day N, Byar D, Green S. Overadjustment in case-control studies. *Am J Epidemiol* 1980; 112:696–706.
32. Desmeueles M, Mikkelsen T, Mao Y. Increasing incidence of primary malignant brain tumors: influence of diagnostic methods. *J Natl Cancer Inst* 1992;84:442–445.
33. Dickerson K. The existence of publication bias and risk factors for its occurrence. *JAMA* 1990;263:1385–1389.
34. Dohrmann GJ, Farwell JR, Flannery JT. Astrocytomas in childhood: a population-based study. *Surg Neurol* 1985;23:64–68.
35. Doll R. Lifestyle: an overview. *Cancer Detect Prev* 1990;14:589–595.
36. Easterbrook PJ, Berlin JA, Gopalan R, Matthews DR. Publication bias in clinical research. *Lancet* 1991;337:867–872.
37. Emerson JC, Malone KE, Daling JR, Starzyk P. Childhood brain tumor risk in relation to birth characteristics. *J Clin Epidemiol* 1991;44:1159–1166.
38. Ericsson J L-E, Karnstrom L, Mattsson B. Childhood cancer, Sweden, 1958–1974. I: Incidence and mortality. *Acta Paediatr Scand* 1978;67:425–432.
39. Evans AS. Causation and disease: a chronological journey. *Am J Epidemiol* 1978;108: 249–258.
40. Farwell JR, Dohrmann GJ, Flannery JT. Medulloblastoma in childhood: an epidemiological study. *J Neurosurg* 1984;61:657–664.
41. Farwell J, Dohrmann GJ, Flannery JT. Tumors of the central nervous system in adolescents. *Am Fam Physician* 1984;29:133–139.
42. Farwell J, Flannery JT. Second primaries in children with central nervous system tumors. *J Neurooncol* 1984;2:371–375.
43. Flegal KM, Brownie C, Haas JD. The effects of exposure misclassification on estimate of relative risk. *Am J Epidemiol* 1986;123:736–751.

44. Freudenheim JL, Johnson NE, Wardrop RL. Misclassification of nutrient intake of individuals and groups using one-, two-, three-, and seven-day food records. *Am J Epidemiol* 1987;126:703–713.
45. Fulchiero A, Winston K, Leviton A, Gilles FH. Secular trends of cerebellar gliomas in children. *J Natl Cancer Inst* 1977;58:839–843.
46. Giuffre R, Liccardo G, Pastore FS, Spallone A, Vagnozzi R. Potential risk factors for brain tumors in children: an analysis of 200 cases. *Childs Nerv Syst* 1990;6:8–12.
47. Gjerris F. Clinical aspects and long-term prognosis of intracranial tumours in infancy and childhood. *Dev Med Child Neurol* 1976;18:145–159.
48. Gold E, Gordis L, Tonascia J, Szklo M. Increased risk of brain tumors in children exposed to barbiturates. *J Natl Cancer Inst* 1978;61:1031–1034.
49. Gold E, Gordis L, Tonascia J, Szklo M. Risk factors for brain tumors in children. *Am J Epidemiol* 1979; 109:309–319.
50. Gold EB, Leviton A, Lopez R, et al. Parental smoking and risk of childhood brain tumors. *Am J Epidemiol* 1993;137:620–628.
51. Goldgar DE, Green P, Parry DM, Mulvihill JJ. Multipoint linkage analysis in neurofibromatosis type I: an international collaboration. *Am J Hum Genet* 1989;44:6–12.
52. Goldwein JW, Leahy JM, Packer RJ, et al. Intracranial ependymomas in children. *Int J Radiat Oncol Biol Phys* 1990;19:1497–1502.
53. Gordis L. Should dead cases be matched to dead controls? *Am J Epidemiol* 1982;115:1–5.
54. Gori GB. Adjudicating cancer causation: scientific, political and legal conflicts. *Regul Toxicol Pharmacol* 1991;13:309–325.
55. Greenberg RS, Shuster JL Jr. Epidemiology of cancer in children. *Epidemiol Rev* 1985; 7:22–48.
56. Greenland S. Limitations of the logistic analysis of epidemiologic data. *Am J Epidemiol* 1979;110:693–698.
57. Greenland S, Robins JM. Confounding and misclassification. *Am J Epidemiol* 1985;122: 495–506.
58. Greenwald P, Friedlander B, Lawrence C, Heame T, Earle K. Diagnostic sensitivity bias: an epidemiologic explanation for an apparent brain tumor excess. *J Occup Med* 1981;23: 690–694.
59. Grieg NH, Ries LG, Yancik R, Rapoport SI. Increasing annual incidence of primary malignant brain tumors in the elderly. *J Natl Cancer Inst* 1990;82:1621–1624.
60. Hansen ES. International Commission for Protection Against Environmental Mutagens and Carcinogens. ICPEMC Working Paper 7/1/2. Shared risk factors for cancer and atherosclerosis—a review of the epidemiological evidence. *Mutat Res* 1990;9:163–179.
61. Hurst HW, McIlhenny J, Park TS, Thomas WO. Neonatal craniopharyngioma: CT and ultrasonographic features. *J Comput Assist Tomogr* 1988;12:858–861.
62. Iolascon A, Lania A, Badiali M, et al. Analysis of N-ras gene mutations in medulloblastomas by polymerase chain reaction and oligonucleotide probes in formalin-fixed, paraffin-embedded tissues. *Med Pediatr Oncol* 1991;19:240–245.
63. Izuora GI, Ikerionwu S, Saddegi N, Iloeje SO. Childhood intracranial neoplasms, Enugu, Nigeria. *West Afr J Med* 1989;8:171–174.
64. James CD, He J, Carlbom E, et al. Loss of genetic information in central nervous system tumors common to children and young adults. *Genes Chromosom Cancer* 1990;2:-102.
65. Janisch W, Haas JF. Epidemiologic investigations on brain tumors in the GDR: possibilities and limits. *Arch Geschwulstforsch* 1984;54:243–247.
66. Jenkins RB, Kimmel DW, Moertel CA, et al. A cytogenetic study of 53 human gliomas. *Cancer Genet Cytogenet* 1989;39:253–279.
67. Jennings MT. Pediatric neuro-oncology: controversies in current therapy. *Indian J Pediatr* 1990;57:461–468.
68. Jooma R, Hayward RD, Grant DN. Intracranial neoplasms during the first year of life: analysis of one hundred consecutive cases. *Neurosurgery* 1984;14:31–41.
69. Keith HM, Craig WM, Kernohan JW. Brain tumors in children. *Pediatrics* 19;3:839–844.
70. Kernohan JW. Tumors of congenital origin. In: Minkler J, ed. *Pathology of the nervous system.* New York: McGraw-Hill; 1971:1927–1937.
71. Kim JH, Duncan C, Manuelidis EE. Congenital cerebellar medulloblastoma. *Surg Neurol* 1985;23:75–81.

72. Knudson AG Jr. The genetics of childhood cancer. *Cancer* 1975;35:1022–1026.
73. Koos WT, Miller MH. Intracranial tumors of infants and children. Stuttgart: Georg Thieme Verlag; 1971.
74. Kuijten RR, Bunin GR, Nass CC, Meadows AT. Gestational and familial risk factors for childhood astrocytoma: results of a case-control study. *Cancer Res* 1990;50:2608–2612.
75. Lannering B, Marky I, Nordborg C. Brain tumors in childhood and adolescence in west Sweden 1970–1984: epidemiology and survival. *Cancer* 1990;66:604–609.
76. Lashley PM, Clarke H, Archer EY. Primary pediatric brain tumors in Barbados: 10-year analysis (1978–1988). *J Trop Pediatr* 1991;37:64–66.
77. Ledbetter DH, Rich DC, O'Connel P, et al. Precise localization of NF1 to 17q11.2 by balanced translocation. *Am J Hum Genet* 1989;44:20–24.
78. Lee J, Kolonel LN. Nutrient intakes of husbands and wives: implications for epidemiologic research. *Am J Epidemiol* 1982;115:515–525.
79. Lellouch-Tubiana A, Pfister A, DaLage C. Classification histologique et prevalence de tumeurs du systeme nerveux central chez le nourrisson. Etude de cent pieces d'exerese. *Ann Pathol* 1989;9:195–198.
80. MacMahon B, Newill VA. Birth characteristics of children dying of malignant neoplasms. *J Natl Cancer Inst* 1962;28:231–244.
81. Marley JE, McMichael AJ. Principles behind practice. 6: Disease causation—the role of epidemiologic evidence. *Med J Aust* 1991;155:95–101.
82. Mortimer E, Lepow M, Gold E, Robbins FC, Burton GJ, Fraumeni J. Long term follow-up of persons inadvertently inoculated with SV40 as neonates. *N Engl J Med* 1981;305:1517–1518.
83. Nasca PC, Baptiste MS, MacCubbin PA, et al. An epidemiologic case-control study of central nervous system tumors in children and parental occupational exposures. *Am J Epidemiol* 1988;128:1256–1265.
84. National Institutes of Health Consensus Development Conference. Neurofibromatosis: conference statement. *Arch Neurol* 1988;45:575–578.
85. Nishio S, Takeshita I, Fujii K, Fukui N. Brain stem glioma: the role of a biopsy. *Br J Neurosurg* 1991;5:265–273.
86. Niswander KR, Gordon M. *The women and their pregnancies*. DHEW Publication No (NIH), U.S. Government Printing Office; 1972:73–79.
87. Ogasawara H, Inagawa T, Yamamoto M, Kaniya E, Yano T, Utsunomiya H. Medulloblastoma in infancy associated with omphalocele, malrotation of the intestine, and extrophy of the bladder. *Childs Nerv Syst* 1988;4:108–111.
88. Ohry A, Brooks ME, Rozin R. Is the polio virus responsible for late central nervous system tumors? *Med Hypotheses* 1978;4:44–49.
89. Oi S, Kokunai T, Matsumoto S. Congenital brain tumors in Japan (ISPN Cooperative Study): specific clinical features in neonates. *Childs Nerv Syst* 1990;6:86–91.
90. Olshan AF, Breslow NE, Daling JR, Weiss NS, Leviton A. Childood brain tumors and paternal occupation in the aerospace industry. *J Natl Cancer Inst* 1986;77:17–19.
91. Peacock WJ, Lazareff JA, Levin CV. Childhood brain tumors in Cape Town. *S. Afr Med J* 1987;71:5–8.
92. Pierre-Kahn A, Hirsch JF, Roux FX, Renier D, Sainte-Rose C. Intracranial ependymomas in children: survival and functional results of 47 cases. *Childs Brain* 1983;10:145–156.
93. Pitor H, Goldsworthy T, Moran S. The natural history of carcinogenesis: implications of experimental carcinogenesis in the genesis of human cancer. *J Supramol Struct Cell Biochem* 1981;17:133–146.
94. Preston-Martin S, Yu MC, Benton B, Henderson BE. N-nitroso compounds and childhood brain tumors: a case-control study. *Cancer Res* 1982;42:5240–5245.
95. Preston-Martin S. The epidemiology of primary nervous system tumors in children. *Ital J Neurol Sci* 1985;6:403–409.
96. Preston-Martin S. Epidemiological studies of perinatal carcinogenesis. *IARC Sci Publ* 1989;96:289–314.
97. Raskind R, Beigel F. Brain tumors in early infancy: probably congenital in origin. *J Pediatr* 1964;65:727–732.
98. Roberts RO, Lynch CH, Jones MPJ, Hart MN. Medulloblastoma: a population-based study of 532 cases. *J Neuropathol Exp Neurol* 1991;50:134–144.

99. Ron E, Modan B, Boice JD Jr, et al. Tumors of the brain and nervous system after radiotherapy in childhood. *N Engl J Med* 1988;319:1033–1039.
100. Roos KL, Dunn DW. Neurofibromatosis. *CA* 1992;42:241–254.
101. Rorke LB. The cerebellar medulloblastoma and its relationship to primitive neuroectodermal tumors. *J Neuropathol Exp Neurol* 1983;42:1–15.
102. Rubinstein LJ. Presidential address: cytogenesis and differentiation of primitive central neuroepithelial tumors. *J Neuropathol Exp Neurol* 1972;31:7–26.
103. Sackett D. Bias in analytic research. *J Chronic Dis* 1979;32:51–63.
104. Salonen T, Saxen L. Risk indicators in childhood malignancies. *Int J Cancer* 1975;15: 941–946.
105. Savitz DA, John EM, Kleckner RC. Magnetic field exposure from electric appliances and childhood cancer. *Am J Epidemiol* 1990;131:763–773.
106. Sorva R, Heiskanen O. Craniopharyngioma in Finland: a study of 123 cases. *Acta Neurochir (Wien)* 1986;81:85–99.
107. Stein Z, Susser M. Miscarriage, caffeine, and the epiphenomena of pregnancy: the causal model. *Epidemiology* 1991;2:163–167.
108. Starr MA. Tumors of the brain in childhood. *Med News* 1889;54:29–37.
109. Stratton MR, Darling J, Lantos PL, Cooper CS, Reeves BR. Cytogenetic abnormalities in human ependymomas. *Int J Cancer* 1989;44:579–581.
110. Sussman A, Leviton A, Allred EN, et al. Childhood brain tumor: presentation at younger age is associated with a family tumor history. *Cancer Causes and Control* 1990;1:75–79.
111. Takakura K, Inoya H, Nagashima K, Ikeda K, Tomonaga M, Kondo K. Viral neurooncogenesis. *Prog Exp Tumor Res* 1987;30:10–20.
112. Teppo L, Salonen T, Hakulinen T. Incidence of childhood cancers in Finland. *JNCI* 1975; 55:1065–1067.
113. The Childhood Brain Tumor Consortium. A study of childhood brain tumors based on surgical biopsies from ten North American institutions: sample description. *J Neurooncol* 1988;6:9–23.
114. Tokuriki Y, Handa H, Yamashita J, Okumura T, Paine JT. Brainstem glioma: an analysis of 85 cases. *Acta Neurochir* 1986;79:67–73.
115. Tomita T, McLone DG. Brain tumors during the first twenty-four months of life. *Neurosurgery* 1985;17:913–919.
116. Tomlinson FH, Schettauer BW, Jenkins RB. Medulloblastoma. II: A pathobiologic overview. *J Child Neurol* 1992;7:240–252.
117. Tsunematsu Y, Watanabe S, Inoue R, et al. Multiple primary malignancies in childhood cancer. *Jpn J Clin Oncol* 1985;15:223–233.
118. Turgut N, Ozcan OG, Saglam S. Central neurofibromatosis: case report and review of the literature. *Eur Neurol* 1991;31:188–192.
119. Undjian S, Marinov M. Intracranial ependymomas in children. *Childs Nerv Syst* 1990;6: 131–134.
120. Vagnozzi R, Liccardo G, Spallone A, Operamolla P, Castello MA, Giuffre R. Epidemiology of primary brain tumors in childhood. Perinatal risk factors: analysis of 200 cases. *J Pediatr Neurosci* 1987;3:261–268.
121. van Hoff J, Schymura MJ, Curnen MG. Trends in the incidence of childhood and adolescent cancer in Connecticut, 1935–1979. *Pediatr Oncol* 1988;16:78–87.
122. Vitali R, Amici A, Crupi S, Minelli A, Mastrandrea V. Incidence of childhood cancer in the province of Perugia (Italy). *Zentralbl Bakteriol Mikrobiol Hyg* 1984;179:300–307.
123. Weed DL, Selmon M, Sinks T. Links between categories of interaction. *Am J Epidemiol* 1988;127:17–27.
124. Weiss NS. Inferring casual relationships: elaboration of the criterion of "dose-response." *Am J Epidemiol* 1981;113:487–490.
125. Werler MM, Pober BR, Nelson K, et al. Reporting accuracy among mothers of malformed and nonmalformed infants. *Am J Epidemiol* 1989; 129:415–421
126. West CG. Parental occupation and occurrence of brain tumors in children. Doctoral thesis, Harvard School of Public Health, Boston, 1988.
127. Wilkins JR 3rd, Sinks T. Parental occupation and intracranial neoplasms of childhood: results of a case-control overview study. *Am J Epidemiol* 1990;132:275–292.

128. Wilkins JR 3rd, McLaughlin JA, Sinks TH, Kosnik EJ. Parental occupation and intracranial neoplasms of childhood: anecdotal evidence from a unique occupational cancer cluster. *Am J Ind Med* 1991;19:643–653.
129. Winston K, Gilles FH, Leviton A, Fulchiero A. Cerebellar gliomas in children. *J Natl Cancer Inst* 1977;58:833–838.
130. Wyke J. Oncogenic viruses. *J Pathol* 1981;135:39–85.

3

Principles of Neuropathology

Reid R. Heffner, Jr.

CLASSIFICATION OF PEDIATRIC CNS TUMORS

It may be possible in the future to develop a classification of tumors, including those arising in the CNS, based on etiology. Data continue to accumulate suggesting an association between human cancers of the nervous system and viral infections with such agents as polyomavirus. There is also evidence, particularly in animals, that chemical carcinogens are responsible for the development of neoplasia in the brain. Many viral and chemical mutagens appear to induce neoplasia by producing genetic alterations in target cells, which then undergo neoplastic transformation. Some of these genetic changes will probably become diagnostic markers for specific neoplasms before the actual mutagen is known. The emergence of recombinant technology to identify oncogenes and other genomic abnormalities is a potentially powerful means of diagnosing and eventually classifying CNS neoplasms on the basis of discrete changes at the molecular level.

In the meantime, current classifications are descriptive, based primarily on morphology, and depend heavily on two pillars of pathologic information—tumor location and cytoplasmic differentiation. Location, while not as widely applicable, is fundamental in the definition of some tumors. Hence, medulloblastomas arise in the cerebellum and schwannomas arise within cranial or peripheral nerves, but neither of these lesions, by definition, is located in the cerebral parenchyma. Tumor location is derived from the venerable concept of cell of origin. That is, a tumor in a specific location arises from the cells indigenous to that site. For example, in the case of meningiomas, these tumors in theory can arise only from cells comprising the meninges—fibroblasts and arachnoidal cells. The cell-of-origin concept is best demonstrated in epithelial carcinomas where in situ lesions can be monitored as they progress to invasive cancer. In the nervous system parenchyma, tracing the lineage of cells from premalignant to malignant is much more problematical. Consequently, the cell of origin cannot really be proven and tumors are more likely to be described in terms of their resemblance to a normal cell type. Therefore, astrocytomas are composed of cells that histo-

Brain Tumors in Children: Principles of Diagnosis and Treatment, 2/e, edited by M.E. Cohen and P.K. Duffner, Raven Press, Ltd., New York, 1994.

logically resemble astrocytes. This principle leads to a consideration of the second pillar—the reliance on cytoplasmic differentiation of neoplastic cells to diagnose and classify tumors. Early studies were derived from the examination of paraffin-embedded tissues, sometimes subjected to elegant but largely outmoded staining procedures such as the phosphotungstic acid hematoxylin (PTAH) and silver impregnation methods. This kind of information has been supplemented in modern times by electron microscopy and immunocytochemistry, which provide more sophisticated and precise insights into cytoplasmic differentiation.

The first comprehensive classification was proposed by Bailey and Cushing (1) in 1926. This system was founded on the science of embryology, a discipline that was on the frontier of medicine in its day. Each category of tumor was considered to have an embryological cell of origin or its architecture was reminiscent of a stage of embryogenesis. The Bailey and Cushing nosology still represents the framework of most brain tumor classifications, although many modifications have been made. A major refinement was the introduction of tumor grading for the purposes of assigning prognosis by Kernohan et al. (2). One of the most popular classifications, particularly among neuropathologists in America and Britain, was developed by Russell and Rubinstein (3). Finally, the World Health Organization (WHO) classification (4) published in 1979 has attempted to incorporate several classifications into a single system. Despite a number of limitations, a majority of neuropathologists recognize this classification as preferable to previous systems.

Current classifications of pediatric CNS tumors are limited by the fact that they have been dependent on classical histopathology, which is largely descriptive. Diagnosis, on which these classifications are based, has been somewhat subjective and variable, particularly in unusual and difficult cases, even among expert observers. Moreover, classical morphology, because it is static rather than dynamic, provides only indirect evidence of cell proliferation rates and capacity to invade and spread. Classifications have also had to conform to established brain tumor nosology. Not uncommonly, pediatric tumors cannot be easily assigned to an existing diagnostic category within the adult tumor nomenclature. New efforts at classification will need to use emerging technologies, including molecular biology, to provide more accurate information about natural history, biological behavior, and prognosis. Ultimately, the premise of an ideal classification will be an understanding of etiology and oncogenesis, so that prevention as well as improved therapy may be possible.

SPECIMEN ACQUISITION

Inadequate sample size, because of restricted surgical access to the lesion or forfeiture of tissue as a casualty to the laser, cavitron, or suction apparatus, often compromises diagnosis. Tumors of the CNS are often histologically heterogeneous, so that a small sample may not accurately represent the entire neoplasm. Heterogeneity is axiomatic in many tumors of glial origin, which are characterized by benign and malignant components, as illustrated in a recent study of 1000 samples from 50 gliomas (5). Heterogeneity is also expressed by the variable chromosomal numbers and fragments found in cells cloned from the same tumor.

In an era when stereotactic biopsies are almost certain to be used with increasing frequency, the pathologist will not always be able to rely on traditional sample size to render a diagnosis. To a considerable extent, the neurosurgeon can counterbalance the reduced sample size by obtaining a truly representative specimen. The use of modern scanning methods (CT or MRI) in combination with precision stereotactic instruments and needles designed to minimize bleeding is becoming the essential prerequisite to representative sampling. The practice of obtaining multiple biopsies of the lesion and consultating intraoperatively with the pathologist can be effective in eliminating many inadequate specimens. The combination of all of the above modalities may actually increase diagnostic accuracy when the efforts of the experienced neurosurgeon and pathologist are properly coordinated (6,7).

Collection and preparation artifacts may also interfere with accurate interpretation. Fixed tissue should be submitted to supplement material that has been frozen, if at all possible, since freezing causes considerable distortion of the tissue even after proper fixation. Interhospital consultations represent special problems when microscopic slides are exchanged between institutions. The tissue may be improperly fixed, sectioned, or stained. Consultation slides are frequently unaccompanied by blocks or wet tissue, on which additional diagnostic studies such as electron microscopy or immunohistochemistry could be performed. Clinical information is often unavailable or incomplete.

INTRAOPERATIVE CONSULTATION

The interpretation of cryostat sections is more challenging than that of permanent specimens, and consequently diagnoses may be provisional or deferred (8). The shortcomings of frozen section diagnosis are partly offset by the tendency for intraoperative consultations to increase the chances of obtaining a representative sample for permanent sections. The opportunity to prepare touch imprints from the fresh specimen is an additional benefit. So-called "touch preps" are not significantly different from ordinary cytological specimens, except that as the tumor tissue comes into direct contact with the slide, a larger number of neoplastic cells usually remain on the glass surface. Touch preparations also provide better cellular detail than tissue sections. However, because of a loss of architecture in imprints, they are only an adjunct to frozen sections.

HISTOPATHOLOGICAL TERMINOLOGY

The terminology that follows is frequently used in the description and diagnosis of tumors involving the nervous system in routine microscopic sections. Many of the terms are part of the vocabulary of the general pathologist. Other terms are unique to neuropathology and have not been totally accepted by the surgical pathology community, in part because of confusion regarding definition and usage.

Reactive versus Neoplastic

Reactive changes occur in response to injury from trauma, infection, vascular disease, and even tumor. The cells that participate in the reactive process, while not neoplastic, are stimulated and proliferating so that they can stimulate neoplasia histologically. One of the most difficult diagnostic problems involves the distinction between reactive gliosis and glioma. As a rule, in gliosis the architecture of the nervous system is preserved, while in glioma it is effaced by infiltrating neoplastic cells. A review of the CT or MRI examination is often helpful, since gliomas tend to expand, producing a mass lesion, whereas reactive gliosis, which is usually in relation to a destructive lesion, contracts. Moreover, the amounts of cellularity, pleomorphism, and atypia are less in a reactive process, and mitoses are rarely encountered. Nevertheless, in the evaluation of a specific case, all these criteria may fail and a definitive diagnosis cannot be made.

Malignant versus Benign

The terms *malignant* and *benign* have different meanings to physicians in different specialties. A tumor may be described as benign or malignant depending on its location, neuroimaging appearance, histologic properties, grade, or biological behavior. When applied to organs outside the nervous system, malignancy usually refers to lesions that can or have metastasized. Within the neuraxis, tumor metastases are rare, even in the most aggressive neoplasms, and metastatic potential is less meaningful. Particularly in the brain, many tumors are apt to be lethal despite the absence of histological evidence of malignancy.

The criteria on which malignancy is judged are cellularity, pleomorphism, nuclear atypia, and mitotic activity. In addition to these criteria, which refer to nuclear characteristics, anaplasia (described below) is a feature of malignant cells. Cellularity is determined by the nuclear density or number of tumor nuclei per unit area of tumor as seen on the microscopic slide. Pleomorphism refers to a variability in nuclear size and shape. In contrast to normal cells, which tend to have nuclear uniformity, atypical nuclei are generally greater than normal in size and have a higher density of nuclear chromatin. Mitoses are usually more numerous in tumors with aggressive behavior. The number of mitoses can be expressed as the mitotic count (number of mitoses per high-power field).

Seeding, Spread, and Metastases

Tumors may spread by local invasion from a primary site or by seeding, which is the spread of tumor through existing spaces such as the meninges or along parenchymal surfaces. On gross inspection, the seeded surface of the brain, spinal cord, or ventricle may appear cloudy or opaque. More extensive seeding expands the subarachnoid space, which can be studded or filled with a granular or shaggy, exudate-like infiltrate. Seeding is more common in aggressive tumors that originate in the parenchyma, such as medulloblastoma and ependymoma, and generally signifies a poor prognosis.

Within the brain, tumors tend to spread along the pathways of lesser resistance, particularly in the loose, acellular subpial and subependymal regions, along fiber tracts such as the corpus callosum, and in the spaces around vessels and neurons. These collections of infiltrating neoplastic cells seen microscopically adjacent to the leptomeninges and ventricles, surrounding the perivascular Virchow-Robin spaces, and enveloping neurons (satellitosis) came to the attention of Scherer (9), who described these signs of spreading tumor as "secondary structures." Metastatic disease occurs when there is discontinuous spread of a primary tumor to distant sites beyond the central nervous system. The spread of tumor cells into the adjacent dura mater or bone should not be considered evidence of a metastatic process.

Encapsulation and Invasion

By definition, when surrounded by a capsule, tumors exhibit indolent growth and relatively benign behavior. Dermoids, epidermoids, and some lipomas are among those benign tumors that are truly encapsulated. Most benign tumors compress rather than invade the parenchyma and are surrounded by a false or pseudocapsule composed of reactive CNS tissue. Meningiomas and nerve sheath tumors are the most common lesions to form a pseudocapsule. The majority of CNS tumors are not well circumscribed and are invasive due to the elaboration of tissue-destructive enzymes, such as collagenases and hydrolases, by the tumor cells. On the other hand, metastatic tumors with great potential for invasion are paradoxically well demarcated from the surrounding CNS tissue, particularly when they are small. Glioblastomas may appear to be well circumscribed grossly, although usually malignant foci can be found histologically outside the boundary between the tumor and normal brain.

Anaplasia

Anaplasia, which means "backward growth," implies that tumor cells have undergone retrogression from a more highly differentiated state to a lower level of differentiation. Anaplastic tumors are composed of primitive cells in which there is poor cytoplasmic differentiation. For example, anaplastic astrocytes seem to be unable to synthesize adequate numbers of intermediate filaments. Therefore, techniques such as electron microscopy and immunohistochemistry that are used to demonstrate cytoplasmic constituents are of limited value in the evaluation of anaplastic tumors. The cytoplasmic abnormalities of anaplasia are frequently accompanied by nuclear abnormalities such as pleomorphism, nuclear atypia, and increased nuclear size, which is reflected in a higher nuclear:cytoplasmic ratio.

Metaplasia

In contrast to anaplasia, metaplasia is a nonneoplastic, reactive, and reversible change during which a normal cell appears to differentiate into another cell type. Metaplasia commonly represents an adaptive change that allows cells to cope with an unfavorable environment. In patients who smoke, the bronchial epithelium undergoes squamous metaplasia as an adaptation to a hostile airway. In tumors, the reasons for metaplasia do not appear to be adaptive, but the underlying mechanisms are unknown.

Necrosis

Necrosis in neoplasms is mediated by tumor necrosis factors, which are produced by macrophages and other mononuclear elements, other cytokines, and a variety of enzymes liberated by tumor cells which degrade the surrounding normal tissues. Necrosis is generally synonymous with rapid growth, but its importance relative to outcome varies with tumor type. In meningiomas, necrosis may reflect a somewhat more aggressive behavior, while in astrocytomas it is regarded by many as a definite malignant criterion.

Pseudopalisading

As opposed to true palisading, which is characteristic of nerve sheath tumors, pseudopalisading is a type of necrosis in which nonviable tumor cells are surrounded on one or more sides by rows of neoplastic cells, which assume the appearance of a palisaded or picket fence. The pathogenesis of pseudopalisading is unknown, but it is a constant feature of glioblastoma multiforme. Pseudopalisading may also be seen in other malignant tumors, particularly those of glial origin.

Rosettes

A rosette (imitation rose) is an organoid structure resembling a flower that has been cross sectioned. Many types of rosettes have been described, but for diagnostic purposes only two are important. The Homer Wright rosette is formed by a circle of tumor cells from which delicate fibrillary processes converge toward a central point. Some of the processes may be argentophilic, like neuronal axons, supporting the idea that Homer Wright rosettes represent neuroblastic differentiation. As a diagnostic criterion, these rosettes are not always reliable, since they are frequently few in number and difficult to locate. Even when present, Homer Wright rosettes are often abortively formed. They are typically observed in primitive neuroectodermal tumors including medulloblastoma, neuroblastoma, and pineoblastoma. Perivascular rosettes are arranged around thin-walled blood vessels that appear to be venous in origin. Between the ring of tumor cells and the vascular channel is a so-called nuclear free zone, which contains the cytoplasmic processes of tumor cells that attach to the vessel wall. Perivascular rosettes are characteristic of ependymomas.

Desmoplasia

An exuberant proliferation of mesenchymal tissue composed mainly of fibroblasts and collagen may be stimulated by a neoplasm confined to the CNS parenchyma or, more commonly, by invasion of tumor cells into normal structures containing mesenchymal elements such as the meninges. Desmoplasia is a reactive rather than a neoplastic process, although histologically the proliferating mesenchymal tissue appears to be part of the tumor itself. A desmoplastic response is common in such tumors as medulloblastoma and ganglioglioma.

Endothelial Proliferation and Neovascularity

In order to expand, tumors require their own blood supply. Histologically, many tumors, such as meningioma, are extremely vascular and contain a plethora of new blood vessels. The individual blood vessels within an area of neovascularity may be larger than those normally found in the nervous system parenchyma. They are also tortuous, with a lumen that varies in diameter along its course. Endothelial proliferation often occurs in capillaries or in small venules, which become filled with endothelial cells so that they resemble renal glomeruli. Endothelial proliferation and neovascularity are under the influence of tumor angiogenesis factors that are produced by most, if not all, malignant neoplasms. Endothelial proliferation is an indication of aggressive behavior in tumors of the nervous system in most instances. It is most commonly found in glioblastoma multiforme, anaplastic astrocytoma, and metastatic tumors.

Tumor Grading versus Staging

The basic concept of tumor grading is that biological behavior can be forecast on the basis of a semiquantitative analysis of histologic parameters. Grading attempts to stratify tumors in terms of such malignant criteria as cellularity, nuclear changes, and overall anaplasia. In the typical grading system, a numerical value is assigned to each grade, with lower grades (grades I and II) being more benign than higher grades (grades III and IV). For many decades, such a system has been widely used to grade astrocytomas. Essentially the same system was originally proposed, and has recently been revived, to grade other gliomas (10,11). Some investigators are also applying these principles to nonglial tumors. Grading, which is determined by microscopic criteria, is not to be confused with tumor staging, which is based on gross tumor attributes such as location and size and on the extent of tumor spread. Staging of CNS tumors to determine prognosis has received greater attention in recent years with the availability of advanced techniques such as computed tomography (CT) and magnetic resonance imaging (MRI), which permit tumor staging in living patients.

ELECTRON MICROSCOPY

Electron microscopy, a time-honored technique in the pathological investigation of many diseases, requires considerable space, expensive equipment, and experienced personnel. It is also comparatively time-consuming and may delay turnaround time by at least a week. Many applications of electron microscopy are gradually being replaced by other technologies that require less manual dexterity and technical expertise, provide better information, and are not only faster but also cheaper. Nevertheless, electron microscopy is still a valuable asset when reserved for the investigation of certain tumors. Because the sample viewed ultrastructurally is quite small, random sampling of the specimen is not recommended. Prior to the preparation of ultrathin sections, the area to be examined ultrastructurally should be carefully selected from multiple thick, 1-μm plastic sections previewed under the light microscope. From a diagnostic standpoint, electron microscopy is most useful to evaluate cytoplasmic differentiation or cell specialization. This evaluation involves an ultrastructural search for the basement membranes, desmosomes, and microvilli at the cell surface as well as neurofilaments, neurosecretory granules, and other organelles in the cell cytoplasm.

IMMUNOHISTOCHEMISTRY

Immunohistochemical procedures rely on the availability of antibodies to cellular constituents such as epitopes of glial and neuronal proteins. In order to visualize the immunologic reaction microscopically, the antibody molecule is attached to a marker. It is essential that high-quality antibodies that have an affinity for a target cell antigen are used. Depending on the type of immunologic reagent, antibodies are produced in the research laboratory or, in many instances, are commercially available. Polyclonal antibodies are typically obtained from immunized animals and are often contaminated by antibodies against antigens other than the target immunogen. The advent of monoclonal antibody technology, which provides a more pure antibody reagent, has encouraged the expansion of immunohistochemistry as a diagnostic tool. Once an antibody attaches to an epitope in a tumor cell, the labeled antibody can be identified at the site of antigen binding. For many years, fluorescent markers, such as fluorescein isothiocyanate, were employed. However, immunofluorescence microscopy, which is still widely used, has several significant disadvantages. Since fresh tissue is necessary, retrospective studies utilizing fixed tissue or paraffin-embedded blocks are virtually impossible. Moreover, fluorescence, which wanes as time elapses, must be photographed if a permanent record is required. Also, the laboratory must maintain a fluorescence microscope and appropriate photographic equipment.

Immunoperoxidase techniques overcome many of the deficiencies inherent in immunofluorescence methods (12). Fixed or paraffin-embedded tissue can be used; the staining reaction is stable; and the reaction is visible under ordinary light microscopy. In the prototype method, an antibody directed against the target tissue antigen is coupled to horseradish peroxidase. Following antigen–antibody binding, peroxidase is allowed to react with its substrate, peroxide, in the presence of an indicator such as diaminobenzidine (DAB). As a consequence of the reaction, the indicator is converted to a visible precipitate in the tissue, at the antigenic sites. The original procedure has been modified to improve the quality of antigen detection. The peroxidase–antiperoxidase (PAP) method and the avidin–biotin (ABC) method are examples of newer refinements. Immunoperoxidase techniques are theoretically simple but are fraught with a number of practical difficulties. Some commercial antibodies must be carefully tested before use, due to their lack of specificity. Preservation of tissue antigen is imperative for the reaction to be valid. Improper fixation and excessive heating during processing can destroy the antigenicity of some cellular constituents. False-positive interpretations may result from nonspecific background staining. Parallel testing in control specimens can prevent this problem to some extent. The use of high-quality monoclonal antibodies and proper training of laboratory personnel can be instrumental in eliminating background staining and other artifacts.

A host of experimental and commercial antibodies have been applied to the study of neoplasms, including CNS tumors in children (13) (Table 3-1). Immunohistochemical methods demonstrate cellular antigens in both normal and neoplastic cells. At present, diagnosis of most neoplasms on the basis of detection of tumor-specific antigens is not possible. It should also be obvious that immunoreactivity in a neoplasm is meaningful only if the observer can distinguish between neoplastic cells that are positively stained and normal or reactive cells. In some tumors, this distinction is relatively easy, but in gliomas and other tumors having an antigen that is normally found in brain, the staining reaction may be particularly troublesome to interpret.

Perhaps the most widely used immunohistochemical method in the investigation of brain tumors is the glial fibrillary acidic protein (GFAP) technique. In normal cells, GFAP is located in glial cells, particularly astrocytes or astrocyte progenitors. GFAP is an intermediate filament, with a diameter of 10 to 12 nm, that is antigenically distinct from other fibrous proteins such as neurofilaments and cytokeratins found in epithelial cells. In neoplastic lesions, strong GFAP staining is observed in most well-differentiated astrocytomas (14) (Fig. 3-1). Less intense staining is seen in some astrocytomas that lack large numbers of cytoplasmic filaments, and in more anaplastic

TABLE 3-1. *Immunohistochemistry of common CNS neoplasms*

	GFAP	Vimentin	S-100 protein	Neurofilaments/ synaptophysin	Cytokeratin/ EMA
Astrocytoma	+ + +	+	+	−	−
Oligodendroglioma	+/−	+/−	+	−	−
Ependymoma	+	+/−	+	−	+
Ganglioglioma	+	+	+	+ + +	−
PNET	+	+/−	+	+	−
Meningioma	−	+ +	−	−	+
Schwannoma	−	+ +	+ + +	−	−
Metastatic carcinoma	−	+/−	+/−	−	+ + +

Histochemical reactions represent general staining characteristics of each tumor category. Staining reactions may vary among tumors, so that in the diagnosis of individual tumors a profile of histochemical stains is advisable.

Staining is denoted by + or −: weakly positive (+), moderately positive (+ +), strongly positive (+ + +), negative staining (−).

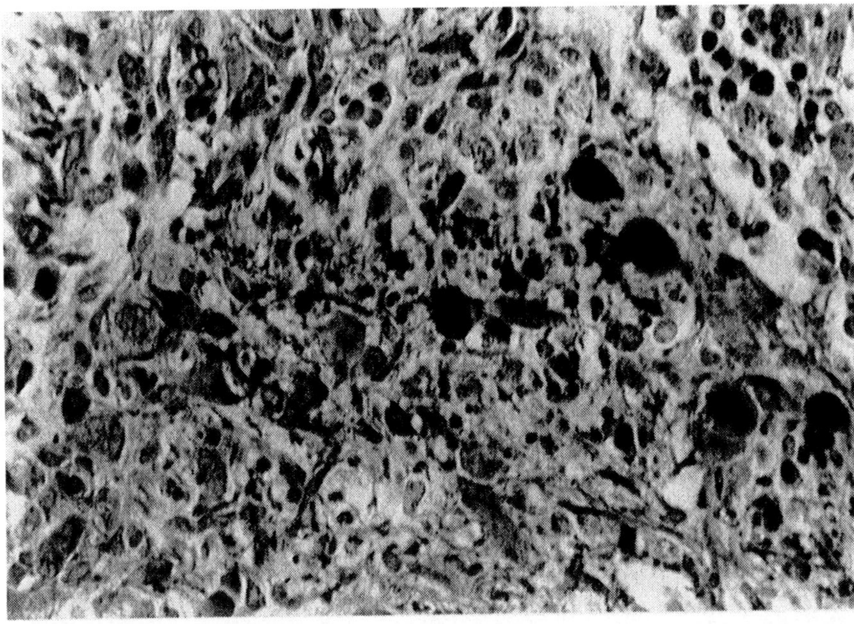

FIG. 3-1. Astrocytoma. The cytoplasm, which is abundant in several neoplastic cells, as well as astrocytic fibrillary processes, are heavily stained for GFAP. (Immunoperoxidase method for GFAP.)

astrocytomas. A weaker staining reaction is observed in ependymomas, choroid plexus tumors, and olidendrogliomas.

Vimentin is a 57-kD filament protein that is ultrastructurally indistinguishable from glial filaments. In the developing nervous system, vimentin is relatively abundant in immature glial cells. As myelination progresses, its expression is decreased while GFAP becomes more apparent. Vimentin and GFAP coexist in mature astroglia, both normal and neoplastic. In tumors of nonglial origin, vimentin is reported to be present in meningiomas, schwannomas, carcinomas, sarcomas, melanomas, and lymphomas (15). Because cells of varying histogenesis contain vimentin, the demonstration of this intermediate filament protein in neurooncologic diagnosis is somewhat limited.

The intermediate filament, desmin, is reported to exist in cardiac muscle, skeletal muscle, visceral smooth muscle, and smooth muscle of blood vessels. This 53-kD acidic protein is composed of a nonhelical N-terminal head and a C-terminal tail, which are at opposite ends of an alpha helical middle portion containing approximately 300 amino acids. The synthesis of desmin begins early in myoblastic differentiation and is intimately associated with the Z bands of skeletal muscle and with dense bodies in smooth muscle. Desmin is expressed in benign and malignant tumors of smooth and skeletal muscle origin, such as leiomyoma and rhabdomyosarcoma (16). Despite the presence of smooth muscle in vascular structures, desmin is generally not present immunohistochemically in tumors of vascular histogenesis. The presence of desmin in neoplasms arising from nonmuscular tissues is generally accepted as evidence for muscle differentiation. In tumors of the nervous system, desmin is occasionally found in medulloblastomas (myomedulloblastomas) and in tumors of Schwann cell derivation (triton tumors).

Cytokeratins, a class of intermediate filaments with molecular weights ranging from 40 to 67 kD, are located in epithelial cells of various origin. Anticytokeratin antibodies are generally used in diagnosis of carcinomas. Cytokeratins are also easily demonstrated in craniopharyngiomas and meningiomas. Epithelial membrane antigen (EMA) is a nonfibrous glycoprotein that is found in most normal and neoplastic epithelial cells. In the nervous system, EMA is an excellent marker for metastatic carcinoma and chordomas. Many meningiomas are also positively stained for EMA. In normal neuroectodermal tissues, EMA is visualized in ependymal cells and choroid plexus epithelium. Glial neoplasms such as astrocytoma are reportedly EMA negative.

Neurofilaments are exclusively located in neurons and their processes. These cytoskeletal elements are heteropolymers composed of three subunits with molecular weights of 68, 160, and 200 kD. Each of the triplet proteins is immunochemically distinct; and its synthesis, which occurs in the neuronal perikaryon, is regulated by a different gene. Antineurofilament antibodies decorate normal nerve cells and tumors containing neurons including gangliogliomas, differentiating medulloblastomas, and neuroblastomas. Neurofilament proteins may also be detected immunohistochemically in retinoblastomas, particularly in cells forming Flexner-Wintersteiner rosettes.

In addition to neurofilament protein, other markers of neuronal cells are gaining attention. Immunohistochemical methods for the demonstration of synaptophysin have perhaps been the most promising. Synaptophysin, a glycosylated polypeptide with a molecular weight of 38 kD, is a component of the presynaptic vesicle membrane. In the nervous system, synaptophysin is considered to be an oligomeric protein that avidly binds calcium within the neurotransmitter vesicles and appears to be important in the calcium ion-dependent release of neurotransmitters. Synaptophysin may be emerging as a reliable marker of neuroectodermal differentiation. It has been demonstrated across the entire spectrum of neuroectodermal tumors, from those containing neurons, such as gangliogliomas and neuroblastomas, to neuroendocrine tumors, such as carcinoid and paragangliomas (17). Neuron-specific enolase (NSE) is a dimeric enzyme that catalyzes the conversion of 2-phosphoglycerate to phosphoenolpyruvate. The gamma subunit of NSE is expressed in a variety of neural and nonneural tissues including lymphocytes, smooth muscle cells, and renal tubular epithelium. Central nervous system NSE is not specific for neurons and can be detected in reactive astrocytes as well as in gliomas, meningiomas, schwannomas, and choroid plexus papillomas. In normal cells intense NSE immunoreactivity is characteristic of neurons and neuroendocrine cells, but in neoplastic cells NSE is not a specific marker of neuronal elements. Some evidence suggests that the increased expression of NSE in reactive and neoplastic cells may reflect the increased metabolic demands of these conditions.

Myelin basic protein (MBP) and myelin associated glycoprotein (MAG) are myelin-specific proteins that can be found in the myelin sheath of the central and peripheral nervous system. Using immunohistochemical methods, MBP has been visualized in developing and mature oligodendrocytes. MAG is particularly abundant in developing oligodendrocytes and in schwann cells. Oligodendrocytes are known to express large amounts of MBP and MAG during demyelination and remyelination. In theory, MBP and MAG should be ideal markers in the diagnosis of neoplastic disease of the nervous system, but in practice neither of these myelin-associated proteins appears to be consistently expressed in tumors. In the diagnosis of oligodendroglioma, wherein the presence of these myelin-associated proteins would be most useful, most investigators have been unable to find a staining pattern that is reliable and consistent.

S-100 protein with a molecular weight of 21 kD is a calcium- binding protein composed of alpha and beta subunits having three antigenically distinct portions. While earlier publications indicated that S-100 protein was restricted to schwann cells, S-100 protein and its subunits have subsequently been demonstrated in a variety of neuroectodermal cells including melanocytes and glia. As a diagnostic marker in CNS tumors, S-100 protein is probably of little value. However, in the diagnosis of spindle cell tumors of the peripheral nerve, intense immunoreactivity distinguishes nerve sheath tumors from those of mesenchymal origin such as fibrosarcoma. Fibroblastic meningiomas are generally more weakly stained than nerve sheath tumors.

METHODS OF ASSESSING CELL PROLIFERATION

For many decades, a crude approximation of cell proliferation was obtained from the mitotic index. Routine histologic sections were evaluated for the number of mitoses, a laborious procedure with inherent inaccuracies (18). The identification of mitotic figures is somewhat subjective, and it is often difficult, for example, to distinguish mitoses from pyknotic nuclei. Moreover, the cells undergoing mitosis comprise only a minute proportion of cycling cells so that the enumeration of mitoses is often unreliable due to sample size. Newer staining techniques allow improved identification of mitotic figures for the calculation of the mitotic index, which is the number of mitoses per 1,000 tumor cell nuclei (19).

The metaphase arrest technique has been used primarily in experimental situations to determine cell proliferation rates. Cells in culture are exposed to agents such as vincristine which will arrest the cell cycle in mitosis, accentuating the number of metaphase mitotic figures. Mitotic rate is estimated as a function of vincristine concentration and incubation time. The technique is hampered by a number of technical difficulties, including significant distortion of metaphase-arrested mitoses, which can be difficult to interpret. The use of tissue culture precludes the adoption of this technique in most surgical pathology laboratories.

Genes situated on the short arms of the five acrocentric chromosomes are involved in the transcription of ribosomal RNA. This group of genes and their associated proteins comprise the nucleolar organizer regions. After staining with silver, nucleolar organizer regions (AgNOR) can be recognized in the interphase nuclei of tumor cells from tissue that has been routinely fixed in formaldehyde. In studies (20) of a variety of tumor types, there has been relatively good correlation between the number of AgNOR per nucleus and the proliferative activity of the tumor. However, in metallic impregnation methods, the staining can be inconsistent, particularly if reagents are not prepared with utmost care. Also, there is concern that increased AgNOR counts may be due, in some cases, to amplification of ribosomal RNA genes or a hyperdiploid state.

Flow cytometry (FCM) is a technique in which individual cells suspended in fluid are directed in a single-file stream past sensors with the ability to measure their physical and/or chemical characteristics (21). Available techniques allow the assessment of tumors using mainly fresh or frozen tissues as well as body fluids. The most widely used system passes individual cells from cytologic specimens or tissue that has been disrupted through a beam of laser light. Individual cells scatter light in various directions. The angles of deflected light are collected by sensors and converted to electronic signals, which are tabulated and analyzed. The data are most frequently expressed as a histogram, and a common approach to tumor analysis involves the interpretation of DNA histograms (Fig. 3-2). The process begins with the staining of individual nuclei by fluorescent dyes that bind to DNA stoichiometrically. The DNA histogram of normal cells is characterized by two peaks. The dominant peak represents the majority of cells in the resting (G_0) phase as well as cycling presynthetic (G_1) phase cells that contain the same quantity of DNA. Opposite this peak on the right side of the histogram is a smaller peak composed of G_2 and cells undergoing mitosis(M). Cells within the G_2/M peak are tetraploid. These cells may be in the postsynthetic phase of the cell cycle prior to mitosis (G_2) or in the process of mitosis before actual division (M). The signal activity above baseline between the left and right peaks represents the S-phase fraction of the cell cycle, when DNA synthesis occurs. DNA content abnormalities are compared to the DNA fluorescence of diploid cell standards (22). The ratio of the DNA fluorescence intensity of the G_0/G_1 peak in the tumor sample to the standard is defined as the DNA index (DI). A diploid sample with a normal DNA content has a DI of one. A

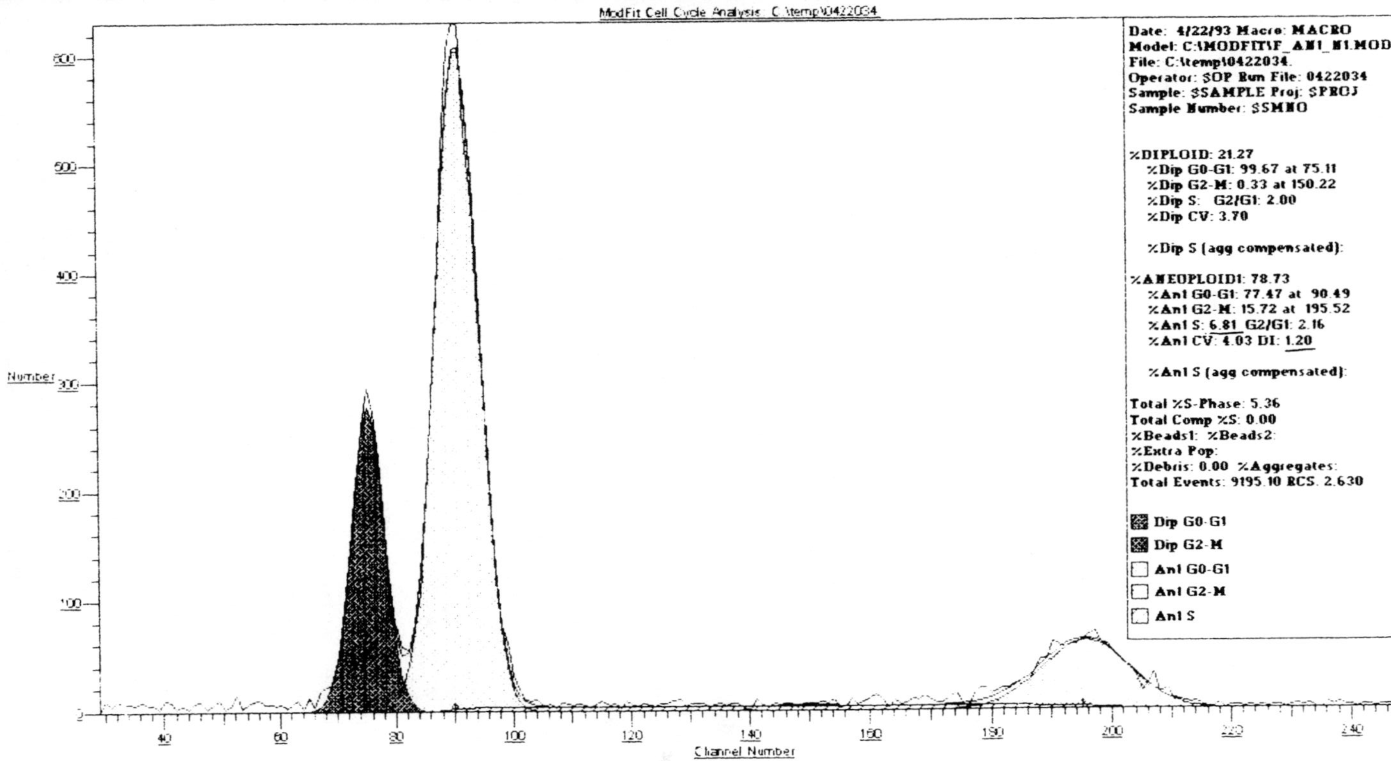

FIG. 3-2. DNA Histogram. Three peaks are seen. The left peak represents the reference diploid peak (G_0/G_1 fraction). The large central peak represents the aneuploid component from a breast carcinoma. The DNA index was calculated to be 1.20. The right peak represents the G_2/M fraction of tumor cells. The area under the curve between the second and third peaks is the S-phase fraction. (Provided by Jan Errick, M.D., SUNY-Buffalo Department of Pathology.)

DI less than or greater than one is considered abnormal, but is not necessarily indicative of malignancy, since such indices are reported in benign tumors. Malignant cells are commonly aneuploid with an increased or decreased amount of DNA. Aneuploid tumors display additional G_0/G_1 peaks that correspond to tumor cells having a DNA content that is different from the diploid standard.

Most malignant tumors have chromosomal abnormalities, but the sensitivity of FCM measurement of DNA is dependent on a significant quantitative DNA abnormality approximating at least 5% of total DNA content. Tumors having a near-diploid cytogenetic disturbance are appraised by FCM as having diploid DNA content. Tumors with chromosomal deletions and duplications that counterbalance each other, in that net DNA content is normal, are not distinguishable from the diploid state by FCM. In the majority of benign brain tumors associated with favorable prognosis, FCM has revealed a diploid histogram and a low percentage of S-phase cells. Of greater clinical value are studies that complement or surpass histopathologic diagnosis. FCM has the potential to be a predictive indicator of biological behavior where histologic evaluation fails. This potential has not been fully realized in pediatric brain tumors and would be particularly critical in predicting prognosis of patients with the same histologic diagnosis. The future of FCM is illustrated in a recent study (23) of patients with aneuploid medulloblastoma who enjoyed longer survival than those with diploid tumors.

One of the most exciting applications of FCM is the characterization of cell subpopulations, which depends on flow sorting and multiparameter analysis. In flow sorting, cellular elements with preselected characteristics are diverted from the main stream so that a homogeneous population of cells can be isolated. In multiparameter analysis, information regarding cell subpopulations can be obtained without physically isolating the cells. These techniques require intact cells in which a marker is attached to the cell surface or the cytoplasm of sectioned cells. Markers are typically antibodies to cellular constituents, and the labeling procedures are essentially modifications of those employed in immunohistochemistry. These techniques have great potential for studies along several lines of investigation. One obvious path involves the determination of DNA content in subpopulations of tumor cells defined by the presence of specific cell surface markers. This concept has become very sophisticated in studying non-CNS tumors, involving the simultaneous analysis of several subpopulations of cells that are distinguished by separate immunophenotypic markers for each cell type. Several advantages of FCM are worthy of emphasis. These include the capacity to study large numbers of cells in a short amount of time, providing quantitative and statistically significant data. A major advantage of FCM is the ability to sort different subpopulations of cells and to measure multiple parameters simultaneously. A significant disadvantage of FCM is the requirement for individual cell preparations. The preparation of single-cell suspensions from certain

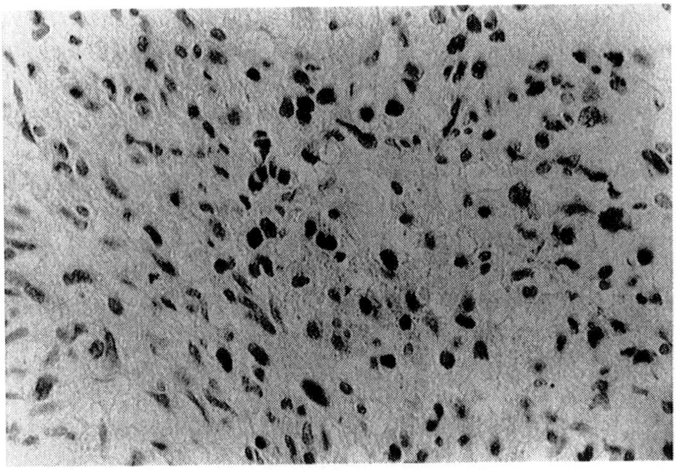

FIG. 3-3. Astrocytoma. In contrast to the lack of staining in noncycling neoplastic astrocytes, the nuclei of many actively proliferating tumor cells are positively stained for proliferating cell nuclear antigen. (Immunoperoxidase method for PCNA.)

types of tissue is difficult, particularly in collagen-containing neoplasms such as meningiomas and schwannomas. Although it is possible to suspend cells from a tissue biopsy after enzyme digestion of the collagenous framework, the results of analysis may be uninterpretable in the absence of morphologic correlation.

PROLIFERATION ANTIGENS

The majority of proliferation antigens are nuclear antigens that increase or appear during one or more proliferative phases in the cell cycle, allowing the recognition of cycling cells. Techniques to identify proliferation antigens permit an estimation of the growth fraction in both normal and neoplastic cells, although they do not provide information regarding the duration of the cell cycle, which reflects the doubling time of cell proliferation. Most proliferation antigens are unstable and are denatured by formalin. Because unfixed specimens submitted for cryostat examination are generally small, a limited sample may be available for analysis. Techniques to fix tissue in acetone for paraffin sections are currently under investigation. The murine monoclonal antibody Ki-67 reacts with human nuclear protein in the growth fraction (G_1, S, G_2, and M phases of the cell cycle), but not in the G_0 phase. The precise nature of the Ki-67 antigen is unknown, although recent work suggests that it is a nonhistone protein that, during immunoblot analysis, appears as a double band with molecular weights of 345 kD and 395 kD(24). As might be expected, in most tumors including brain neoplasms, Ki-67 expression is found in histologically malignant lesions. In a specific tumor type, the variation of expression found within tumor grades might be useful therapeutically, since proliferating cells are most affected by irradiation and chemotherapy. When brain tumors are studied using antibodies to Ki-67, not surprisingly glioblastoma multiforme has the greatest growth fraction (>16%), while meningioma, ependymoma, oligodendroglioma, and schwannoma exhibit growth fractions of less than 2% (25). More recently a second antigen, proliferating cell nuclear antigen (PCNA), has received considerable attention (Fig. 3-3). PCNA is an auxiliary protein of DNA polymerase, a nuclear enzyme involved in DNA repair. This 36-kD antigen was first discovered in systemic lupus erythematosus patients, some of whom produce an autoantibody to this nuclear protein. PCNA studies may offer increased flexibility since these antigens may be demonstrated in both S-phase cells and the growth fraction of the cell cycle. Other proliferation antigens under investigation are P53, P105, ribonucleotide reductase, and DNA polymerase-α. The data derived from studies using proliferation antigens in pediatric CNS tumors are of a preliminary nature at present. Further studies are necessary to ascertain whether these antigens will be advantageous in assessing treatment and prognosis. Studies that involve the use of statin identification may eventually complement those based on the demonstration of proliferation antigens. In contrast to proliferation-associated antigens, statin is a nuclear protein located in noncycling cells.

MARKERS OF DNA SYNTHESIS

Bromodeoxyuridine (BUDR) and other halogenated pyrimidines are thymidine analogs that compete with thymidine and are incorporated into DNA that is being synthesized in the S phase of the cell cycle. The development of antibodies to halogenated pyrimidines was a major advance. This permitted the identification of halopyrimidines by immunohistochemistry instead of by autoradiography, which requires the use of tritiated thymidine. A second significant advance has been the ability to label fresh tumor tissue in vitro, obviating the need to administer halopyrimidines to the patient during surgery. After cells are exposed to BUDR, the fraction of cells in the tumor that are in the S phase of the cell cycle can be counted and expressed as a percentage of the total cell population. This ratio represents the labeling index (LI), which is the percentage of positive-staining cells. The data obtained from studies of pediatric CNS tumors are incomplete but suggest that an increased LI is associated with histologic malignancy. A presumed benefit of S-phase evaluation is the opportunity to distinguish between two or more groups of patients who will have a different prognosis, although the histology of the tumor in all cases is identical.

GROWTH FACTORS

In normal tissues and organs, there is a necessity for coordination of cell differentiation and proliferation, which is regulated by messenger molecules or growth factors. Certain pathologic processes such as wound healing are also mediated by growth factors. Abnormalities in growth-factor signaling pathways may lead to premature cell death or uncontrolled cellular proliferation, which ultimately may culminate in neoplasia. Growth factors may function in a paracrine manner in which they are synthesized by one cell type and influence a second cell species. On the other hand, the target cell to be influenced by the growth factor may also synthesize the messenger molecules (autocrine secretion). The prototype growth factor is a peptide molecule that causes cells in the resting (G_0) phase to enter and continue through the cell cycle. Sustained stimulation by growth factor over a period of several hours is necessary for a transition through the G_1 phase. If the signal is interrupted during this time, the cell may return to the G_0 state. A number of naturally occurring substances antagonize the proliferative effects of growth factors. Some of these inhibitors are cytokines such as tumor necrosis factor, interferons, and transforming growth factor β. The role of growth factors in the induction and maintenance of neoplasia is extremely complicated but probably operates at several levels (26). Many growth factors are known to be under the control of proto-oncogenes. There is considerable evidence that oncogene activation and other genetic aberrations with the production of excessive or inappropriate growth factor occur, as reported in a number of neoplasms. Alterations in growth-factor receptors on target cells has been implicated in carcinogenesis. For example, increased numbers of epidermal growth-factor receptors have been found in epidermoid carcinomas and gliomas. Many growth-factor receptors are also governed by oncogenes that appear to become amplified in certain types of neoplasms. Finally, tumors may arise as a result of disregulation by inhibitory growth factors (27). Normal inhibitory signals may be reduced or lost. Alternatively, transformed cells may lack the ability to respond to inhibitory growth factors.

An ever-enlarging list of growth factors is under investigation, including platelet-derived growth factor, brain-derived neurotrophic factor, insulin-like growth factors, and a number of cytokines with growth-factor activity. We will concentrate our discussion on three growth factors with considerable implications for neoplasia of the central nervous system—epidermal growth factor, fibroblast growth factor, and nerve growth factor. Epidermal growth factor (EGF) is derived from a transmembrane precursor composed of 160 amino acids. When the precursor is exposed to specific proteases, active epidermal growth factor composed of approximately 53 amino acids is produced. Epidermal growth factor, originally purified from submaxillary glands of mice, is probably produced by many types of cells, although the specific cellular sites of synthesis have been difficult to identify. A variety of cells appear to respond to EGF, the effects of which include gastric secretion, hair follicle development, and angiogenesis. Epidermal growth-factor receptor (EGFR) is a large glycoprotein with a molecular weight of 175 kD. The EGFR gene is a homologue of the viral oncogene, v-erb, which is associated with avian erythroblastosis. In normal cells, EGF binds to its receptor to stimulate an intrinsic tyrosine kinase that phosphorylates the receptor. This event is followed by RNA synthesis and eventual DNA synthesis, but the precise mechanism of this signal transmission is not understood. Amplification of the EGFR gene has been reported (28) in squamous carcinomas and in a significant proportion of malignant astrocytomas. Amplification of the EGFR gene also correlates with a higher histologic grade of astrocytoma. EGFR-gene amplification is frequently accompanied by structural gene deletions and the production of altered, truncated EGFR proteins. Antibodies against the abnormal receptor have recently been developed. It may be possible to use this antibody as a diagnostic tool to identify a tumor-specific marker in astrocytomas.

Fibroblast growth factors (FGF) are a family of structurally similar proteins with myriad biological properties (29). FGF are involved in wound healing and tissue repair and are potent stimulants of angiogenesis. They also possess neurotrophic properties and modulate both glial and neuronal maturation. Two closely related factors, acidic FGF (aFGF) and basic FGF (bFGF), can be distinguished by their differing isoelectric properties. These growth factors, produced by macrophages and endothelial cells, have a high affinity for heparin and glycosaminoglycans, which are important components of basement membranes. The first fibroblast growth factor to be described in detail was bFGF, a potent mitogen for fibroblasts and neuroectodermal cells. bFGF has been found in numerous organs including peripheral nerve, retina, and brain, as well as in tumors such as breast carcinoma, hepatoma, and gliomas. Among the many functions of bFGF is the stimulation of increased DNA synthesis and cell division in mesodermal and neuroectodermal cells. The observation that FGF proteins are overexpressed in certain types of neoplastic cells suggests that they may play a yet-undefined role in oncogenesis. The control of angiogenesis by bFGF also suggests that fibroblastic growth factors may have a strong influence on tumor growth.

Nerve growth factor (NGF) has been studied more extensively than other neurotrophic molecules. NGF is synthesized by target cells such as dorsal root ganglia and sympathetic neurons as well as by nontarget cells such as schwann cells. Unlike like FGF, NGF is not considered to be a powerful mitogen, although some mitogenic activity has been seen in adrenal chromaffin cells. NGF binds to both high- and low-affinity receptors. According to recent studies (30), the high-affinity receptor (P140) is a 140-kD protein tyrosine kinase encoded by the trk proto-oncogene. The low-affinity receptor (P75) is composed of 427 amino acids with a molecular weight of 75 kD. Several monoclonal antibodies have been developed against the glycoprotein receptor, NGFR (P75), which has been demonstrated on sympathetic and sensory neurons as well as tumors of neural crest origin such as melanoma, neuroblastoma, and pheochromocytoma (31). Investigations using immunocytochemistry reveal that low-affinity NGFR is present in nerve sheath tumors (32) and perhaps in medulloblastomas (31). NGFR (P75) is not associated with gliomas.

MOLECULAR PATHOLOGY

Diagnostic molecular pathology is a subspecialty with increasing importance and promise. This discipline applies the principles of molecular biology to clinical diagnosis and research (33–35). It begins with the use of so-called probes or sequences of nucleic acid that can be used to recognize a complementary sequence in a cell or tissue sample to be tested. Since the complementary target is composed of many nucleotide bases, the binding or hybridization is highly specific and is considered to represent the most tenacious interaction between two macromolecules occurring in nature. For example, the affinity is much stronger than that of the antigen–antibody binding in immunohistochemical reactions. Moreover, while immunohistochemistry is used to demonstrate cellular protein product if it is present in sufficient quantity, hybridization technology depends only on the presence of target genetic material or its messenger RNA. Probes, therefore, are ideal diagnostic tools when gene product is absent or below the detection level of immunohistochemical or other methods. Once the molecular probe is produced, often in bacterial cells, the nucleic acid fragment must be labeled in order to be identified. Radioisotopic and nonisotopic labels can be used. Labeled molecular probes are commonly employed in three systems—southern blot, northern blot, and in situ hybridization. In the southern blot, large fragments of DNA are cut into different-sized pieces during exposure to endonuclease enzymes. During gel electrophoresis, the restriction fragments are separated according to size. Because larger fragments move more slowly than shorter fragments, the DNA pieces are separated into a series of bands. After transfer to a membrane that serves as a support for the nucleic acid fragments, the hybridization reaction with a molecular probe is carried out. Northern blot analysis is similar to southern blot, except that the system is used for the detection and quantification of messenger RNA. In a general sense, southern blot analysis is designed to study gene structure, whereas northern blot analysis is designed to study gene expression. In situ hybridization, derived from southern and northern blot technology, is modified to detect nucleic acid sequences in tissue sections or cells. In southern or northern blot analysis, several million cells are required for adequate signal generation, but in situ hybridization is theoretically capable of detecting signal in a single cell. Earlier in situ hybridization systems used radioisotopically labeled probes because of the sensitivity of this type of detection system. However, radioactive probes have several disadvantages for the laboratory devoted to clinical diagnosis. Radioisotopes are expensive and present a radiation risk to laboratory personnel. Many isotopes have a brief half life and hence a short shelf life. Perhaps most important, autoradiography may take several days or even weeks, requiring a turnaround time generally unacceptable in clinical diagnosis. A number of nonradioactive labels have replaced isotopes, including several that utilize the technology of immunohistochemistry. Presently, the most popular technique involves the conjugation of probes with biotin to form biotinylated compounds. The major drawback of biotinylated probes is their weaker sensitivity as compared to radio-labeled probes, but biotin-labeled probes have a superior shelf life since they are not subject to radioactive decay.

A relatively new development that has greatly expanded the applications of molecular pathology is a technique known as the polymerase chain reaction (PCR) (36). This technique has the ability to amplify target DNA or RNA sequences up to a million- fold. In contrast to conventional southern and northern blots, which require comparatively large quantities of nucleic acid, PCR can be performed on a limited number of cells. The technique is subject to automation, and testing can be rapidly completed. In order for PCR to be successful, the target nucleotide sequence must be identified, so that complementary oligonucleotide primers to both ends of the molecule can be synthesized. When primers are added to the sample containing target DNA, they bind or anneal to sequences of DNA flanking the segment designated for amplification. The primers are added in excess, favoring the annealing of primer to DNA rather than the formation of DNA-DNA complexes. The third step in the cycle culminates in the synthesis of a complementary strand of DNA in the presence of the enzyme, DNA polymerase. When the reaction is completed, the sample is heated to denature and separate the double strands of DNA, and the cycle is then repeated. Typically about 30 cycles are needed to achieve the desired amplification.

Molecular biologic techniques are being applied with increasing success in the investigation of cancer. One of the earliest applications involved the detection of oncogenic viruses. Viral agents may contribute to the development of neoplasia by acting as an oncogene or a promotor, by modifying the host genome, by influencing the expression of host cell proteins during viral DNA integration, or by causing immunosuppression, as in HIV infection (37). Viruses that have been most closely associated with human cancers are Epstein-Barr, hepatitis B, HIV, and human papilloma (HPV) viruses. In situ hybridization and other molecular techniques continue to be employed, not only to investigate the etiology of various cancers but also to identify viral agents as possible diagnostic markers of certain tumors. Moreover, if human papilloma viruses can be used as a model, since several HPV subtypes are known to occur in lesions which tend to progress to invasive cancer, it may be feasible in the future to identify nervous system tumors with similar histological and other parameters as more malignant, based on the presence of specific viral agents or subtypes.

Tumor markers are amenable to detection with the aid of molecular techniques. The most familiar example is represented by the problem of tumor-specific proteins that are present in trace amounts, if at all, in poorly differentiated neoplasms. These gene products, when evaluated by immunohistochemistry, are frequently insufficient to generate a detectable signal. A molecular probe can be used to detect increased mRNA that encodes the gene product. Anaplastic tumors, in particular, might be expected to transcribe elevated levels of mRNA without further translation into protein. This approach has already been proven in the diagnosis of endocrine tumors (i.e., prolactin mRNA in prolactinomas) and should also be valuable in nervous system tumors (38). Other gene products such as proliferation antigens, growth factors, and their receptors might also be elucidated using this methodology.

Finally, molecular probes are ideally suited to the study of structures that are central in the development of neoplasia—chromosomes and genes. Many tumors are associated with cytogenetic abnormalities such as chromosomal translocations and deletions (39). As an illustration, meningiomas are commonly associated with deletions in chromosome 22. Some chromosomal abnormalities seem to be relatively tumor-specific, while others are shared by multiple tumors. Many genetic changes are too subtle or minute to be appreciated in cytogenetic preparations. Abnormalities at the submicroscopic or molecular levels include some gene rearrangements and single gene defects affecting oncogenes and tumor suppressor genes.

Gene rearrangements have been extensively studied in lymphomas. Normal lymphocytes undergo a variety of gene rearrangements in order to produce different antigen-receptor proteins—immunoglobulins and T cell receptors. In other words, specific genes contained in the c, d, j, and v region sequences are combined in a multiplicity of ways, resulting in an almost infinite variety of antigen-receptor proteins. Inasmuch as cancer is considered to be a clonal process, in which all cells comprising a given tumor arise from a single cell, the gene rearrangement in a lymphoma would be identical in every tumor cell. The monoclonal proliferation can be demonstrated as a distinct, nongerm line band of DNA in southern blot analysis (40). Gene rearrangement studies are also helpful in detecting residual disease during clinical relapse or remission and in determining the relationship between the clonality of the original neoplastic cells and a recurrence. The capacity to investigate gene rearrangements has not been exploited in tumors of the nervous system.

Genes responsible for cell differentiation and proliferation have been under intense investigation during the past decade. Although these proto-oncogenes have normal biological functions, they may be genetically transformed into oncogenes that have been strongly implicated in some human cancers (41). Oncogenes may arise under a number of circumstances including translocations or inversions, deletions or insertions, and point mutations. An oncogene may be transcriptionally activated to produce elevated mRNA levels or amplified due to an increased copy number. Of special importance is the fact that particular oncogenes are associated with certain types of tumors. Burkitt's lymphoma represents a classic illustration of chromosomal translocation resulting in oncogene activation. The translocation moves the c-myc proto-oncogene situated at band q24 on chromosome 8 next to the immunoglobulin heavy chain locus (IgH) on chromosome 14. In the process, the sequence of the c-myc transcript is altered and, perhaps because of greater stability, the c-myc gene is deregulated, becoming an oncogene. The excessive production of abnormal c-myc gene product leads to uncontrolled proliferation of lymphoid cells and eventually to lymphoma. The presence of c-myc has also been reported (42) in medulloblastomas in which there is oncogene amplification (duplication). Amplification of a nucleotide sequence that shares structural homology with c-myc occurs in about 20% of neuroblastomas and correlates with an increased population of tumor cells in the S phase of the cell cycle. This oncogene, N-myc, is associated with rapid tumor progression and poor prognosis, especially when the number of gene copies per tumor cell becomes excessive (43). As already mentioned, amplification of the EGFR gene is reported in approximately 40% of malignant gliomas, but not in lower grade tumors. Although small numbers of gliomas in the pediatric age group have been studied and further evaluation is needed, the correlation of EGFR gene amplification with histologic malignancy has so far been confirmed (44). Thus, it seems that in several tumor types, oncogene amplification is indicative of more aggressive tumor behavior.

Whereas the presence or enhanced activity of oncogenes is found in many tumors, other genes are now being discovered, the loss of which contributes to neoplastic transformation (45). These genes are categorized as tumor suppressor genes or antioncogenes, whose normal function is to suppress cellular proliferation. Such genes are recessive so that both copies must be inactivated in order for malignancy to develop. The most thoroughly studied of these is the Rb gene, which controls growth in normal cells in the G_1/S interval of the cell cycle. In retinoblastoma there is a deletion of the q14 region on chromosome 13, resulting in a loss of the Rb gene (46). More recently, type 1 neurofibromatosis has been shown (47) to occur with a loss of the NF-1 gene, a tumor-suppression gene that maps to the 17q 11.2 chromosome region. The gene product protein of NF-1 is similar in structure to p21 ras, suggesting that NF-1 is a partner in the complex signaling network involving p21 ras proteins that interact with gene products of the ras proto-oncogene. It is postulated that NF-1 downregulates p21 ras and inhibits ras-mediated mitogenic messages.

FUTURE DIRECTIONS

A major effort during the next decade will involve the application of those techniques described above, which have been focused primarily on adult tumors, to the study of nervous system tumors in children. Refinements and improvements in those techniques can also be forecast for the near future. Better means of assessing proliferative capacity of tumors will await the discovery of proliferation antigens yielding more information than those currently known and improvements in flow cytometry. Flow cytometry has mainly been used to analyze cells in suspension. The technology is now emerging that will permit flow cytometry to be adapted to the study of fixed and paraffin-embedded tissue (48). Because of this advance, correlation between flow cytometric and microscopic findings in tissue sections, as well as retrospective reviews of archival materials, will be possible. A more comprehensive understanding of growth factors and their receptors may provide additional insight into how tumors proliferate and spread. However, the key to a more enlightened approach to the diagnosis and to the biology of tumors will be an expanded use of molecular technologies. Recombinant DNA technology will be more extensively used as additional oncogenes and tumor suppressor genes are isolated and probes with greater sensitivity and increased signal are developed. In situ hybridization is now becoming automated, making this modality faster and more precise. Other molecular techniques such as DNA extraction and purification, oligonucleotide synthesis, and DNA amplification (PCR) will soon be available in diagnostic laboratories in automated form. Methods are also under development to extract DNA from fixed tissue samples, allowing analysis of stored archival specimens by southern blot and other procedures. Although immunocytochemistry will remain a mainstay in diagnosis and new antibody reagents will be developed to yet undiscovered nuclear and cytoplasmic proteins, molecular techniques will begin to assert themselves as superior tools to identify gene products such as tumor markers, proliferation antigens, growth factors, and their receptors. The growing body of knowledge regarding molecular mechanisms will also be a basis for predicting tumor behavior. Currently, prognostic indicators such as N-myc in neuroblastoma are few in number and limited in scope. Gene rearrangements, already applicable to lymphomas, and perhaps other molecular alterations will be used to identify residual or recurrent tumor in tissues that may appear reactive or even normal.

A second thrust will involve exploiting underutilized existing technology and emerging technology. Morphometric analysis of histologic and ultrastructural characteristics in tissue sections has thus far not been widely applied to the investigation of nervous system tumors. Morphometry permits a three-dimensional reconstruction of the tumor specimen from microscopic sections and could provide a detailed picture of the arrangement and architecture of tumor cells. The impact of morphometric analysis in the evaluation of nerve and muscle specimens points to the potential of this approach. Another quantitative method that uses computerized image analysis, cytophotometry, measures the amount of DNA in tumor cells. Differences in transmitted light emanating from specially stained cells or tissue sections viewed under a microscope are recorded and analyzed. With cytophotometry, subpopulations of tumor cells can be isolated for study. In anaplastic astrocytomas, the neoplastic elements have been shown to be aneuploid, while areas of endothelial proliferation are diploid (49). Cytophotometry has advantages over flow cytometry, in that small cell samples can be analyzed and tissue architecture is preserved. However, the reduced sample size interferes with the ability to distinguish each separate phase of the cell cycle.

A new area of investigation has focused on tumor progression and the interaction of cells with each other and with their environment. Cell separation due to lack of adhesion may facilitate tumor spread and metastasis. Cell-to-cell interaction is influenced by a family of adhesion molecules that can be induced and enhanced on cell surfaces by various mediators such as cytokines. Also, certain tumor suppressor genes may regulate adhesion molecule production to keep cells attached to each other. Recently, the gene product DCC, an antioncogene that is deleted in colon cancer, was shown to be a protein similar to neural adhesion molecule (N-CAM) (50). On the other hand, fibronectin, a 440-kD glycoprotein constituent of extracellular matrix including basement membrane, is an important binding site for invading tumor cells. Some neoplastic cells appear to suffer a disregulation of fibronectin genes. Further work will be necessary to elucidate the defects in genes that regulate the interactions between cells and between the extracellular matrix and cells. Finally, neoplastic cells may acquire tolerance to cytotoxic drugs. The first indication of drug resistance may be amplification of certain chromosomal regions called homogeneously staining regions. These regions have been associated with amplification of the mdr (multiple drug resistance) gene. Molecular probes to identify mdr and similar genes may become valuable in devising therapeutic strategies.

REFERENCES

1. Bailey P, Cushing, H. *A classification of the tumors of the glioma group on a histogenetic basis with a correlated study of prognosis*. Philadelphia: JP Lippincott; 1926.
2. Kernohan JW, Mabon RF, Svien HJ, et al. A simplified classification of the gliomas. *Proc Staff Meet Mayo Clin* 1949:24:71–75.

3. Russel DS, Rubinstein LJ. *Pathology and tumors of the nervous system*. Baltimore: Williams & Wilkins; 1977.
4. Zulch KJ. *Histological typing of tumors of the central nervous system*. Geneva: World Health Organization; 1979.
5. Paulus W, Peiffer J. Intratumoral histologic heterogeneity of gliomas: a quantitative study. *Cancer* 1989;64:442–447.
6. Chandrasoma PT, Apuzzo MLJ. *Stereotactic brain biopsy*. New York: Igaku-Shoin; 1989.
7. Taratuto AL, Sevlever G, Piccardo P. Clues and pitfalls in stereotactic biopsy of the central nervous system. *Arch Pathol Lab Med* 1991;115:596–602.
8. Burger PC, Vogel FS. Frozen section interpretation in surgical neuropathology. I: Intracranial lesions. II: Intraspinal lesions. *Am J Surg Pathol* 1977;1:323–347 and 1978;2:81–95.
9. Scherer HJ. Structural development in gliomas. *Am J Cancer* 1938;34:333–351.
10. Mørk SJ, Løden AC. Ependymoma:a follow-up study of 101 cases. *Cancer* 1977;40:907–915.
11. Smith MT, Ludwig CL, Godfrey AD, Armbrustmacher VW. Grading of oligodendrogliomas. *Cancer* 1983;52:2107–2114.
12. Mason DY, Gatter KC. The role of immunocytochemistry in diagnostic pathology. *J Clin Pathol* 1987;40:1042–1054.
13. Perentes E, Rubinstein LJ. Recent applications of immunoperoxidase histochemistry in human neuro-oncology. *Arch Pathol Lab Med* 1987;111:796–812.
14. Cosgrove M, Fitzgibbons PL, Sherrod A, Chandrasoma PT, Martin SE. Intermediate filament expresssion in astrocytic neoplasms. *Am J Surg Pathol* 1989;13:141–145.
15. Franke FE, Schachenmayr W, Osborn M, Altmannsberger M. Unexpected immunoreactivities of intermediate filament antibodies in human brain and brain tumors. *Am J Pathol* 1991; 139:67–79.
16. Truong LD, Rangdaeng S, Cagle P, Ro JY, Hawkins H, Font RL. The diagnostic utility of desmin. *Am J Clin Pathol* 1990;93:305–314.
17. Gould VE, Lee I, Wiedenmann B, Moll R, Chejfec G, Franke WW. A novel marker for neurons, certain neuroendocrine cells, and their neoplasms. *Hum Pathol* 1986;17:979–983.
18. Baak JPA. Mitosis counting in tumors. *Hum Pathol* 1990;21:683–684.
19. Woosley JT. Measuring cell proliferation. *Arch Pathol Lab Med* 1991;115:555–557.
20. Derenzini M, Pession A, Trere D. Quantity of nucleolar silver-stained proteins is related to proliferating activity in cancer cells. *Lab Invest* 1990;63:137–140.
21. Coon JS, Landay AL, Weinstein RS. Advances in flow cytometry for diagnostic pathology. *Lab Invest* 1987;57:453–478.
22. Zarbo RJ. Flow cytometric DNA analysis of effusions. *Am J Clin Pathol* 1991;95:2–4.
23. Tomita T, Yasue M, Engelhard HH, McLone DG, Gonzalez-Crussi F, Bauer KD. Flow cytometric DNA analysis of medulloblastoma: prognostic implication of aneuploidy. *Cancer* 1988;61:744–749.
24. Gerdes J, Li L, Schlueter C, et al. Immunobiochemical and molecular biologic characterization of the cell proliferation-associated nuclear antigen that is defined by monoclonal antibody Ki-67. *Am J Pathol* 1991;138:867–873.
25. Böker DK, Stark HJ, Gullotta F, Nadstawek J, Schultheiss R. Immunohistochemical demonstration of the Ki-67-antigen in paraffin-embedded tumor biopsies. *Clin Neuropathol* 1990;9:51–54.
26. Aaronson SA. Growth factors and cancer. *Science* 1991;254:1146–1153.
27. Marx JL. The yin and yang of cell growth control. *Science* 1986;232:1093–1095.
28. Wong AJ, Bigner SH, Bigner DD, et al. Increased expression of the epidermal growth factor receptor gene in malignant gliomas is invariably associated with gene amplification. *Proc Natl Acad Sci* 1987;84:6899–6903.
29. Snider WD, Johnson EM Jr. Neurotrophic molecules. *Ann Neurol* 1989;26:489–506.
30. Kaplan DR, Hempstead BL, Martin-Zanca D, Chao MV, Parada LF. The trk proto-oncogene product: a signal transducing receptor for nerve growth factor. *Science* 1991;252: 554–558.
31. Thompson SJ, Schatteman GC, Gown AM, Bothwell M. A monoclonal antibody against nerve growth factor receptor. Immunohistochemical analysis of normal and neoplastic human tissue. *Am J Clin Pathol* 1989;92:415–423.
32. Perosio PM, Brooks JJ. Expression of nerve growth factor receptor in paraffin-embedded soft tissue tumors. *Am J Pathol* 1988;132:152–160.

33. Fenoglio-Preiser CM. Technology transfer: the new molecular pathology, opportunities for the future. *Mod Pathol* 1988;1:251–255.
34. Hilborne LH, Grody WW. Diagnostic applications of recombinant nucleic acid technology: basic techniques. *Lab Med* 1991;22:849–856.
35. Wolfe HJ. DNA probes in diagnostic pathology. *Am J Clin Pathol* 1988;90:340–344.
36. Remick DG, Kunkel SL, Holbrook EA, Hanson CA. Theory and applications of the polymerase chain reaction. *Am J Clin Pathol* 1990;93[Suppl 1]:S49-S54.
37. Hausen HZ. Viruses in human cancers. *Science* 1991;254:1167–1172.
38. Lloyd RV, Cano M, Chandler WF, Barkan AL, Horvath E, Kovacs K. Human growth hormone and prolactin secreting pituitary adenomas analyzed by *in situ* hybridization. *Am J Pathol* 1989;134:605–613.
39. Solomon E, Borrow J, Goddard AD. Chromosome aberrations and cancer. *Science* 1991; 254:1153–1160.
40. Arnold AJ, Cossman J, Bakhshi A, Jaffe ES, Waldman TA, Korsmeyer SJ. Immunoglobulin-gene rearrangements as unique clonal markers in human lymphoid neoplasms. *N Engl J Med* 1983;309:1593–1599.
41. Cline MJ. Molecular diagnosis of human cancer. *Lab Invest* 1989;61:368–380.
42. Friedman HS, Burger PC, Bigner SH, et al. Phenotypic and genotypic analysis of a human medulloblastoma cell line and transplantable xenograft (D341 Med) demonstrating amplification of c-myc. *Am J Pathol* 1988;130:472–484.
43. Seeger, RC, Brodeur GM, Sather H, Dalton A, Siegel SE, Wong KY, Hammond D. Association of multiple copies of the N-myc oncogene with rapid progression of neuroblastomas. *N Engl J Med* 1985;313:1111–1116.
44. Wasson JC, Saylors RL III, Zeltzer P, et al. Oncogene amplification in pediatric brain tumors. *Cancer Res* 1990;50:2987–2990.
45. Studzinski GP, Moore DC, Carter DL. Suppressor genes: restraint of growth or of tumor progression? *Lab Invest* 1990;63:279–281.
46. Friend SH, Bernards SR, Weinberg RA, Rapaport JM, Albert DM, Dryja TP. A human DNA segment with properties of the gene that predisposes to retinoblastoma and osteosarcoma. *Nature* 1986;323:643–646.
47. Weinberg RA. Tumor suppressor genes. *Science* 1991;254:1138–1146.
48. Coon JS, Landay AL, Weinstein RS. Flow cytometric analysis of paraffin-embedded tumors:implications for diagnostic pathology. *Hum Pathol* 1986;17:435–437.
49. Davenport RD, McKeever PE. Ploidy of endothelium in high grade astrocytomas. *Anal Quant Cytol Histol* 1987;9:25–29.
50. Fearon ER, Cho KR, Nigro JM, et al. Identification of a chromosome 18q gene that is altered in colorectal cancers. *Science* 1990;247:49–56.

4

Principles of Neurosurgery

Adam N. Mamelak and Michael S.B. Edwards

Widespread advances in tumor biology and molecular genetics have substantially increased our understanding of the principles of oncogenesis in pediatric brain tumors (6). In addition, better understanding of the effects of radiation and chemotherapy on a variety of cell types has allowed us to deliver more effective and safer treatments to children (12). Despite these advances, and partially because of them, surgery continues to play a central role in the treatment of pediatric brain tumors. Surgery is safer and more efficacious than ever before because of advances in surgical techniques and developments in neuroanesthesia and pediatric critical care.

The goal of this chapter is to familiarize the non-neurosurgeon with some of the capabilities and limitations of surgery for treating brain tumors in children. It emphasizes the role of recent advances in surgical techniques, and, for children with malignant tumors of the CNS, the importance of proper referral to medical centers where pediatric neurosurgeons work as part of a multidisciplinary team of pediatric specialists to assure the best care possible.

OBJECTIVES OF SURGERY

There are three primary goals of surgery: (a) to establish a tissue diagnosis; (b) to reduce a mass effect or obstruction of CSF flow caused by a tumor; and (c) to potentially cure the disease. Each one of these goals is equally important in deciding whether to operate and what surgical approach to use on a suspected tumor.

Tissue Diagnosis

Establishing a tissue diagnosis is obviously important because accurate histological classification of a tumor, and its benign or malignant nature, is crucial for planning therapy and determining prognosis. For example, determining that a mass in the pineal region is a benign dermoid or teratoma, rather than a germinoma, pinealoblastoma, or malignant germ cell tumor,

Brain Tumors in Children: Principles of Diagnosis and Treatment, 2/e, edited by M.E. Cohen and P.K. Duffner, Raven Press, Ltd., New York, 1994.

significantly alters the surgical approach, postoperative treatment planning, and prognosis. Radiation and/or chemotherapy are imperative for treating malignant tumors, but surgical excision is the single most important treatment for curing benign tumors.

Recently, the intravenous administration of cell-cycle specific labeling agents bromodeoxyuridine (BUDR) and iododeoxyuridine (IUDR) has also allowed tumors to be characterized on the basis of their rate of cell division, which is represented by the labeling index (LI) of BUDR or IUDR (17). The LI measures the percentage of cells in a microscopic field that are stained with BUDR or IUDR, indicating that these cells were actively dividing at the time of surgery. Regardless of histological grade, a tumor with a high LI is more likely to act aggressively, although the converse statement is not necessarily true (22). Therefore, LI information can influence the decision about how aggressively to treat a tumor.

Surgery is almost always used to establish a tissue diagnosis. One notable exception is in the case of a diffuse brain stem glioma, in which tissue diagnosis is not always necessary because the characteristic appearance of this lesion on magnetic resonance (MR) images, coupled with the morbidity of even stereotactic biopsy in this region, are felt to obviate the need for histological verification (3,10). Another exception is with widely disseminated germ cell tumors that have elevated CSF markers of alpha fetoprotein or beta human chorionic gonadotropin (β-HCG). Finally, recurrent tumors that have no significant mass effect are not always verified histologically, although this practice varies among medical centers.

Reducing Mass Effect and Obstruction of CSF Flow

The reduction of mass effect and tumor burden (cytoreduction) is important because the cranial vault is essentially a rigid container of fixed volume in children above the age of 2, and any increase in intracranial volume or mass secondary to tumor growth or hydrocephalus increases intracranial pressure. Compensatory mechanisms such as reduction of CSF production or accessory CSF drainage pathways are extremely limited in their ability to counteract increased intracranial pressure (ICP). Pressure on normal brain structures results in ischemia, due to vascular compression (13), destruction of parenchyma via infiltration, and shift of intracranial contents. For patients with supratentorial and infratentorial lesions, the risks of transtentorial herniation and herniation through the tentorium or downward through the foramen magnum can become significant when ICP is uncontrolled (27). Therefore, prompt and effective cytoreduction can be lifesaving, even when a tumor is only subtotally resected. This is one reason most pediatric neurosurgeons prefer open craniotomy over stereotactic biopsy in the majority of children, even when only a subtotal resection is anticipated preoperatively.

Potentially Curing Tumors

Surgery alone is increasingly able to cure pediatric tumors of the CNS. In contrast to adults, for whom even gross total resection of tumors is rarely curative, some childhood tumors can be cured or the chances for cure greatly enhanced by a complete surgical resection (26,30). The prognosis for children is excellent after complete excision of benign nonglial tumors such as craniopharyngioma, teratoma, epidermoid and dermoid tumors, and choroid plexus papilloma. Glial tumors such as the cystic juvenile pilocytic astrocytoma of the cerebellum can also be cured by surgical excision (29). In the case of cerebellar astrocytoma, surgery is so effective that if the postoperative MR image reveals accessible residual tumor, we believe the treatment of choice is immediate reoperation to remove the residual tumor (Fig. 4-1). Other tumors, such as gangliogliomas, dysembryoplastic neuroepithelial tumors, low-grade oligodendrogliomas, and some focal low-grade astrocytomas, can also be cured or kept in extended remission after complete resection (8).

Secondary Goals of Surgery

Reestablishing CSF flow pathways, either by relieving obstruction or by shunting CSF flow to alternative sites of absorption, is another surgical goal.

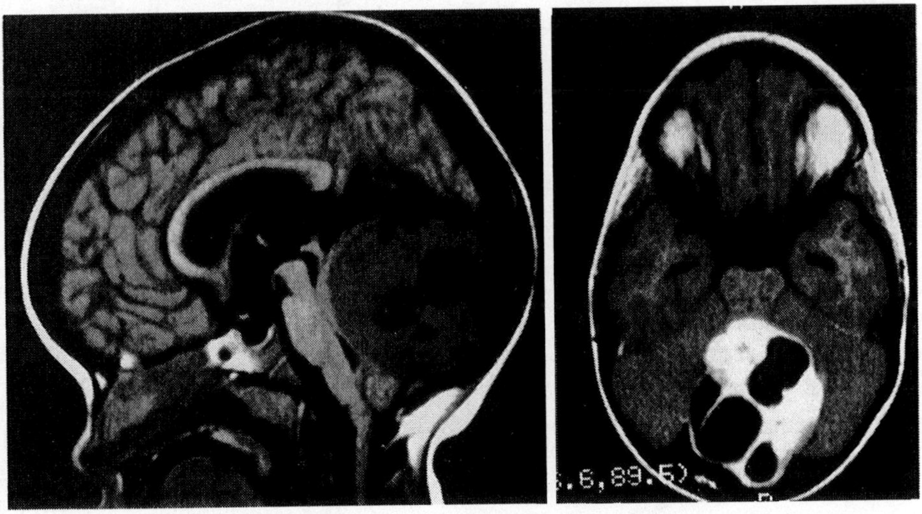

FIG. 4-1. Sagittal and axial magnetic resonance images of a large cystic cerebellar astrocytoma compressing the fourth ventricle and brain stem, with associated hydrocephalus. Intraoperative ventriculostomy followed by total resection of this lesion resulted in a surgical cure without the need for permanent ventriculoperitoneal shunting.

Hydrocephalus is more common in children than in adults, probably because of the prevalence of posterior fossa lesions that obstruct the fourth ventricle. Hydrocephalus can cause rapid head growth, spasticity, ataxia, cranial nerve palsy, and intellectual deterioration. Because these consequences can be devastating to the developing brain, prompt correction of increased intracranial pressure is of the utmost importance. Debulking or totally excising a tumor may restore normal flow of CSF; however, ventriculoperitoneal shunting or another CSF diversionary procedure is often needed.

PLANNING THE OPTIMAL SURGICAL APPROACH

The surgical goals mentioned above must be tempered by consideration of many issues. To plan the optimal surgical approach for each patient, consideration of the anatomical location of the tumor is important. Tumors that invade deep gray nuclei, such as the hypothalamus, thalamus, or basal ganglia in the dominant hemisphere, and tumors that are intrinsic to the brain stem cannot be totally resected without significant risk of devastating neurological sequelae. In some cases, the infiltrative nature of the tumor or the surgeon's inability to differentiate the tumor from normal brain tissue tempers surgical aggressiveness, resulting in either a subtotal resection or biopsy. However, many lesions on the surface of the brain, including those in eloquent areas (motor, sensory, visual, speech cortex), can often be resected with minimal risk when cortical mapping is used during an "awake" craniotomy, which is performed under local anesthesia in children over 12 years of age.

Knowledge of tumor type (obtained by frozen section) and patient age is crucial in anticipating the need for postoperative adjuvant therapy, and therefore influences the surgeon's decision to attempt a more complete resection at the risk of damaging other vital structures. In addition, the general functional status of the child and chances for a viable quality of life after aggressive resection must be considered. These decisions are often best made by a team of physicians, nurses, and social workers, with input from family members or custodians before surgery. However, the intraoperative findings usually determine the final decision with regard to surgical aggressiveness.

Neurosurgeons vary considerably in their opinions about and experience with specific types of tumor surgery, both of which influence how aggressively they approach a particular tumor. If the surgeon believes that the entire tumor cannot or should not be removed, then he or she is likely to perform a biopsy or subtotal resection regardless of the operative findings. The confident surgeon who is experienced in totally resecting similar tumors will most often attempt a gross total resection. For example, many neurosurgeons do not attempt gross total resection of craniopharyngiomas, owing to the endocrine morbidities and presumed low cure rates associated with such aggressive surgery. However, some neurosurgeons, including ourselves, have long advocated aggressive surgery for these tumors (15). Knowing that surgeons vary in their approach may help the referring physician to inquire about expected outcome and morbidity. Awareness of the potential risks and benefits associated with a more or less aggressive resection helps the referring physician counsel family members about morbidity, chances of cure, and other related issues.

PREPARATION FOR SURGERY AND PREOPERATIVE ASSESSMENT

Psychological Preparation

Preoperative psychological preparation is important to ready children for an operation. For younger children, play therapy (i.e., acting out the procedure with dolls and models) can help dispel fears of the operating room and postoperative intensive care unit (ICU). This approach allows the child to ask questions important to him or her that the surgical team may not have been aware of during initial discussions. For older children, tempered truthfulness is imperative, especially in adolescents, who must be made to feel they are playing a role in the surgical decision-making process.

Controlling ICP and Seizures

The risks of surgery must be minimized before the operation takes place. In the majority of patients with intracranial masses, elevated ICP poses a potentially life-threatening risk both preoperatively and intraoperatively. The use of corticosteroids to reduce cerebral edema is a mainstay of perioperative management. Dexamethasone is particularly useful in this regard, although methylprednisolone has also been used successfully. Diuretics such as mannitol or furosemide can rapidly reduce critical increases in ICP, and forestall impending disasters such as transtentorial herniation. However, the effects of diuretics are short-lived, and they should be used only as temporizing measures just before surgery, ventriculostomy placement, or diagnostic imaging studies. Intraoperative diuretics and steroids are also used extensively to reduce brain swelling before the dura mater is open and to prevent herniation of brain tissue through the dural opening (13).

Anticonvulsants are a standard part of the perioperative management of children with supratentorial tumors. They are not routinely used in patients with posterior fossa tumors because the risk of seizure from masses or surgery in this region is exceedingly small. Even in children without a history of seizures before diagnosis, anticonvulsants are recommended because surgical manipulation, edema, and blood products can be irritating to the cortex after surgery. Postoperative seizures have been known to exacerbate cerebral edema and occasionally produce neurological deficits. In general, we prefer to give anticonvulsants to all children with supratentorial lesions at the time of diagnosis, regardless of previous seizure history. In children who require surgery almost immediately after diagnosis, anticonvulsants are administered in a loading dose during surgery.

Imaging Studies and Laboratory Tests

Once a child is stabilized, appropriate imaging studies and laboratory tests should be obtained. MR imaging has replaced computed tomography (CT) as the standard of care for neuroimaging, and a multiplanar MR image with and without gadolinium should be obtained on every patient to define the extent and anatomy of the tumor. If risks of spinal seeding or foci are high, as in patients with medulloblastoma, pineal germ cell tumor, or malignant ependymoma, a complete spinal MR image should be performed preoperatively. Unless contraindicated, a lumbar puncture to obtain CSF cytological for analysis, cell counts, and tumor markers should also be considered. Angiography can also be very useful in planning surgery for children, especially in suprasellar tumors, which potentially distort the normal vascular anatomy of the cerebral vessels at the circle of Willis and skull base (Fig. 4-2). Magnetic resonance angiography (MRA), which is rapidly becoming commonplace in the preoperative workup of patients, is particularly useful in children because it is a minimally invasive way to image the vascular anatomy of the

A

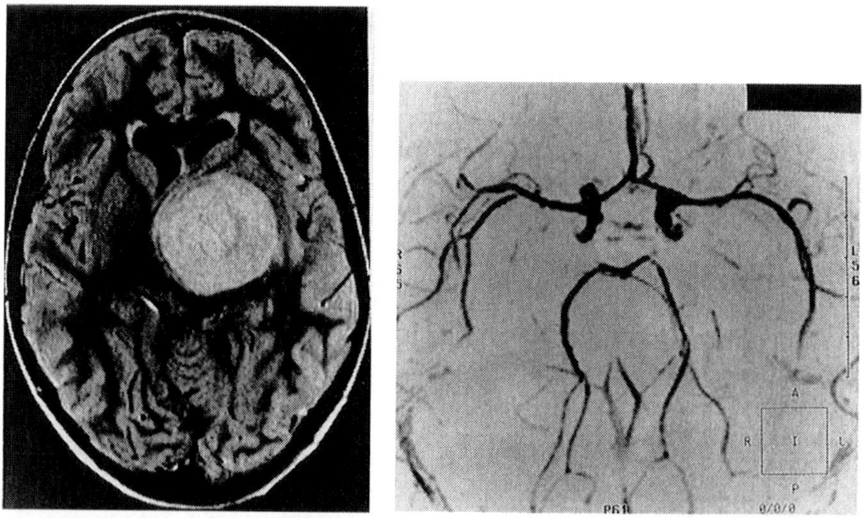

B

FIG. 4-2. A, Axial T1-weighted magnetic resonance image demonstrating a large suprasellar astrocytoma extending into the left frontal lobe. **B,** Magnetic resonance angiogram demonstrating stretching and compression of left middle cerebral artery by tumor.

brain. Finally, preoperative endocrine and neuro-ophthalmologic evaluations to document existing defects and correct underlying endocrine disorders are imperative for all children with suprasellar, optic pathway, hypothalamic, pituitary, or diencephalic tumors.

Patients with lesions affecting speech should undergo preoperative neuropsychological testing. The intracarotid sodium amytal (Wada) test should be included in the older child and adolescent, to determine cerebral dominance. If seizures are present, preoperative electroencephalogram (EEG) and video (CCTV) monitoring may be necessary to determine seizure foci (5).

THE ROLE OF PREOPERATIVE SHUNTING

Whether patients with obstructive hydrocephalus should receive preoperative shunts or a ventriculostomy is still somewhat controversial. Proponents of preoperative shunting argue that it reduces ICP and ventriculomegaly, thereby reducing the risks of herniation or a sudden shift of intracranial contents during surgery (1). Adversaries argue that over 60% of patients with preoperative ventriculomegaly do not require a permanent shunt, that the risk of upward herniation from a shunt is 15% (11,23,27), and that a ventriculostomy placed intraoperatively will function just as well as preoperative shunting in treating elevated ICP during surgery and the immediate postoperative period (8). Intraoperative ventriculostomy lets the decision about permanent shunting be made after surgery. Tumor seeding along CSF pathways has also been mentioned as a potential risk of permanent shunting, but methods to avoid these risks have been proposed (16), and the true risk of dissemination via shunt pathways appears to be very small (4). Another reason to avoid permanent shunting lies in the potential for shunt failure and infection in children. A recent study indicated a 30% chance of shunt failure in the first postoperative year, and an 80% chance of shunt failure over 12 years (28). Because there appears to be a near linear relationship between rate of shunt infection and decrease in intelligence quotient (24), we believe that permanent shunting in children should be avoided if at all possible. Therefore, we do not routinely place a preoperative shunt. Instead, all patients with hydrocephalus have a ventriculostomy placed as the first step in their operation. CSF is removed after the bone over the operating site is removed. Only enough CSF to allow the dura to pulsate normally is drained in order to minimize the risk of upward or transtentorial herniation or ventricular collapse. The ventriculostomy is used postoperatively to monitor and control ICP. Uncontrolled ventricular drainage is never used; all children are placed on an ICP monitor and have CSF drained to a predetermined intracranial pressure.

THE SURGICAL TEAM

To ensure optimal success in caring for children who undergo surgery, an established full-time team devoted to the care of pediatric patients is mandatory. A recent study comparing the outcome from pediatric neurosurgery between academic and private institutions found that while outcomes for children with benign lesions were comparable, children with malignant tumors fared much better in academic centers (9,21). This finding is attributable to the complex and multidisciplinary issues involved in caring for these patients, in which input from a range of highly specialized experts is beneficial.

The surgical team should include a pediatric anesthesiologist—if possible, one who specializes in neuroanesthesia—because of the risks of anesthesia in children. Inhalational anesthetics increase cerebral blood flow and ICP (13), which can be devastating in patients with a mass lesion and associated cerebral edema or hydrocephalus. Adequate hyperventilation, temperature regulation, and use of diuretics can greatly reduce the attendant risks of surgery under these conditions. In addition, familiarity with anesthetic agents that do not suppress cortical electrical activity is essential when electrocorticography and speech or motor mapping are performed. The surgical team should also include a highly skilled neuropathologist with years of clinical experience diagnosing childhood tumors.

ISSUES IN SURGICAL TECHNIQUE

Patient positioning and surgical approach require consideration of the unique physiology of children. Because 60% of childhood tumors are located in the posterior fossa, the prone position using the Concorde modification is preferred (20), as it reduces the risk of air embolism associated with the sitting position. Although intrasellar lesions such as pituitary tumors and intrasellar craniopharyngiomas are rare in children, familiarity with the transsphenoidal approach is useful in these cases. While most brain stem lesions can be approached through the floor of the fourth ventricle, familiarity with the various lateral and anterior skull base approaches to the brain stem and posterior fossa expands the repertoire of ways in which a tumor can be resected, thereby limiting morbidity while achieving a total resection.

INTRAOPERATIVE AND POSTOPERATIVE MANAGEMENT

A pediatric intensive care unit with devoted staff who have neurosurgical expertise is extremely helpful in the postoperative management of children. The use of osmolar fluids, careful dehydration, and frequent monitoring of electrolytes and hematocrit is particularly critical in infants. The judicious use of high doses of corticosteroids, hyperosmolar therapy, and high therapeutic levels of anticonvulsants can reduce the chances of postoperative complications caused by cerebral edema, seizures, or electrolyte imbalances. ICP monitoring and CSF drainage to maintain normal ICP is preferred over increased dehydration and/or hyperosmolar agents. CSF lost secondary to ICP drainage in infants must be replaced milliliter for milliliter with normal saline to prevent hyponatremia and subsequent seizures.

Children have smaller blood volumes than adults. Therefore, to minimize blood loss and replace it rapidly, children more frequently need blood transfusions during and after surgery than do adults. Autologous blood is preferable, but often the immediate need for surgery or the child's physical condition precludes this option. Children weighing over 45 kg (100 lb) are able to donate their own blood. For smaller children, we prefer to obtain at least one unit of donor designated blood from immediate family members. If necessary, we use banked blood, since there is no evidence to suggest that blood donated by family members is safer than banked blood.

Arterial lines are valuable in the postoperative care of most children. Patients are not routinely intubated or hyperventilated after surgery, unless they are at high risk for medullary dysfunction or are unable to maintain adequate respiration. Arterial blood gas monitoring is used to manage ventilatory status and ensure adequate oxygenation, while preventing hypercapnia and its attendant rise in ICP. Arterial blood gas monitoring is aided by the use of pulse oximetry and an apnea monitor. Arterial lines are also used to draw blood, thereby preventing multiple venous punctures, which are both painful and difficult, especially in younger children.

Steroids should be withdrawn slowly to prevent development of aseptic meningitis, particularly after posterior fossa surgery. If symptoms of meningitis appear, a lumbar puncture should be performed. After bacterial meningitis is ruled out, reinstituting higher doses of steroids is usually curative.

Enhanced and unenhanced postoperative MR images should be obtained within 48 hours of surgery to differentiate residual tumor from postoperative changes such as surgical scarring, thereby greatly assisting in decisions about further management.

Controlling pain in children is often easier than in adults. Intravenous morphine is preferable, because it gives prompt analgesia and can be rapidly reversed with naloxone if a child's neurological or respiratory status deteriorates. Intramuscular injections should be avoided in children because they are painful. In older children, patient-controlled analgesia can be used with great success. Oral analgesia with acetaminophen or codeine is useful after the immediate postoperative period.

RECENT ADVANCES IN SURGICAL TECHNIQUES

The surgical microscope and self-retaining brain retractors have greatly improved the neurosurgeon's ability to perform extensive microdissection of tumors and safely explore deep brain structures while reducing morbidity and mortality. Improved illumination and magnification have also allowed small residual pieces of tumor to be removed, assuring better outcome. However, even with the most advanced microsurgical techniques, infiltrating tumors such as astrocytomas cannot be completely resected. Even when a "gross total" resection is obtained in a less infiltrating tumor such as a medulloblastoma or ependymoma, it is assumed that a significant number of residual cells exist, and the need for adjuvant therapy and tumor staging still remains.

The surgical laser has improved the ability to safely resect tumor in critical areas, while reducing the risk of damage to adjacent tissues. Lasers are useful if the surgical approach is narrow and the tumor is firm or moderately vascularized. Most neurosurgeons use the carbon dioxide laser. This tool has been particularly useful for intrinsic spinal cord tumors and tumors of the pineal or tentorial regions. Similarly, the Cavitron ultrasonic aspirator (CUSA) has made removal of firm tumors safer and faster. This device uses a combination of suction and vibration at ultrasonic frequencies at the tip of a hand-held wand to remove tumor tissue that is quite adherent, while minimizing injury to surrounding structures. The CUSA is particularly useful in removing the center portion of radiation-damaged masses and firm tumors. Good surgical judgment about using the laser and the CUSA is extremely important.

Stereotactic methods, including MR imaging and CT-guided biopsy, have also permitted access to deep brain lesions while minimizing morbidity. Stereotactic techniques do not usually permit significant tumor resection but do avoid the risks of craniotomy when only a tissue diagnosis is desired, as in the case of a deep brain stem or thalamic lesion (2,25). Stereotactic craniotomy can also be performed. This technique is especially powerful when MR images or CT scans are superimposed onto the operating field by projection through the surgical microscope (18,19). This sophisticated method allows precise localization of deep-seated tumors within critical structures and permits removal of substantial portions of tumor while causing minimal trauma to surrounding parenchyma. Even more sophisticated techniques using frameless stereotaxy and robotic enhanced surgery are being developed.

Intraoperative neurophysiological monitoring of cranial nerves, brain stem auditory evoked responses, and other evoked potentials have increased the safety of brain stem, cerebellopontine angle, and skull base surgery (5). Monitoring allows the surgeon greater confidence in resecting tumors that involve the cranial nerves and corticospinal pathways. Cortical mapping is a technique that records the cortical EEG while stimulating the peripheral nerves and the cortical and subcortical surfaces with small electrical currents. It permits the surgeon to map primary motor (Fig. 4-3), sensory, speech, or visual cortex (5,7,31). As a consequence, the surgeon can resect substantial portions of tumors invading the dominant hemisphere or eloquent cortex, while greatly reducing the chance of causing functional deficits. Epileptogenic foci can also be identified and resected, thereby potentially eliminating

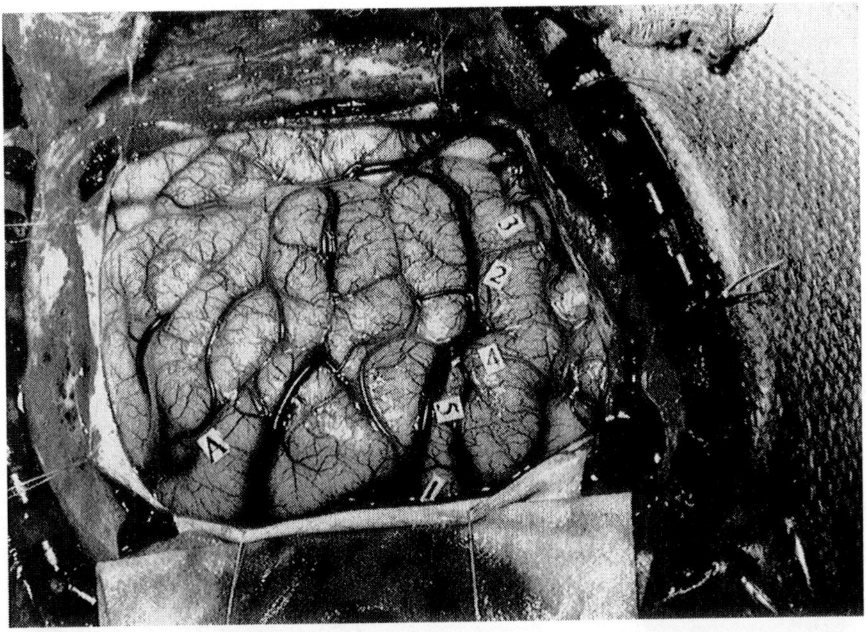

FIG. 4-3. Cortical mapping of primary motor cortex using intraoperative cortical stimulation and electrocorticography. The numbers on the surface of the cortex define locations that produced a motor response following electrical stimulation. *A* corresponds to an epileptogenic focus, which was incorporated into the surgical resection to cure this patient of seizures.

or ameliorating seizure disorders. In children over 12 years of age, "awake" craniotomy under local anesthesia with short-acting sedation has improved functional mapping of language.

Recent developments and refinements of the endoscope for ventriculoscopic use have increased the popularity of endoscopic techniques. The ventriculoscope is ideally suited for surgical approaches to intraventricular tumors such as choroid plexus papilloma, ependymoma, giant cell astrocytoma, and colloid cyst. It is also well suited for fenestration of the third ventricle (third ventriculostomy) before surgery to remove posterior fossa tumors, fenestration of complex ventricular cysts or the septum pellucidum, and identification and repair of ventricular pathologies that are causing shunt obstruction or malfunction (14). Because much of pediatric neurosurgery is concerned with the treatment of hydrocephalus and shunt malfunctions, it is not surprising that the ventriculoscope has gained popularity among us first; however, its use is presently evolving.

Interventional neuroradiology and endovascular therapy have significantly reduced the risks of excising vascularized tumors. Preoperative embolization of vascular feeders or obliteration of arteriovenous shunts helps to shrink the tumor and limit the potential risks of intraoperative blood loss. In highly vascularized tumors such as meningiomas, preoperative embolization can often mean the difference between an easy total resection and a life-threatening hemorrhage.

Improvements in neuroimaging have substantially increased the safety of surgical resection. MR imaging helps to define the full extent of the tumor and associated edema. MRA depicts the vascular supply to a tumor and the relation of normal cerebral vasculature to tumor. MRA may avoid the need for conventional angiography, thereby minimizing exposure of the child, especially the infant, to the potentially harmful side effects of radiation and anesthesia during angiography. We find MRA to be particularly useful for tumors involving the suprasellar area or circle of Willis because it depicts critical vascular anatomy, which must be protected during surgery.

A recent treatment approach is to administer chemotherapy after the biopsy to diagnose the tumor, but before surgical resection. Chemotherapy reduces tumor size and vascularity, making resection safer. This approach is especially beneficial for infants with vascularized tumors, for whom the surgical mortality rate has been reported to be as high as 30%. Another recent approach is second-look surgery, which has been a common procedure in general pediatric oncology. It is beginning to play a role in some infants with CNS tumors. A tumor may completely resolve after an initial surgical debulking, followed by chemotherapy. After chemotherapy is completed, and MR images are obtained, the decision to administer radiation therapy should be made. A second-look operation to determine if an abnormality seen on MR imaging is tumor or scar is often less risky than administering radiation therapy for presumed tumor recurrence—therapy that would not be necessary if the second-look operation failed to reveal residual tumor.

ILLUSTRATIVE CASES

Case 1

A 14-year-old right-handed boy began having complex partial seizures at age 8 that were poorly controlled with anticonvulsants. An MR image obtained at age 13 revealed a diffuse, heterogeneous, nonenhancing lesion of the left temporal area. Preoperative EEG and CCTV monitoring of seizures revealed a left medial temporal focus to be the source of his seizure disorder. Preoperative Wada testing revealed left-hemispheric language. A left frontotemporal craniotomy was performed under local anesthesia while he was awake. Intraoperative speech and motor mapping were performed; the results defined the posterior and superior limits of a safe tumor resection. Intraoperative electrocorticography confirmed a medial temporal epileptogenic focus. An extensive anterior temporal lobectomy extending 4.5 cm back from the temporal tip was performed. Postresection electrocorticography failed to reveal epileptogenic activity. One day after surgery, the patient was seizure-free, and an MR image revealed an extensive near-total resection. The pathological diagnosis was oligodendroglioma B; the BUDR LI was 1.2%, suggesting high risk for regrowth. There were no complications and the patient received external beam radiation therapy to a total dose of 5400 cGy, followed by adjuvant chemotherapy with procarbazine, CCNU, and vincristine to treat the residual tumor. Eight years later he remains seizure-free with no evidence of tumor recurrence.

Case 2

An 8-year-old girl began to get headaches 2 months before admission. Her headaches became progressively more severe and she developed morning nausea and vomiting. Two weeks before admission she developed blurred vision and an unsteady gait. An MR image revealed a large enhancing mass filling the fourth ventricle and producing hydrocephalus and a partial palsy of the right sixth nerve. A posterior fossa craniectomy was performed; a medulloblastoma arising from the midline cerebellar vermis was completely resected and a ventriculostomy was placed. The BUDR LI of the tumor was 3.4%. Postoperatively she required ventricular drainage for 5 days, after which her ventriculostomy was removed. A postoperative MR image showed no macroscopic evidence of residual tumor. A spinal MR image and a CSF cytological exam were negative for evidence of tumor dissemination. She was treated with hyperfractionated craniospinal radiation therapy (3000 cGy to the whole brain and spine, 7200 cGy to the posterior fossa, in 100 cGy fractions twice a day), and has been free of disease for 6 years.

Case 3

A 4-year-old boy was noted by his parents to be small for his age. He complained of frequent headaches and squinted to watch television. An endocrine workup revealed growth hormone deficiency. A neuro-ophthalmologic examination demonstrated a bitemporal hemianopsia. MR imaging revealed a large enhancing suprasellar mass lesion compressing the optic chiasm. MRA demonstrated tumor encasing the right internal carotid and anterior cerebral arteries. A right frontotemporal craniotomy was performed and a juvenile pilocytic astrocytoma was subtotally resected. The CUSA was used to debulk the central portion of approximately 40% of the tumor; the carotid, middle cerebral, and anterior cerebral arteries were preserved. Postoperatively the patient developed the syndrome of inappropriate antidiuretic hormone, and was minimally arousable for 7 days, during which time he was carefully monitored and supported in the pediatric intensive care unit. He made a good recovery and was discharged after 2 weeks. He then received radiation therapy to a total dose of 5400 cGy. His disease has stabilized, and he is continuing to undergo follow-up evaluations.

CONCLUSIONS

Surgery is a major component in the treatment of children with brain tumors. Advances in almost every aspect of the surgical management of pediatric tumors have led to more complete surgical resections and reduced morbidity and mortality. While the majority of childhood brain tumors still cannot be cured by surgery alone, more complete initial resections and repeat debulkings have clearly resulted in increased survival and disease-free periods for many children. A variety of techniques and tools are now readily available to help the neurosurgeon, including improved imaging methods, better surgical tools and microscopes, and sophisticated electrophysiologic and anesthetic techniques to protect the surrounding structures from unnecessary damage during surgery. In order to ensure the best care for children with malignant brain tumors, a multidisciplinary team of pediatric specialists including neurosurgeons, neurologists, neuroanesthesiologists, intensivists, and oncologists is essential. Prompt referral to an academic center in which these new treatment modalities are both available and frequently performed will likely improve the outcome of any patient suspected of having a malignant brain tumor.

ACKNOWLEDGMENTS

The authors thank Cheryl Christensen for manuscript preparation and Pamela Derish for editing the manuscript.

REFERENCES

1. Albright L, Reigel DH. Management of hydrocephalus secondary to posterior fossa tumors. *J Neurosurg* 1977;46:52–55.
2. Apuzzo MLJ, Chandrasoma PT, Cohen D, Zee CS, Zelman V. Computed imaging stereotaxy: experience and perspective related to 500 procedures applied to brain masses. *Neurosurgery* 1987;20:930–937.
3. Artigas J, Ferszt R, Brock M, Kazner E, Cervos-Navarro J. The relevance of pathological diagnosis for therapy and outcome of brain stem gliomas. *Acta Neurochir [Suppl] (Wien)* 1988;42:166–169.
4. Berger MS, Baumeister B, Geyer JR, Milstein J, Kanev PM, LeRoux PD. The risks of metastases from shunting in children with primary central nervous system tumors. *J Neurosurg* 1991;74:872–877.
5. Berger MS, Ojemann GA, Lettich E. Neurophysiological monitoring during astrocytoma surgery. *Neurosurg Clin North Am* 1990;1:65–80.
6. Bishop JM. The molecular genetics of cancer. *Science* 1987;235:305–311.

7. Black PM, Rosner SF. Cortical mapping for defining the limits of tumor resection. *Neurosurgery* 1987;20:914–919.
8. Daumas-Duport C, Scheithauer BW, Chodkiewicz JP, Laws ER, Vedrenne C. Dysembryoplastic neuroepithelial tumors: a surgically curable tumor of young patients with intractable partial seizures. *Neurosurgery* 1988;23:545–556.
9. Duffner PK, Cohen ME, Flannery JT. Referral patterns of childhood brain tumors in the State of Connecticut. *Cancer* 1982;50:1636–1640.
10. Edwards MS, Prados M. Current management of brain stem gliomas. *Pediatr Neurosci* 1987;13:309–315.
11. Epstein F, Murali R. Pediatric posterior fossa tumors: hazards of the "preoperative shunt." *Neurosurgery* 1978;3:348–350.
12. Finlay JL, Goins SC, Vteg R, et al. Progress in the management of childhood brain tumors. *Hematol Oncol Clin North Am* 1987;1:753–776.
13. Fisher DM. Anesthetic techniques for neurovascular treatment of vascular malformations in children. In: Edwards MSB, Hoffman HJ, eds. *Cerebrovascular disease in children and adolescents*. Baltimore: Williams & Wilkins; 1989:159–177.
14. Heilman CB, Cohen AR. Endoscopic ventricular fenestration using a "saline torch." *J Neurosurg* 1991;74:224–229.
15. Hoffman HJ. Craniopharyngiomas. *Can J Neurol Sci* 1985;12:348–352.
16. Hoffman HJ, Hendrick EB, Humphreys RP. Metastasis via ventriculoperitoneal shunt in patients with medulloblastoma. *J Neurosurg* 1976;44:562–566.
17. Hoshino T, Ito S, Asai A, et al. Cell kinetic analysis of human brain tumors by in situ double labelling with bromodeoxyuridine and iododeoxyuridine. *Int J Cancer* 1992;50:1–5.
18. Kelly P. Stereotactic biopsy and resection of thalamic astrocytoma. *Neurosurgery* 1989; 25:185–195.
19. Kelly PJ. Image directed tumor resection. *Neurosurg Clin North Am* 1990;1:81–95.
20. Kobayashi S, Sugita K, Tanaka Y, Kyoshima K. Infratentorial approach to the pineal region in the prone position: Concorde position. *J Neurosurg* 1983;58:141–143.
21. Kramer S, Meadows AT, Pastore G, Jarrett P, Bruce D. Influence of place of treatment on diagnosis, treatment, and survival in three pediatric solid tumors. *J Clin Oncol* 1984;2: 917–923.
22. McDermott MW, Krouwer HGJ, Asai A, Ito S, Hoshino T, Prados M. A comparison of CT contrast enhancement and BUDR labeling indices in moderately and highly anaplastic astrocytomas of the cerebral hemispheres. *Can J Neurol Sci* 1992;19:34–39.
23. McLaurin RL. On the use of precraniotomy shunting in the management of posterior fossa tumors in children: a cooperative study. In: Chapman P, ed. *Concepts in pediatric neurosurgery*, vol 6. Basel: Karger; 1985:1–5.
24. McLone DG, Czyzewski D, Raimondi AJ, et al. Central nervous system infections as a limiting factor in children with myelomeningocele. *Pediatrics* 1982;70:338–342.
25. Pattisapu JV, Walker ML, Heilbrun MP. Stereotactic surgery in children. *Pediatr Neurosci* 1989;15:62–65.
26. Raimondi AJ, Tomita T. Medulloblastoma in childhood: comparative results of partial and total resection. *Childs Brain* 1978;5:310–328.
27. Raimondi AJ, Tomita T. Hydrocephalus and infratentorial tumors. *J Neurosurg* 1981;55: 174–182.
28. Saint-Rose C, Piatt JH, Renier D, et al. Mechanical complications in shunts. *Pediatr Neurosurg* 1991–92;17:2–9.
29. Wallner KE, Gonzales MF, Edwards MSB, Wara WM, Sheline GE. Treatment results of juvenile pilocytic astrocytoma. *J Neurosurg* 1988;69:171–176.
30. Warnick RE, Edwards MSB. Pediatric brain tumors. *Curr Probl Pediatr* 1991;21:129–173.
31. Wood CC, Spencer DD, Alison T, McCarthy G, Williamson PD, Goff WR. Localization of human sensorimotor cortex during surgery by cortical surface recording of somatosensory evoked potential. *J Neurosurg* 1988;68:99–111.

5

Principles of Radiation Therapy

Larry E. Kun

Irradiation is frequently indicated in the management of children with brain tumors. In most childhood tumors, irradiation after either surgical resection (partial or complete) or simple biopsy contributes substantially to the duration of survival and the chance for a cure. Details and techniques of irradiation vary depending on the tumor histology and location, and the age of the child.

RADIOBIOLOGIC PRINCIPLES

The use of irradiation is predicated on a differential effect on tumor and normal tissues: a *therapeutic ratio*. As a medical discipline, radiation oncology seeks to use ionizing radiation in ways that maximize this ratio. One must demonstrate both the efficacy of irradiation in diminishing or destroying the potential for clonogenic growth of residual tumor cells and the relative tolerance of adjacent normal tissues. In broad terms, one may enhance the therapeutic ratio either *biologically* (by altering the total dose or intensity of treatment, defined by the time–dose relationship, or by the combined use of chemical radiosensitizers or radioprotective agents) or *physically* (by selecting specific treatment techniques capable of more precisely localizing the radiation dose to the desired volume).

The goal of therapeutic irradiation is to achieve selective death of tumor cells. Biologically, ionizing radiation interacts ultimately with cellular DNA. DNA may be affected directly or, more frequently, indirectly after intracellular ionization, which produces highly reactive free radicals, in turn causing DNA damage. Cell death only rarely occurs immediately, primarily in lymphocytes or other peculiarly sensitive cells that demonstrate intermitotic death. Cell death results largely from the inability of damaged cells to reproduce continually. Cellular death is seen during the first or subsequent attempts at division, implying a lack of clonogenic survival, eliminating potential for tumor growth or metastasis.

After radiation exposure, there is an exponential decline in cell survival;

Brain Tumors in Children: Principles of Diagnosis and Treatment, 2/e, edited by M.E. Cohen and P.K. Duffner, Raven Press, Ltd., New York, 1994.

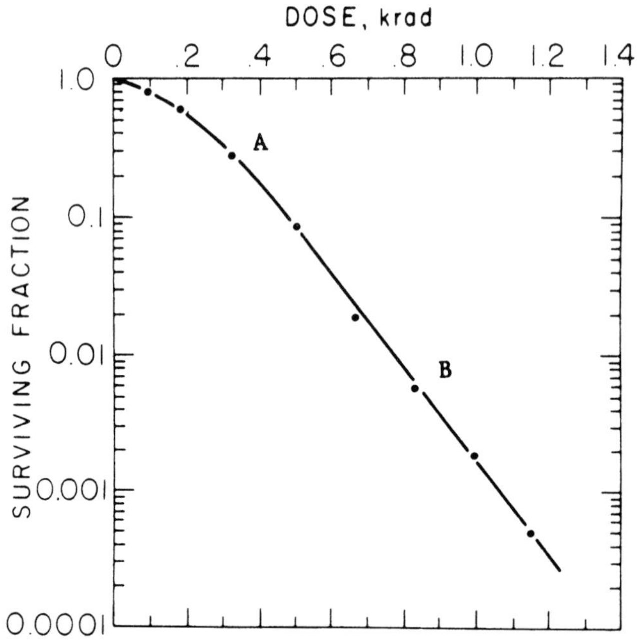

FIG. 5-1. Typical cell survival curve demonstrating clonogenic survival as a function of dose after a single exposure to photon irradiation (x rays). Note the shoulder (*A*) at lower doses followed by exponential decline associated with higher doses (*B*). (From Hall EJ. Cell survival curves: radiosensitivity and cell age in the mitotic cycle. In: Hall EJ, ed. *Radiobiology for the Radiologist.* 2nd ed. New York: Harper & Row; 1978:36,82.)

i.e., a given dose of radiation will produce the same proportion of cell death (Fig. 5-1). Typically, a shoulder in the survival curve (Fig. 5-1A) represents the ability of irradiated cells to accumulate and repair *sublethal damage* after small doses of irradiation. Increasing doses beyond these amounts results in exponential cell death (Fig. 5-1B). The rate of exponential cell destruction is a measure of the *radiosensitivity* of the irradiated cell population. Classical radiobiologic theory identified little variation in true radiosensitivity among different tumor cell lines or between normal and neoplastic cell lines. Recent observations link the initial shoulder and early exponential slope as *inherent radiosensitivity* parameters. Proportional survival after doses of 1.5 to 2 Gy (150 to 200 cGy, or rad) in cultured cell lines characterize different tumors and normal tissues. The SF 2 Gy (surviving fraction after 2 Gy exposure in vitro) correlates with observed radiocurability, differentiating, for example, the more sensitive medulloblastoma from the clearly less responsive glioblastoma (12,39,44). Repair capabilities responsible for the shoulder include repair of both *sublethal damage* and *potentially lethal damage*. The latter represents a component of cellular damage influenced by the environmental conditions affecting cell growth and cycling after irradiation.

One of the factors influencing the shape of the survival curve after irradiation is the oxygen concentration. The reduction of oxygen tension below that normally present in tissue leads to substantial reduction in cell kill (Fig. 5-2). The oxygen enhancement ratio (OER) is the dose necessary to produce a given survival fraction in the reduced-oxygen population, divided by that required to produce the same effect in the normally oxygenated environment. The OER for most human cell lines is 2 to 3; that is, hypoxic cells require 2 to 3 times the radiation dose to achieve the same degree of cell kill noted in normally oxygenated tissue. Thomlinson and Gray (67) demonstrated zones of necrosis within tumors thought to represent hypoxic areas of viable tumor cells in locations between the normally oxygenated tissues surrounding tumor vessels and the more distant, necrotic foci. The survival and later repopulation of the relatively resistant hypoxic cells represent one mechanism of resistance to irradiation, or ultimate failure to achieve tumor control. One of the advantages of fractionated irradiation is the relative reoxygenation in tumors during a protracted course of therapy. Tumor cell kill following a single large photon fraction (e.g., radiosurgery) is theoretically limited by the

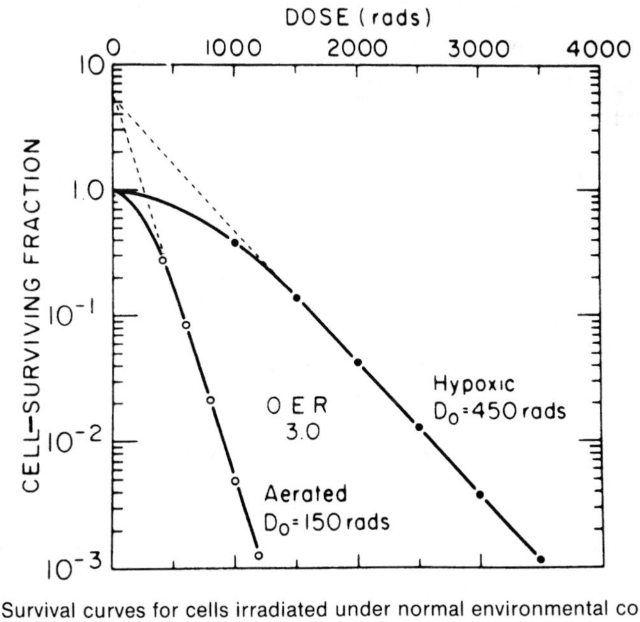

FIG. 5-2. Survival curves for cells irradiated under normal environmental condition (aerated) and under hypoxic conditions. D_0 refers to the slope of the exponential portion of the survival curve. (From Hall EJ. Cell survival curves: radiosensitivity and cell age in the mitotic cycle. In: Hall EJ, ed. *Radiobiology for the radiologist.* 2nd ed. New York: Harper & Row; 1978:36, 82.)

relatively resistant hypoxic cell component in comparison to the continually diminished proportion of hypoxic cells during fractionated delivery.

Sensitivity to irradiation varies also with the position of the cell in the mitotic cycle. Although this variation is only relatively constant in different cell lines, sensitivity appears to be greatest for cells in mitosis (M) and early synthesis (S) and less for cells in late S and early G_2. Irradiation of a population of cells randomly distributed in the cell cycle will preferentially affect cells in the more sensitive portions of the cycle, relatively synchronizing surviving cells in the less sensitive cycle positions. After a brief delay, surviving cells resume the normal cell cycle and progress naturally along the cycle. Attempts to use synchronization by prior irradiation or chemical exposure to increase the proportion of cells in sensitive phases of the cycle have been unsuccessful in clinical settings.

The most fundamental variable influencing the therapeutic ratio in clinical radiation oncology is the *time–dose relationship*. The application of radiation therapy rapidly evolved to *fractionated, protracted* treatment 60 years ago with the pioneering efforts of early radiobiologic experiments and empiric clinical observations by Coutard and del Regato (6,57). *Fractionated* treatment using multiple, relatively small doses of irradiation, *protracted* over several weeks' time, achieves relative sparing of normal tissues while permitting alterations in tumor kinetics and/or infrastructure capable of enhancing tumor cell kill. Multiple small fractions (typically 100 to 200 cGy) separated by at least 6 hours (and typically 24 to 48 hours) permit repair of sublethal damage and achieve a cell survival curve representing the addition of doses just beyond the shoulder region (Fig. 5-3). Biologically, the effects of fractionation and protraction include *repair* of sublethal or potentially lethal damage, *redistribution* through the cell cycle (including the progression of surviving cells into more sensitive phases of the cycle), *reoxygenation* (noting an experimentally verified relative reduction in hypoxic cell proportions during a course of fractionated irradiation), and potential *repopulation* (both of normal tissues and tumor cells, dependent on the protraction of treatment).

The effect of fraction size is tissue-dependent. Early-responding tissues (e.g., bone marrow stem cells and the repopulating basal epidermal and intestinal crypt cells) are relatively less dependent on fraction size than the late-responding tissues (e.g., glial or neuronal cells in the CNS; visceral and endothelial cell components in lung, liver, kidney, soft tissue, or bone) (65,76). Reduction in the dose per fraction preferentially spares late-responding tissues, allowing potentially more effective higher total doses (re: tumor cell kill) while anticipating equivalent or reduced dose-limiting late normal tissue reactions (66). Differences in the response of early- and late-responding tissues are quantified in α/β ratios, derived from the linear quadratic equation that describes the cell survival curve: $S = e-(\alpha D+BD^2)$, where S = surviving fraction, D = total dose, α = constant describing single-hit cell kill or irreparable damage, and B = constant describing accumulation

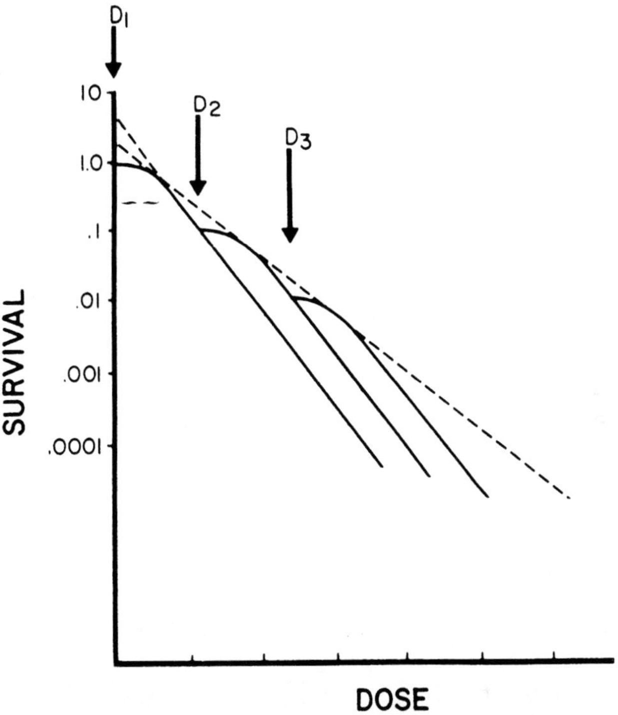

FIG. 5-3. The effect of fractionation is shown in an idealized composite model of serial exposures to photon irradiation. Note the summated curve (*dotted line*) represents survival as modified by serial repair of sublethal damage (repeating the shoulder portion of each curve). (From Cox JD. The rational application of radiotherapy. In: Copeland EM III, ed. *Surgical oncology.* New York: John Wiley; 1983:649–668.)

of sublethal damage. A high α/β ratio (associated with tumor and acutely responding tissues) indicates relatively less ability of the tissue to repair sublethal damage, predicting a less pronounced change in survival with reduced dose per fraction. Tissues with a low α/β ratio (typified by the CNS) are much more dependent on dose per fraction, showing maximal sparing with reduced dose per fraction (65,66). A series of clinical trials in children with brain stem gliomas has established tolerance to high, hyperfractionated doses (66 to 72 Gy), with uncertain benefit in tumor control (18,19,56). Whether dose levels of 75.6 to 78 Gy are associated with increased subacute toxicity is yet unclear (19).

In practice, irradiation is usually delivered once daily 4 to 6 days per week, now considered *standard fractionation*. *Hyperfractionation* implies division of the daily dose into more than one treatment, delivering approximately the same total dose per day but in 2 or 3 fractions, each separated by a minimum of 6 hours (a time shown to permit most cellular repair). Hyperfractionation maximizes sparing of the late-responding, low α/β normal CNS (66,76). Maintaining roughly the same overall treatment time minimizes the potential adverse effect of tumor cell repopulation during therapy (77). *Accelerated fractionation* utilizes multiple daily fractions, each at dose levels close to those used in standard fractionation, thereby multiplying the total daily dose by the number of fractions delivered each day and accordingly diminishing the overall treatment time. For rapidly proliferating tumors (e.g., Burkitt's lymphoma in children) or tumors exhibiting accelerated repopulation during a several-week course of therapy (potentially apparent in malignant gliomas), accelerated fractionation offers a potential benefit. The lack of clinical data substantiating CNS tolerance with conventional fraction sizes delivered in less than 24-hour intervals limits trials of accelerated fractionation in children with CNS tumors (11).

On the basis of prior experience with standard fractionation, the radiation dose can be shown to correlate with the likelihood of achieving local tumor control. A sigmoid curve (Fig. 5-4) defines this relationship, demonstrating significant improvement in tumor control with small increments of dose in the midportion of the curve. The relative effect on normal tissue is shown to vary similarly with dose, implying an "ideal" dose level of maximal tumor

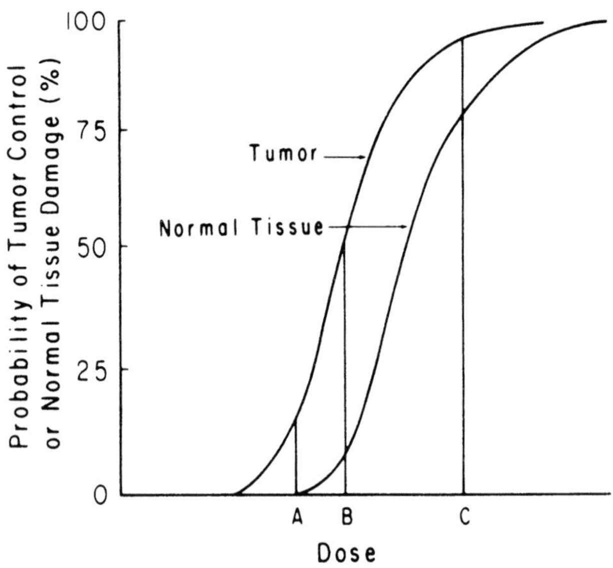

FIG. 5-4. Idealized curves relating probabilities of tumor control and normal tissue damage to total doses of irradiation. Significant improvement in tumor control is shown with small increments of dose in the midrange of the sigmoid curve (*B*). The slope and relative location of the two curves vary in different clinical situations. (From Withers HR, Peters LJ. Biological aspects of radiation therapy. In: Fletcher GH, ed. *Textbook of radiotherapy.* 3rd ed. Philadelphia: Lea & Febiger; 1980:103–179.)

control at minimal or acceptable levels of toxicity. The total dose required to achieve a given proportion of tumor control depends on both fractionation and tumor size as noted. Limited information relating total dose to local control or survival is available for certain CNS tumors. Direct correlations between survival (or cure) and irradiation dose to the posterior fossa have been demonstrated for medulloblastoma (2).

PHYSICAL PRINCIPLES

The dose absorbed in the tissue is expressed in units of *gray* (Gy), specifically defined as 1 joule energy absorbed in 1 kg mass. One Gy is equal to 100 rad in the older system; common practice includes the *centigray* (cGy); 1 cGy = 1 rad.

In standard practice, irradiation for CNS tumors is delivered by *external beam* techniques. A defined beam of energy is directed toward a *target volume* including the known tumor and potential sites of microscopic involvement. *Photon* beam irradiation uses x rays or γ rays produced by linear accelerators [x rays or ^{60}Co teletherapy equipment (γ-rays)]. Increasing the energy of the photon beam delivers relatively greater dose at depth and increases the depth at which maximal dose is delivered, the latter varying from 0.5 cm for ^{60}Cobalt to 4 cm for 20-MeV photons. The greater depth to maximal dose implies increased entrance field skin sparing with higher energies.

A single beam of x or γ rays delivers diminishing dose with increasing distance from the plane of maximal dose just below the surface. Beams entering from opposite directions focused at the same volume are termed parallel opposed beams (e.g., right and left lateral or anterior and posterior), which add together, providing a homogeneously irradiated volume.

Electron beam irradiation provides controlled doses to superficial treatment volumes; there is little electron applicability in CNS tumors. Other types of external beam irradiation include neutrons and charged particles produced by high-energy cyclotrons or specially designed linear accelerators. *Neutrons* possess depth dose characteristics similar to ^{60}Co but interact biologically in a way different from photons. Photons produce ionization within tissue which is sparsely distributed along the path of the entering beam. Neutrons ionize more densely, possessing a higher linear energy transfer (LET). The potential advantage of high LET irradiation is a relative lack of oxygen dependence: the OER for neutrons is only 1.3 to 1.5, compared with 2 to 3 for photons. High LET radiations produce little if any shoulder in cell survival curves, indicating little if any capability of repair.

The concept of relative biologic effect (RBE) compares the physical dose of different modalities resulting in a given biologic effect. The RBE for standard photon beams is approximately 1. The RBE for neutrons is 2 to 3; that is, a given physical dose of neutrons will produce 2 to 3 times the biologic effect of an equal dose of photons. The RBE for neutrons is dependent on the size of the fraction used; smaller fractions exhibit greater RBE because of the larger proportion of photon dose still along the shoulder of the cell survival curve. Early clinical experiments with neutrons resulted in unacceptable late effects owing to a lack of understanding of the relative dependency of the RBE on the fraction size (64). Similarly, recent clinical experiments using neutrons in CNS tumors appear to show a greater RBE than anticipated, due to an apparent increase in RBE measured for neurologic tissue compared with connective tissues. Despite rather remarkable "sterilization" of malignant gliomas in clinical neutron trials, severe damage to white matter has limited survival outcome to levels virtually identical to those achieved with photons (32,33).

Other modalities include heavy charged particles (e.g., protons and helium ions) and pi-mesons. Such particles offer both a biologic advantage (with high LET characteristics similar to those described for neutrons) and unique physical interactions, producing relative concentrations of dosages at depths that can be intentionally varied by the energy of the incident beam (Fig. 5-5). Such "peaks" of energy are used clinically for treating localized, central lesions such as pituitary adenomas or basisphenoid chordomas (31).

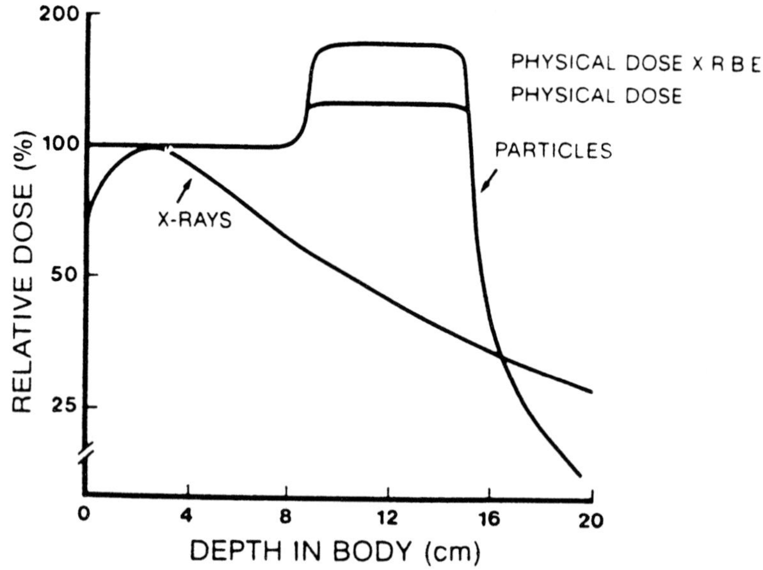

FIG. 5-5. Schematic representation of "biologically effective dose" comparing high-LET charged particles (e.g., protons and pi-mesons) to photons (x rays). (From CROS [The Committee for Radiation Oncology Studies]. Proposed for a program in particle-beam radiation therapy in the United States. *Cancer Clin Trials* 1978;1(3):153–208.)

Interstitial irradiation involves direct implantation of radioactive substances within target volume. The dose administered in interstitial implants is quite confined relative to external beam irradiation, delivering high doses with acceptable inhomogeneity within the target volume. The dose falls off rapidly, to less than 50% dose beyond 1 to 2 cm of the implant. The major advantage of radioactive implants is the physical limitation of the high dose volume to a precisely preplanned target volume (1). Dose rates within the implant are nominally 30 to 100 cGy/per hour continuously. In comparison to standard external beam irradiation (dose rates = 100 to 400 cGy/per minute), the continuous low dose rate delivery in implants results in diminished oxygen dependency, a potentially important advantage in often necrotic malignant gliomas (1,27).

MODIFIERS OF RADIATION RESPONSE

Attempts physically to increase the oxygen tension in hypoxic tumor cells predated trials of chemical sensitizers. Irradiation under controlled *hyperbaric oxygen* has never shown clinically meaningful gain in CNS tumors. Recent trials of a perfluorochemical emulsion (Fluosol) suggest potential efficacy in delivering increased oxygen to otherwise necrotic foci in malignant gliomas (13).

Chemical modifications to reduce the oxygen dependency noted with photon irradiation have also been sought. Experimental data in hypoxic systems have shown increased tumor response and improvement in the therapeutic ratio with electron-donating chemical agents apparently capable of mimicking the intracellular effects of oxygen during photon irradiation (11). Primary adult CNS tumors have provided an ideal model for studying radiosensitizers due to the high frequency of local failure after irradiation and the relative lack of distant dissemination influencing response and survival data. Effective hypoxic cell sensitizers have been elusive. Promising results with metronidazole in malignant gliomas were not duplicated after extensive trials using the analogue compound misonidazole (46). Trials of halogenated pyrimidines are ongoing, with marginal if objective benefit in malignant gliomas (48).

Other chemical modifiers seek to alter the therapeutic ratio by changing the availability of intracellular glutathione (GSH), an indigenous radioprotective sulfhydryl compound. Experiments in xenograft models of human glioblastoma indicate preferential depletion of intratumor glutathione following systemic administration of buthionine sulfoximine (61). The potential for selective increased sensitivity in neoplastic tissue is suggested by the lack of similar GSH depletion in normal CNS tissue (61).

The use of *cytotoxic radiosensitizers* has been suggested by documented radiosensitization in laboratory investigations focused primarily on platinum compounds (9). Clinical studies indicate both the feasibility of achieving radiosensitizing drug levels in human brain tumors *in vivo* and tolerance of concomitant cisplatinum and irradiation (15,63). Trials of concurrent cisplatinum and irradiation are ongoing in pediatric brain stem gliomas (30).

TECHNIQUES OF RADIATION THERAPY FOR BRAIN TUMORS

In practice a course of irradiation begins with the definition of the *tumor volume* and the broader *target volume*, the latter including the known tumor site and margins of potential subclinical extensions. The target volume coincides with the tumor volume in localized, benign lesions (e.g., low-grade gliomas, ependymomas, meningioma, craniopharyngioma). With infiltrating tumors (e.g., anaplastic astrocytoma, glioblastoma multiforme, anaplastic oligodendroglioma) the target volume will exceed the known tumor, including large volumes of the brain. For tumors capable of seeding the subarachnoid space (e.g., medulloblastoma, other embryonal tumors including primitive neuroectodermal tumors, pineoblastoma, and cerebral neuroblastoma; and malignant intracranial germ cell tumors), the initial target volume includes the entire neuraxis (i.e., craniospinal irradiation).

Technically, one must first assure patient positioning to provide both immobilization during treatment and daily reproducibility. Various devices as-

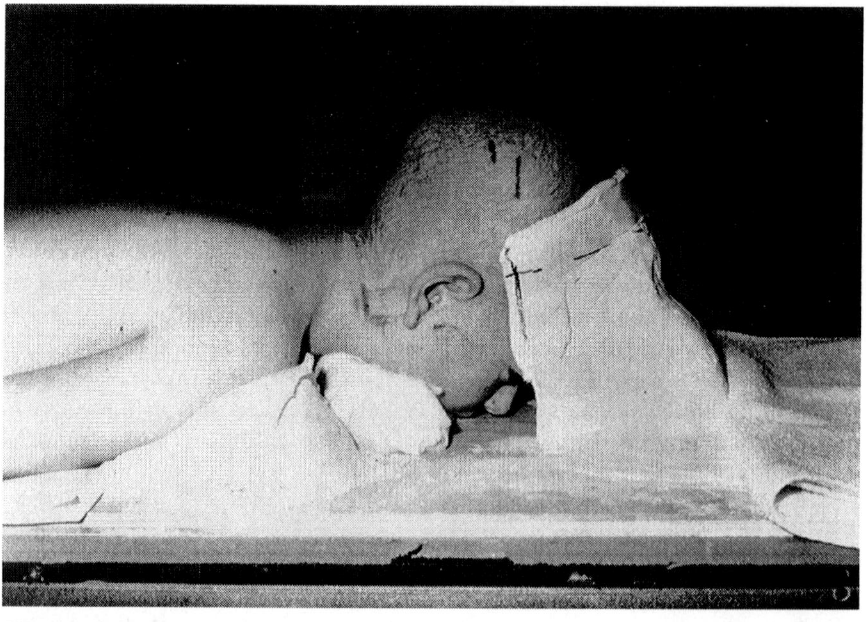

FIG. 5-6. Daily positioning is facilitated by a head-holding device. Custom-designed blocks (*arrow*) define the irradiation field.

sist in maintaining such factors, frequently employing sedation for youngsters between 6 months and 3 years. For craniospinal irradiation, casts or similar means of positioning are required to accurately reproduce daily alignments in the prone position (Fig. 5-6). Because external irradiation beams diverge, the matching of lateral fields, including the cranium and upper cervical spine, to adjoining posterior spinal fields is particularly critical. Painstaking efforts of precision localization and use of "moving junctions," which anatomically divide potential sites of underdosage or overdosage, are necessary to optimize homogeneity in administering craniospinal irradiation (Fig. 5-7).

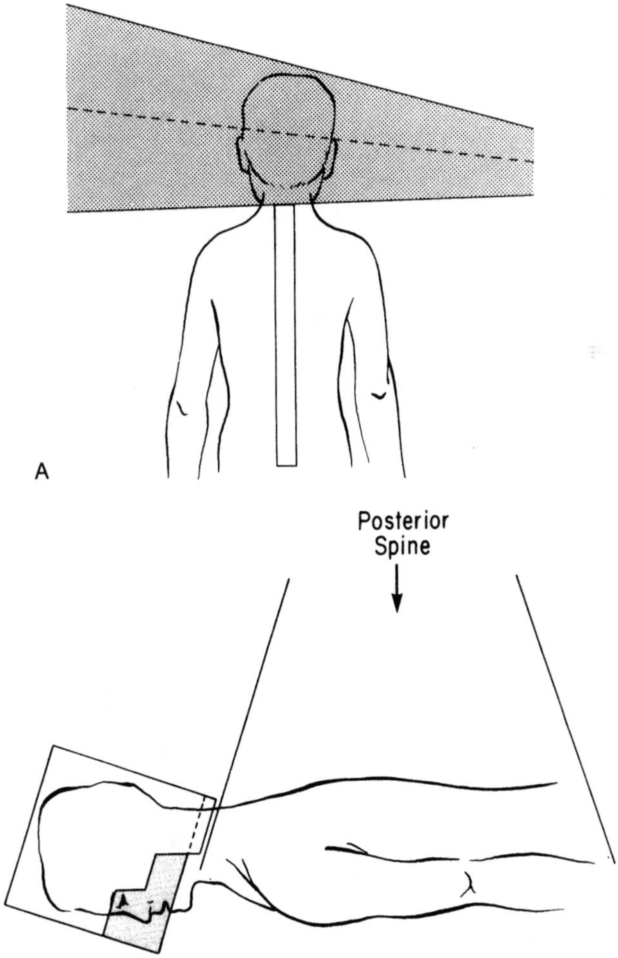

FIG. 5-7. The three-field technique of craniospinal irradiation showing **(A)** beam divergence and **(B)** field positions to achieve homogeneous irradiation to the entire neuraxis.

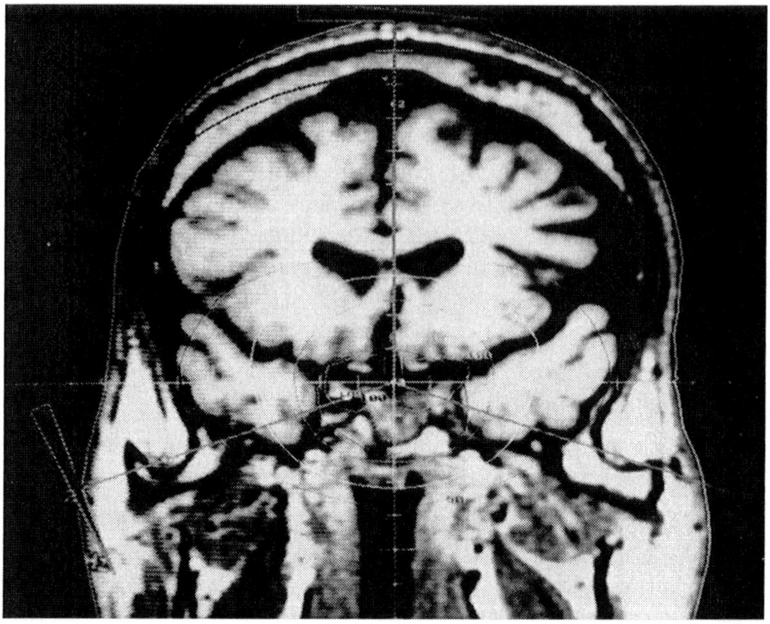

FIG. 5-8. Computerized isodose distribution for coronal arc technique used for parasellar tumors. The complex field arrangement achieves high dose delivery relatively confined to the central target volume.

Conventional treatment techniques utilize two or more treatment fields to concentrate the dose on the target volume and minimize incidental irradiation to the brain and other adjacent normal tissues. Relatively simple techniques, including arcs and multiple stationary fields, provide improved concentration of the desired dose. Coronal positioning and use of wide coronal arcs in tumors of the parasellar region (e.g., craniopharyngioma, hypothalamic astrocytoma) provide excellent dose localization (Fig. 5-8). Evolving three-dimensionally planned *conformal techniques* use three-dimensional imaging to identify multiplanar approaches, using existent linear accelerator technology to achieve improved tumor: normal tissue ratios while providing greater accuracy and assurance of target volume coverage (68).

Precision Volume Techniques

Highly focused, stereotactically delivered irradiation is increasingly used as a component of radiation therapy for brain tumors. Stereotactic *interstitial brain implants* have shown apparent efficacy in malignant gliomas in adults and, more recently, in children. Resurgent interest in the United States has followed clinical and laboratory studies at the University of California, San Francisco (1,21). Removable high-dose-rate applications generally employ high-activity radioiodine-125 inserted into stereotactically placed afterloading catheters. Alternative techniques include (a) 3 to 5 catheters geometrically placed around and within the central, enhancing component of the tumor, and (b) a geometric array of 15 to 25 catheters uniformly placed within and around the target volume (25) (Fig. 5-9). Both methods seek to deliver 40 to 50 cGy per hour, usually to a total of 50 to 60 Gy over 5 to 6 days (25,37). Tumor selection is usually limited to peripheral hemispheric lesions less than 5 cm in greatest dimension. Acknowledging the selection bias identifying relatively small tumors in patients with reasonable functional levels, both adult and pediatric data suggest improved survival in malignant gliomas (especially glioblastoma) with interstitial implants as a part of initial management or at the time of recurrence (17,24,38,49,54). Anticipated in the high-dose-rate delivery is a roughly 40% incidence of *intralesional necrosis*, often requiring surgical intervention and arguably contributing to a more favorable outcome (17,25,34).

An alternative approach based primarily on experience in Heidelburg, Germany, uses permanent or lengthy temporary (>2 to 4 months) implants of low-activity ^{125}Iodine to deliver 55 to 75 Gy over a protracted interval (12,71). The low-dose-rate technique, averaging 60 to 85 cGy per day, has been used

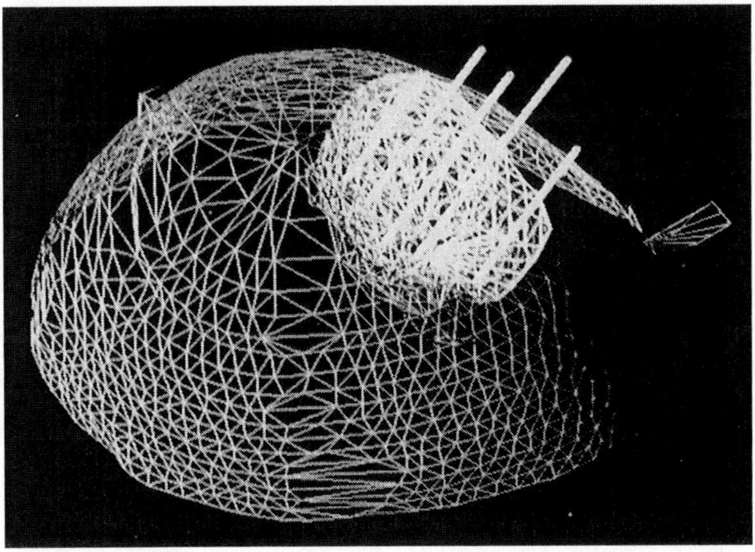

FIG. 5-9. Three-dimensional display of localized dose distribution from a six-catheter stereotactic brain implant using ^{125}Iodine. High dose volume is well confined to the tumor region.

in central (e.g., thalamic or brain stem) low-grade and high-grade lesions, on the basis of the lower incidence of implant-associated necrosis (12). Whether low-dose-rate brachytherapy is efficacious in malignant gliomas is yet uncertain (23,71).

Stereotactic radiosurgery is a highly sophisticated three-dimensional technique employing multiple focused beams to concentrate irradiation in a precisely defined volume. The *gamma knife* incorporates over 200 separate ^{60}Cobalt sources in a helmet designed to focus each beam at the isocenter, allowing variation in collimator size to select spherical volumes of less than 1 cm to approximately 5 cm (36,41). More recent experience has centered on modifications of *linear accelerator* delivery to achieve comparable precision and focused dose delivery through multiple noncoplanar arcs (38). Available data in adults and children reflect single large fractions (typically 8 to 30 Gy) for recurrent tumors of various types or a 15- to 18-Gy "stereotactic boost" for newly diagnosed malignant gliomas (34,38,39). Preliminary data for initial management of malignant gliomas suggest the "stereotactic boost" can substitute for interstitial implantation in selected and, potentially, most presentations (39,74).

The availability of linear accelerator–based technology and development of repeat fixation devices are just now introducing capabilities for fractionated stereotactic radiosurgery, combining the volume precision of stereotactic delivery with the biologic advantages of fractionation. Limited experience to date suggests excellent tolerance and potential efficacy with a "paucifractionated" approach: 42 Gy administered in 6 fractions of 7 Gy over 2 weeks (62). Questions regarding indications for stereotactic radiosurgical boost versus interstitial implant in initial management of malignant CNS tumors, identification of a biologically acceptable yet practical fractionation scheme that may substitute for surgery in certain deep-seated, benign lesions, and relative evolution of stereotactic and conformal beam techniques provide ample clinical investigations of a powerful new modality uniquely applicable to brain tumors (39,74).

TISSUE EFFECTS

The effects of irradiation on neoplastic and normal tissues vary with the treatment factors discussed above and the kinetics of the target tissue. Rapidly dividing tissues, generally poorly differentiated tumors or the proliferating stem cells of the normal skin, gastrointestinal tract, or bone marrow, will show fairly rapid cell loss after irradiation. Such rapidly responding tissues evidence clinically apparent changes within days of initial exposure. Direct visceral effects (e.g., changes in the more slowly proliferating oligodendrocytes and astrocytes) are often apparent months after irradiation, reflecting the delay in apparent cellular disruption of more slowly replicating tissues.

Indirect radiation effects are mediated by endothelial changes in small arterial vessels, also detected only months postirradiation.

Irradiation effects on normal tissue are temporally defined as acute (during and immediately after treatment), subacute (within 1 to 6 months), and late (usually beyond 6 months) reactions. Acute effects of CNS irradiation include those on extraneural tissue as well as the target organ. Anticipated cutaneous changes (hyperpigmentation, erythema) and alopecia are usually seen during the third week of fractionated irradiation. There is relative reduction in skin sparing effects where the beam enters tangentially, explaining permanent alopecia seen in such areas as the forehead, vertex, or posterior occipital scalp. During irradiation to the entire neuraxis one sees varying degrees of bone marrow suppression, including lymphopenia (immediately), neutropenia and thrombocytopenia (during the second and third weeks of treatment), and anemia (1 to 2 months after irradiation).

Acute CNS changes are uncommon. The issue of associated brain edema has been discussed for decades. Only recently has it been possible experimentally to document acute edematous changes in the normal brain after relatively large single fractions (2,000 to 5,000 cGy) (4,22). Clinically, neurologic deterioration is seen with conventional treatment techniques. Transient increase in neurologic symptoms and signs are rarely apparent at the initiation of treatment, particularly with residual posterior fossa lesions in children. More severe, sometimes fatal neurologic deterioration has attended high-dose irradiation: after large single fractions of 750 to 1,000 cGy for metastatic tumors, immediate neurologic deteriorations have been reported in up to 50% of cases (78). Nausea and vomiting inconstantly associated with cranial irradiation are less well explained. Such nonspecific effects may be troublesome even with well fractionated treatment, particularly in adolescents.

Subacute effects after brain irradiation are common. The somnolence syndrome, noted commonly after cranial irradiation for acute leukemia, is observed as mild encephalopathic or focal neurologic changes after treatment of intracranial tumors (3,20). Temporally similar reactions 1 to 2 months after spinal cord irradiation present as Lhermitte's sign. The pathophysiology of subacute alterations is believed to be secondary to effects on the replicating oligodendrocytes (70). White matter changes are often discernible by CT or MR imaging (5,69). It is important to recognize subacute alterations as transitory, treatment-related phenomena not to be confused with tumor progression (28,40).

Late effects are the most serious potential consequences of CNS irradiation. Alterations occurring 6 months to several years after treatment include morphologic (atrophy, calcification, white matter degeneration, or necrosis) and functional (encephalopathy, neuropsychologic deterioration, or focal neurologic deficits) changes. Specific factors related to late complications include host factors (tumor, age, diabetes mellitus, or hypertension), techniques of irradiation (particularly individual fraction size, potential dose inhomogeneity, and treatment volume), and associated treatments (chemotherapy and surgery).

Probably the most serious, if uncommon, late CNS alteration is postirradiation cerebral necrosis. Most often reported 6 months to 2 years posttreatment, focal necrosis has been noted both as an incidental effect after treatment of extracranial tumors and most often after irradiation of primary brain tumors. The pathophysiology of late necrosis is believed to be secondary to direct effects on the replicating glial cells and indirect effects due to capillary endothelial changes resulting in narrowing of small vessels (70). Symptoms and signs of postirradiation necrosis are not specific, presenting as neurologic signs associated with focal neurologic lesions, usually related to the tumor region or associated volume of highest irradiation dose. Changes detected by CT or MRI are reported to correlate with the dose distribution and usually the primary tumor site (35,44).

The incidence of postirradiation necrosis is a dose-related phenomenon. Both total dose and fraction size affect the frequency of this occurrence. Necrosis in this setting is virtually unreported after doses up to 50 to 55 Gy given with standard fractionation at 180 to 200 cGy daily (35,60). A threshold level of 5.4 Gy (at 180 cGy daily) has been described; necrosis has only rarely been noted below this level (43). Larger daily increments in excess of 220 to 250 cGy are associated with an increasing risk of late necrosis at total doses approximating 50 Gy (43,60). Both clinical and laboratory reports demonstrate the impact of fraction size in relation to late CNS changes. CNS effects, as reported for the brain, spinal cord, and optic nerves, are relatively more dependent on fraction size than other tissues (60,73).

The effect of age on CNS tolerance is poorly documented. Experimentally, one can detect changes of focal necrosis in young nonhuman primates after doses of irradiation that are tolerated in the adult (4). Clinically, children under 1 to 2 years show greater morbidity after irradiation, with both neurologic and neuropsychologic alterations (2). It has been postulated that the developing brain is more sensitive to radiation until myelin production and potential neuronal division are complete at 1 to 2 years (2,55). Posttreatment neuroimaging changes in white matter are more prominent at younger ages (5,69). Standard procedure in most instances requires a 10% reduction in total dose, preferably accompanied by increased fractionation, for children under 2 years of age.

Particularly in young children, the likelihood of altered neuropsychologic function is a major area of continued investigation, as outlined in Chapter 23 (29,45). Endocrine dysfunction is similarly of greatest concern in young children, as reviewed in Chapter 23. Radiation effects on the spinal cord are comparable temporally to those described for the brain. Acute effects are virtually unknown. Lhermitte's sign occurs 1 to 3 months after spinal irradiation in up to 25 to 40% of patients receiving over 35 to 40 Gy to significant lengths of the cord. This transitory subacute phenomenon does not appear to be related to the later development of progressive myelopathy.

Late postirradiation myelopathy is a well-described occurrence noted between 4 months and 1 to 2 years after doses above the 4.5- to 5.0-Gy level at standard fractionation (58). The pathophysiology appears to be analogous to that noted in brain tissues, with both parenchymal white matter lesions and late vascular changes in the white matter (58). As with brain necrosis, one may correlate individual fraction size most directly with the occurrence of postirradiation myelopathy, as modified by the total dose and length of cord irradiated (1,58). The latent interval between irradiation and myelopathy appears to correlate directly with age, animal models documenting shorter intervals in the young (21). An unexpected incidence of myelopathy in children with parameningeal sarcomas suggests an interaction between intrathecal chemotherapy and irradiation that has otherwise been difficult to identify (50,58). Techniques necessitating the joining of two or more fields in areas adjacent to or directly involving the spinal cord require specific attention to minimize the risk of overlap producing excessive doses to the cord.

The risk of secondary carcinogenesis after CNS irradiation includes incidental exposure of the thyroid and soft tissues plus the brain and meninges (53). Intracranial tumors arising after therapeutic irradiation are rare. Most such tumors have been sarcomatous neoplasms arising in the supporting structures around and within the brain (52,59,72). Secondary gliomas are increasingly recognized following cranial irradiation and chemotherapy for childhood leukemia. The incidence may be as high as 10% in subsets of patients with "high-dose" irradiation and intrathecal chemotherapy; the overall incidence appears to be limited to 1 to 2% (52).

CONCLUSIONS

An understanding of the basic principles of radiation therapy, both physical and biological, is important for those managing children with CNS tumors. Radiation therapy is at a crucial point in developing new therapeutic approaches based on three-dimensional neuroimaging and treatment planning. Rapidly evolving capabilities in conformal techniques, dynamic treatment approaches, and stereotactic delivery of both interstitial implants and radiosurgery have focused on CNS tumors, an ideal model demanding the greatest precision in dose distribution. Further progress in tumor control and enhancement of the therapeutic ratio is sought through investigations of cytotoxic radiosensitizers, high-LET irradiation, and altered fractionation.

Although systematic control of primary CNS tumors remains elusive, current techniques assure sufficient proportions of long-term survivors to warrant attention to the late effects of irradiation. Knowledge of the timing, frequency, and apparent modifying treatment factors is critical in following such patients. Progress in identifying more ideal techniques of irradiation are oriented both toward precision volume coverage to homogeneously encompass the tumor volume and, equally, toward minimizing the dose to adjacent normal brain.

REFERENCES

1. Berstein M, Gutin PH. Interstitial irradiation of brain tumors: a review. *Neurosurgery* 1981; 9:741–750.
2. Bloom HJG, Wallace ENK, Henk JM. The treatment and prognosis of medulloblastoma in children. *AJR* 1969;105:43–62.
3. Boldrey E, Sheline G. Delayed transitory clinical manifestations after radiation treatment of intracranial tumors. *Acta Radiol Ther* 1966;5:5–10.
4. Caveness WF. Experimental observations: delayed necrosis in normal monkey brain. In: Gilbert HA, Kagen AR, eds. *Radiation damage to the nervous system*. New York: Raven Press; 1980:1–38.
5. Constine LS, Konski A, Ekholm S, McDonald S, Rubin P. Adverse effects of brain irradiation correlated with MR and CT imaging. *Int J Radiat Oncol Biol Phys* 1988;15:319–330.
6. Coutard H. Principles of X-ray therapy of malignant disorders. *Lancet* 1934;2:1–12.
7. Cox JD. The rational application of radiotherapy. In: Copeland EM III, ed. *Surgical oncology*. New York: John Wiley; 1983:649–668.
8. CROS (The Committee for Radiation Oncology Studies). Proposal for a program in particle-beam radiation therapy in the United States. *Cancer Clin Trials* 1978;1(3):153–208.
9. DeWitt L. Combined treatment of radiation and cis-diamminodichloro platinum (II): a review of experimental and clinical data. *Int J Radiat Oncol Biol Phys* 1987;13:403–426.
10. Dische S. Hypoxic cell sensitizers in radiotherapy. *Int J Radiat Oncol Biol Phys* 1978;4: 157–160.
11. Dische S, Saunders MI. Continuous hyperfractionated accelerated radiotherapy (CHART): an interim report upon late morbidity. *Radiother Oncol* 1989;16:67–74.
12. Etou A, Mundinger F, Mohadjer M, et al. Stereotactic interstitial irradiation of diencephalic tumors with iridium 192 and iodine 125: 10 years follow-up and comparison with other treatments. *Childs Nerv Syst* 1989;5:140–143.
13. Evans R, Kimler B, Morantz R, et al. A phase I/II study of the use of Fluosol as an adjuvant to radiation therapy in the treatment of primary high-grade brain tumors. *Int J Radiat Oncol Biol Phys* 1990;19:415–420.
14. Fertil B, Malaise EP. Intrinsic radiosensitivity of human cell lines is correlated with radioresponsiveness of human tumors: analysis of 101 published survival curves. *Int J Radiat Oncol Biol Phys* 1985;11:1699–1707.
15. Feun LG, Steward DJ, Maor M, et al. A pilot study of CDDP and radiation therapy in patients with high grade astrocytomas. *J Neurooncol* 1983;1:109–113.
16. Florell RC, MacDonald DR, Irish WD, Bernstein M, Leibel SA, Gutin PH, Cairncross JG. Selection bias, survival, and brachytherapy for glioma. *J Neurosurg* 1992;76:179–183.
17. Fontanesi J, Muhlbauer M, Heideman RL, et al. High-activity ^{125}I interstitial irradiation in the treatment of pediatric central nervous system tumors: a pilot study. *J Neurosurg* 1993 (in press).
18. Freeman CR, Krischer J, Sanford RA, et al. Hyperfractionated radiation therapy in brain stem tumors. Results of treatment at the 7020 cGy dose level of Pediatric Oncology Group Study #8495. *Cancer* 1991;68:474–481.
19. Freeman CR, Krischer JP, Sanford RA, et al. Final results of a study of escalating doses of hyperfractionated radiotherapy in brain stem tumors in children. *Int J Radiat Oncol Biol Phys* 1993 (*in press*).
20. Freeman JE, Johnston PGB, Voke JM. Somnolence after prophylactic cranial irradiation in children with acute lymphoblastic leukaemia. *Br Med J* 1973;4:523–525.
21. Geyer JR, Taylor EM, Milstein JM, Shaw CM, Hubbard BA, Geraci JP, Bleyer WA. The effect of age on the latency of radiation myelopathy. *J Neurooncol* 1991;10:141–151.

22. Gregersen MI, Pallavicini C, Chien S. Studies on the chemical composition of the CNS in relation to the effects of x-irradiation and of disturbances in water and salt balance. *Radiat Res* 1962;17:209–225.
23. Gutin PH, Phillips TL, Hosobuchi Y, et al. Permanent and removable implants for the brachytherapy of brain tumors. *Int J Radiat Oncol Biol Phys* 1981;7:1371–1381.
24. Gutin PH, Edwards MSB, Wara WM, et al. Preliminary experience with ^{125}I-brachytherapy of pediatric brain tumors. *Concepts Pediatr Neurosurg* 1985;5:187–206.
25. Gutin PH, Leibel SA, Wara WM, et al. Recurrent malignant gliomas: survival following interstitial brachytherapy with high-activity iodine-125 sources. *J Neurosurg* 1987;67: 870–873.
26. Hall EJ. Cell survival curves: radiosensitivity and cell age in the mitotic cycle. In: Hall EJ, ed. *Radiobiology for the radiologist*. 2nd ed. New York: Harper & Row; 1978:36, 82.
27. Hall EJ. The dose-rate factor in radiation biology. *Int J Radiat Oncol Biol Phys* 1991;59: 595–610.
28. Hoffman WF, Levin VA, Wilson CB. Evaluation of malignant glioma patients during the postirradiation period. *J Neurosurg* 1979;50:624–628.
29. Jannoun L, Bloom H. Long-term psychological effects in children treated for intracranial tumors. *Int J Radiat Oncol Biol Phys* 1990;18:747–753.
30. Kadota RP, Mandell LR, Fontanesi J, Kovnar EH, Krischer J, Kun LE, Friedman HS. Hyperfractionated irradiation and concurrent cisplatin in brain stem tumors: a Pediatric Oncology Group Pilot Study (9139). *Pediatr Neurosurg* 1993 (in press).
31. Kjellberg RN. A system of therapy of pituitary tumors: Bragg peak proton hypophysectomy. In: Seydel HG, ed. *Tumors of the nervous system*. New York: John Wiley; 1975:145–168.
32. Laramore GE, Diener-West M, Griffin TW, et al. Randomized neutron dose searching for malignant gliomas of the brain: results of an RTOG study. *Int J Radiat Oncol Biol Phys* 1988;14:1093–1102.
33. Laramore GE. Neutron radiotherapy for high grade gliomas: the search for the elusive therapeutic window. *Int J Radiat Oncol Biol Phys* 1990;19:493–495.
34. Leibel SA, Gutin PH, Wara WM, et al. Survival and quality of life after interstitial implantation of removable high-activity iodine-125 sources for the treatent of patients with recurrent malignant gliomas. *Int J Radiat Oncol Biol Phys* 1989;17:1129–1139.
35. Leibel SA, Sheline GE. Tolerance of the brain and spinal cord to conventional irradiation. In: Gutin P, Leibel S, Sheline G, eds. *Radiation injury to the nervous system*. New York: Raven Press; 1991:239–256.
36. Leksell L. The stereotaxic method and radiosurgery of the brain. *Acta Chir Scand* 1951; 102:316–319.
37. Loeffler JS, Alexander E III, Wen PY, et al. Results of stereotactic brachytherapy used in the initial management of patients with glioblastoma. *J Natl Cancer Inst* 1990;82:1918–1921.
38. Loeffler JS, Rossitch E Jr, Siddon R, Moore MR, Rockoff MA, Alexander E III. Role of stereotactic radiosurgery with a linear accelerator in treatment of intracranial arteriovenous malformations and tumors in children. *Pediatrics* 1990;85:774–782.
39. Loeffler JS, Alexander E III, Shea WM, Wen PY, Fine HA, Kooy HM, Black P McL. Radiosurgery as part of the initial management of patients with malignant gliomas. *J Clin Oncol* 1992;10:1379–1385.
40. Longee DC, Friedman HS, Djang WT. Transient late magnetic resonance imaging changes suggesting progression of brain stem glioma: implications for entry criteria for phase II trials. *Neurosurgery* 1988;23:248–253.
41. Lunsford LD, Flickinger J, Coffey RJ. Stereotactic gamma knife radiosurgery: initial North American experience in 207 patients. *Arch Neurol* 1990;47:169–175.
42. Malaise EP, Fertil B, Chavaudra N, Guichard M. Distribution of radiation sensitivities for human tumor cells of specific histological types: comparison of in vitro to in vivo data. *Int J Radiat Oncol Biol Phys* 1986;12:617–624.
43. Marks JE, Baglan RJ, Prassad SC, Blank WF. Cerebral radionecrosis: incidence and risk in relation to dose, time, fractionation and volume. *Int J Radiat Oncol Biol Phys* 1981;7: 243–252.
44. Mikhael MA. Radiation necrosis of the brain: correlation between computed tomography, pathology, and dose distribution. *J Comput Assist Tomogr* 1978;2:71–80.
45. Mulhern RK, Hancock J, Fairclough D. Neuropsychological status of children treated with brain tumors: a critical review and integrative analysis. *Med Pediatr Oncol* 1992;20:181–191.

46. Nelson DF, Curran WJ, Nelson JS. Hyperfractionation in malignant glioma, report on a dose searching phase I/II protocol of the Radiation Therapy Oncology Group (RTOG). *Proc ASCO* 1990;9:90.
47. Peters LJ. Inherent radiosensitivity of tumor and normal tissue cells as a predictor of human tumor response. *Radiother Oncol* 1991;17:177–190.
48. Phillips TL, Levin VA, Ahn DK, et al. Evaluation of bromodeoxyuridine in glioblastoma multiforme: a Northern California Cancer Center phase II study. *Int J Radiat Oncol Biol Phys* 1991;21:709–714.
49. Prados MD, Gutin PH, Phillips TL, et al. Interstitial brachytherapy for newly diagnosed patients with malignant gliomas: the UCSF experience. *Int J Radiat Oncol Biol Phys* 1992; 24:593–597.
50. Raney B, Tefft M, Heyn R, Newton W, Jones PM, Haeberlen V, Maurer H. Ascending myelitis after intensive chemotherapy and radiation therapy in children with cranial parameningeal sarcoma. *Cancer* 1992;69:1498–1506.
51. del Regato JA. Historical changes in time-dose relationship in therapeutic radiology. *Front Radiat Ther Oncol* 1958;3:1–5.
52. Rimm IJ, Frederick CL, Tarbell NJ, Winston KR, Sallan SE. Brain tumors after cranial irradiation for childhood acute lymphoblastic leukemia. A 13-year experience from the Dana-Farber Cancer Institute and the Children's Hospital. *Cancer* 1987;59:1506–1508.
53. Roggli VL, Estraka R, Fechner RE. Thyroid neoplasia following irradiation for medulloblastoma. *Cancer* 1979;43:2232–2238.
54. Scharfen CO, Sneed PK, Wara WM, et al. High activity iodine-125 interstitial implant for gliomas. *Int J Radiat Oncol Biol Phys* 1992;24:583–591.
55. Schjeide OA, Yamazaki J, Haack K, Ciminelli E, Clemente CD. Biochemical and morphological aspects of radiation inhibition of myelin formation. *Acta Radiol Ther Phys Biol* 1966; 5:185–203.
56. Schrieve DC, Wara WM, Edwards MSB, et al. Hyperfractionated radiation therapy for gliomas of the brain stem in children and in adults. *Int J Radiat Oncol Biol Phys* 1992;24: 599–610.
57. Schultheiss TE, Stephens LC. Pathology radiation myelopathy, widening the circle. *Int J Radiat Oncol Biol Phys* 1992;10:1109–1115.
58. Schultheiss TE, Stephens LC. Permanent radiation myelopathy. *Br J Radiol* 1992;65: 737–753.
59. Shapiro S, Mealey J. Late anaplastic gliomas in children previously treated for acute lymphoblastic leukemia. *Pediatr Neurosci* 1989:15:176–180.
60. Sheline GE, Wara WM, Smith V. Therapeutic irradiation and brain injury. *Int J Radiat Oncol Biol Phys* 1980;6:1215–1228.
61. Skapek SX, Colvin OM, Griffith OW, et al. Buthionine sulfoximine-mediated depletion of glutathione in intracranial human glioma-derived xenografts. *Biochem Pharmacol* 1988;37: 4313–4317.
62. Souhami L, Olivier A, Podgorsak EB, Villemure J-G, Sadikot AF. Fractionated stereotactic radiation therapy for intracranial tumors. *Cancer* 1991;68:2101–2108.
63. Stewart DJ, Leavans M, Maor M, et al. Human CNS distribution of cis-diamminodichloroplatinum and its use as a radiosensitizer in malignant brain tumors. *Cancer Res* 1982;42: 2474–2479.
64. Stone RS. Neutron therapy and specific ionization. Janeway Memorial Lecture. *AJR* 1948; 59:771–785.
65. Thames HD Jr, Peters LJ, Withers HR, Fletcher GH. Accelerated fractionation vs. hyperfractionation: rationales for several treatments per day. *Int J Radiat Oncol Biol Phys* 1983; 9:127–138.
66. Thames HD, Bentzen SM, Turesson I, Overgaard M, Van den Bogaert W. Time-dose factors in radiotherapy: a review of the human data. *Radiother Oncol* 1990;19:219–235.
67. Thomlinson RH, Gray LH. The histological structure of some human lung cancers and the possible implications for radiotherapy. *Br J Cancer* 1955;9:539–549.
68. Thornton AF Jr., Hegarty TJ, Ten Haken RK, et al. Three-dimensional treatment planning of astrocytomas: a dosimetric study of cerebral irradiation. *Int J Radiat Oncol Biol Phys* 1991;20:1309–1315.
69. Valk PE, Dillon WP. Radiation injury of the brain. *AJNR* 1991;12:45–62.

70. van der Kogel, AJ. Central nervous system radiation injury in small animal models. In: Gutin PH, Leibel SA, Sheline GE, eds. *Radiation injury to the nervous system*. New York: Raven Press; 1991:91–112.
71. Voges J, Sturm V, Berthold F, Pastyr O, Scylegel W, Lorenz WJ. Interstitial irradiation of cerebral gliomas in childhood by permanently implanted 125-Iodine: preliminary results. *Klin Padiatr* 1990;202:270–274.
72. Waga S, Handa H. Radiation-induced meningioma: with review of literature. *Surg Neurol* 1976;5:215–219.
73. Wigg DR, Koschel K, Hodgson GS. Tolerance of the mature human central nervous system to photon irradiation. *Br J Radiol* 1981;54:787–798.
74. Wilson CB. Radiosurgery: a new application? *J Clin Oncol* 1992;10:1373–1374.
75. Withers HR, Peters LJ. Biological aspects of radiation therapy. In: Fletcher GH, ed. *Textbook of radiotherapy*. 3rd ed. Philadelphia: Lea & Febiger; 1980:103–179.
76. Withers HR, Peters LJ, Thames HD, Fletcher GH. Hyperfractionation. *Int J Radiat Oncol Biol Phys* 1982;8:1807–1809.
77. Withers HR, Taylor JMG, Maciejewski B. The hazard of accelerated tumor clonogen repopulation during radiotherapy. *Acta Oncologica* 1988;27:131–146.
78. Young DF, Posner JB, Chu F, Nisce L. Rapid-course radiation therapy of cerebral metastases: results and complications. *Cancer* 1974;34:1069–1076.

6

Principles of Chemotherapy

Martin L. Brecher

DEVELOPMENT OF MODERN CHEMOTHERAPY

At one time, most solid cancers were considered to be localized tumors that metastasized only after the primary tumor had grown to considerable size. Surgery was directed at removal of the bulk tumor, and treatment failures were blamed on inadequate surgery. After the recognition that regional spread of tumor cells occurred via lymphatic channels, emphasis was placed on more radical surgical procedures. The development of radiation therapy (RT) as a therapeutic modality has substantially increased survival, and in some tumors has provided cure. By the late 1950s, there was increasing support for the concept that many cancers metastasized early in their course, and thus required treatment with drugs that could reach and kill tumor cells wherever they may have spread (161).

A host of agents capable of bringing about remission of clinical cancers has been known for at least two millennia, but it was not until the 1940s that drugs such as nitrogen mustard (a derivative of mustard gas used in World War I), the folic acid antagonists, and cortisone were discovered to have specific oncolytic effects (32,160). In the decade following World War II, approximately 20,000 compounds were submitted for evaluation as cancer chemotherapeutic drugs. Most testing was confined to animal systems because few centers were geared for clinical trials (47). Investigators were aided by the development of new animal models, including the carcinogen-induced mouse leukemia L1210, which remains one of the most useful and predictable models available. The antitumor effects of drugs in rodents subsequently led to their trials in humans. The chemotherapeutic agents initially demonstrated their effectiveness against systemic tumors such as the acute leukemias and lymphomas. The results of early trials in the treatment of solid tumors were much less dramatic than those seen in hematologic malignancies (159).

In 1955, the Cancer Chemotherapy National Service Center was organized under the auspices of the National Cancer Institute (NCI). Over the next 10 years, the NCI set in motion the elements of a drug development program,

---

Brain Tumors in Children: Principles of Diagnosis and Treatment, 2/e, edited by M.E. Cohen and P.K. Duffner, Raven Press, Ltd., New York, 1994.

including screening, toxicology, pharmacology, formulation, clinical trials, and supportive care.

By the late 1950s, it was possible to cure systemic cancer in humans by chemotherapeutic drugs (CTD). In 1956, Li et al. (90) began their studies of methotrexate (MTX) in metastatic choriocarcinoma. In 1962, the NCI founded the Acute Leukemia Task Force, which, working together with cooperative groups and the Southern Research Institute, laid out curative strategies for acute lymphoyctic leukemia (ALL) (160). In 1968, the Wilms' tumor trials demonstrated the efficacy of chemotherapy in treating micrometastases (22). Also in the 1960s, clinical trials in the treatment of breast cancer indicated that even a slowly growing tumor could respond to adjuvant chemotherapy (16,52).

During the early 1960s, only sporadic individual efforts were reported with chemotherapy in the treatment of brain tumors. Representatives from five university neurosurgical departments, the NCI, and the National Institute of Neurologic Diseases and Blindness met in 1966 to form the Brain Tumor Chemotherapy Study Group, with the purpose of formulating cooperative group protocols and pooling results in order to complete studies within a reasonable time.

NEW AGENT TRIALS

Once the structure–activity relationships of a drug in current clinical use are identified, efforts are directed toward synthesis of analogous known structures. In addition, new classes of agents are sought in light of the increased understanding of the biochemical and kinetic mechanisms of cancer cell growth.

New chemotherapeutic drugs are first tested in vivo in animal tumor systems. Antitumor activity is generally identified on the basis of increased life span in treated animals as compared with a control group (47). The toxicity of these agents is then determined in monkeys and dogs, because the qualitative and quantitative effects on various organ systems in these large animals appear to parallel those in humans (58).

Next, promising new chemotherapeutic agents are put through *phase I* trials in humans, which are essentially toxicity studies in which drug dosages are pushed to their toxic limits. Dosage guidelines and limitations are established, and toxic effects in humans are delineated. Phase I studies are not intended to monitor antitumor activity, because the drug is administered by varying schedules to a heterogeneous population of cancer patients. The drug then enters *phase II* trials to identify the spectrum of activity against human neoplasms and response rates in specific cancers. If significant activity is noted, the drug is then incorporated into *phase III* trials, which are controlled, prospective studies. Phase I and II studies delineate an optimal dose schedule and establish antitumor activity. The purpose of the phase III trial is to determine if the use of this drug improves therapeutic results when used in an adjuvant fashion with other drugs and/or other modalities of therapy such as RT and/or surgery.

BASIC PRINCIPLES OF CHEMOTHERAPY

The Cell Cycle

Knowledge of cell-cycle kinetics (Fig. 6-1) is basic to our understanding of current theories of the mechanism of action of most modern chemotherapeutic agents, and is thus crucial for the logical design of chemotherapeutic protocols. The cell cycle can be defined as the interval between the midpoint of mitosis and the midpoint of the subsequent mitosis in one or both daughter cells. The cycle is divided into four phases: G_1 is the phase during which cells synthesize RNA, enzymes, and proteins in preparation for the beginning of DNA synthesis. The G_1 phase is the most variable in duration, with slowly growing populations containing cells that have long G_1 periods (5). The S phase is the period during which the DNA replicates and chromosomal proteins are laid down on the newly synthesized DNA (153). During this phase, several critical enzymes, including thymidine-kinase, DNA polymerase, dihydrofolate reductase, and ribonucleotide reductase, increase (18,70,84,137). The G_2 phase is the interval between the completion of DNA synthesis and mitosis. In this period, the substrates necessary for the two daughter cells are produced. The M phase is the period of mitosis. In any tumor cell population, some cells may be cycling continuously while others may be in the G_0, or resting, state. Cells in the G_0 phase, although not actively proliferating, have the potential to reenter the proliferating pool and cell cycle. In addition, certain cells differentiate and will die without dividing

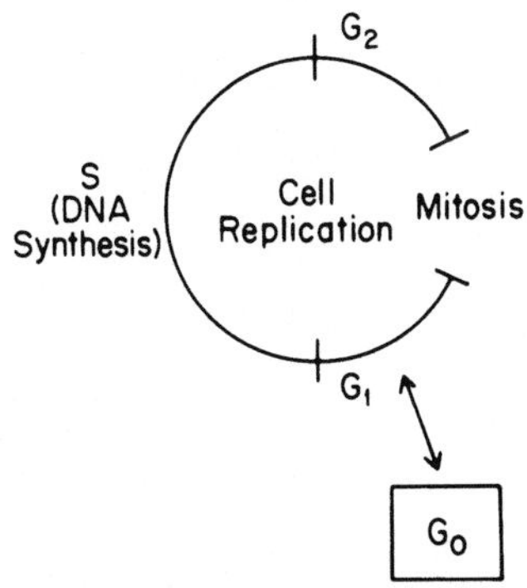

FIG. 6-1. The cell cycle.

again. This last group of cells is generally not of concern to the chemotherapist.

Kinetics of Tumor Growth

Theoretically, cancer arises when one normal cell changes into a malignant or neoplastic cell either by natural mutation or after chemical, viral, or radiation induction (125). Subsequent tumor growth has been described by the mathematical model of Gompertz (Fig. 6-2), which states that tumor growth is at every instant exponential, but with a growth constant that is simultaneously decreasing exponentially (85). By the time a lesion measures 1 cm in diameter, which represents roughly the smallest clinically detectable lesion, it has undergone approximately 30 doublings (131) (Fig. 6-3). Thus, although the diagnosis of cancer may be made at an early stage clinically, all tumors are recognized relatively late in their biological growth. Metastatic disease may well have occurred by the time of diagnosis. At late stages, relatively few doublings have a dramatic impact on tumor size. The increasing doubling time, which occurs as the tumor grows in size, is due in part to a lengthening of the generation time of the dividing tumor cells (123,135). With increasing tumor size, a progressively increasing proportion of the viable cell population enters a nonproliferative state (G_0). There is also increasing cell loss from the tumor by exfoliation and/or cell death (125).

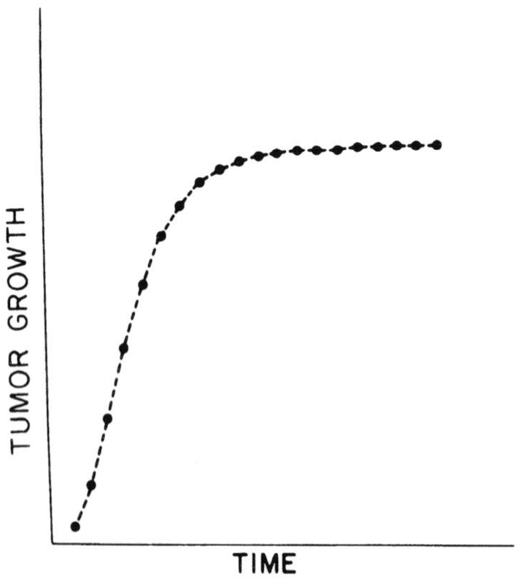

FIG. 6-2. The Gompertzian curve.

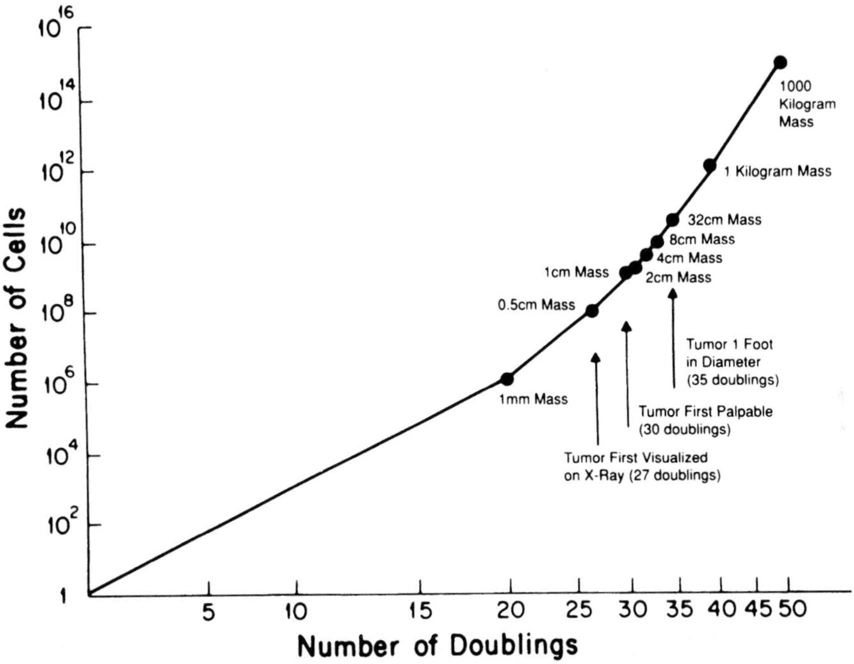

FIG. 6-3. Theoretical tumor growth curve.

Mechanisms of Action of Chemotherapeutic Agents

Skipper et al. (136) first demonstrated that the ability of chemotherapeutic drugs to kill tumor cells followed first-order kinetics; i.e., a constant percentage, rather than a constant number of cells, is killed by a given therapeutic maneuver. Bacteriologists have long recognized the first-order kinetics of germicidal kill of bacteria in vitro. As with microbiology, the knowledge of the influence of a log kill influences our understanding of cancer chemotherapy. For example, a child with advanced ALL might harbor 10^{12} or about 1 kg of leukemic cells. A drug capable of killing 99.99% of these cells would reduce the mass to 10^8 cells, or approximately 0.1 mg, resulting in a complete clinical remission. However, the remaining cells could obviously regrow and cause a relapse in disease. Unfortunately, remission and cure are not the same, as cure in all probability requires a total cell kill. In experimental models, for example, a single cancer cell injected into a susceptible host can kill that animal (68,124). In addition, it is known that myelomas in humans and animals probably arise from a single cell because they produce a single clone-specific immunoglobulin (125). Likewise, chronic myelocytic leukemia (CML) is thought to arise from a single clone (49). Therefore, at present, the most important role of chemotherapy in the treatment of solid tumors is in eradicating subclinical metastases after debulking of disease by surgery and/or RT (147). As a generalization, first-order kinetics characterize effective drug kill of tumor cells. Efficacy of the best currently known anticancer drugs is not only variable but also generally limited in tumor cell kill potential. Thus, for eradication of disease and cure, drug treatment of micrometastasis should be started as soon as possible when the cancer burden is at its nadir.

CLASSIFICATION OF CHEMOTHERAPEUTIC AGENTS

Those chemotherapeutic agents (Fig. 6-4) that act at any stage in the life of the cell are called cell-cycle-nonspecific agents (CCNS). Cell-cycle-specific (CCS) agents, unlike CCNS drugs, are effective only during active proliferation (146). Some CCS agents have activity that is not restricted to a specific phase of the cell cycle, while other agents are phase specific. Theoretically, because of their broader spectrum of action, CCNS agents have a biologic advantage over CCS agents. However, these agents, because of their ability to destroy noncycling cells, have a lower therapeutic index than CCS drugs, and are more likely to damage normal cells.

Alkylating Agents

The alkylating agents are a group of CCNS drugs whose toxic effect results from the replacement of a hydrogen atom in the DNA chain by an alkyl group (147). Cross-linking of DNA is the primary mechanism of antitumor action of the alkylating agents.

The nitrosoureas, including BCNU, CCNU, and methyl-CCNU, act as alkylating agents but, in addition, have an isocyanate metabolite that inhibits DNA repair (71). As they are lipid-soluble, these drugs readily diffuse into the central nervous system (CNS). For this reason, they are of particular interest in the therapy of brain tumors.

The oxazaphosphorines, cyclophosphamide and ifosfamide, inactive prodrugs that require biotransformation by hepatic microsomal oxidative enzymes before expressing alkylating activity, are finding increasing use in the treatment of pediatric brain tumors. A steep dose-response curve has been demonstrated for these agents. The availability of mesna, a synthetic sulfhydryl compound that protects the urinary tract epithelium from the toxic effects of their metabolites, and the use of hematopoietic growth factors to ameliorate myelotoxicity, have permitted significant dose escalation of these agents.

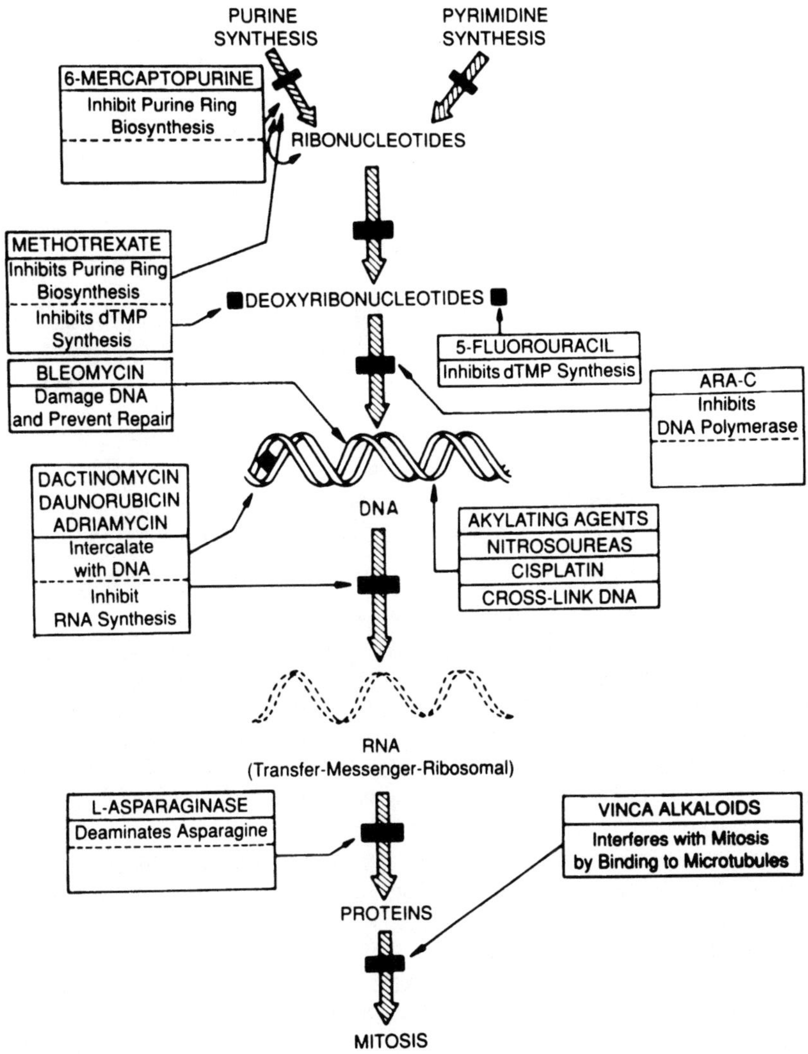

FIG. 6-4. Mechanisms of action of commonly used chemotherapeutic agents (modified from reference 24).

Antibiotics

The antibiotic anticancer agents are also cell-cycle-nonspecific and include adriamycin, daunomycin, actinomycin-D, and bleomycin. Adriamycin and daunomycin intercalate with the major groove of the DNA helix, preventing both DNA transcription and replication. Actinomycin-D intercalates with the minor groove of the DNA helix inhibiting RNA transcription. Bleomycin probably exerts its lethal effect by binding to DNA, causing fission and fragmentation of the helix. Unfortunately, as these agents do not readily cross into the CNS from the bloodstream, their use in the treatment of brain tumors has been limited. However, some clinical trials from Japan have shown some response to bleomycin in patients with malignant gliomas (73,141).

Mitotic Inhibitors

Vincristine (VCR) and vinblastine are phase-specific agents derived from the periwinkle plant, *vinca rosea*. They bind to the subunit protein of the microtubules that are thought to be important for spindle formation during cytokinesis. This results in mitotic arrest and bizarre mitotic formations (147). VCR also produces axonal damage by disruption of the neurotubules responsible for axoplasmic transport (44). Single agent reports using VCR in the treatment of brain tumors have been encouraging but somewhat limited. Good phase III data are presently not available (48).

Antimetabolites

The antimetabolites are CCS agents that interfere with purine and pyrimidine synthesis. MTX, the most widely studied antimetabolite in the treatment of CNS tumors, is an inhibitor of dihydrofolate reductase (13). This results in reduced availability of folates needed for thymidylate and purine synthesis (25). Free MTX is necessary to produce maximal inhibition of DNA synthesis. In addition, this agent may interfere with the synthesis of several putative neurotransmitters. The therapeutic and toxic effects of MTX on target tissues are a function of both the level of drug and duration of exposure (158).

The effectiveness of intrathecal (IT) MTX in the treatment of meningeal leukemia raises the possibility that similar results can be achieved in primary brain tumors (150). Studies with IT MTX alone have shown suggestive, but limited, responses in a few patients with medulloblastomas (105,152) (see Chapter 9).

Steroids

Steroids primarily act by reducing the vasogenic edema associated with intracranial masses. There is some additional evidence that these agents may also have a direct cytotoxic effect. Steroids are believed to act on cell membranes. It is possible that this activity may potentiate or inhibit the entry of chemotherapeutic agents across the cell membrane (157). In animals, steroids have been shown to decrease the incorporation of tritiated thymidine into tumor DNA when compared to controls (130). Others have shown inhibition of experimental glial tumors in tissue cultures (98). Nonetheless, evidence for a direct antitumor activity of steroids remains inconclusive.

Cis-platin

The platinum compounds are among the most active CTD in the treatment of pediatric brain tumors. While the mechanisms of action of these agents remain to be fully elucidated, cis-platin (CDDP) appears to have alkylating agent activity, exerting its effect primarily in the G_1 phase of the cell cycle (42). Cis-platin binds to defined double-stranded decanucleotides, causing kinking of the DNA helix (82). Cis-platin induced local alterations in DNA confirmation may inhibit the function of many enzymes that act on DNA, including a variety of DNA repair enzymes. Favorable responses to single-agent therapy with CDDP have been reported in small numbers of patients (75). Cis-platin has produced objective responses when administered as an intracarotid infusion to patients with recurrent glioma (46).

Carboplatin (CBDCA) is a second-generation platinum complex that is less nephrotoxic and ototoxic than the parent compound, although it has greater myelotoxicity. It appears to retain the same antitumor effects (80). Walker et al. (149) have reported that CBDCA has significant activity in recurrent childhood brain tumors, including brain stem glioma and malignant astrocytoma.

Epipodophyllotoxins

The epipodophyllotoxins, including etoposide (VP-16) and teniposide (VM-26), are thought to exert their antitumor effects by the formation of DNA-topoisomerase II cleavable complexes, which are converted to DNA single- and double-stranded breaks upon treatment with protein denaturants (40). Clinical observations that protracted infusions of low-dose VP-16 may provide greater antitumor activity, without dramatic change in toxicity, as compared with the same total dose given in bolus fashion suggest that the antitumor effect may be cell-cycle-phase specific (40). If drugs that block DNA synthesis are given before epipodophyllotoxins, an antagonistic effect can be anticipated (35).

Laboratory studies have indicated a supra-additive effect for VP-16 in combination with cis-platin (43). In a phase II trial at SJCRH, there were two complete responses and nine partial responses in 13 patients with newly diagnosed medulloblastoma, pinealblastoma, and cerebral neuroblastoma (81).

CHEMOTHERAPY TOXICITY

The therapeutic ratio for cancer CTD is narrow, because the drugs affect normal as well as malignant cells. One cannot increase the dose of chemotherapeutic agents greatly without significantly increasing toxicity to normal tissue. Indeed, in a number of mouse models, doubling the chemotherapeutic dose that causes the toxic deaths of 10% of animals will result in the death of 90% of such animals. On the other hand, decreasing the drug dosage may eliminate the antitumor effect. Thus, a modest change in drug concentration reaching the tumor cells, or the host tissue, may result in either inadequate therapeutic effect or excessive toxicity (56).

In general, normal tissues that are turning over rapidly are most susceptible to the side effects of CTD. This includes the GI tract (the lining of the upper duodenum turns over in 1.8 days), bone marrow, and skin with its appendages, such as the hair follicles. Oral ulcerations are commonly seen with drugs such as MTX, cytosine arabinoside (ARA-C), and actinomycin-D. There may occasionally be ulcerations throughout the GI tract, which may be difficult to document during life but may act as a portal of entry for organisms leading to septicemia.

Bone marrow suppression is the most common and worrisome complication, and is usually the dose-limiting toxicity. Chemotherapy may lead to neutropenia, resulting in increased susceptibility to bacterial infection, and thrombocytopenia, resulting in significant blood loss. The nitrosoureas result in a delayed nadir of bone marrow suppression approximately 4 weeks after drug administration. Procarbazine is also known to cause marked bone marrow suppression. Thus, with the use of any of these drugs, hematologic parameters should be frequently monitored.

VCR causes minimal to no bone marrow suppression. Toxicity relates primarily to that affecting peripheral nerves. Constipation is believed due to toxicity of VCR on the nerves supplying the GI tract. This agent is also associated with alopecia.

Cis-platin's (CDDP) primary toxicities are nausea, vomiting, neurosensory hearing loss, and peripheral neuropathies. The drug is also a potent nephrotoxin. Increased auditory toxicity has been noted when CDDP is given after cranial irradiation.

There is some evidence that chemotherapy may be administered prior to cranial irradiation without increasing the neurotoxicity associated with the subsequent radiotherapy (111). This approach has the additional advantage of providing a phase II "window" permitting evaluation of response in patients who are previously untreated except for surgery. Radiation may also be more effective in chemotherapy-sensitive patients who have experienced reduction of the residual tumor mass.

Some cytotoxic drugs, including alkylating agents, are themselves potential carcinogens. Recent reports have suggested that the epipodophyllotoxins

TABLE 6-1. *Neurotoxicity of chemotherapeutic drugs*

Agent	Incidence	Type	Reversibility	Comments
L-asparaginase	25–50%	Encephalopathy, somnolence and confusion, OBS (organic brain syndrome, seizures, stroke-like syndrome, abnormal EEGs)	Generally reversible	L-asp does not cross the BBB, but may deplete the brain of semiessential amino acids, such as asparagine, which may cause these effects
5-fluorouracil	1%	Cerebellar	Reversible	
Methotrexate IT MTX	10–50%	Headache, vomiting, meningismus, CSF pleocytosis	Reversible	
	Rare	Paraplegia	Transient or permanent	
	Rare	Convulsion	Reversible	No apparent neurological residium
Intraventricular MTX	?	Leukoencephalopathy	Irreversible	Periventricular necrosis seen in the presence of CSF flow obstruction
IV MTX	Rare	Leukoencephalopathy	Irreversible	Generally seen when total dose of MTX is over 5 g, and is more common if cranial RT is administered
Nitrogen mustard	Rare	Tinnitus/hearing loss	Reversible	With higher doses, but no toxicity seen with standard doses
Procarbazine	10–40%	Drowsiness/stupor, peripheral neuropathy	Reversible	
	Rare	Hallucinations/agitation	Reversible	
	Rare	Ataxia		
Vincristine	Up to 100%	Peripheral neuropathy includes depressed DTR/weakness/cranial neuropathies/abdominal pain and constipation/bladder distention/impotence/orthostatic hypotension	Reversible	Degeneration of spindle fiber axons
	1%	Seizures/peripheral neuropathy/quadriplegia	Nonreversible	
Cis-platin	Rare	Peripheral neuropathy/encephalopathy	Reversible	Similar to heavy metal toxicity (lead), may be related to cumulative dose
High-dose cytosine arabinoside	?	Stupor to coma	Likely reversible	More commonly seen in those with prior CNS insult such as pre-existing CNS leukemia, prior CRT, or IT CTD

TABLE 6-2. *Psychiatric side effects of chemotherapeutic drugs*

Drug			
Prednisone	+ + + to + + +	Psychosis/Mood/Changes/ Irritable	Dose-related
Imidazole carboxamide	+	Organic brain syndrome/ depression	
Methotrexate	+ to + +	OBS	Much more common in association with whole brain irradiation
Vinblastine	+ + +		
L-asparaginase	+ to + +	Depression OBS Depression Psychosis	
Procarbazine	+	OBS (Including manic psychosis & hallucinations)	

[a] These toxicities are reversible.

may be associated with the development of secondary myeloid leukemias. The risk of leukemogenesis appears to depend on both dose and schedule (115,117).

Virtually all CTD employed have a wide spectrum of side effects. Knowledge of the various toxicities is mandatory when planning treatment protocols. Several of these drugs, when used in combination, may potentiate one another and thus lead to myelosuppression and life-threatening infections. As a general rule, a patient who is in good nutritional status, without infection or metabolic abnormalities, will tolerate chemotherapy better than a debilitated patient. The CNS toxicities of commonly used CTD are listed in Tables 6-1 and 6-2.

DRUG–DRUG INTERACTIONS

It is well known that the interaction of one drug with another can measurably alter the expected pharmacologic effect. Over 60% of non-chemotherapeutic agents are known to influence the action and/or the toxicity of CTD. In a study performed at the Sidney Farber Cancer Institute (56), an average 5.6 drugs per patient was administered on any one day. Many of these agents are bound to serum albumin, and thus are not available at the cellular level until they are released in their free form. For example, MTX is 60% bound to albumin. A weak acid such as aspirin can displace free MTX from protein-bound sites and thus increase its bioavailability.

Microsomal enzymes of the liver may be induced by barbiturates, antidepressants, and anticoagulants. These drugs, in general, decrease the toxicity of chemotherapeutic agents that are metabolized, activated, or bound to protein in the liver. Examples of such drugs are the anthracycline antibiotics, daunomycin, adriamycin, cyclophosphamide, and imidazole carboxamide (DTIC). Conversely, those drugs that inhibit microsomal enzyme induction, such allopurinol, Darvon, and phenylbutazine, may potentially increase the toxicity of CTD.

Those drugs that alter renal function, such as diuretics, aminoglycoside antibiotics, and probenecid, are capable of increasing the toxicity of chemotherapeutic agents such as MTX and CDDP, or other agents that are primarily excreted by the kidney.

EFFECT OF RENAL AND HEPATIC DISEASE ON ANTICANCER DRUGS

Methotrexate

Renal excretion is the major route for elimination of MTX; over 80% of an intravenously administered dose is excreted unchanged in the urine (27,67). Freeman-Narrod et al. (54) reported a prolonged MTX plasma half life of 6 to 8 hours in patients with depressed renal function (creatinine clearance less than 80 ml/min) compared with a half life of 90 minutes in patients with normal renal function. Reduction of MTX dosage in patients with known renal dysfunction is particularly important in limiting MTX toxicity to normal tissue. Toxicity of MTX relates to both duration of exposure and suprathreshold concentrations. Thus, in patients with reduced renal function, or when high doses of the drug are used, plasma MTX blood levels must be obtained in order to identify patients at high risk for the development of toxicity, and who may benefit from supplemental leucovorin rescue and alkalinization of the urine (15,103,138,139).

Cis-platin

Cis-platin (CDDP) binds to serum protein (36,69). The disappearance of platinum from plasma is biphasic, with reported half lives of 20 to 49 minutes for the initial phase and 17 to 73 hours for the terminal phase (33,36,62,63). The long terminal phase of elimination is associated with the slow removal of that platinum which is tightly bound to plasma protein (66). Alteration in renal function may prolong elimination of free unbound platinum in plasma (63,114). Patients with decreased renal function have an increased sensitivity to nephrotoxic drugs. As toxicity increases with decreasing plasma clearance, patients with known renal disease should have the dose of platinum reduced (126).

Nitrosoureas

Despite the central role of the liver in the metabolism of nitrosoureas, there have been no clinical reports on the effect of hepatic disease on the pharmacokinetics of the chloroethyl nitrosoureas.

Vinca Alkaloids

Because VCR is extensively metabolized, biliary excretion plays a major role in its elimination. After intravenous administration of ^{3}H-VCR, up to 72% of the radioactive dose is found in the feces by 72 hours, half as metabolites (8,9). The toxicity of VCR is known to increase in patients with impaired liver function (99).

DRUG RESISTANCE

Drug resistance is one of the principle causes for chemotherapy failures (19). The mechanisms of resistance include inability of the drug to cross cell membranes, lack of intracellular drug activation, increased breakdown of the drug in the cell, rapid repair of the lesion caused by the drug, or increase in the target substrate. Resistance to a particular drug may result from an intrinsic property of the cell or may be acquired after one or more exposures to the agent. Relatively little is known about the intrinsic resistance to chemotherapeutic agents of normal structures of the CNS that may give rise to malignant tumors. Acquired drug resistance may result from the loss of normal cell properties, such as intracellular transport or essential activating enzymes, or by the amplification of existing cell properties, including increased drug-deactivating enzymes and repair enzymes (112). Drug-resistant cells may arise by mutation (28,92,132). The most widely accepted theory is that when a cancer is large enough to be diagnosed, resistant clones are already present. These clones may then be "selected" by a drug as the sensitive cells are removed by CTD (134). New tumor growth will contain cells of the resistant clone. A mathematical model relating tumor size to the spontaneous mutation rate of tumor cells has been developed by Goldie and Coldman (60). They point out that the probability of resistant clones increases in a parallel fashion with the size of the tumor. It has been recognized for many years that small tumors, or those that are completely resected, respond best to therapy and have the best chance for cure. Unfortunately, human cancers are biologically far advanced by the time of diagnosis. A tumor burden of 10^8 to 10^9 cells must be present before a mass becomes detectable either clinically or roentgenographically (38). As such, it is likely that cells resistant to a particular drug regimen are present at the time of diagnosis.

TABLE 6-3. *Mechanisms of drug resistance*

Drug	Resistance mechanism
Cisplatin	Transport ↓ Glutathione ↑ Glutathione S-transferase ↑ Metallothionein ↑ DNA repair ↑
Cyclophosphamide	Aldehyde dehydrogenase ↑ Glutathione ↑ Glutathione S-transferase ↑
Nitrogen mustard	Transport ↓ Glutathione ↑ Glutathione S-transferase ↑ DNA repair ↑
Melphalan	Transport ↓ Glutathione ↑
Nitrosoureas	O^6-alkylguanine-DNA-alkyltransferase Glutathione S-transferase ↑
Actinomycin D Bleomycin Etoposide Daunorubicin Doxorubicin Teniposide Vinblastine sulfate Vincristine sulfate	Multidrug resistant (P-170) ↑

From Phillips PC. Antineoplastic drug resistance in brain tumors. In: Cohen ME, Duffner PK, eds. *Neurologic clinics. Brain tumors in children.* Philadelphia: WB Saunders; 1991: 386. Reprinted with permission.

The expression of drug resistance may be specific to a particular agent, or may represent multidrug cross resistance. Some of the mechanisms of specific drug resistance are listed in Table 6-3 (126). The term *multi-drug resistance* has been applied to the phenomenon by which exposure to a single drug results in the development of resistance to multiple, chemically unrelated chemotherapeutic agents. One mechanism by which this may occur is by increased expression of the MDR 1 gene, which encodes a 170-kD protein (P-170) that functions as an energy-dependent efflux pump, reducing intracellular drug concentration (7,110). Increased expression of P-170 has been associated with amplification of the MDR 1 gene (53,119).

P-glycoprotein is found in a variety of normal tissues, as well as in tumors, even in the absence of prior drug therapy. It is speculated that it may serve an important function in the elimination of natural toxins present in many foods. Not surprisingly, the anticancer drugs that exhibit MDR cross-resistance are predominantly those isolated from natural sources, including antibiotics such as doxorubicin and actinomycin D; mitotic inhibitors, including VCR and vinblastine; and the podophyllotoxins.

The significance of MDR in the therapy of brain tumors is unknown at this time. Matsumato and his colleagues (97) demonstrated overexpression of the MDR 1 gene, without evidence of MDR 1 gene amplification, in a human glioma cell line expressing the MDR phenotype. Teshler et al. (144) identified P-170 glycoprotein in 2 of 16 pediatric primitive neuroectodermal tumors, although MDR 1 gene amplification was not detected in either tumor. Further studies are required to determine the frequency of MDR in various pediatric brain tumors.

Multiple drug resistance may occur without increased expression of P-170 glycoprotein. Cross-resistance has been reported between topoisomerase II inhibitors (e.g., etoposide, teniposide) and drugs such as doxorubicin, daunorubicin, and vindesine (127). It is hypothesized that the cytotoxicity of a subgroup of antineoplastic drugs is mediated via an interaction with topoisomerase II, and that drug resistance results from an alteration in either topoisomerase II or cellular modulation of the enzyme (74). In addition, cross-resistance between radiation and a variety of antineoplastic agents has been associated with elevated intracellular levels of glutathione (GSH) (109).

A variety of approaches have been used to circumvent the problem of drug resistance. Most chemotherapy protocols rapidly cycle non-cross-resistant drug combinations in an effort to prevent the emergence of drug-resistant cell clones (122). The use of high-dose chemotherapy, with or without autologous bone marrow rescue, may increase drug uptake and exceed the capacity of the neoplasm to deactivate a drug or repair cellular injury (6,57). In addition, pharmacologic approaches to circumventing or reversing drug resistance are being investigated. Butathione sulfoxamime has been used to lower intracellular GSH, which may reverse resistance to some alkylating agents (120). Calcium channel blockers, such as verapamil and cyclosporin A, have been found to reverse MDR in resistant cell lines. They appear to inhibit the binding of antineoplastic agents to p-glycoprotein, by either competitive displacement or inactivation, thereby inhibiting their efflux from the cell (29,145). Several trials are currently evaluating the ability of pharmacologic agents to reverse MDR in the clinical setting. Dose escalation may be another method of overcoming drug resistance. Alkylating agents, in particular, have a steep dose–response curve. Several clinical trials (6,57) have demonstrated responses to myeloablative doses of chemotherapy, followed by autologous bone marrow reconstitution, in patients with solid tumors refractory to conventional therapy. There are few trials to date on the efficacy of this approach in the treatment of childhood brain tumors. However, patients with recurrent brain tumors are rarely cured with conventional dose therapy, and those with newly diagnosed high-grade astrocytomas, including glioblastoma multiforme, have a relatively low cure rate with the standard approach of surgical resection, RT, and chemotherapy.

Finlay (50,51) recently reviewed a series of 61 children and young adults, 53 of whom had recurrent disease, treated with myeloablative therapy and autologous marrow rescue, and reported responses in 23% of children with malignant astrocytoma. Toxicity was significant, with 21% of patients suffering toxic deaths. Additional studies are required to determine if this approach will increase survival for patients with high-risk or recurrent brain tumors. The availability of hematopoietic growth factors, including granulocyte colony stimulating factor (G-CSF) and granulocytic-macrophage colony stimilating factor (GM-CSF), may permit dose intensification by decreasing the duration of profound neutropenia following high-dose chemotherapy treatment, thereby reducing the risk of infectious complications. Earlier recovery of marrow function might also allow for more rapid cycling of drug combinations, decreasing the period for tumor regrowth between treatments and, perhaps, preventing the emergence of drug resistant clones. To date, there has been no convincing evidence that the cytokines studied have enhanced the growth of the underlying solid tumors (129).

In Vitro Chemosensitivity Testing

Several techniques have been developed to evaluate the chemosensitivity of tumor cells in vitro. The double-layer soft-agar method reported by Hamberger and Salmon (64) in 1977, commonly referred to as the "clonogenic assay," has been the most extensively studied. Bertelsen et al. (12) reviewed their experience with in vitro chemosensitivity testing in over 1500 solid tumors, and found this assay to be 57% reliable for predicting in vivo sensitivity, and 92% reliable for in vivo resistance. Predictive accuracy varied with tumor histology. Similar results have been reported using the clonogenic assay with human tumor xenografts, which would permit verification of results in the same tumor lines in vivo in athymic mice (11). Although the clonogenic assay has proven quite useful for screening new anti-cancer drugs, it is premature to predict whether in vitro testing may permit the individualization of primary chemotherapy regimens in the future.

Radiosensitizers

Since the report by Adams and Dewey (2) in 1963 that N-ethylmaleinide enhances the radiation damage of hypoxic cells, the radiosensitizing abilities of various electron-affinic organic compounds have been studied. Aromatic and heterocyclic nitro compounds, especially nitro-imidazole derivatives such as misonidazole and metronidazole, are effective for radiosensitizing hypoxic cells (140). This results from repair inhibition of damaged intracellular molecules by the electron-affinic compounds (1).

It has also been shown that misonidazole is capable of sensitizing tumors in mice to a variety of alkylating agents (26). Three likely mechanisms for this chemosensitization are (a) depletion of the intracellular protector GSH, (b) increased intracellular uptake of drug, and (c) increased efficacy of DNA interstrand cross-link formation (21).

More recently, cis-platin has been found to be a radiosensitizing agent when administered as an infusion during radiation treatments (72,142). It has been postulated that the cis-platin may cause increased intracellular formation of reactive-free radicals or may directly damage DNA binding (41,148). Radiosensitization has been demonstrated at cis-platin concentrations as low as 1 μg/ml (41,72,142). Myelosuppression has been the primary toxicity associated with infusional cis-platin, while gastrointestinal, renal, and ototoxicity has been less than that encountered with standard bolus administration (30,121). The Pediatric Oncology Group (POG) conducted a phase I trial of infusional cis-platin in combination with hyperfractionated radiotherapy in children with brain stem glioma, and found acceptable toxicity with a dose level of cis-platin of 100 mg/m^2/120-hour course. The group is currently conducting a phase III trial of this combination in children with newly diagnosed brain stem gliomas.

PROBLEMS UNIQUE TO THE TREATMENT OF TUMORS OF THE CNS

To date, progress in the chemotherapy of brain tumors has lagged behind that of other neoplasms of childhood. Reasons for this include (a) the relative inaccessibility of the CNS to drugs administered systemically, (b) the lack of accrual of large numbers of patients with specific tumor types at individual centers, (c) the difficulty in quantifying objective responses, (d) the fear of drug toxicity, and (e) the concern about a poor quality of life resulting from the effects of aggressive treatment.

Paul Ehrlich (45) was the first to suggest the presence of a blood–brain barrier (BBB) that prohibited passage of materials from blood into the brain. Anatomically, the barrier is the result of an alteration of the structure of the cerebral capillary endothelium, which differs from the capillary endothelium in other locations. In the brain, tight junctions occur between adjacent cells of the cerebral capillary endothelium. These junctions limit transport across the capillary wall. In addition, cerebral capillaries contain fewer cytoplasmic pinocytic vesicles, have a relative lack of fenestration, and have a perivascular glial sheath, all of which restrict passage across the capillary lumen.

Rall and Zubrod (116) have summarized the biochemical qualities needed to permit passage of a drug into the CNS. These attributes include lipid solubility, low molecular size (less than 200 mol wt for water-soluble drugs), weak ionization in plasma, and poor protein binding (34). Furthermore, the presence or lack of a specific transport system can significantly influence penetration into the CNS (151).

In malignant tumors of the brain there is frequently a disruption of the anatomical basis of the BBB (94). This results in increased permeability of normally excluded agents in the central area of the tumor (86,87,89). Nonetheless, in brain tumors, the BBB still appears to play a substantial role. For example, in tumors that are sensitive to adriamycin, progression in the size of brain metastases has been observed at the same time that systemic tumors are responding to this form of chemotherapy (10).

An additional complicating factor in preventing drug entry into the CNS is the concept of the brain-adjacent tumor (BAT). The advancing edge of the tumor, which contains cells with the greatest growth fraction (4,143), is least likely to respond to treatment, because cells found at the periphery, unlike those found in the necrotic center of the tumor, are associated with an intact BBB. The presence of this intact barrier effectively limits access of most CTD to that area of the neoplasm with the highest growth fraction (86–89).

Another major obstacle to the successful treatment of brain tumors with chemotherapy is that total gross surgical resection is generally not possible because of the intimate presence of vital structures. Therefore, CTD may be employed at a time when the tumor burden remains high.

Many brain tumors have been shown to have a low mitotic index, with growth fractions of 10 to 30% (86). Therefore, only a relatively small proportion of the tumor cell population will be susceptible to CCS drugs. In addition, the individual tumors are often not homogeneous and may contain many subpopulations of cancer cells that differ in characteristics, such as karyotype, morphology, and rate of growth, and therefore in their response to chemotherapy (23,24).

TREATMENT CONSIDERATIONS

Adjuvant therapy should begin immediately after surgery and/or RT, when cell numbers are relatively small and growth fraction is highest. To optimize treatment, CCS agents, which do not readily cross cell membranes, should be combined with CCNS agents, which, because of their lipophilic properties, have the potential of crossing the BBB and penetrating the BAT.

The kinetics of cell recruitment is important in formulating treatment protocols. The size of the growth fraction of a tumor is inversely related to mass. Consequently, CCNS agents, with their potential for reducing mass by destroying G_0 as well as cycling cells, increase the likelihood of returning nonproliferating cells into the cell cycle where they may be responsive to CCS agents. CCS agents are most effective when used in an adjuvant fashion to treat microscopic residual or micrometastases, because of the higher growth fraction associated with the smaller mass of cells. Unfortunately, the therapeutic benefits of this approach may be limited when treating slowly growing solid tumors, because CCS agents may be more injurious to normal renewing tissue than to the tumor itself. Nonetheless, on balance, combinations of CCNS and CCS agents have proven to be the most effective.

Because resistance to chemotherapeutic agents may be induced when cells are exposed to low concentrations of drugs for a long period of time, or when drug dosage is gradually escalated, intermittent high-dose therapy is apt to be most effective (14). Several authors have demonstrated that intermittent high-dose therapy, repeated at intervals, when toxicity has subsided, provides the best results (61,136).

When using phase-specific agents, duration of exposure of the tumor cells to the drug may be as important as the peak level. Maintaining prolonged effective levels results in maximum cell kill by allowing tumor cells to cycle through that part of the cell cycle which is affected by the phase-specific agent. Alternating cycles of effective agents or groups of effective agents, which are non-cross-resistant, decreases the likelihood of resistant cell lines emerging and further increases the potential of combination chemotherapy (60,133).

Thus, knowledge of the biochemical mechanisms by which drugs act, the mechanisms by which malignant cells acquire resistance, patterns of cross-sensitivity and resistance of chemotherapeutic agents, the kinetics of tumor growth, and the pharmacologic and toxic effects of drugs all aid in the design of effective and tolerable drug combinations. When these principles have been applied, cures of disseminated cancers, such as ALL, Hodgkin's disease, non-Hodgkin's lymphoma, and testicular cancer have been obtained (162).

As many brain tumors will spread throughout the cerebral spinal fluid (CSF), design of brain tumor protocols may include administration of a drug directly into the spinal fluid. It has recently been suggested that up to one-third of patients with medulloblastomas will have detectable spinal metastases by myelography (37). Although seeding of the spinal fluid is most common with medulloblastomas and ependymomas, it is recognized to a lesser degree with virtually all CNS neoplasms.

Drugs may be administered directly into the CSF either via lumbar puncture (LP) or directly into the lateral ventricle with an implantable device. When a drug is injected IT, substantial concentrations are not obtained in the ventricles or over the convexities of the brain unless 25% of the CSF volume is exchanged (118). Unfortunately, this is an impractical maneuver. Although giving drugs via the intraventricular route may circumvent this distribution problem, there must be a free flow of the CSF, or severe toxicity may result. MTX given via an intraventricular catheter in the presence of CSF obstruction may result in severe and even fatal leukoencephalopathy (128). IT chemotherapy may be given simultaneously with the same drug intravenously, leading to higher levels and a more even distribution of the drug for a longer period of time. This was first demonstrated by Oldendorf and Davson (107) using C-labeled sucrose, by Bourke et al. (17) with labeled 5-FU, and subsequently by Freeman et al. (55) using MTX.

Despite the various obstacles, administration of CTD directly into the CSF can achieve high levels in adjacent brain tissue, which may not be achievable by systemic drug administration. Because the ependyma and pia-arachnoid appear to present little restriction to the movement of molecules between CSF and brain extracellular space, the IT route of administration offers significant therapeutic advantage for molecules too large to pass the BBB, and may avoid systemic toxicity (20,87).

The steep dose–response curve of bifunctional alkylating agents, coupled with their known activity against a variety of pediatric brain tumors, suggest the need for strategies to achieve high levels of these drugs in the CSF. Recent trials have demonstrated that agents such as thiotepa and 4-hydroxyperoxy-cyclophosphamide (4-HC) can be safely administered into the CSF and may produce responses in leptomeningeal neoplasia (3,59).

EVALUATION OF RESPONSE

To evaluate the effectiveness of therapy, parameters must be objective, consistent, and reproducible. The use of computed tomography (CT) has allowed the identification and measurement of tumor size. This is particularly important in phase II studies, where the efficacy of new agents is being evaluated. Magnetic resonance imaging (MRI) has further increased our ability to visualize structural abnormalities in the CNS. The role of PET scanning in the evaluation of CNS lesions has yet to be fully defined. CT scans and MRI are not infallible, as changes after surgery may be associated with spurious findings. Overall evaluation of treatment response can be loosely divided into five areas (a) objective measurable tumor shrinkage followed by radiographic imaging, (b) changes in neurological status, (c) changes in functional status, (d) duration of remission, and (e) overall survival.

PROJECTIONS FOR THE FUTURE

Targeted Drug Delivery

There is a theoretical advantage to giving CTD by direct installation into the carotid artery, thereby increasing the drug concentration delivered to the brain tumor. This is currently being investigated in the treatment of adult brain tumors. Both BCNU and platinum have been infused with encouraging results (95). Liposomes are multicentric lipid vesicles capable of carrying CTD toxins or radionucleotides in a protected environment. They are natural, biodegradable, and have little toxicity. The intact CNS is not one of the preferential sites for entrapment of liposomes. However, pharmacokinetic studies in monkeys and rodents of drugs carried on liposomes have shown drug levels in the brain several-fold higher than after injection of free drugs. Intracranial L1210 leukemic-bearing mice were treated with liposomal MTX and compared with those treated with free MTX and with liposomes alone. Results from liposomal MTX were significantly superior to free drugs in prolonging survival. Thus, liposomes potentially represent a new tool for the neurooncologist (39,76,77).

In 1975, Kohler and Milstein (79) described the hybridoma technique to develop monoclonal antibodies. Monoclonals are exceedingly specific and can be targeted to a single antigen, including tumor antigens or specific cancers. In theory, monoclonals can be used in both diagnosis and therapy. Monoclonals contain few binding sites and so are not suitable to act as a direct carrier for many substances. At present, the plant toxins, abrin and ricin, and diphtheria toxoid have been bound to monoclonals and are being tested for their antitumor effect in animal models. Because monoclonal antibodies have few binding sites, monoclonals cannot be effectively bound directly to CTD but can be bound to liposomes, which in turn can be "packed" with CTD. Monoclonals could act as a "homing device," delivering liposomes filled with an active CTD, toxin or radionucleide, to the target tissue. This would result in a much higher dose of drug delivered to the target area with a resultant greater tumor cell kill. Simultaneously, systemic toxicity would be decreased because less drug would reach normal tissue.

BIOLOGIC RESPONSE MODIFIERS

Both interferon-α (IFN − α) and IFN-β have been reported to inhibit the growth of glioma cell lines (83,101). In addition, histologic studies suggest that IFN-β has a maturation-inducing effect on anaplastic cells. It is generally thought that the antitumor activity of IFN is a result of its antiproliferative effects, but it may also be related to immunomodulation (83). IFN may be a useful adjunct when combined with radiation and chemotherapy in the treatment of brain tumors (100). Yoshida et al. (154) observed four complete responses and one partial response in nine patients with newly diagnosed brain tumors treated with radiotherapy, chemotherapy, and interferon. In addition, several other series (96,100) have shown activity of IFN in recurrent brain tumors. There have been several phase I and phase II studies of adoptive cellular therapy utilizing lymphokine-activated killer (LAK) cells and interleukin-2 (IL-2) in the treatment of refractory brain tumors in adults (104,155,156). Although some clinical responses have been reported, a major limitation of adoptive therapy is the difficulty in identifying, isolating, and expanding cells from an autologous or allogeneic source that will specifically mediate an antitumor response in vivo.

The use of biologic response modifiers in combination with chemotherapy is being evaluated in a number of malignant diseases (78,106). It remains to be determined if they will have a role in the treatment of tumors of the CNS (see Chapters 7 and 8).

The one group of cytokines that appears to play a clearly defined role in aggressive chemotherapy programs is the hematopoietic growth factors. G-CSF is now being included in many intensive chemotherapy protocols. In addition to stimulating the production of neutrophils, it has been reported to enhance neutrophil function (108), and has been shown in a multicenter randomized trial (31) to shorten significantly the incidence, severity, and duration of neutropenia. The use of G-CSF may allow for further dose intensification of chemotherapy protocols both by allowing dose escalation of myelosuppressive agents and decreasing the time interval between treatments. It is hoped that such dose intensification may improve response rates and, ultimately, survival, although these potential benefits are as yet unproven.

GM-CSF results in a dose-dependent rise in the number of neutrophils, monocytes, and eosinophils (91). The use of GM-CSF following bone marrow transplantation has been associated with accelerated engraftment and definite patient benefit (65,93,102,113). Unfortunately, despite intensive investigation, no single factor has so far been identified as the physiologic thrombopoietin, and therefore thrombocytopenia remains a dose-limiting toxicity of many chemotherapeutic agents.

CONCLUSIONS

In summary, the chemotherapy of brain tumors has all the problems inherent in the treatment of any cancer, plus the added dimensions unique to the brain: (a) the inability to remove a tumor completely without serious neurologic residual—hence the problem of remaining tumor volume, (b) the problem of the pharmacological sanctuary, (c) the difficulty in quantifying responses, and (d) the long-term and irreversible toxicities that may result from treatment (see Chapters 22 and 23). Nevertheless, significant response rates have been reported for a number of pediatric brain tumors. Since it does not appear that the near future offers great promise for improving the cure rate of brain tumors with either surgery or radiotherapy alone, the search must continue for identification of new and better agents and the development of more effective delivery mechanisms for these agents.

REFERENCES

1. Adams GE, Cooke MS. Electron-affenic sensitization. I: A structural basis for chemical radiosensitizers in bacteria. *Int J Radiat Biol* 1969;15:457–477.
2. Adams GE, Dewey DL. Hydrated electrons and radiobiological sensitization. *Biochem Biophys Res Commun* 1963;12:473–477.
3. Arndt CAS, Colvin UM, Balis FM, et al. Intrathecal administration of 4-hydroxy-peroxy-cyclophosphamide in rhesus monkeys. *Cancer Res* 1987;47:5832–5934.
4. Barendsen GW, Broerse JJ. Experimental radiotherapy of a rat rhabdomyosarcoma with

15 MeV neutrons and 300 kV x rays. I: Effects of single exposures. *Eur J Cancer* 1969; 5:373–391.
5. Baserga R. The cell cycle. *New Engl J Med* 1981;304(8):453–459.
6. Baumgartner C, Bleker EA, Bucher U, et al. Autologous bone marrow transplantation in the treatment of children and adolescents with advanced malignant tumors. *Med Pediatr Oncol* 1984;12:104–111.
7. Beck WT. The cell biology of multiple drug resistance. *Biochem Pharmacol* 1987;36: 2879–2887.
8. Belt RJ, Patton TF, Himmelstein KJ, Taylor S, Repta A, Sternson LA. Pharmacokinetics of cis-platinum in humans. *Proc AACR* 1980;21:193(abst).
9. Bender RA, Castle MC, Margileth DA, and Oliverio VT. The pharmacokinetics of (^{3}H)-vincristine in man. *Clin Pharmacol Ther* 1977;22:430–438.
10. Benjamin RS, Wiernick PH, Bachur NR. Adriamycin chemotherapy: efficacy, safety and pharmacological basis of an intermittent single high-dose schedule. *Cancer* 1974;33:19–27.
11. Berger DP, Henss H, Winterhalter BR, Fiebig HH. The clonogenic assay with human tumor xenografts: evaluation, predictive value, and application for drug screening. *Ann Oncol* 1990;5:333–341.
12. Bertelsen CA, Sondak VK, Mann BD, Korn EL, Kern DH. Chemosensitivity testing of human solid tumors: a review of 1582 assays with 258 clinical correlations. *Cancer* 1984; 53:1240–1245.
13. Bertino JR. Folate antagonists, antineoplastic and immunosuppressive agents. In: Sartorelli AC, Johns DG, eds. *Handbook of experimental pharmacology*. Vol 38, Part II. New York: Springer-Verlag; 1974:468–483.
14. Bertino JR. Toward improved selectivity in cancer chemotherapy: The Richard and Hinda Rosenthal Foundation Award Lecture. *Cancer Res* 1979;39:293–304.
15. Bleyer WA. The clinical pharmacology of methotrexate: new applications of an old drug. *Cancer* 1978;41:36–51.
16. Bonnadonna G, Valagussa P, Rossi A, et al. CMF adjuvant chemotherapy in operable breast cancer. In: Jones SF, Salmon SE, eds. *Adjuvant therapy in cancer. II*. New York: Grune & Stratton; 1979:227–235.
17. Bourke RS, West CR, Chheda G, Tower DB. Kinetics of entry and distribution of 5-fluorouracil in cerebrospinal fluid and brain following intravenous injection in a primate. *Cancer Res* 1973;33:1735–1746.
18. Brent TP, Butler JAV, Crathorn AR. Variations in phosphokinase activities during the cell cycle in synchronous populations of HeLa cells. *Nature* 1965;207:176–177.
19. Brockman RW. Resistance to therapeutic agents. In: Burchenal JH, Oettgen H, eds. *Cancer achievements, challenges and prospects for the 1980s*. Vol 2. New York: Grune & Stratton; 1981:55–66.
20. Brodie BB, Kurz H, Schanker LS. The importance of dissociation constant and lipid solubility in influencing the passage of drugs into the cerebrospinal fluid. *J Pharmacol Exp Ther* 1960;130:20–25.
21. Brown JM. Electron-affenic agents: development of the optimum radiosensitizer and chemosensitizer for clinical application. In: Tsutomu Sugahara, ed. *Modification of radiosensitivity in cancer treatment*. Tokyo: Academic Press; 1984:139–176.
22. Burgert EO, Glidewell O. Dactinomycin in Wilms' tumor. *JAMA* 1967;199:464–468.
23. Calabresi P, Dexter DL, Heppner GH. Clinical and pharmacological implications of cancer cell differentiation and heterogeneity. *Biochem Pharmacol* 1941;28:1933–1941.
24. Calabresi P, Parks RE Jr. Chemotherapy of neoplastic diseases. In: Gilman A, Goodman LS, Gilman A, eds. *The pharmacological basis of therapeutics*. 6th ed. New York: Macmillan; 1980.
25. Chabner BA, Myers CE, Coleman CN, Johns DG. The clinical pharmacology of antineoplastic agents: first of two parts. *New Engl J Med* 1975;292:1107–1112.
26. Clement JJ, Gorman MS, Wodensky I, Catane R, Johnson RL. Enhancement of antitumor activity of alkylating agents by the radiation sensitizers musoni, dazole. *Cancer Res* 1980;40:4165.
27. Christophidis N, Louis WJ, Lucas I, Moon W, Vajda FJE. Renal clearance of methotrexate in man during high-dose oral and intravenous infusion therapy. *Cancer Chemother Pharmacol* 1981;6:59–64.

28. Clements GB. Selections of biochemically variant, in some cases mutant, mammalian cell in culture. In: Klein G, Weinstrause S, Haddara A, eds. *Advances in cancer research*. Vol 21. New York: Academic Press; 1975:273–290.
29. Cornwell MM, Pastan I, Gottesman HM. Certain calcium channel blockers bind specifically to multidrug-resistant human KB carcinoma membrane vesicles and inhibit drug binding to P-glycoprotein. *J Biol Chem* 1987;262:2166–2170.
30. Costello M, Dominic C, Clerico A. A pilot study of 5 day continuous infusion of high-dose cisplatin and pulsed etoposide in childhood solid tumors. *Am J Pediatr Hematol Oncol* 1988;10:103–108.
31. Crawford J, Ozer H, Stoller R. Reduction by granulocyte colony-stimulating factor of fever and neutropenia induced by chemotherapy in patients with small cell lung cancer. *New Engl J Med* 1991;325:164–170.
32. Creasey WA. Anti-neoplastic and immunosuppressive agents. In: Sartorelli AC, Johns DG, eds. *Handbook of experimental pharmacology*. XXXVII/2. Berlin: Springer-Verlag; 1975:670–694.
33. Crom WR, Evans WE, Pratt CB, et al. Cisplatin disposition in children and adolescents with cancer. *Cancer Chemother Pharmacol* 1981;6:95–99.
34. Crone C. The permeability of brain capillaries to non-electrolytes. *Acta Physiol Scand* 1956;64:417–17.
35. Damon LE, Christensen S, Rochlitz C, Cadman EC. Sequence dependent synergistic cytotoxicity between etoposide and fluoropyrimidines. *Anticancer Res* 1989;9:1761–1768.
36. DeConti RC, Toftness BR, Lange RC, Creasey WA. Clinical and pharmacological studies with cis-diamminedichloroplatinum (II). *Cancer Res* 1973;33:1310–1315.
37. Deutsch M, Reigel D. Myelography and cytology in the treatment of medulloblastoma. *Int J Radiat Oncol Biol Phys* 1981;7:721–725.
38. DeVita VT, Young RC, Canellos GP. Combination versus single agent chemotherapy: a review of the basis for selection of drug treatment of cancer. *Cancer* 1975;35:98–110.
39. Dillipane DP, Woo SY, Rahman A, et al. Enhancement of chemotherapeutic efficacy of methotrexate entrapped in liposomes against murine intracranial L1210 leukemia. Personal communication.
40. D'incalci M, Garattini S. Podophyllotoxin derivatives. In Pinedo HM, Longo DL, Chabner BA, eds. *Cancer chemotherapy and biological response modifiers*. Annual 13. New York: Elsevier; 1992:77–82.
41. Douple EB. Keynote Address. Platinum–radiation interactions. *NCI Monograph* 1988;6: 315–319 (abst).
42. Drewinko B, Gottlieb JA. Action of cis-dichlorodiammineplatinum (II) (NSC-119875) at the cellular level. *Cancer Chemother Rep* 1975;59:665–673.
43. Durand RE, Goldie JH. Interaction of etoposide and cisplatin in an in vitro tumor model. *Cancer Treat Rep* 1987;71:673–679.
44. Dyck PJ, Kiely JM. Differential diagnosis of neuropathy associated with cancer. In: Thompson RA, Green JR, eds. *Advances in neurology: neoplasia in the central nervous system*. Vol 15. New York: Raven Press; 1976:149–161.
45. Ehrlich P. Das sauertoffbedurfnis des organismus. In: *Eine Frbenanalytische Studie*.Berlin: Herschwald; 1885:69.
46. Feun LG, Wallace S, Stewart DJ, et al. Intracarotid infusion of cis-diamminedichloroplatinum in the treatment of recurrent malignant brain tumors. *Cancer* 1984;54:794–799.
47. Fewer D. History and general considerations. In: Fewer D, Wilson CB, Levin VA, eds. *Brain tumor chemotherapy*. Springfield, IL: Charles C Thomas; 1976:3–15.
48. Fewer D. Specific agents in brain tumor chemotherapy. In: Fewer D, Wilson CB, Levin VA, eds. *Brain tumor chemotherapy*. Springfiled, IL: Charles C Thomas; 1976:123–156.
49. Fialkow PJ. Use of glucose-6-phosphate dehydrogenase markers to study human myeloproliferative disorders. In: Neth R, Gallo RC, Hoffschneider P, Mannweiler K, eds. *Modern trends in human leukemia III*. New York: Springer-Verlag; 1979:53.
50. Finlay JL. High dose chemotherapy with bone marrow rescue in children and young adults with malignant brain tumors. *Proc AACR* 1991;32:A1078 (abst).
51. Finlay JL, August C, Packer R, et al. High-dose multi-agent chemotherapy followed by bone marrow "rescue" for malignant astrocytomas of childhood and adolescence. *J Neurooncol* 1991;9(3):239–248.

52. Fisher B, Slack N, Katrych D, et al. Ten-year follow-up results of patients with carcinoma of breast in a cooperative clinical trial evaluating surgical adjuvant chemotherapy. *Surg Gynecol Obstet* 1975;140:528–534.
53. Fojo AT, Whang-Peng J, Gottesman MM, Pastan I. Amplification of DNA sequences in human multi-drug resistant KB carcinoma cells. *Proc Natl Acad Sci USA* 1985;82: 7661–7665.
54. Freeman-Narrod M, Gerstley BJ, Treat C, Engstrom PF, Bornstein R. Variation in the half-life of methotrexate in man. *Proc AACR* 1974;15:49 (abst).
55. Freeman AI, Wang JJ, Sinks LF. High-dose methotrexate in acute lymphocytic leukemia. *Cancer Treat Rep* 1977;61(4):727–731.
56. Frei E III, ed. *Pharmacology of cancer, achievements, challenges and prospects for the 1980s*. New York: Grune & Stratton; 1981:31–122.
57. Frei E, Antiman K, Teicher B, Eder P, Schnipper L. Bone marrow autotransplantation for solid tumors: prospects. *J Clin Oncol* 1989;7:515–526.
58. Freireich E, Gehan E, Rall D, Schmidt L, Skipper H. Quantitative comparison of toxicity of anticancer agents in mouse rat and hamster, dog, monkey and man. *Cancer Chemother Rep* 1966;50:219–245.
59. Friedman HS, Oakes WJ. New therapeutic options in the management of childhood brain tumors. *Oncology* 1992;6(5):27–36.
60. Goldie JH, Coldman AJ. A mathematic model for relating the drug sensitivity of tumors to their spontaneous mutation role. *Cancer Treat Rep* 1979;63:1727–1733.
61. Goldin A, Venditti J, Humphreys S, Mantel N. Modification of treatment schedules in the management of advanced mouse leukemia with amethopterin. *J Natl Cancer Inst* 1956; 17:201–212.
62. Gormley PE, Bull JM, LeRoy AF, Cysyk R. Kinetics of cis-dichlorodiammineplatinum. *Clin Pharmacol Ther* 1979;25:351–357.
63. Hall S, Salem P, Benjamin RS, et al. Continuous intravenous infusion of cis-diamminedichloroplatinum. II: A clinical, toxicologic and pharmacologic study. *Proc AACR* 1978;19: 417 (abst).
64. Hamburger AW, Salmon SE. Primary bioassay of human tumor stem cells. *Science* 1977; 197:561–563.
65. Herrmann F, Schulz G, Wieser M, et al. Effect of granulocyte macrophage colony-stimulating factor on neutropenia and related morbidity induced by myelotoxic chemotherapy. *Am J Med* 1990;88:619–624.
66. Himmelstein KM, Patton TF, Belt RN, Taylor S, Repta AJ, Sternson LA. Clinical kinetics of intact cisplatin and some related species. *Clin Pharmacol Ther* 1981;29:658–664.
67. Huffman DH, Wan SH, Azarnoff DL, Hoogstraten B. Pharmacokinetics of methotrexate. *Clin Pharmacol Ther* 1973;14:572–579.
68. Ishibashi K. Studies on number of cells necessary for transplantation of Yoshida sarcoma. *Gan No Rinsho* 1950;41:1–14.
69. Jacobs C, Kalman SM, Tretton M, Weiner MW. Renal handling of cis-diamminedichloroplatinum (II). *Cancer Treat Rep* 1980;64;1223–1226.
70. Johnson LF, Fuhrman CL, Wiedmemann LM. Regulation of dihydrofolate reductase gene expression in mouse fibroblasts during the transition from the resting to growing state. *J Cell Physiol* 1978;97:397–406.
71. Kahn HE Jr, Kohn KW, Lyles JM. Inhibition of DNA repair by the 1,3-Bis(2-chlorethyl-) 1-nitrosourea breakdown product, 2-chlorethyl isocyanata. *Cancer Res* 1974;34:398–402.
72. Kanazawa H, Rapucchietto D, Kullmen RF. Schedule-dependent therapeutic gain from the combination of fractionated irradiation and cis-diamminedichloroplatinum (II) in C3H/Km mouse model systems. *Cancer Res* 1988;48:3158–3164.
73. Kanno T, Nakazawa T, Kudo T. *Study of bleomycin on brain tumors*. Tokyo: School of Medicine, Keio University. Japan; 1970.
74. Kessel D. Resistance to teniposide and etoposide. In: Kessel D, ed. *Resistance to antineoplastic drugs*. Boca Raton: CRC Press; 1989:207–231.
75. Khan A, McCullough D, Borts F, Sinks LF. Update on use of cis-platinum in CNS malignancies. *Proc ASCO* 1980;21:390 (abst).
76. Kimelberg HK, Atchison MA. Effects of entrapment in liposomes on the distribution, degradation and effectiveness of methotrexate in vivo. *Ann NY Acad Sci* 1978;308: 395–410.

77. Kimelberg HK, Tracy TF, Watson RE, Kung D, Reiss FL, Bourke RS. Distribution of free and liposome-entrapped (3-H) methotrexate in the central nervous system after intracerebroventricular injection in a primate. *Cancer Res* 1978;38:706–712.
78. Kirkwood JM, Ernstoff MS. Interferons in the treatment of human cancer. *J Clin Oncol* 1984;2:336–352.
79. Kohler G, Milstein C. Continuous cultures of fused cells secreting antibody of predefined specificity. *Nature* 1975;256:495–497.
80. Kornblith PL, Walker M. Chemotherapy for malignant gliomas. *J Neurosurg* 1988;68: 1–17.
81. Kovnar EH, Kellie SJ, Horowitz ME, et al. Pre-irradiation cisplatin and etoposide (VP-16) in the treatment of high-risk medulloblastoma and other malignant embryonal tumors of the central nervous system: a phase II study. *J Clin Oncol* 1990;8:330–336.
82. Kozelka J, Chottard JC. How does cisplatin alter DNA structure? A molecular mechanics study on double-stranded oligonucleotides. *Biophys Chem* 1990;35:165–178.
83. Korosue K, Takeshita I, Mannoji H, Fukui M. Interferon effects on multiplication, cytoplasmic protein, and GFAP content, and morphology in human glioma cells. *J Neurooncol* 1983;1:69–76.
84. Larsson A. Ribonucleotide reductase from regenerating rat liver. *Eur J Biochem* 1969;11: 113–121.
85. Laster WR Jr, Mayo JG, Simpson-Herren L, et al. Success and failure in the treatment of solid tumors. II: Kinetic parameters and "cell cure" of moderately advanced carcinoma 755. *Cancer Chemother Rep* 1969;53:169–188.
86. Levin VA. A pharmacoligic basis for brain tumor activity. *Semin Oncol* 1975;2:57–61.
87. Levin VA, Clancy TP, Ausman JI, Raul DP. Uptake and distribution of ^{3}H-methotrexate by the murine ependymoblastoma. *J Natl Cancer Inst* 1972;48:875–883.
88. Levin VA, Freeman-Dove M, Landahl HD. Permeability characteristics of brain adjacent to tumors in rats. *Arch Neurol* 1975;32:785–791.
89. Levin VA, Landahl H, Patlak CS. Considerations in selecting effective brain tumor agents: capillary permeability and sequestered cell populations. *Proc AACR* 1976;17:202 (abst).
90. Li MC, Hertz R, Spencer DB. Effect of methotrexate upon choriocarcinoma and chorioadenoma. *Proc Soc Exp Biol Med* 1956;93:361–366.
91. Lieschke GJ, Maher D, O'Connor M, et al. Phase I study of intravenously administered bacterially synthesized granulocyte-macrophage colony-stimulating factor and comparison with subcutaneous administration. *Cancer Res* 1990;50:606–614.
92. Ling V, ed. Genetic aspects of drug resistance in somatic cells. In: *Fundamentals in cancer chemotherapy, antibiotics and chemotherapy*. Vol 23. Basel: Karger; 1978:191–199.
93. Link H, Boogaerts M, Carella A, et al. Recombinant human granulocyte-macrophage colony stimulating factor (rh-GM-CSF) after autologous bone marrow transplantation for acute lymphoblastic leukemia and non-Hodgkin's lymphoma: a randomized double blind multicenter trial in Europe. *Blood* 1990;76[Suppl 1]:152a (abst).
94. Long DM. Capillary ultrastructure and the blood brain barrier in human malignant brain tumors. *J Neurosurg* 1970;32:127–144.
95. Madiewicz S, West CR, Avellanosa AM, et al. Phase II studies of intra-arterial 1,3-bis (2,chloroethyl-)-1-nitrosourea (BCNU): therapy for metastatic brain tumors. *Proc ASCO* 1980;21:473 (abst).
96. Mahaley M, Urso M, Whaley R, et al. Malignant glioma treatment with interferon. *Proc ASCO* 1984;3:65 (abst).
97. Matsumoto T, Tani E, Kaba K, et al. Amplification and expression of a multidrug resistance gene in human glioma cell lines. *J Neurosurg* 1990;72:96–101.
98. Mealey J, Chen TT, Schanz GP. Effects of dexamethasone and methylprednisolone on cell cultures of human glioblastomas. *J Neurosurg* 1971;34:324–334.
99. Mueller JM, Flaherty MJ. Vincristine-induced quadriparesis. *South Med J* 1978;71: 1310–1311.
100. Nagai M, Arai T, Kohno S, Iizuka E. Current status of interferon therapy in malignant brain tumors. *Gan No Rinsho (Japan)* 1983;29:608–615.
101. Nederman T, Benediktsson G. Effects of interferon on growth rate and radiation sensitivity of cultured human glioma cells. *Acta Radiol Oncol* 1982;21:231–234.
102. Nemunaitis J, Rabinowe SN, Singer JW, et al. Recombinant granulocyte-macrophage colo-

ny-stimulating factor after autologous bone marrow transplantation for lymphoid cancer. *New Engl J Med* 1991;324:1773–1778.
103. Nirenberg A, Mosende C, Mehta BM, Gisolfi A, Rosen G. High-dose methotrexate with citrovorum factor rescue: predictive value of serum methotrexate concentrations and corrective measure to avert toxicity. *Cancer Treat Rep* 1971;61:779–783.
104. Nitta T, Sato K, Yagita H, et al. Preliminary specific targeting therapy against malignant glioma. *Lancet* 1990;335:368–371.
105. Norrell H, Wilson C. Brain tumor chemotherapy with methotrexate given intrathecally. *JAMA* 1967;201:15–17.
106. Ochs J, Brecher ML, Mahoney D, et al. Recombinant interferon-alpha given before and in combination with standard chemotherapy in children with acute lymphoblastic leukemia in first marrow relapse: a Pediatric Oncology Group pilot study. *J Clin Oncol* 1991;9(5): 777–782.
107. Oldendorf WH, Davson H. Brain extracellular space and the sink action of cerebrospinal fluid. *Arch Neurol* 1967;17:196–205.
108. Ohsaka A, Kitagawa S, Sakamoto S, et al. In vivo activation of human neutrophil functions by administration of recombinant human granulocyte colony-stimulating factor in patients with malignant lymphoma. *Blood* 1989;74:2743–2748.
109. Ozols RF, Masudo H, Hamilton TC. Mechanisms of cross-resistance between radiation and antineoplastic drugs. *Natl Cancer Inst Monogr* 1988;6:159–165.
110. Pastan I, Gottesman M. Multiple-drug resistance in human cancer. *New Engl J Med* 1987; 316:1388–1393.
111. Pendergrass TW, Milstein JM, Geyer JR, et al. Eight drugs in one day chemotherapy for brain tumors: experience in 107 children and rationale for pre-radiation chemotherapy. *J Clin Oncol* 1987;5:1221–1231.
112. Phillips PC. Antineoplastic drug resistance in brain tumors. In: Cohen ME, Duffner PK, eds. *Neurologic clinics: brain tumors in children*. Philadelphia: WB Saunders; 1991: 383–404.
113. Powles R, Smith C, Milan S, et al. Human recombinant GM-CSF in allogenic bone-marrow transplantation for leukaemia: double-blind placebo-controlled trial. *Lancet* 1990;336: 1417–1420.
114. Prestayko AW, Luft FC, Einhorn L, Crooke ST. Cisplatin pharmacokinetics in a patient with renal dysfunction. *Med Pediatr Oncol* 1978;5:183–188.
115. Pui C-H, Behm FG, Raimondi SC, et al. Secondary acute myeloid leukemia in children treated for acute lymphoid leukemia. *New Engl J Med* 1989;321:136–142.
116. Rall DP, Zubrod CG. Mechanism of drug absorption and excretion passage of drugs in and out of the central nervous system. *Ann Rev Pharmacol* 1962;2:109–128.
117. Ratain MJ, Kaminer LS, Bitran JD, et al. Acute nonlymphocytic leukemia following etoposide and cisplatin combination chemotherapy for advanced non-small-cell carcinoma of the lung. *Blood* 1987;70:1412–1417.
118. Reiselbach RE, DiChiro G, Freireich EJ, Rall DP. Subarachnoid distribution of drugs after lumbar injection. *New Engl J Med* 1962;267:1273–1278.
119. Roninson IB, Abelson HT, Housinan DE, Howell N, Varshavsky A. Amplification of specific DNA sequences correlates with multi-drug resistance in Chinese hamster cells. *Nature* 1984;309:626–628.
120. Russo A, DeGraff W, Friedman N, Mitchell J. Selective modulation of glutathione levels in human normal versus tumor cells and subsequent differential response to chemotherapy drugs. *Cancer* 1986;46:2845–2848.
121. Salem P, Khalyl M, Jabbouy K, Hashim L. Cis-diamminedichloroplatinum (II) by 5-day continuous infusion. *Cancer* 1984;43:837–840.
122. Santoro A, Bonnadonna G, Bonfont U, Valagussa P. Alternating drug combinations in the treatment of advanced Hodgkin's disease. *New Engl J Med* 1982;306:770–775.
123. Schabel FM Jr. The use of tumor growth kinetics in planning "curative" chemotherapy of advanced solid tumors. *Cancer Res* 1969;29:2384–2389.
124. Schabel FM Jr. Concept and practice of total tumor cell kill. In: Clark RL, Cumley RW, McCay JE, Copeland MM, eds. *Oncology 1970. Proceedings of the Tenth International Cancer Congress. Vol 2. Experimental cancer therapy*. Chicago: Yearbook Medical Publishers; 1970:35–45.

125. Schabel FM Jr. Concepts for systemic treatment of micrometastases. *Cancer* 1975;35: 15–24.
126. Schreiner GE, Maher JF. Toxic nephropathy. *Am J Med* 1965;38:409–449.
127. Seeber S, Osieka R, Schmidt CG, Achterrah SW, Crooke ST. In vivo resistance towards anthracyclines, etoposide, and cis-diamminedichloroplatinum (II). *Cancer Res* 1982;42: 4719.
128. Shapiro WR, Young DF, Mehta BM. Methotrexate: distribution in cerebrospinal fluid after intravenous, ventricular and lumbar injections. *New Engl J Med* 1975;293:161–166.
129. Shepro DS, Sullivan R. Clinical use of recombinant hematopoietic colony-stimulating factors. In: Stollerman GH, ed. *Advances in internal medicine*. St Louis: Mosby–Year Book; 1991:329–362.
130. Sherbert GV, Lakshmi MS, Haddah SK. Does dexamethasone inhibit the growth of human gliomas? *J Neurosurg* 1977;47:864–870.
131. Silver RT, Young RC, Holland JF. Some new aspects of modern cancer chemotherapy. *Am J Med* 1977;63:772–878.
132. Siminovitch L. On the nature of heritable variation in cultured somatic cells. *Cell* 1976; 7:1–11.
133. Skipper HE. Concurrent comparisons of some 2-,3-, and 4-drug combinations delivered simultaneously and sequentially (1210 and P388 leukemia systems). In: *Cancer chemotherapy*. Vol 9. Ann Arbor: University Microfilms International; 1980.
134. Skipper HE. Reasons for success and failure in treatment of murine leukemias with the drugs now employed in treating human leukemias. In: *Cancer chemotherapy*. Vol 1. Ann Arbor: University Microfilms International; 1978.
135. Skipper HE, Schabel FM Jr. Quantitative and cytokinetic studies in experimental tumor models. In: Holland J, Frei E III, eds. *Cancer medicine*. Philadelphia: Lea & Febiger; 1973:629–650.
136. Skipper HE, Schabel FM Jr, Wilconx WS. Experimental evaluation of potential anticancer agents. XII: On the criteria and kinetics associated with "curability" of experimental leukemia. *Cancer Chemother* 1964;35:3–111.
137. Spadari S, Weissbach A. The interrelation between DNA synthesis and various DNA polymerase activities in synchronized HeLa cells. *J Molec Biol* 1974;86:11–20.
138. Stoller RG, Drake JC, Jacobs SA. Monitoring high dose methotrexate: value of serum creatinine and plasma methotrexate. *Proc ASCO* 1976;17:255 (abst).
139. Stoller RG, Hande KR, Jacobs SA, Rosenberg SA, Chabner BA. Use of plasma pharmacokinetics to predict and prevent methotrexate toxicity. *New Engl J Med* 1977;297:630–634.
140. Stratford IJ. Mechanism of hypoxic radiosensitization and the development of new sensitizers. *Int J Radiat Oncol Biol Phys* 1982;8:391–398.
141. Takeuchi K. Effects of bleomycin on brain tumors. Presented at the 31st Meeting of Kano District of Japan Neurologic Society. November 29, 1969.
142. Tanabe M, Godat D, Kallmen RF. Effects of fractionated schedules of irradiation combined with cis-diamminedichloroplatinum II on the SCCVII/ST tumor and normal tissues of the C3H/KM mouse. *Int J Radiat Oncol Biol Phys* 1987;13:1523–1532.
143. Tannock IF. The relation between cell proliferation and the vascular system in a transplanted mouse mammary tumor. *Br J Cancer* 1968;22:258–273.
144. Teshler MD, Nolta AJ, Raffel C. Multiple drug resistance gene (MDR-1) expression in childhood PNET. *Pediatr Neurosci* 1990;15:143 (abst).
145. Tsuuruo T. Circumvention of drug resistance with calcium channel blockers and monoclonal antibodies. In: Ozols RF, ed. *Drug resistance in cancer therapy*. Boston: Kluwer Academic Publishers; 1989:73–95.
146. Valeriote F, Vietti T. Cellular kinetics and conceptual basis of chemotherapy. In: Sutow W, Vietti T, Feinbach D, eds. *Clinical pediatric oncology*. New York: CV Mosby; 1977: 182–186.
147. Vietti TJ, Valeriote FA. Conceptual basis for use of chemotherapeutic agents and their pharmacology. *Pediatr Clin North Am* 1976;23(1):67–92.
148. Vokes E, Weichelsbaum RR. Concomitant chemoradiotherapy: rationale and clinical experience in patients with solid tumors. *J Clin Oncol* 1990;8:911–934.
149. Walker R, Allen J. Carboplatinum in the treatment of recurrent childhood brain tumors. *J Clin Oncol* 1988;6:62–67.

150. Whiteside JA, Phillips FS, Dargeon HW, Burchenal JH. Intrathecal amethopterin in neurologic manifestations of leukemia. *Arch Intern Med* 1958;101:279–285.
151. Wilbrandt W, Rosenberg T. The concept of carrier transport and its corollaries in pharmacology. *Pharmacol Rev* 1961;13:109–183.
152. Wilson CB, Norell HA. Brain tumor chemotherapy with intrathecal methotrexate. *Cancer* 1969;23:1038–1045.
153. Wolff JA, Krivit W, Newton WA Jr, D'Angio GJ. Single versus multiple dose dactinomycin therapy of Wilms'tumor. *New Engl J Med* 1968;279:290–294.
154. Yoshida J, Wakabayashi T, Kato K, et al. Combination therapy with interferon P, ACNV, and radiation, in malignant brain tumors. *Gan To Kagakeur Ryoho* (*Japan*) 1986;13: 520–524.
155. Yoshida S, Tanaka R, Takai N, Ono K. Local administration of autologous lymphokin-activated killer cells and recombinant interleukin-2 to patients with malignant brain tumors. *Cancer Res* 1988;48:5011–5016.
156. Yoshida S, Tanaka R, Takai N, Ono K. Adoptive immunotherapy with LAK cells and interleukin-2 in the treatment of recurrent malignant gliomas. *Curr Ther Res* 1990;47: 654–664.
157. Zager RF, Frisby SA, Oliverio VT. Cellular transport and antitumor activity of methotrexate (MTX) in combination with clinically useful drugs. *Proc AACR* 1972;13:33 (abst).
158. Zaharko DS, Dedrick RL, Peale AL, Drake JC, Lutz RJ. Relative toxicity of methotrexate in several tissues of mice bearing Lewis lung carcinoma. *J Pharmacol Exp Ther* 1974;189: 585–592.
159. Zubrod CG. Development of anti-cancer therapy. In: Burchenal JH, Oettgen H, eds. *Cancer achievements, challenges and prospects for the 80s*. Vol 2. New York: Grune & Stratton; 1981:1–10.
160. Zubrod CG. Historic milestones in curative chemotherapy. *Semin Oncol* 1979;6:490–505.
161. Zubrod CG. Present status of cancer chemotherapy (mini-review). *Life Sci* 1974;14: 809–818.
162. Zubrod CG. Selective toxicity of anticancer drugs. Presidential Address. *Cancer Res* 1978; 38:4377–4384.

7

Advances in Molecular Genetic Treatment of Cancer

Steven J. Greenberg

The striking and unprecedented array of achievements in molecular biological research over the last decade has ushered in an exciting new era of human gene therapeutics. The strategies involved in therapeutic genetic manipulation reflect as much ingenuity as they do diversity. Conceptually, however, the approaches thus far employed fall into two general categories. Reconstitution of defective genes or supplementation of certain gene products in order to enhance a desired biological response has been achieved by the process of gene transfer technology (17,36,38,44,53,74). On the other hand, downmodulation or inhibition of unwanted gene product expression has been accomplished by antisense technology. Although these distinctions are useful for the purpose of introducing background information and basic concepts, the strategies employed in these two research fields are commingled, producing a hybrid technology.

One area that promises to benefit significantly from the advent of gene transfer and antisense technologies is cancer treatment. Indeed, the early pioneering studies that have advanced from benchtop to bedside have focused on the quest to augment cancer killing properties through supplemental induction of bioactive cytokines and by neutralization of oncogene transcripts by gene transfer and antisense therapies, respectively. For more thorough treatment of molecular biological and molecular genetic techniques, the interested reader is referred to excellent texts and manuals on these subjects (1,41,64,71). This chapter will review the emergence and application of these areas of human gene therapeutics, with special emphasis on cancer treatment.

GENE TRANSFER THERAPY

In the past several years, a gene transfer technology has emerged that is vastly superior to previous techniques because of its ability to transfer DNA

Brain Tumors in Children: Principles of Diagnosis and Treatment, 2/e, edited by M.E. Cohen and P.K. Duffner, Raven Press, Ltd., New York, 1994.

into eukaryotic hematopoietic cells. Previously, molecular biologists were able to incorporate small bits of genetic information by one of three standard procedures: transfection, transformation, and infection. The transfer of naked DNA into a cell, termed *transfection*, may be accomplished by a variety of techniques, including calcium phosphate or DEAE Dextran precipitation, electroporation, or microscopic injection of DNA directly into a cell, such as an oocyst. Alternatively, the genetic information encoded by a single gene first may be engineered into a vector. *Vectors* are autonomously replicating DNA units into which DNA fragments are inserted for gene cloning and, depending on the size of the DNA fragment to be inserted, may be a plasmid, lambda phage, or cosmid. Genes taken up by these vectors are multiplied or cloned as the vector replicates. Transfer of plasmid DNA into bacteria for the purposes of cloning is a process called *transformation*. Other physical methods that have been devised to transfer a functional gene into a cell include protoplast fusion, liposomal transfer, and receptor-mediated delivery. Finally, the transfer of genetic information, as may occur between a structurally competent infectious particle and a host cellular genome, is called *infection*. Efficient gene transfer therapy is accomplished by gene-incorporation into a molecularly engineered *expression* vector that preferentially results in expression of the inserted gene and, subsequently, the gene–vector construct is assembled into a vehicle, usually a highly infectious viral particle, which efficiently transports the genetic information into a eukaryotic cell.

The proper expression of a gene transferred into a cell is regulated by multiple, spatially related genetic sequences found upstream and downstream from the gene of interest. These genetic modulators are termed *cis*-acting DNA elements. Thus, each gene is accompanied by promoter and enhancer sequences, splice signals, polyadenyation signals, and elements that determine the messenger RNA half life. Normally these elements exert their influence in concert in a manner specific to cell type, orchestrating regional and temporal gene expression throughout the organism. These elements may be manipulated experimentally to cause the induction and expression of a particular gene inserted within a given recombinant construct. Such systems of recombinant elements are called *expression vectors*, and the most widely used systems for the purpose of gene transfer are the retroviral-mediated expression vectors and recombinant retroviruses (reviewed in 22,44,52,54,55,56,59,66).

Retroviral vectors provide a highly efficient method for gene transfer into eukaryotic cells. These features include stable provirus integration into the host chromosome of the infected cell (normally not achieved by double-stranded DNA viruses), a defined and predictable proviral structure, a wide infectivity and expression host range, a flexible genome capacity, higher levels of constitutive or inducible gene expression (compared to transfection techniques), and the ability to produce high-titer infectious recombinant retrovirus that permits the stable transformation of an entire population of cells.

Retroviral-mediated gene transfer is divided into two components. The first is the retroviral vector itself, which does not encode viral proteins but is constructed with unique cloning sites for insertion of complementary DNA (cDNA). The extreme efficiency by which the retroviral vector promotes insertion of genetic material into the host genome is remarkable. Comparable DNA material lacking the retroviral insertion sequences is vastly inferior in its ability to incorporate into the chromosome. The inserted cDNA is the gene of interest to be expressed that is driven either by the retroviral long terminal repeat (LTR) promoter, or by other promoters of eukaryotic gene expression, such as the immediate early promoter of human cytomegalovirus, or the simian virus early promoter. These vectors can carry, in addition, the neomycin phosphotransferase (neo) gene expressed from an alternate promoter and useful as a selectable marker (Fig. 7-1). By replacing the viral genes with the gene of interest and retaining the efficient viral integration process, DNA is both inserted and expressed in the host cellular genome.

What is thereby created is a replication-defective retrovirus missing its own genes that encode for the viral proteins, such as the core proteins, polymerase/reverse transcriptase, and envelope glycoprotein. However, these *trans* genes, which were removed, can be supplied by another virus, a *defective* virus that contains the trans functions missing in the vector. Thus, the second component of this system is a retrovirus packaging cell line that provides the viral proteins necessary for vector transfer (Fig. 7-1). This mechanism for obtaining viability by combining the activities of two defective components is called *complementation*. By this series of manipulations the retroviral vector carrying the gene of interest is assembled into a virion, and the recombinant virions are harvested from the packaging cell line and then used to infect the target cells. Through the cis functions retained in the vector, the foreign gene is transferred into a chromosome of the cell and expressed as if it were a viral gene.

The first human genetic engineering experiment was performed in 1989 by a group of medical scientists at the National Institutes of Health (28). This epochal event was not an attempt at therapy, but rather focused on a gene marking experiment. In order to track and study the fate of tumor infiltrating lymphocytes (TIL) (62) in patients with advanced malignant melanoma, a marker gene (the neomycin resistance gene Neo obtained from the bacterium *Escherichia coli*) was inserted into a retroviral expression vector and transferred into TIL extracted from patients. The marked cells were grown with unmarked cells, harvested, and infused back into the patient. The initial five patients receiving the genetically engineered Neo marker in this manner have established the safety of human gene transfer methodology and validated the feasibility of recovering viable genetically rearranged cells with the trans-

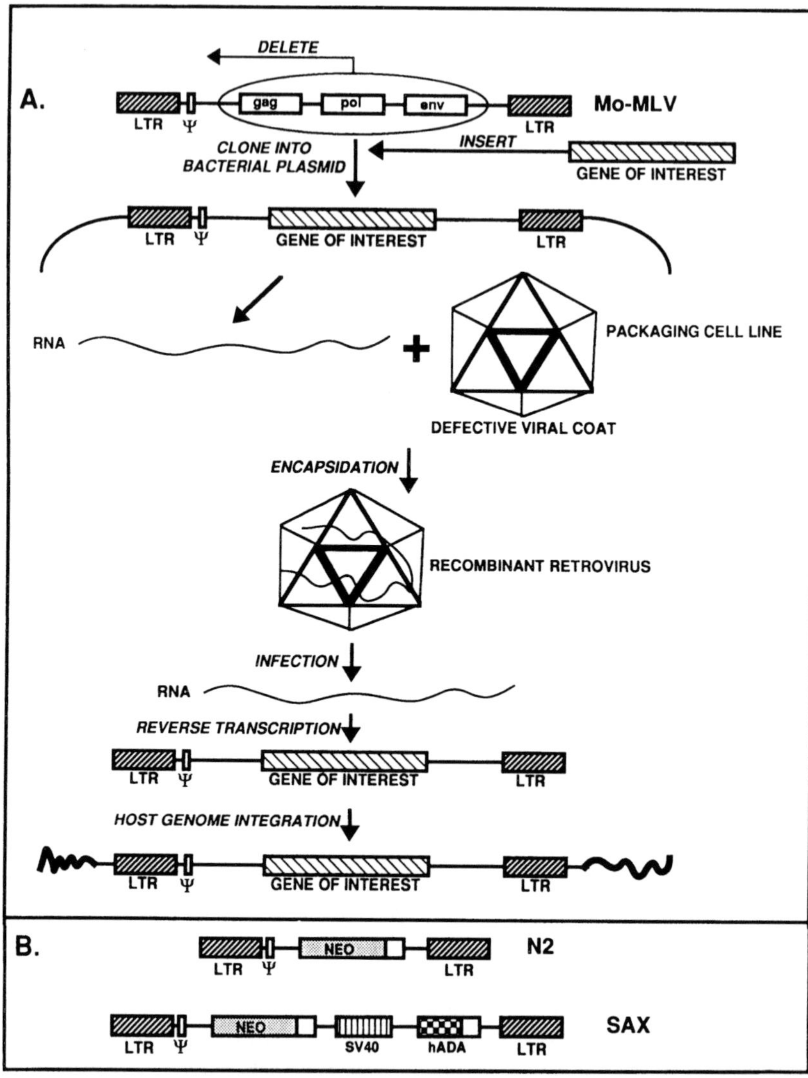

FIG. 7-1. Construction of retroviral vectors and gene transfer. **A,** In the schematic representation of the prototype Moloney-murine leukemia virus (Mo-MLV), viral trans functions (i.e., genes that encode for core protein, polymerase, and envelope glycoprotein) are removed and replaced by a cDNA encoding a gene of interest. Ψ, the encapsidation signal required for virus packaging, and the LTR (long terminal repeat), necessary for proviral integration and RNA transcription, are retained. The retroviral expression vector is cloned into *E. coli* and the DNA then transfected into a packaging cell line. By complementation, recombinant vector-containing viral particles are produced. Eukaryotic cells subsequently infected by virus stably incorporate vector provirus and then express the inserted gene. **B,** Schematic representation of the N2 expression vector carrying the neomycin-resistance gene, and SAX, carrying, in addition, the human adenosine deaminase gene under its separate SV40/early promoter.

ferred gene intact, both in the bloodstream and from tumor in which TIL have a propensity to migrate (62).

Gene marking protocols are now also underway for the study of adult chronic myelogenous leukemia (33), acute lymphocytic leukemia (31), and childhood acute myelogenous leukemia (32). In the course of autologous bone marrow transplantation for treatment of these diseases, cells in the marrow are gene-marked. These molecularly engineered markers are used to discriminate between relapse that arises from systemic disease remaining after preparative therapy and relapse due to residual cells in the marrow. The source of relapse is of fundamental clinical importance, since the results dictate whether future therapy will include either more aggressive marrow purging or more strenuous systemic ablation techniques.

In contrast to gene marking, the first gene therapy experiments were designed to reconstitute the function of the immune system by the administration of autologous lymphocytes transduced with a normal human adenosine deaminese (ADA) gene that provided the enzymatic activity lacking in patients with ADA-deficient severe combined immunodeficiency (SCID)(29). According to this protocol, patients' mature mononuclear cells are first isolated from whole blood and expanded in vitro by stimulation with OKT3 antibody and interleukin-2. During the growth phase, T cells are cocultured with the retroviral vector (Fig. 7-1) containing the human ADA gene and the Neo marker gene. After a few days in culture the cells are infused into the patient, and the process can be repeated monthly. Two young ADA-deficient SCID patients have thus far received enzyme-corrective gene therapy and have shown clinical improvement, no significant adverse side effects, and a steady increase in ADA level approaching nearly 25% of normal levels after repeated infusions (14). These early successes have already fostered second-generation ADA replacement gene therapies designed to transduce progenitor-enriched bone marrow cells and thereby, it is hoped, to expand the corrected T-cell repertoire and prolong expression of the functional gene indefinitely. The prospects of gene therapy have attracted the attention of the international scientific medical community, and gene therapy protocols for ADA deficiency have recently been adopted and implemented in Italy and the Netherlands (6,69).

Human cancer gene therapy was inaugurated in 1991 as an extension of the Neo gene marker experiments with TIL (30). However, the goal in these experiments was to enhance the killing capabilities of TIL against cancer (in this case malignant melanoma) by adding the human gene for tumor necrosis factor (TNF) to the retroviral expression vector. TNF possesses potent anticancer effects. In humans, toxic levels are reached at 8 μg/kg of body weight (4). By the gene transfer strategy, reconstituted TIL would migrate to the cancer and secrete into the microenvironment constitutively expressed TNF. Delivered in this manner, effective high doses of TNF would be provided at specific tumor sites and systemic side effects would be avoided. It is unclear if TIL hone to the central nervous system, and a cellular delivery system for TNF to tumors of the brain awaits development. Since TIL are also sequestered in liver, spleen, and lung, there was, however, the potential for TNF-induced toxicity in these organs, independent of tumor burden. An early review of a number of patients currently under treatment suggest that there have been no side effects from the gene transfer therapy or TNF-related organ toxicity (3). This is a phase I trial, and further studies are necessary to assess whether this procedure is effective as a cancer therapy.

A variation in this form of cancer gene transfer therapy targets the cancer cells as recipients of molecularly engineered cytokine genes. This approach is based on the premise that the elaboration of certain cytokines boost the host's T-lymphocyte antitumor immune-mediated response (47). Accordingly, the TNF gene has been inserted into patients' tumor cells that were first surgically extracted and cultured in vitro. Thereafter, the transduced, TNF-secreting tumor cells were used as a cell vaccine and transferred back into the patient's thigh by subcutaneous and intradermal injections (34). Three weeks following autologous tumor vaccination, the injection sites and draining lymph nodes are surgically excised, and the putative tumor-reactive T-cells recruited in this manner are expanded in vitro and ultimately reinfused into the patient. Alternatively, to improve TIL immunotherapy, the interleukin-2 (IL-2, formerly T-cell growth factor) gene was inserted into tumor cells that were isolated from a patient, grown in culture, and transplanted back to the patient (35). It is proposed that the antitumor cell mediated response will be augmented by the secretion of IL-2 by tumor. Subsequently, the immunoreactive cells derived from tumor and draining lymph nodes are expanded and reinfused into the patient. These early studies on the immunization of cancer patients using autologous cancer cells modified by insertion of various cytokine genes are an exciting overture to a full score of molecular genetic protocols to enhance the body's intrinsic cancer-fighting mechanisms.

ANTISENSE THERAPY

Several major developments in molecular biology have made the selective inhibition of gene expression feasible. It is now recognized that single-stranded oligo RNA and DNA sequences can act as specific inhibitors of gene expression. Simply stated, an antisense nucleic acid sequence is one that interacts with a complementary nucleic acid sequence to block a biological effect mediated by the target sequence (reviewed in 5,23,26,45,57,67).

Technologically, the application of antisense as modulators of gene expression has evolved along two divergent pathways. In the transcript-targeted approach, an antisense oligomer with nucleotide sequences complementary to the protein coding or *sense* sequence is employed and results in arrest of translation. Theoretically, inhibition of one copy of mRNA should be more efficient than inhibiting a protein product, since a single mRNA molecule engenders multiple peptide copies. Early experiments using natural, i.e., phosphodiester-linked, antisense oligoribo-and oligodeoxiribonucleotides indicated that relatively short oligonucleotides were effective in inhibiting gene expression (remember that a 15-base oligonucleotide should impart uniqueness within the human genome of approximately 3×10^9 base pairs). Unfortunately, native oligonucleotides display short half lives in serum and media and intracellularly due to nuclease activity. Further, due to the charged phosphate backbone, native oligomers are poorly permeable into cells. Several classes of phosphate-modified oligonucleotides have been synthesized, including oligo-alkylphosphotriesters, oligomethylphosphonates, and oligophosphorothioates, that are nuclease resistant and thus more resilient and that enhance permeability into cells.

A second approach in antisense technology has been to target sequence-specific sites in double-stranded genomic DNA by triple-helix formation. Triplex DNA is permitted to form at corresponding homopyrimidine–homopurine tracts in which a third-strand homopyrimidine oligodeoxyribonucleotide binds. The additional pyrimidine strand is bound by Hoogsteen hydrogen bonds in the major grove to the complementary purine strand in the Watson-Crick duplex. Triple helix formation may effectively suppress DNA replication at this site, inhibit transcription, or by occupying a binding site, prevent recognition of a nuclear transcription factor. The antisense function of both RNA- and DNA-targeting analogues can be enhanced by the incorporation of ribozyme sequences capable of producing chain scission and intercalating, cross-linking, or metal chelating agents.

Antisense may function via a number of mechanisms that include inhibition of DNA replication and transcription, interference with pre-mRNA processing, impedance to RNA nuclear membrane transport, decreased cytoplasmic RNA stability, and interruption of translation. Although the field of antisense molecular biology is in its infancy, the challenge of introducing simple antisense molecules into complex cellular systems and eliciting specific responses is compelling. Already antisense technology has been applied to specifically down-regulate oncogene expression and is actively being used as a modality for the inhibition of retroviral replication.

The transfer and processing of external stimuli via cytoplasmic messengers to influence nuclear events are fundamental to the physiologic responses of growth and proliferation. Protooncogenes are cellular genes normally found in the genome and are thought to encode proteins that are involved in the cascade of events by which growth factors stimulate normal cell division (reviewed in 9). Protooncogene expression can be subverted by gene amplification, chromosomal translocation or deletion, or point mutation; and, not unexpectedly, when altered, protooncogenes may contribute to the induction or progression of cancer. Dominant, mutated forms of these endogenous genes are called oncogenes and were originally ascribed to retrovirally encoded tumor producing genes. They encode proteins with diverse functions, including growth factors (e.g., *v-sis*), growth factor receptors (e.g., *v-fms, v-erb B, V-kit*), transducers of growth factor responses (e.g., *v-src, v-ras*, and *v-raf*), and nuclear transcription factors, (e.g., *v-jun* and *v-fos*). In a reciprocal fashion, oncogenesis may be facilitated by recessive mutation of genes termed *antioncogenes*, or *tumor suppression genes*, also normal components of the genome, that serve to attenuate protooncogene functions. The activation of dominant oncogenes and the inactivation of tumor suppressor genes are genetic events that form central tenets in our understanding of the molecular basis of cancer.

The prediction that the activities of these genes that promote and control cellular growth patterns would correlate with cancer activity has been confirmed in breast and ovarian cancer by amplification of *erb-B2* (7), in neuroblastoma by *N-myc* amplification (8), and by mutations in *ras* in adenocarcinoma of the lung (65). Consequently, oncogenes and tumor suppressor genes have become the targets, figuratively and literally, for antisense-directed gene therapy.

Indeed, a number of provocative studies now attest to the validity of the use of antisense oligonucleotides to down-modulate oncogene-regulated growth. For example, antisense oligomers to *c-myc* inhibit cell differentiation (18,24) and have an antiproliferative effect when cocultured with human Burkitt lymphoma cell lines (48) and leukemic cell lines (25,73) or murine erythroleukemia cells (61); similarly, antisense to *N-myc* inhibits growth of neuroectodermal cell lines (72). The protooncogene *c-myb* is believed to encode a nuclear protein involved in hematopoietic differentiation and proliferation. A *c-myb* antisense oligodeoxynucleotide has been shown to inhibit normal human hematopoiesis *in vitro* (20), to block peripheral blood mononuclear cell response to mitogen or antigen stimulation (21), and to effectively inhibit proliferation of a colonic adenocarcinoma cell line (49). Antisense oligomers to *c-raf* and related receptor protein kinases in *ras*-transformed cells has been shown to suppress the tumorigenic phenotype in some systems (2,12,37,40) but not in others (63). Targeting the nuclear transcription factor *c-fos* by antisense analogues has been used to analyze cell transformation (51) and differentiation of embryonal carcinoma cells (16,39). Antisense to the *bcr-abl* translocation in chronic myeloid leukemia blast cells causes a selective antiproliferative effect (68), and antisense to the oncogene growth factor *v-sis* is capable of reversing in vitro cell transformation (10). By contrast, by reversal of antioncogenic effects, the tumor-suppressing properties of other genes may be confirmed using antisense technology. Thus, an antisense oligomer constructed to target a putative metastasis-suppressor gene, such as E-cadherin, results in a more malignant invasive tumor cell type (70). The mounting evidence that in vitro reversion of malignant morphology can be achieved by antisense targeting of specific oncogene sequences leaves little doubt as to the validity of future experiments whereby antisequences will be loaded into expression vector cassettes for the purpose of modulating oncogene expression in cancer.

Another cancer-related gene target within the sights of the antisense molecular scientist involves the phenomenon of multiple drug resistance (11,58). The overproduction of certain proteins that confers drug-resistance to multiple cytotoxic drugs may severely hinder attempts to develop effective chemotherapeutic protocols within the limitations of toxic side effects (19). Just as it is possible now to confer methotrexate resistance to stem cells by genetic transfer of the dihydrofolate reductase gene (13), it is reasonable to assume it may be feasible to circumvent unwanted multiple drug resistance in cancer cells by the antisense down-modulation of the MDRI gene.

In contradistinction to the promotion of oncogenesis and transformation by the subversion of normal physiology due to oncogene expression, the induction and expression of other genes results in suppression of a malignant phenotype. The prototype genes with tumor-suppressor properties are the retinoblastoma and p53 alleles, although an increasing number of other anti-oncogenes or tumor-suppressor genes are being uncovered. The replacement of defective suppressor genes would be an intriguing form of cancer therapy that could be achieved by gene transfer therapy.

For example, the retinoblastoma tumor suppressor gene transfected into retinoblastoma, prostate carcinoma, or osteosarcoma cells that display inactive suppressor gene function causes reversal of the neoplastic nature of the cells both in vitro and in vivo (27). The wild type p53 gene has also been shown to induce cell differentiation and inhibit proliferation. Transferred into a variety of cancer cell lines that lack normal p53 expression, including colorectal, breast, and ovarian carcinoma, osteosarcoma, and glioblastoma, p53 causes suppression of proliferation (50). The demonstration that replacement of lost or defective tumor-suppressor genes can limit tumor formation and invasiveness and promote differentiation is an encouraging development in the field of genetic research that will form the foundation of future molecular strategies to treat cancer.

EXOGENOUS VIRAL AND VIRAL GENE THERAPY

One of the fundamental principles distinguishing neoplasia from normal tissue is the sustained and unregulated growth of cancer cells. This essential feature forms the basis of new molecular genetic cancer therapies in which the cancer cell is selectively targeted by virtue of its proliferating phenotype.

The contrast between a dividing tumor cell population and normal somatic cells is perhaps greatest with regard to gliomas versus the surrounding nervous system tissue composed of neurons and glia. Certain herpes simplex viral mutants are able to replicate in dividing cells only, yet they retain herpetic-induced cytopathic effects. This bias in viral replication was used selectively to kill human gliomas inoculated into nude mice (46). Thymidine kinase deficient herpes simplex viral mutants injected directly into gliomas significantly reduced tumor growth and prolonged survival in mice harboring systemic and intracerebral tumors. In these early studies, the potential for coincident killing of normal dividing cells was not realized, although some evidence of encephalitis with scattered foci of lymphocytic infiltration in the meninges and brain was noted. Nonetheless, it appears that genetically altered viruses are worthy of further exploration for use in tumor therapy, especially with regard to certain tumors of the central nervous system.

The ineffectiveness of some viruses to infect and replicate in nondividing cells also extends to a basic disadvantage in using retroviral vectors. The retroviral-mediated gene transfer systems that are currently in use stably integrate their genes in eukaryotic cells actively dividing, with very limited success for gene integration in quiescent cells. Again, retroviral gene transfer would tend to target delivery into dividing tumor cells and spare nondividing tissue. In an elegantly devised set of experiments (15), the herpes simplex thymidine kinase gene (the converse of the experiment above) was inserted into a retroviral expression vector, and the kinase gene was subsequently transduced in murine fibroblasts. Mice were inoculated with a mixture of fibrosarcoma cells and cells transduced with murine fibroblasts expressing herpes simplex thymidine kinase. Subsequently, mice were treated with the antiherpes drug ganciclovir. Cells modified to contain the herpes simplex thymidine kinase gene become sensitive to treatment with the antiviral agent ganciclovir. Tumors produced from a mixture of tumor cells and herpes simplex thymidine kinase retroviral vector-producing fibroblasts regressed rapidly and completely with ganciclovir treatment. In subsequent experiments, it was shown that rats carrying intracerebral gliomas, subsequently injected intratumorally with the thymidine kinase retroviral vector-producing murine fibroblasts, and thereafter treated with ganciclovir, responded with complete macroscopic and microscopic tumor regression in 11 of 14 animals treated.

The use of genetically modified viruses and retroviral-mediated viral gene transfer in these studies is striking in terms of the relative effectiveness of the therapies and the lack of overt undesirable effects in cancers with an otherwise universally fatal outcome. These approaches will form the framework of future molecular genetic approaches to the treatment of brain tumors in humans by exogenous viral and viral gene therapy.

SUMMARY

Future historians may view the decade preceding the next century as prologue to a new chapter in applied molecular biology wherein our greater understanding of the basic mechanisms that control and regulate genetic expression has led to the development of an array of new weaponry with which to battle cancer. The armamentarium will include improved genetic transfer vehicles to convey an assortment of genes to the tumor site and to augment the immune system's inherent cancer-fighting ability. In addition, neoplastic tissue will be transduced to express histocompatibility and chemoattractant genes, leading to exposure and enhanced recognition of the cancer cells by the host defense system. Subverted oncogene expression will be suppressed by loading cassettes of antisense sequences into retroviral-mediated expression vectors that, in turn, are packaged into recombinant retroviruses for delivery into the host. Cells with mutated or lost tumor suppressor genes will be supplemented via gene transfer therapy with functional antioncogenes. Finally, tumors will be selectively targeted to express suicide genes that, when activated, encode for products fatal to the cancer cell. These radically different approaches, mere intellectual scientific fantasies only a few years ago, are heralding an exciting and encouraging new era in the treatment of cancer.

REFERENCES

1. Alberts B, Bray D, Lewis J, Raff M, Roberts K, Watson JD, eds. *Molecular biology of the cell*, 2nd ed. New York: Garland; 1989.
2. Anderson SK, Stankova J, Roder JC. Decreased p21 levels in antisense *ras* transfectants augments NK sensitivity. *Mol Immunol* 1989;26:985–991.
3. Anderson WF. Human gene therapy. *Science* 1992;256:808–813.
4. Asher AL, Mule JJ, Reichert CM, Shiloni E, Rosenberg SA. Studies on the antitumor efficacy of systemically administered tumor necrosis factor against several murine tumors *in vivo*. *J Immunol* 1987; 138:963–974.
5. Beaucage SL, Caruthers MH. A new class of key intermediates for deoxypolynucleotide synthesis. *Tetrahedron Lett* 1981;22:1859–1862.
6. Bordignon C, Yu SF, Smith CA, Hentzopoulos P. Retroviral vector-mediated high-efficiency expression of adenosine deaminase (ADA) in hematopoietic long-term cultures of ADA deficient marrow cells. *Proct Natl Acad Sci USA* 1989;86:6748–6752.
7. Borg A, Baldetorp B, Ferno M, Killander D. *Erb-B2* amplification in breast cancer with a high risk of proliferation. *Oncogene* 1991;6:137–143.
8. Brodeur G, Seeger RC, Schwab M, Varmus HE, Bispho JM. Amplificiation of *N-myc* in untreated neuroblastoma correlates with advanced disease stage. *Science* 1984;224: 1121–1124.
9. Cantley LC, Auger KR, Carpenter C, Duckworth B, Granziani A, Kapeller R, Soltoff S. Oncogenes and signal transduction. *Cell* 1991;64:281–302.
10. Carpenter PM, Mercola M, Mercola D. Reversible transformation by *v-sis*: a model cell line for analysis of transformation by antisense methods. *Antisense Res Dev* 1991;1:289–295.
11. Cart GA, Clendennia NJ, Chabner B. Drug resistance in cancer. *Cancer Treat Rep* 1984; 68:87–99.
12. Cho-Chung YS, Clair T, Tortora G, Yokozaki H, Pepi S. Suppression of malignancy targeting the intracellular signal transducing proteins of cAMP: the use of site selective cAMP analogs antisense strategy and gene transfer. *Life Sci* 1991;48:1123–1132.
13. Corey CA, DeSilva AD, Holland CA, Williams DA. Serial transplantation of methotrexate-resistance bone marrow: protection of murine recipients from drug toxicity by progeny of transduced stem cells. *Blood* 1990;75:337–343.

14. Culver KW, Anderson WF, Blaese RM. Lymphocyte gene therapy. *Hum Gene Ther* 1991; 2:107–109.
15. Culver KW, Ram Z, Wallbridge S, Ishii H, Oldfield EH, Blaese RM. *In vivo* gene transfer with retroviral vector-producer cells for treatment of experimental brain tumors. *Science* 1992;256:1550–1552.
16. Edwards SA, Rundell AY, Adamson ED. Expression of *c-fos* antisense RNA inhibits the differentiation of F9 cells to parietal endoderm. *Dev Biol* 1988;129:91–102.
17. Eglitis MA, Kantoff P, Gilboa E, Anderson WF. Gene expression in mice after high efficiency retroviral-mediated gene transfer. *Science* 1985;230:1395–1898.
18. Freytag, SO. Enforced expression of the *c-myc* oncogene inhibits cell differentiation by precluding entry into a distinct predifferentiation state in G_0/G_1. *Mol Cell Biol* 1988;8: 1614–1624.
19. Galski H, Sullivan M, Willingham M, et al. Expression of a human multidrug resistance cDNA (MDRI) in the bone marrow of transgenic mice. *Mol Cell Biol* 1989;9:4357–4363.
20. Gewirtz AM, Calabretta B. A *c-myb* antisense oligodeoxynucleotide inhibits normal human hematopoiesis *in vitro*. *Science* 1988;242:1303–1306.
21. Gewirtz AM, Anfossi G, Ventorelli D, Valpreda S, Sims R, Calabretta B. G_1/S transition in normal human T-lymphocytes requires the nuclear protein encoded by *c-myb*. *Science* 1989;245:180–183.
22. Gilboa E, Eglitis MA, Kantoff PW, Anderson WF. Transfer and expression of cloned genes using retroviral vectors. *Biotechniques* 1986;4:504–512.
23. Green PJ, Pines O, Inouye M. The role of antisense RNA in gene regulation. *Ann Rev Biochem* 1986;55:569–597.
24. Heikkila R, Schwab G, Wickstrom E, Loke SL, Pluznik DH, Watt R, Neckers LM. A *c-myc* antisense oligodeoxynucleotide inhibits entry into S phase but not progress from G_0 to G_1. *Nature* 1987;328:445–449.
25. Holt JT, Redner RL, Nienhuis AW. An oligomer complementary to *c-myc* mRNA inhibits proliferation of HL-60 promyelocytic cells and induces differentiation. *Mol Cell Biol* 1988; 8:963–973.
26. Houba-Herin N, Inouye M. Antisense RNA. In: Eckstein F, Lilley DMJ, eds. *Nucleic acids and molecular biology Vol 1*. Berlin: Springer-Verlag; 1987:210–220.
27. Huang HJS, Yee JK, Shew JY, et al. Suppression of the neoplastic phenotype by replacement of the RB gene in human cancer cells. *Science* 1988;242:1563–1566.
28. [Anonymous] Treatment of patients with advanced cancer using cyclophosphamide, interleukin-2, and gene-marked tumor infiltrating lymphocytes. [Protocol] *Hum Gene Ther* 1990;1:73–86.
29. [Anonymous] The ADA human gene therapy clinical protocol. [Protocol] *Hum Gene Ther* 1990;1:327–362.
30. [Anonymous] Gene therapy of patients with advanced cancer using tumor infiltrating lymphocytes transduced with the gene coding for tumor necrosis factor. [Protocol] *Hum Gene Ther* 1990;1:441–480.
31. [Anonymous] Retroviral-mediated gene transfer of bone marrow cells during autologous bone marrow transplantation for acute leukemia. [Protocol] *Hum Gene Ther* 1990;3: 305–318.
32. [Anonymous] Autologous bone marrow transplant for children with AML in first complete remission: use of marker genes to investigate the biology of marrow reconstitution and the mechanism of relapse. [Protocol] *Hum Gene Ther* 1991;2:137–159.
33. [Anonymous] Autologous bone marrow transplantation for CML in which retroviral markers are used to discriminate between relapse which arises from systemic disease remaining after preparative therapy versus relapse due to residual leukemia cells in autologous marrow. A pilot trial. [Protocol] *Hum Gene Ther* 1991;2:359–376.
34. [Anonymous] Immunization of cancer patients using autologous cancer cells modified by insertion of the gene for tumor necrosis factor. [Protocol] *Hum Gene Ther* 1992;3:57–73.
35. [Anonymous] Immunization of cancer patients using autologous cancer cells modified by insertion of the gene for interleukin-2. [Protocol] *Hum Gene Ther* 1992;3:75–90.
36. Joyner A, Keller G, Phillips RA, Bernstein A. Retrovirus transfer of a bacterial gene into mouse hematopoietic progenitor cells. *Nature* 1983;305:556.
37. Kasid U, Pfeifer A, Brennan T, Beckett M, Weischelbaum RR, Dritschilo A, Mark GE.

Effect of antisense *c-raf*-1 on tumorigenicity and radiation sensitivity of a human squamous carcinoma. *Science* 1989;243:1354.
38. Keller G, Paige C, Gilboa E, Wagner F. Expression of a foreign gene in myeloid and lymphoid cells derived from multipotent haematopoietic precursors. *Nature* 1985;318: 149–154.
39. Kerr LD, Holt JT, Matrisian LM. Growth factors regulate transin gene expression by *c-fos*-dependent and *c-fos*-independent pathways. *Science* 1988;242:1424–1427.
40. Kolch W, Heidecker G, Lloyd P, Rapp UR. Raf-1 protein kinase is required for growth of induced NIH/313 cells. *Nature* 1991;349:426–428.
41. Kriegler M. Assembly of enhancers, promoters, and splice signals to control expression of transferred genes. In: Goeddel DV, ed. *Gene expression technology, Methods in enzymology*: Academic Press; 1990 vol 185.
42. Levi BZ, Ozato K. Constitutive expression of *c-fos* antisense RNA blocks *c-fos* gene induction by interferon and by phorbol ester and reduces *c-myc* expression in F9 embryonal carcinoma cells. *Genes Dev* 1988;2:554–566.
43. Levi BZ, Kasik JW, Ozato K. *C-fos* antisense RNA blocks expression of *c-fos* gene in F9 embryonal carcinoma cells. *Cell Differ Dev* 1988;25:95–101.
44. Mann R, Mulligan RC, Baltimore D. Construction of a retrovirus packaging mutant and its use to produce helper-free defective retrovirus. *Cell* 1983;33:153–159.
45. Marcus-Sekura CJ. Techniques for using antisense oligodeoxyribonucleotides to study gene expression. *Anal Biochem* 1988;172:289–295.
46. Martuza RL, Malick A, Marker JM, Ruffner KL, Coen DM. Experimental therapy of human glioma by means of a genetically engineered virus mutant. *Science* 1991;252:854–856.
47. Mastrangelo MJ, Schultz S, Kane M, Berd D. Newer immunologic approaches to the treatment of patients with cancer. *Semin Oncol* 1988;15:589–594.
48. McManaway ME, Neckers LM, Loke SL, et al. Tumour specific inhibition of lymphoma growth by an antisense oligodeoxynucleotide. *Lancet* 1990;335:808–811.
49. Melani C, Rivoltini L, Parmiani G, Calabretta B, Colombo MP. Inhibition of proliferation by *c-myb* antisense oligodeoxynucleotides in colon adenocarcinoma cell lines that express *c-myb*. *Cancer Res* 1991;51:2897–2901.
50. Mercer WE, Shields MT, Lin D, Appella E, Ulrich SJ. Growth suppression induced by wild-type p53 protein is accompanied by selective down-regulation of proliferating-cell nuclear antigen expression. *Proc Natl Acad Sci USA* 1991;88:1958–1962.
51. Mercola D, Westwick J, Rundell AY, Adamson ED, Edwards SA. Analysis of a transformed cell line using antisense *c-fos* RNA. *Gene* 1988;72:253–265.
52. Miller AD, Buttimore C. Redesign of retrovirus packaging cell lines to avoid recombination leading to helper virus production. *Mol Cell Biol* 1986;8:2895–2902.
53. Miller AD, Jolly DJ, Friedmann T, Verma IM. A transmissible retrovirus expressing human hypoxanthine phosphoribosyltransferase (HPRT): gene transfer into cells obtained from humans deficient in HPRT. *Proc Natl Acad Sci USA* 1983;80:4709–4713.
54. Miller AD, Rosman GJ. Improved retroviral vectors for gene transfer and expression. *Biotechniques* 1989;7:980–990.
55. Miller CK, Temin HM. Insertion of several different DNAs in reticuloendotheliosis virus strain T suppresses transformation by reducing the amount of subgenomic mRNA. *J Virol* 1986;1:75–80.
56. Mogli MC, Dick JE, Huszar D, Bernstein A, Phillips RA. Modulation of gene expression in multiple hematopoietic cell lineages following retroviral vector gene transfer. *Proc Natl Acad Sci USA* 1987;84:789–793.
57. Moser HE, Dervan PB. Sequence-specific cleavage of double helical DNA by triple helix formation. *Science* 1987;238:645–650.
58. Myers C, Cowan K, Sinha B, Chabner B. The phenomenon of pleoitropic drug resistance. In: Devita VT, Hellman S, Rosenberg SA, eds. *Important advances in oncology*. New York: Marcel Dekker; 1987:39–52.
59. Osborne WRA, Miller AD. Design of vectors for efficient expression of human purine nucleoside phosphorylase in skin fibroblasts from enzyme-deficient humans. *Proc Natl Acad Sci USA* 1988;85:6851–6855.
60. Prasolov VS, Chumakov PM. Antisense RNA p53 inhibits proliferation of normal and transformed cells. *Mol Biol (Mosk)* 1989;22:1371–1374.

61. Prochownik EV, Kukowska J, Rodgers C. *C-myc* antisense transcripts accelerate differentiation and inhibit G_1 progression in murine erythroleukemia cells. *Mol Cell Biol* 1988;8: 3683–3695.
62. Rosenberg SA, Packard BS, Aebersold PM, et al. Use of tumor-infiltrating lymphocytes and interleukin-2 in the immunotherapy of patients with metastatic melanoma. *N Engl J Med* 1988;319:1676–1680.
63. Salmons B, Groner B, Friis R, Meullener D, Jaggi R. Expression of anti-sense mRNA in *H-ras* transfected NIH/3T3 cells does not suppress the transformed phenotype. *Gene* 1986; 45:215–220.
64. Sambrook J, Fritsch EF, Maniatis T, eds. *Molecular cloning: a laboratory manual*, 2nd ed. Cold Spring Harbor Laboratory: Cold Spring Harbor Laboratory Press; 1989.
65. Slebos RT, Kiberlaar RE, Paledio O, et al. *K-ras* oncogene activation as a prognostic marker in adenocarcinoma of the lung. *N Engl J Med* 1990;323:561–565.
66. Smith LJ, Benchimol S. Introduction of new genetic material into human myeloid leukemic blast stem cells by retroviral infection. *Mol Cell Biol* 1988;8:974–977.
67. Stein CA. Cohen JS. Oligodeoxynucleotides as inhibitors of gene expression: a review. *Cancer Res* 1988;48:2659–2668.
68. Szczylik C, Skorski T, Nicolaides NC, et al. Selective inhibition of leukemia cell proliferation by BCR-ABL antisense oligodeoxynucleotides. *Science* 1991;253:562–568.
69. van Beusechem VW, Kukler A, Heidt PJ, Valerio D. Long-term expression of human adenosine deaminase in rheusus monkeys transplanted with retrovirus-infected bone marrow cells. *Proc Natl Acad Sci USA* 1992;89:7640–7644.
70. Vleminck K, Vakaet L, Mareel M, Fiers W, Van Roy F. Genetic manipulation of E-cadherin expression by epithelial tumor cells reveals an invasion suppressor role. *Cell* 1991;66: 107–119.
71. Watson JD, Hopkins NH, Roberts JW, Steitz JA, Weiner AM, eds. *Molecular biology of the gene*, 4th ed. Menlo Park, CA: Benjamin/Cummings; 1987.
72. Whitesell L, Rosolen A, Neckers LM. Episome-generated *N-myc* antisense RNA restricts the differentiation potential of primitive neuroectodermal cell lines. *Mol Cell Biol* 1991;11: 1360–1370.
73. Wickstrom EL, Bacon TA, Gonzalez A, Freeman DL, Lyman GH, Wickstrom E. Human promyelocytic leukemia HL-60 cell proliferation and *c-myc* protein expression are inhibited by an antisense pentadecadeoxynucleotide targeted against *c-myc* mRNA. *Proc Natl Acad Sci USA* 1988;85:1028–1032.
74. Williams DA, Lemischka IR, Nathan DG, Mulligan RC. Introduction of new genetic material into pluripotent hematopoietic stem cells of the mouse. *Nature* 1984;310:476–480.

8

Selected Immunotherapy Studies of the Interferons and IL-2/LAK

Jeffrey C. Allen and Roberta Hayes

THE INTERFERONS

The interferons are a diverse family of glycoprotein cytokines that share similarities in structure, antigenicity, and biologic effects. They have been extensively studied in both preclinical and clinical settings for their antiviral, immunomodulatory, and antineoplastic effects. The three classes of interferon (α, β, and γ) are distinguished by the method of production of their natural products, the cell receptors with which they interact, and to some extent their biologic effects. The α species is derived from leukocytes, the β from fibroblasts, and the γ from activated lymphocytes (1). The interferon gene cluster is located on the short arm of chromosome 9, an area frequently deleted in glioma cells lines and malignant gliomas (2).

The interferons are of interest as antineoplastic agents because in preclinical testing they exhibited biologic effects that should impact on cancer growth. For example, interferon-γ is a potent immunostimulant. It can induce the presentation of major histocompatibility complex (MHC) antigens on the surface of cancer cells, thereby making them more susceptible to immune recognition and cellular immune killing (3). In an in-vitro study of murine glioma cell lines, interferon-α upregulated class I MHC antigen expression (H-2K/D, the murine equivalent of the human HLA-A,B, and C) and interferon-γ upregulated the expression of class II MHC (H-2IA/E, the murine equivalent of the human HLA- DR) as well as class I antigens (4). All of the interferons can influence the activity of cellular genes, especially oncogenes, and may function as tumor-suppressor genes (5). Thus, the interferons, as antineoplastic agents, contribute not only immunomodulatory but also direct inhibitory effects on cancer growth.

In the formative period of cancer immunotherapy, investigators conceived its optimum application in the elimination of a very small tumor cell burden

Brain Tumors in Children: Principles of Diagnosis and Treatment, 2/e, edited by M.E. Cohen and P.K. Duffner, Raven Press, Ltd., New York, 1994.

either in a presymptomatic period or after major cytoreductive therapy. Immunotherapy, which included several biologic-response modifiers such as the interferons, was originally used after major cytoreductive therapies such as intensive chemotherapy, surgery, or radiotherapy. With increasing clinical experience and knowledge of their biologic effects, it has become appreciated that the interferons, as single agents or in combination with chemotherapy or radiotherapy, can cause major regressions of relatively large tumor burdens during the clinically symptomatic period (6).

One of the major handicaps in designing clinical trials with the interferons in brain tumor patients is the lack of knowledge of the precise mechanism of action of their antiproliferative effects. Several concepts have emerged in preclinical studies. The antiproliferative effects of the interferons appear to be dose-related and cytostatic; that is, their antiproliferative effect disappears when they are removed. These effects also vary with cancer type and occur in normal and transformed cells (7). The antimetabolic effects may be greater on resting than on rapidly dividing cells, which may account for the interferons activity on slowly proliferating malignancies. Of considerable interest to the field of neurooncology is the ability of the interferons to induce cellular differentiation in both normal and transformed tissues, frequently in association with inhibition of specific oncogene functions (8).

Clinical research in the field of neurooncology is in its formative stage. A number of questions arise in conducting clinical trials with the interferons. For example, the dose required for an optimum biologic or immunomodulatory effect in patients may differ from the dose required to enhance interferons' cytostatic or cytotoxic effects. When the interferons are used in conjunction with other antineoplastic agents in anticipation of an additive or synergistic cytotoxic effect, it is unclear whether the interferon should be administered before, with, or after chemotherapy or radiotherapy. The optimum dose, route (intravenous, subcutaneous, intratumoral), and schedule (daily, intermittent, continuous) of the various interferon species are unknown.

Other clinical dilemmas have been encountered. Of initial concern was the relative lack of CNS potency of parenterally administered interferon. Several studies using parenteral interferon involving adults with systemic cancer have noted the occurrence of brain metastases in spite of systemic responses (9). Another concern is that one of the dose-limiting toxicities of parenterally administered interferon (α and β) is neurotoxicity. Patients may experience signs of a diffuse encephalopathy with behavioral changes, confusion or disorientation, dementia and occasional seizures. Cognitive changes may linger long after interferon is discontinued (10). Thus, there has been a wide spectrum of clinical trials in cancer patients, studying not only the three recombinant interferon species as single agents in recurrent disease in classic dose-escalation trials, but also in combination with other cytotoxic agents and modalities to search for possible immunopotentiating, antiproliferative, and synergistic effects.

For patients with brain tumors, clinical trials have been conducted with all three interferon species utilizing various routes (SC, IV, intrathecal, and intracavitary) and dose schedules. Most of the clinical trials have been conducted in adults with recurrent malignant astrocytomas. This review will highlight several selective systemic cancer trials and summarize the adult and pediatric single-agent and multiagent brain tumor studies. Interferon-α, the most studied of the three interferon species, has shown dramatic clinical activity in several rare systemic tumors as a single agent and in combination with other chemotherapy agents. Although the percentage of complete responses in patients with hairy cell leukemia is small (10%), over 85% of adult hairy cell leukemia patients acquire disease suppression for long periods and benefit from the therapy as long as it is maintained (11). Approximately 80% of patients with chronic myelogenous leukemia have also experienced hematologic improvement. The response in patients with solid tumors such as melanoma is considerably less impressive (17%) but comparable to other single-agent and multiagent conventional chemotherapy regimens (12). Patients with AIDS-associated Kaposi's sarcoma may have a 30 to 35% objective response rate (13).

Mahaley et al. (14) have performed small clinical trials with all three interferon species in adult glioma patients. Their first clinical trial incorporated a relatively low dose of recombinant interferon-α given subcutaneously during a 3-week period following surgery prior to radiotherapy in newly diagnosed patients. The daily dose was escalated from 10 to 30 mIU/m^2 over 3 weeks. The survival of 9 patients so treated with radiotherapy and adjuvant BCNU was compared retrospectively to 18 conventionally treated patients. No important differences were discerned.

In a subsequent study (15), seven other patients with recurrent malignant gliomas received a course of a recombinant, genetically altered, interferon-β (IFN-β). The IFN-β was administered intravenously on a M/W/F schedule. The initial standard dose was 90 mIU and was escalated every 2 weeks until intolerable side effects occurred. None of the patients experienced a clinical response.

In another phase II trial conducted by Mahaley et al. (16), 14 adult patients with recurrent cerebral gliomas received a course of interferon-γ (2 mg/m^2, IV, twice weekly for 8 weeks). One patient with an oligodendroglioma had an objective response, 3 with high-grade gliomas had stable disease, and the other 10 patients had progressive disease. The authors concluded that interferon-γ had marginal activity. Overall, these trials at Duke Medical Center with the three species of recombinant interferons did not generate much enthusiasm for a role for the interferons in brain tumor protocols, although the trials were too small to draw firm conclusions.

IFN-β has been more extensively studied at other institutions. Different drug formulations, doses, dose schedules, and routes of administration have been employed. In a Japanese study, Nagai and Arai (17) administered natural human IFN-β either intrathecally or intratumorally and documented objective responses in 8 of 20 patients. Duff and co-workers (18) treated 12 adult patients with recurrent gliomas with natural IFN-β administered intravenously (10 mIU/day) and intratumorally (1 mIU every other day) for 10 days via reservoir. The cycle was repeated three times. None of the patients experienced clinical improvement or an objective response. Yung et al. (19) treated 10 evaluable adult patients with recurrent gliomas with recombinant IFN-β (90 mIU, intravenously, M/W/F) until recurrence. Three patients had stable disease and 1 a minor response. Fetell et al. (20) administered intratumoral recombinant IFN-β (5 to 180 mIU) via reservoir twice weekly to 12 evaluable adult glioma patients with recurrent disease. At the end of 6 weeks, 3 had stable disease and the others, progressive disease. Taken collectively, these exploratory adult studies do not enthusiastically encourage the pursuit of further clinical research with the interferons in adult patients with recurrent malignant gliomas, but their activity is comparable to other single agents in prior chemotherapy trials.

There are very few published clinical trials of interferon usage in children with primary brain tumors. A relatively large, multi-institutional study (21) (29 patients) served as a dose-finding trial of recombinant interferon-β (Betaseron, Triton Pharmaceuticals). This study incorporated both intrapatient and interpatient dose escalation steps. The intrapatient dose escalation was included to improve patient tolerance as the intravenous dose was escalated over 6 weeks (induction phase) and then maintained at the final level during the maintenance phase. The acute side effects such as fever, malaise, and myalgia are better tolerated with gradual dose escalation. The first group of patients received a starting dose of 50 mIU/m^2 given intravenously M/W/F, the second 100 mIU/m^2, the third 200 mIU/m^2, and the fourth 300 mIU/m^2. At the conclusion of this trial, it was determined that the maximum tolerable dose schedule began with 200 mIU/m^2. At this dose level, the IFN-β was escalated to 500 mIU/m^2 by the fifth week and maintained at this dose indefinitely during the maintenance phase. The IFN-β therapy was not interrupted while the patient remained on study.

In addition to determining the MTD of intravenous recombinant IFN-β, this study served to identify the dose-limiting organ toxicities and document objective and clinical responses. Typical non-dose-limiting effects of IFN-β were chills, fever, and fatigue. The more serious dose-limiting toxicities were hematologic (neutropenia), hepatic (elevated LFTs), and neurologic (encephalopathy with confusion and seizures). Twenty-one patients were evaluable for response, and 4 had objective (partial) responses (19%) for a median duration of 4 months. The 4 responding patients had high-grade gliomas. Eight other patients had stable disease for over 5 months. Thus, this study served to document the potential therapeutic efficacy of a new type of biologic response modifier in children with recurrent brain tumors. Future studies are exploring IFN-β tolerance as adjuvant therapy following radiotherapy in two newly diagnosed childhood brain tumor populations: brain stem glioma (CSG limited institutional pilot) and cerebral malignant gliomas (NYU Medical Center pilot). The ultimate role of the interferons in patients with primary brain tumors will likely be as part of a multimodality protocol including immunotherapy, radiotherapy, and chemotherapy (22).

ADOPTIVE IMMUNOTHERAPY: THE REGIONAL ADMINISTRATION OF INTERLEUKIN-2 AND LAK CELLS

In addition to the interferons, several other recombinant lymphokine products have been approved for human use and research, including tumor necrosis factor (TNF) and interleukin-2 (IL-2). Normal individuals maintain a population of natural killer (NK) cells that can recognize and destroy cells with non-self antigens that may emerge as a consequence of viral infection or neoplastic transformation. However, some cancer cells, being derived from host cells, may escape this mechanism of immune surveillance.

The molecular cloning of biological agents, such as recombinant interleukin-2, that are naturally produced as part of the host's immune defense mechanism, has fostered several clinical research applications as antitumor therapy. In vitro, high concentrations of IL-2 can activate a subpopulation of peripheral blood leukocytes (PBL), transforming them into cytotoxic cells termed *lymphokine-activated killer* (LAK) cells, which are active in several tumor models (23). LAK cells can be distinguished from NK cells by their ability to lyse NK-resistant, fresh or cultured tumor target cells in vitro, including malignant astrocytomas (24–26) and medulloblastomas (27). Although unactivated PBL from brain tumor patients generally cannot lyse autologous glioma cells in vitro, IL-2-activated PBL, or LAK cells, are capable of lysing autologous as well as allogeneic glioma, but not normal host tissues, including normal brain (28–29). Typically, NK cell function is assayed by the ability to kill the *K-562* human myelogenous leukemia cell line (30), and LAK cells by the lysis of the *Daudi*, B lymphoblastic Epstein Barr virus transformed cell line, derived from a human Burkitt lymphoma (31).

NK cells and LAK cells, as opposed to cytotoxic T lymphocytes (CTL), recognize and lyse target cells unrelated to MHC-antigens (i.e., the HLA system in humans). CTL can attack only other cells that have a similar MHC class I antigen profile (i.e., self-antigens) plus a viral- or tumor-induced foreign antigen. CTL cannot bind soluble antigen such as B lymphocytes. Such CTLs generally express CD/8 (cellular differentiation) antigens. For optimal augmentation of a cytotoxic T cell response, the target or tumor cell has to express both MHC class I (eg., HLA- A, B, or C), and MHC class II (HLA- DR, DQ, and DP) antigens. Another class of T lymphocytes that generally expresses CD4 antigens, known as helper cells, recognizes cells bearing foreign antigen and MHC class II molecules. In response, these helper lymphocytes release several kinds of lymphokine mediators that can activate CD8 positive CTLs, which then can recognize and destroy cells with foreign antigens revealed in contiguity to MHC class I molecules.

Although normal, healthy adults maintain a circulating population of NK cells in peripheral blood, LAK cells are not normally detectable in peripheral blood in the absence of IL-2 stimulation. NK and LAK cells are both capable of cellular immune tumor cell lysis; however, LAK cells are relatively more potent against solid tumors in laboratory studies (32). These LAK cells are produced for human therapy, ex vivo, by incubating peripheral blood mononuclear cells, usually obtained by leukapheresis, for 3 to 7 days in media containing IL-2. Adoptive immunotherapy thus involves the administration of such immune-modified autologous LAK cells into the systemic circulation or a regional cavity such as the brain or lateral ventricles with the intention of inducing a tumorical effect. Insufficient knowledge exists with regard to the mechanism of cellular immune killing and the optimum methods of LAK cell delivery.

The ultimate progenitor of the LAK cell is a matter of debate, but it is suspected that it is derived from NK cell precursors (33). LAK cells require the continued presence of IL-2 to sustain their activity, whereas NK cells do not. Thus, most adoptive immunotherapy protocols provide for protracted administration of IL-2 after LAK cell injection. The potency of LAK cells is diminished by high-dose corticosteroids (34). The concomitant use of high doses of corticosteroids with LAK cells will attenuate their cytotoxic activity. Corticosteroids can be used to ameliorate IL-2/LAK induced life-threatening systemic and CNS toxicity (35).

Clinical research in the United States with IL-2/LAK protocols in brain tumor patients has been conducted primarily in adult patients who have recurrent cerebral malignant gliomas. Adoptive immunotherapy protocols are in a formative stage in this area of clinical research. Advancement as a result of clinical research studies in brain tumor patients is more difficult as a result of several issues.

1. Parenterally administered IL-2/LAK is more effective for systemic cancer than CNS metastases, and patients with CNS metastases may suffer relatively severe neurotoxicity (36). Objective response rates using adoptive immunotherapy regimens combining intravenous IL-2 and LAK cells in adults with metastatic renal cell carcinoma and malignant melanoma have approached 15 to 25% (37,38). A significant number of those patients who responded have remained in remission for several years, some of whom have received only one or two courses of IL-2/LAK therapy. These results are encouraging since melanoma and renal cell carcinoma are relatively refractory to chemotherapy. There is some question as to whether LAK cells, in

addition to IL-2, were required for an optimum biologic effect (39). The dose-limiting toxicity of systemic IL-2/LAK therapy appears to be related to a vascular leak syndrome, and patients suffer primarily from pulmonary edema, hypotension, and impaired renal function. CNS dysfunction, usually transitory, occurs in as many as one-third of patients receiving systemic IL-2, and consists primarily of mild confusion, disorientation, and occasional somnolence (40). Patients with intracerebral metastases experience relatively severe neurotoxicity related in part to cerebral edema and/or progression of intracerebral disease. Presently, contemporary IL-2/LAK protocols for adults with systemic cancer exclude patients with intracerebral metastases. Thus, clinical research using adoptive immunotherapy methods in patients with primary intracerebral tumors has required alternative routes of administration.

2. LAK cells are derived from peripheral blood and have no "homing" behavior. Following intravenous administration, they are diluted in the bloodstream, and the actual number reaching a metastatic cancer is a very small percentage of the total dose administered. Their cytotoxic effect is a direct function of the number of activated cells contacting the target; that is, the greater the number surrounding a cancer cell, the greater the likelihood of a cytotoxic event. Tissue infiltrating lymphocytes (TIL cells) may be a more effective tumoricidal modality than LAK cells (41). They require 4 to 6 weeks of incubation with IL-2, compared to 3 to 4 days for LAK cells, in order to produce comparable cell numbers. However, when reinfused intravenously, they have an ability to localize in metastatic tumors. Although many adult systemic cancer trials are utilizing TIL cells, this is presently impractical for patients with primary brain tumors, in large measure related to the relatively small amount of tumor lymphocytes infiltrating primary brain tumors, although TIL cells have been cultured from primary brain tumors (42). Thus, most adoptive immunotherapy brain tumor trials continue to use LAK cells.

3. The brain tumor population eligible for IL-2/LAK therapy may be relatively immunosuppressed either de novo or as a result of the requirement of high doses of corticosteroid therapy at the time of clinical recurrence. Initial LAK activation studies demonstrated that LAK cells could be obtained from peripheral blood of brain tumor patients, but the generation of these cells was less efficient in patients heavily treated with prior chemotherapy or concomitant high doses of corticosteroids (43). Furthermore, LAK cells and their effectiveness would be greater impaired if administered concomitantly with high-dose corticosteroids.

4. Finally, there is uncertainty about the most effective dose schedule and route of administration for IL-2/LAK therapy for patients with primary brain tumors and whether the addition of other cytokines would increase the beneficial effect of the regimen. Initial systemic trials involved dose-finding studies of IL-2 usually given intravenously daily or on alternate days as a bolus.

Several trials have administered IL-2 as a continuous infusion (44). The concomitant administration of LAK cells has had variable effects on toxicity. The addition of other cytokines such as the interferons in conjunction with IL-2 with or without LAK to augment LAK activity or increase the immunogenicity of the host cancer is an area of active investigation (45). For example, the addition of recombinant interferon-α to an IL-2 cell regimen appears to have increased the response rate in a malignant glioma trial (46).

The clinical paradigms that may provide useful insights as to how to manage brain tumors are the regional systemic adoptive immunotherapy trials, such as those used to treat cancers localized to the peritoneal and pleural cavities or bladder (47). Regional immunotherapy into a body cavity permits the reduction of systemic toxicity and the concentration of the local immunotherapeutic effect where it is needed. Thus, most adult brain tumor adoptive immunotherapy trials have modeled themselves after the regional intracavitary approach. The theoretic attractions include:

1. A method to treat regional or localized brain cancer with intracavitary installation of IL-2/LAK.
2. A method of augmenting an immune response in a relatively immunologically privileged site, i.e., the brain.
3. The ability to avoid systemic IL-2 toxicity.

The technical and theoretical challenges include:

1. Securing a safe and effective method for periodic IL-2/LAK administration into the brain or ventricle.
2. Identifying an optimum population of patients for clinical investigations. Two approaches have been used: (a) an intracavitary protocol for patients with localized, resectable cerebral gliomas in whom corticosteroids can be reduced or eliminated following a radical surgical procedure and (b) an intraventricular protocol in non-shunt-dependent patients with leptomeningeal and/or intraventricular metastases.
3. Determining the optimum dose and schedule of IL-2 and LAK cells for each method of administration.
4. Attempting to augment the tumoricidal effect of IL-2/LAK by using combinations of cytokines (interferons, TNF, and other interleukins).

The early (1986) adoptive immunotherapy human brain tumor trials involved the intraoperative injection of IL-2 with or without LAK cells into the walls of tumor resection cavity on a one-time basis. Jacobs et al. (29) treated 10 patients who had recurrent cerebral malignant gliomas in this phase I study without incurring significant toxicity. In-vitro studies confirmed cellular immune killing of autologous and allogeneic malignant glioma cells in culture by LAK cells from these patients (48). Ingram et al. (49) treated 51 adult patients with recurrent malignant brain tumor with activated

LAK cells embedded in a plasma clot and surgically implanted in a resection cavity. The median survival for the entire group was 60 weeks following initial diagnosis. A report by Lillehei et al. (50) from the Denver Brain Tumor Research Group described treating 11 evaluable patients with surgically implanted lectin-activated LAK cells embedded in a plasma clot who had a resection of a recurrent malignant glioma followed by four daily intracavitary injections of recombinant IL-2 (Hoffman-LaRoche) via reservoir. A subsequent course of IL-2/LAK was given 1 month later via the reservoir. The mean decadron dose at entry was 14 mg/day. No significant responses were observed. The median overall survival was 63 weeks, and the median survival after immunotherapy was 18 weeks. All patients died with progressive disease.

In a study by Barba et al. (51) from the NIH involving nine patients with recurrent cerebral gliomas, intracavitary IL-2/LAK cells were administered on days 1 and 2, followed by three consecutive days of IL-2 (Cetus) alone via reservoir. The LAK cells (a maximum of 10^{10} cells) were suspended in 10 ml of fluid prior to injection. The IL-2 dose ranged from 1 to 6 x 10^4 IU/kg/dose. Five patients received only one course, three patients received two courses, and one who had a partial response had four courses. Although corticosteroids were tapered during immunotherapy, all patients received dexamethasone 10 mg q.i.d. following completion of therapy to avert any serious neurotoxicity. One patient had a partial response for 9 months after initially experiencing an acute neurologic deterioration. Worsening focal neurologic syndromes were encountered in the other eight non-responders related primarily to cerebral edema as revealed by CT/MRI scans, but most were reversible with corticosteroid therapy. Other than local wound problems in four patients, no other significant problems emerged and all patients eventually died of progressive disease.

Merchant and colleagues (52) conducted several adoptive immunotherapy studies at the Medical College of Virginia in Richmond. In studies begun in 1986, 29 patients received injections of IL-2/LAK cells in the brain tissue surrounding the tumor at the time of surgical resection. IL-2 (10^6 IU [Cetus]) alone was injected daily thereafter for 3 more days via reservoir. Ten of these patients received a second course of IL-2/LAK via reservoir 2 to 3 weeks later. Three patients required a second surgical resection for uncontrollable cerebral edema and clinical deterioration; and all IL-2/LAK injection sites revealed necrosis, fibrosis, edema, and tumor. The treatment overall was well tolerated. Although the majority of patients died of progressive disease, 5 patients have experienced long-term survival (>18 months) without disease progression. The authors concluded that this approach was relatively safe, noncurative but with promise.

One could draw several conclusions from these clinical research studies. Intracavitary IL-2/LAK can induce a dramatic localized biologic effect in brain surrounding tumor. Depending on the space avaliable for tissue expansion and the degree of acute edema, focal neurologic symptoms may arise. These symptoms can be rapidly relieved with corticosteroids, but this measure will likely attenuate the tumoricidal effect of IL-2/LAK. A small minority (10 to 20%) of patients appear to benefit from this regimen, especially when they receive interval therapy over several months. The specific tumoral and host factors responsible for a favorable response are poorly understood. The treatment is complex and expensive but no more invasive than other aggressive chemotherapy regimens. Future studies will focus on increasing the potency and number of LAK or TIL cells available for administration, possibly increasing the dose or cumulative exposure to IL-2, giving repeated courses of "maintenance" immunotherapy, and adding other cytokines to augment tumor immunogenicity and LAK potency.

Regional intracavitary therapy has several technical limitations. It excludes patients whose tumors can not be safely debulked and a cavity created. This approach may be less useful for patients with a large amount of residual disease, multifocal disease, callosal extension, or subarachnoid metastases. Because of the concern for the limitations of tissue infiltration of IL-2/LAK cells, methods are needed to induce a tumoricidal immune response throughout the entire CNS by recruiting host mononuclear effector cells from the body.

We (53) have been conducting adoptive immunotherapy studies at NYU Medical Center since 1988. The first protocol sought to determine the maximum tolerable dose of recombinant IL-2 (Cetus) when administered via reservoir into a resection cavity in adult patients with recurrent cerebral malignant gliomas (53). The IL-2 was administered M/W/F for 2 consecutive weeks constituting one cycle of therapy, and LAK cells (0.5 to 1.0 x 10^9) were administered on day 1 as well. A second cycle was repeated after a 2-week interval, and two cycles constituted one course. A course could be repeated every 8 to 12 weeks for stable or responsive disease, for a total of three courses. The initial IL-2 dose was 1.2 mIU/dose (Cetus), and four dose levels were planned in increments of 1.2 mIU. Corticosteroid therapy was completely tapered at the outset of the study. Twenty-seven adult patients with recurrent high-grade cerebral gliomas were evaluated for this protocol, but only 16 remained eligible postoperatively. The histologic diagnoses of the 16 patients were anaplastic astrocytoma (2) and glioblastoma (14). During therapy, the use of corticosteroids was strictly limited. The MTD for repetitive intracavitary IL-2 was determined to be 1.2 mIU/dose, that is, the initial dose level. The long-term toxicity overall has been acceptable. A total of 29 cycles were administered to these 16 patients; 3 patients received one full course of therapy and 4 more than one course. Ten patients have experienced a clinical benefit with prolonged survival. There were 3 objective responses (2 CR and 1 PR) for a median duration of over 22 months and 2 with stable disease for greater than 1.2 and 3.5 years, respectively. The mean total survival for the three groups of glioblastoma patients [protocol responders

(N = 8), protocol nonresponders (N = 6), and protocol ineligible (N = 11)] was 79, 32, and 28 weeks, respectively.

Prior to each IL-2 injection, CSF was removed for analysis. Marked CSF eosinophilia was noted in responders, although peripheral eosinophil levels did not increase. Persistent CSF eosinophilia and cytokine levels (IL-2, IFN) were noted more than 13 weeks after therapy in some patients. Surgical and autopsy material is available on 9 patients following immunotherapy. Upon examination after immunotherapy in autopsy specimens, the tissue nearest the catheter showed marked areas of tumor necrosis with infiltrates of eosinophil and activated T lymphocytes ($CD45R0^{+}$).

A phase II intracavitary pediatric study of comparable design has been recently initiated at our institution. Because of the predilection of childhood brain tumors to metastasize via CSF either within the ventricles or throughout the subarachnoid space, we designed a similar adoptive immunotherapy study in which IL-2/LAK was administered via reservoir directly into lateral ventricles in children with recurrent primary brain tumors with intraventricular and/or leptomeningeal metastases. Patency of the spinal subarachnoid space was confirmed with a metrizamide myelogram. If the patient was shunt-dependent, IL-2/LAK therapy was administered via a spinal reservoir into the cauda equina region.

This was also a phase I/II study where the MTD of intraventricular/intrathecal IL-2 with LAK cells would be determined. The initial IL-2 dose was 3×10^5 IU (Cetus) given on M/W/F for 2 consecutive weeks, constituting one cycle. LAK cells (0.3 to 0.8×10^9) are given with the first two injections. This regimen is repeated in 2 weeks, constituting one complete course. Interval therapy as above is given every 3 months for 1 year as long as the toxicity is tolerable and the tumor is stable or improved. The dose of IL-2 will be increased in 0.3-mIU steps until a MTD has been reached. At least 3 patients will be treated at each dose level. We are presently at our second dose level.

A total of five evaluable patients have been treated since April, 1991 [thalamic glioblastoma-1, brain stem glioma-1, PNET (cerebellar)-1, PNET (cauda equina)-1, germinoma-1]. Three patients were treated at the first dose level with acceptable toxicity, and two have been entered at the second level. Our first patient, a 13-year-old male with a recurrent thalamic glioblastoma with diffuse intraventricular and subarachnoid metastases, has had a remarkable response. His prior therapy included focal radiotherapy, BCNU, and adjuvant recombinant interferon-β. He developed local and diffuse metastases 9 months following diagnosis. He received an IL-2 dose of 3×10^5 IU. The initial intraventricular IL-2/LAK therapy produced relatively severe neurotoxicity with headache, altered sensorium, increased frequency of seizures, high fever, and nuchal rigidity. He improved on his own without corticosteroids 1 week after therapy. A clinical and radiographic response was apparent 2 months after the first course. He has received three courses (six cycles) over the first year and has experienced a complete response that has endured for over 15 months. Although he retains only a small area of contrast enhancement on MRI, an [^{18}F]-deoxyglucose-PET scan was hypometabolic and the metastatic lesions have disappeared. His clinical condition continues to improve.

One child with a recurrent cerebellar PNET developed an intratumoral hemorrhage during the second half of the first course of IL-2/LAK and lapsed into a coma. Surgical resection identified a fresh blood clot, inflammation, tumor, and evidence of old microscopic hemorrhage. She remains alive but severely neurologically damaged 12 months later and has received no more therapy. The three other patients (cauda equina PNET, brain stem glioma, and germinoma) had progressive disease after one course.

The therapy overall has been remarkably well tolerated. Acute headache, fever, malaise, mild nuchal rigidity, and occasional focal seizures have been observed with intraventricular/intrathecal IL-2/LAK therapy. The intratumoral hemorrhage described above may have been related to therapy or disease. We will continue our study to identify the MTD of intraventricular IL-2. Future approaches may include adding other cytokines to IL-2/LAK therapy. We and others have been able to detect biologic changes in the CSF and peripheral blood following intraventricular IL-2/LAK therapy. In our study, in addition to the pleocytosis sustained over 2 weeks, an eosinophilia emerged in the CSF and in the body ranging from 5 to 70%.

List et al. (54) studied the induction of cytokines following the administration of a single intraventricular dose of IL-2 via a reservoir in 11 patients with leptomeningeal carcinomatosis. The doses of IL-2 ranged from 1.25 to 20×10^5 Cetus units per injection. CSF was collected at 0, 1, 2, 4, 6, 12, and 24 hours after injection. The induction of a number of cytokines (TNF-α, IL-1, IL-6, interferon-γ) was detected in this 24-hour period as well as a rapid influx of neutrophilic leukocytes. This occurred in spite of the fact that all the patients were on therapeutic doses of dexamethazone and all had prior systemic chemotherapy. Clinical responses have been observed in 2 patients with leptomeningeal metastases following IL-2/LAK injections via reservoir (55).

Thus, adoptive regional immunotherapy utilizing IL-2/LAK for brain tumor patients remains in its exploratory stage. Its mechanism of action is relatively poorly understood and unpredictable. The procedure is labor-intensive and involves a multidisciplinary approach. The fact that several patients have experienced dramatic and enduring responses encourages a limited number of institutions to continue their clinical and laboratory research studies.

REFERENCES

1. Clark J, Longo D. Interferons in cancer therapy. In: *Updates 1*, Vol 1, No. 4. Philadelphia: JB Lippincott; April 1987:1–16.

2. Olopade O, Jenkins R, Ransom D, et al. Molecular analysis of the short arm of chromosome 9 in human gliomas. *Cancer Res* 1992;52:2523–2529.
3. Giancomini P, Fisher P, Durgou G, et al. Regulation of class II MHC expression interferons: insights into the mechanism of action of interferon. *Anticancer Res* 1988;8:1153–1161.
4. Akbosak A, Oldfield E, Saris S. Expression and modulation of major histocompatibility antigens on murine primary brain tumor *in vitro*. *J Neurosurg* 1991;75:922–929.
5. Muakoshi J, Dobler K, Allolunis-Turner J, et al. Absence of IFN-A and IFN-B1 genes from human malignant glioma cell lines and lack of correlation with sensitivity to interferons. *Cancer Res* 1990;50:278–283.
6. Goldstein D, Laszlo J. Interferon therapy in cancer: from imaginon to interferon. *Cancer Res* 1986;46:4315.
7. Vedanthan S, Gamliel H, Golomb H. Mechanism of interferon actions in hairy cell leukemia: a model of effective cancer biotherapy. *Cancer Res* 1992;52:1056–1066.
8. Rossi G. Interferons and cell differentiation. In Gresser I, ed. *Interferon*. London: Academic Press, London, 1985.
9. Legha S, Papadopoulos N, Plager C, et al. Clinical evaluation of recombinant interferon alfa-2A (*Roferon*-A) in metastatic melanoma using two different schedules. *J Clin Oncol* 1987;5:1240–1246.
10. Quesada J, Tolpaz M, Rios A.Clinical toxicity of interferons in cancer patients: a review. *J Clin Oncol* 1986;4:234–248.
11. Golomb H, Jacobs A, Tefer A. Alpha-2 interferon therapy of hairy cell leukemia: a multicenter study of 64 patients. *J Clin Oncol* 1986;4:900–905.
12. Mahead G, Thomson D, Hersey P. Recombinant interferon alpha-2a in advanced malignant melanoma: a phase I-II study in combination with DTIC. *Int J Cancer*, 1987;[Supp 1]: 31–35.
13. Real F, Oettgen H, Krown S. Kaposi's sarcoma and the acquired immunodeficiency syndrome: treatment with high and low doses of recombinant leukocyte A interferon. *J Clin Oncol* 1986;4:544–550.
14. Mahaley MS, Urso M, Whaley R, et al. Interferon as adjuvant therapy with initial radiotherapy of patients with anaplastic gliomas. *J Neurosurg* 1984;61:1069–1071.
15. Mahaley MS, Dropcho E, et al. Systemic beta-interferon therapy for recurrent gliomas: a brief report. *J Neurosurg* 1989;71:639–641.
16. Mahaley MS, Bertsch L, et al. Systemic gamma-interferon therapy for recurrent gliomas. *J Neurosurg* 1988;69:826–829.
17. Nagai M, Arai T. Clinical effect of interferon in malignant brain tumors. *Neurosurg Rev* 1984;7:55–64.
18. Duff T, Borden E, Bay J, et al. Phase II trial of interferon-B for treatment of recurrent glioblastoma multiforme. *J Neurosurg* 1986;64:408–413.
19. Yung W, Prados M, Lavian V, et al. Intravenous recombinant interferon beta in patients with recurrent malignant gliomas. *J Clin Oncol* 1991;9:1945–1949.
20. Fetell M, Housepian E, Oster M, et al. Intratumor administration of beta-interferon in recurrent malignant gliomas: a phase I clinical and laboratory study. *Cancer* 1990;65:78–83.
21. Allen J, Packer R, Bleyer A, et al. Recombinant beta-interferon (Betaseron[R]): a phase I-II trial in children with recurrent brain tumors. *J Clin Oncol* 1991;9(5):783–788.
22. Wadler S, Schwartz E. Antineoplastic activity of the combination of interferon and cytotoxic agents against experimental and human malignancies: a review. *Cancer Res* 1990;50: 3473–3486.
23. Eberlain TJ, Rosenstein M, Spiess PJ, Wesley R, SA Rosenberg. Adoptive immunotherapy of a syngeneic murine lymphoma using longterm lymphoid cell lines expanded in T cell growth factor. *Cancer Immunol Immunother* 1982;13:5–13.
24. Lotze MT, Grimm EA, Mazumder A, Strausser JL, SA Rosenberg. Lysis of fresh and cultured autologous tumor by human lymphocytes cultured in T-cell growth factor. *Cancer Res* 1981;41:4420–4425.
25. Grimm EA, Mazumder A, Zhang HZ, SA Rosenberg. Lymphokine-activated killer cell phenomenon: lysis of natural-killer killer-resistant fresh solid tumor cells by interleukin 2-activated autologous human peripheral blood lymphocytes. *J Exp Med* 1982;155:1823–1841.
26. Grimm EA, Ramsey KM, Mazumder A, Wilson DJ, Djeu JY, SA Rosenberg. Lymphokine-activated killer cell phenomenon. II: Precursor phenotype is serologically distinct from peripheral T lymphocytes, and natural killer cells. *J Exp Med* 1983;157:884–897.

27. George RE, Loudon WG, Moser RP, Bruner JM, Steck PA, EA Grimm. In vitro cytolysis of primitive neuroectodermal tumors of the posterior fossa (medulloblastoma) by lymphokine-activated killer cells. *J Neurosurg* 1988;69:403–409.
28. Jacobs SK, Wilson DJ, Kornblith PL, EA Grimm. In vitro killing of human glioblastoma by interleukin-2-activated autologous lymphocytes. *J Neurosurg* 1986;64:114–117.
29. Jacobs SK, Wilson DJ, Kornblith PL, EA Grimm. Interleukin-2 and autologous lymphokine activated killer cells in the treatment of malignant glioma. *J Neurosurg* 1986;64:743–749.
30. Ortaldo JR, Oldham RK, Cannon GC, Herberman RB. Specificity of natural cytotoxic reactivity of normal human lymphocytes against a myeloid leukemia cell line. *J Natl Cancer Inst* 1977;59:77–83.
31. Klein E, Klein G, Nadkarni J, et al. Surface IgM-kappa specificity on a Burkitt lymphoma cell in vivo and in derived culture lines. *Cancer Res* 1968;28:1300–1310.
32. Margolin K, Rayner A, Hawkins M, et al. Interleukin-2 and lymphokine-activated killer cell therapy of solid tumors: analysis of toxicity and management guidelines. *J Clin Oncol* 1989;7(4):486–498.
33. Phillips J, Gemlo B, Myers W, et al. In vivo and in vitro activation of natural killer cells in advanced cancer patients undergoing combined recombinant interleukin-2 and LAK cell therapy. *J Clin Oncol* 1987;5(12):1933–1941.
34. Papa M, Vetto J, Ettinghausen S, et al. Effect of corticosteroids on the antitumor activity of lymphokine-activated killer cells and interleukin-2 in mice. *Cancer Res* 1986;46:5618–5623.
35. Vetto J, Papa M, Lotze M, et al. Reduction of toxicity of interleukin-2 and lymphokine-aktivated killer cells in humans by the administration of corticosteroids. *J Clin Oncol* 1987; 5(3):496–503.
36. Mitchell M. Relapse in the central nervous system in melanoma patients successfully treated with biomodulators. *J Clin Oncol* 1989;7(11):1701–1709.
37. Thompson J, Shulman K, Benyunes M, et al. Prolonged continuous intravenous infusion interleukin-2 and lymphokine-activated killer-cell therapy for metastatic renal cell carcinoma. *J Clin Oncol* 1992;10(6):960–968.
38. Bar M, Sznol M, Atkins M, et al. Metastatic malignant melanoma treated with combined bolus and continuous infusion interleukin-2 and lymphokine-activated killer cells. *J Clin Oncol* 1990;8(7):1138–1147.
39. Rosenberg S. The immunotherapy and gene therapy of cancer. *J Clin Oncol* 1992;10(2): 180–199.
40. Bernard J, Ameriso S, Kempf, et al. Transient focal neurologic deficits complicating interleukin-2 therapy. *Neurology* 1990;40:154–155.
41. Rosenberg S, Spress P, Lafreniere R. A new approach to the adoptive immunotherapy of cancer with tumor infiltrating lymphocytes. *Science* 1986;223:1318–1321.
42. Sawamura Y, Abe H, Aida T, et al. Isolation and in vitro growth of glioma-infiltrating lymphocytes, and an analysis of their surface phenotypes. *J Neurosurg* 1988;69:745–750.
43. McVicar D, Davis D, Merchant R. In vitro analysis of the proliferative potential of T cells from patients with brain tumor: glioma-associated immunosuppression unrelated to intrinsic cellular defect. *J Neurosurg* 1992;76:251–260.
44. Geertsen P, Hermann G, von der Maase H, et al. Treatment of metastatic renal cell carcinoma by continuous intravenous infusion of recombinant interleukin-2: a single-center phase II study. *J Clin Oncol* 1992;10(5):753–759.
45. Feruglio C, Zambello R, Trentin L, et al. Cytotoxic in vitro function in patients with metastatic renal cell carcinoma before and after alpha-2b-interferon therapy. *Cancer* 1992;69: 2525–2531.
46. Merchant R, McVicar D, Merchant L, et al.: Treatment of recurrent malignant glioma by repeated intracerebral injections of human recombinant interleukin-2 alone or in combination with systemic interferon-α: results of a phase I clinical trial. *J Neurooncol* 1992;12: 75–83.
47. Van Haelst-Pisani C, Pisani R, Kovach J. Cancer immunotherapy: current status of treatment with interleukin-2 and lymphokine-activate killer cells. *Mayo Clin Proc* 1989;64: 451–465.
48. Jacobs S, Wilson D, Kornblith P, et al. In vitro killing of human glioblastoma by interleukin-2-activated autologous lymphocytes. *J Neurosurg* 1986;64:114–117.
49. Ingram M, Shelton C, Jacques S, et al. Preliminary clinical trial of immunotherapy for malignant glioma. *J Biol Response Mod* 1987;6:489–498.

50. Lillehei K, Mitchell D, Johnson S, et al. Long-term follow-up of patients with recurrent malignant gliomas treated with adjuvant adoptive immunotherapy. *Neurosurgery* 1991;28: 16–23.
51. Barba D, Saris S, Holder C, et al. Intratumoral LAK cell and interleukin-2 therapy of human gliomas. *J Neurosurg* 1989;70:175–182.
52. Merchant R, Ellison M, Young H. Immunotherapy for malignant glioma using human recombinant interleukin-2 and activated autologous lymphocytes. *J Neurooncol* 1990;8: 173–188.
53. Hayes R. The cellular immunotherapy of primary brain tumors. *Rev Neurol* 1992;148(6–7): 454–466.
54. List J, Moser R, Steuer M, et al. Cytokine responses to intraventricular injection of interleukin 2 into patients with leptomeningeal carcinomatosis: rapid induction of tumor necrosis factor α, interleukin 1β, interleukin 6, γ-interferon, and soluble interleukin 2 receptor (M_r 55,000 protein). *Cancer Res* 1992;52:1123–1128.
55. Shimizu K, Okamoto Y, Miyao Y, et al. Adoptive immunotherapy of human meningeal gliomatosis and carcinomatosis with LAK cells and recombinant interleukin-2. *J Neurosurg* 1987;66:519–521.

9

Medulloblastomas

Approximately 20% of all brain tumors of childhood are medulloblastomas. The incidence peaks around 5 years of age (121). Although the tumor has been described in the very young and elderly, some authors have described a bimodal distribution rather than a peak, initially at 3 to 4 years of age and again at 8 to 9 years of age (67). It is generally accepted that the incidence in males exceeds that in females by a small margin. In older children, the sex preference is more nearly equal. Reported male:female ratios vary from 1.3:1 to 4.8:1 (36, 120). Medulloblastomas have been associated with a number of inherited syndromes, the most prominent of which are ataxia telangiectasia (105) and the Li-Fraumeni syndrome (88).

Of all childhood brain tumors, the most dramatic change in survival has occurred with medulloblastomas. In Cushing's series (23) reported in 1930, 1 out of 61 children (1.6%) was alive at the end of 3 years. An 18% 5-year survival rate for medulloblastomas was reported in Connecticut over a 39-year period (1935 to 1968) (36). However, when these data are analyzed by decade and site of treatment, a dramatic change in survival is noted. A 1979 report from the Hospital for Sick Children in London, England (67) underscores the changing prognosis of medulloblastomas. Of 33 cases completing radiotherapy before 1970, there was a disappointing 19% 2-year and 3% 5-year survival rate. However, of 22 cases treated after 1970, survival rates for 2 years were 65%, and for 5 years were 48%. Patients with medulloblastomas treated in the last decade at university cancer centers in the state of Connecticut had a 74% projected 5-year survival (31). Five-year survival rates of approximately 70%, although not the rule, have also been reported by others (6,50,56). In an article by Lefkowitz et al. (62), the 5-year and 10-year survivals were 54% and 41%, respectively; however, for children surviving 5 years, the actuarial survival at 10 years was 75% and at 12 years was 51%.

These encouraging results in all likelihood represent the optimum survival as multiple series continue to suggest 5-year survivals of 50 to 60% (45,81,82,85). Ten-year survivals are closer to 30 to 50% (8,9,10,85). Even when preselecting patients with the best risk factors and excluding those patients not completing either chemotherapy or radiotherapy, 5-year survivals have not exceeded 75%. Although less optimistic, cancer registry data may be a more accurate estimate of overall survival statistics regardless of

Brain Tumors in Children: Principles of Diagnosis and Treatment, 2/e, edited by M.E. Cohen and P.K. Duffner, Raven Press, Ltd., New York, 1994.

the treatment modality (8). For example, our data (31,32) from the Surveillance-Epidemiology-End Result (SEER) registries (1973 to 1980) suggest that survival in a nonselected population is substantially less than 70%. This relates, in part, to where treatment is obtained. Patients who received part or all of their treatment at large referral centers did significantly better than those patients who received treatment at smaller nonuniversity hospitals. In 1985, of the 1,362 children identified with cancer of the nervous system, only 595, or 44%, were being treated by institutions of either the Children's Cancer Study Group or the Pediatric Oncology Group, the two major children's cancer treatment consortiums in the United States (12). It is hoped that in the future, the majority of children with brain tumors will be treated at cancer treatment centers.

The putative congenital nature of medulloblastoma has led some authors to apply Collins' rule in predicting the course of this tumor (8). This rule states that the period of risk for a tumor of embryonal origin is the patient's age at the time of diagnosis plus 9 months. This implies that tumor cells surviving treatment will multiply and reach a clinically similar size in the same time it took for the original tumor to grow to the size recognized at diagnosis. Thus, an individual who has received treatment is at risk for recurrence of a tumor for a period of time equal to his age at presentation plus an in utero time period of 9 months (9,21,90). Unfortunately, this concept

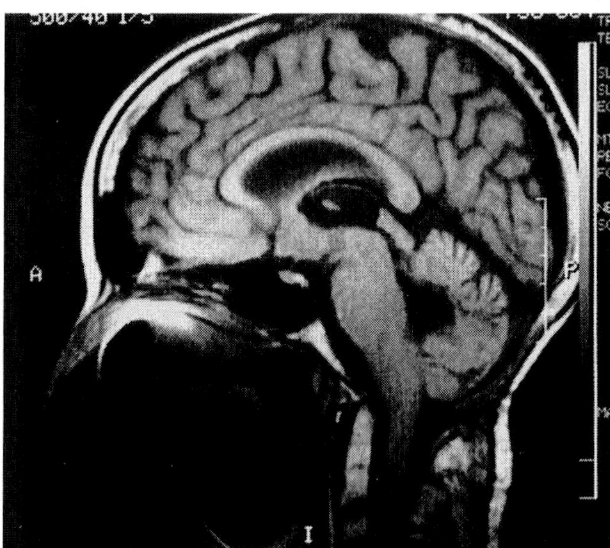

FIG. 9-1. T1-weighted MRI in axial plane. Note metastatic lesion in suprasellar cistern and operative defect in posterior fossa. Metastatic disease presented 5 years following diagnosis. Patient died 10 months following recurrence.

may be misleading. Several groups (10,35,92,110) have reported that recurrence may occur late and that overall survival is poorer in the younger child than in the older child. Lefkowitz et al. (62) reported a number of patients who relapsed beyond the period of risk predicted by Collins' rule. Observation of recurrence years after initial treatment suggests that long-term survivors remain indefinitely at risk (20,62,63) (Fig. 9-1).

PATHOLOGY

In 1925, Bailey and Cushing (3) defined medulloblastoma as a specific entity because of its biologic behavior and distinct histopathologic features. The tumor was called a medulloblastoma by Bailey (1925) because the tumor was believed to be composed of embryonal stem cells with a pluripotential nature. However, the medulloblast as a normally occurring cell capable of differentiating into either glial or neuronal elements has never been satisfactorily identified. Examples of spongioblastic, astrocytic, and oligodendroglial differentiation are well known with this tumor (84). Ependymal differentiation of the tumor, occurring either independently or in association with astrocytic differentiation, has also been described. As such, the findings of Homer-Wright rosettes and perivascular pseudorosettes within the tissue mass of a medulloblastoma are expected. Tissue cultures of tumor cells have confirmed differentiation of medulloblastomas along glial cell lines. Although extremely rare, differentiation of medulloblastomas along neuroblastic rather than glial cell lines has also been described (87,91,99). Evidence of differentiation along varying cell lines supports the concept that a medulloblastoma represents a tumor of stem-cell origin. One theory of origin suggests that the medulloblastoma is unique to the cerebellum and may arise from the fetal external granular layer, rest cells in the posterior medullary velum or internal granular layer of the cerebellum. Another postulate is that the orgin of the medulloblastoma, like that of PNETs, arises from pleuripotential cells found in the subependymal regions or within the pineal anlage (94). Despite this and the recognition that cells of the external granular layer of the cerebellum and neuroepithelial cells lining the neural tube give rise to stem cells from which neuroblasts and spongioblasts originate, evidence supporting the existence of a nonneoplastic embryonic pluripotential medulloblast continues to remain circumstantial.

Prognostic importance of cellular differentiation in medulloblastomas remains an open question. Several studies comparing pathology at diagnosis with that seen following treatment and prolonged survival have not helped to answer the question of the significance of cellular differentiation within medulloblastomas. Packer et al. (83) have suggested that lack of cellular differentiation imparts a favorable prognosis, whereas others (17) have suggested that differentiation has favorable, little, or no effect on prognosis.

Demonstration of a change in character of cell type from time of initial diagnosis until death may validate histologic subcategorization.

GROSS FEATURES

Medulloblastomas, for the most part, present in the midline. Some have suggested that this relates to the location of fetal rest cells. Putatively, the medulloblastoma is derived from remnants of the fetal external granular layer of the cerebellum. Others have postulated that the tumor arises from cell rests in the posterior medullary velum, and possibly the anterior medullary velum of the cerebellum. Embryonic cells arising in the roof of the fourth ventricle migrate superiorly and laterally to form the external layer of the cerebellum. Origin in the medullary velum may account for the midline predilection of the tumor, and origin in the external granular layer accounts for the occasional location in the cerebellum hemispheres (101).

Medulloblastomas tend to be soft, fleshy, and well demarcated. Hemorrhage, cyst formation, and calcification are uncommon. The tumor has a tendency to arise from the vermis, fill the cavity of the fourth ventricle, and, by local extension, infiltrate the floor. The more aggressive tumors may invade contiguous structures, i.e., the cerebellar hemispheres, cerebellar peduncles or brain stem, and/or seed the subarachnoid space. Those medulloblastomas that occur in the lateral hemispheres are more apt to be seen in older children or adults. Infrequently, the tumor may be found en plaque on the surface of the cerebellum. Desmoplastic tumors, i.e., those that excite an intense fibrous reaction, because of their homogeneous nature are thought to be more differentiated medulloblastomas (19).

HISTOLOGIC FEATURES

Microscopically, the classical medulloblastoma is a cellular tumor composed of small round-oval undifferentiated cells with hyperchromatic nuclei in a matrix of poorly defined cytoplasm. Mitotic figures are quite variable. Homer-Wright pseudorosettes are typical of medulloblastomas. Carrot-shaped nuclei are arranged radially around amorphous eosinophilic centers that do not represent a true cavity. Unipolar and occasional bipolar cells are indicative of neuroblast differentiation. Rarely have neurofibrils been demonstrated. Glial differentiation is seen in less than 10% of tumors (16). As a general rule, there is little vascular reaction and, aside from the tendency for the desmoplastic tumor to excite an intense leptomeningeal reaction, the tumor is quite homogeneous (Fig. 9-2) (19,23,99,100). Desmoplastic tumors are characterized by a dense network of intercellular reticulin.

Small-cell tumors that occur throughout the nervous system may look pathologically like medulloblastomas but behave differently. More appropri-

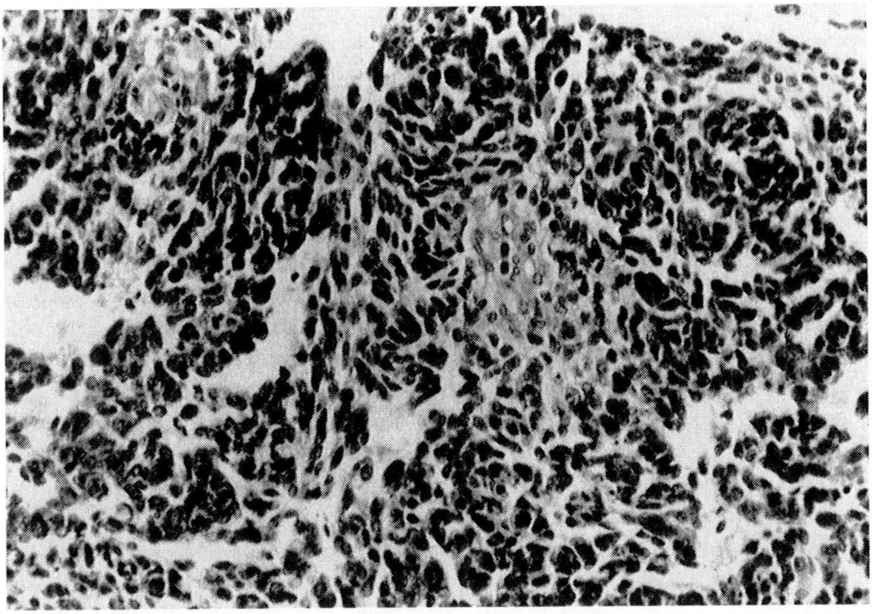

FIG. 9-2. Cellular tumor composed of primitive, small cells with round to oval, hyperchromatic nuclei and scant cytoplasm. The tumor cells are arranged in sheets without a distinctive architecture *(H&F)*.

ately, they should be classified as cerebral neuroblastomas, primitive neuroectodermal tumors, or, if found in the pineal region, pineoblastomas. These tumors have been called primitive neuroectodermal tumors (PNET), the biology and behavior of which are still being actively discussed in the literature (15,95). Because of their marked cellularity, tumors such as malignant ependymomas, pineocytomas, glioblastomas, neurocytomas, and oligodendrogliomas on occasion have been erroneously placed in the category of a small cellular pleomorphic tumor of poor prognosis. Entities such as pineocytomas, neurocytomas, and oligodendrogliomas are small-cell tumors that may in fact have a relatively benign prognosis. In addition, as emphasized by Rubinstein and others (54,68,100), highly anaplastic carcinomas such as oat cell tumors of the lung and lymphosarcoma may be confused with medulloblastomas. The term *PNET* is a stimulating concept that is still being debated.

The medulloblastoma, perhaps more than any other tumor, is known for its tendency to seed the subarachnoid space, both locally and distally. The site of 70 to 80% of first recurrences is the posterior fossa (9,10). The remainder may disseminate throughout the spinal axis and the central nervous system. Subarachnoid extension is common, but subdural involvement is unusual. Supratentorial spread of medulloblastoma, although less common than spinal seeding, is a recognized pattern of treatment failure. Recurrence of the tumor in the cribriform plate region has been ascribed to the failure to irradiate this region adequately. In an effort to avoid radiation to the eye, the eye may be shielded and the radiation port chosen so that the eye lies below the port of planning therapy. Both situations do not allow proper radiation of the frontal areas and thus may account for treatment failure at this site. In addition, if patients are operated on in the prone position, the frontal areas become the most dependent, and hence they become a site where tumor cells might be expected to pool (53).

Extraneural metastases of medulloblastomas are well documented and in some series approach an overall incidence of 5 to 30% (27,30,55) (see Chapter 21). Perhaps as a result of increasing survival, extraneural metastases may be more frequent than previously suspected. Shunting of an obstructed pathway, as well as the surgery itself, is thought to allow tumor to spread beyond the central nervous system. The most common extraneural sites are bone (80%), pelvis (60%), long bone (60%), spine (60%), ribs (30%), and skull and other bones (10%). The second most common site of metastasis is the lymph nodes, although other viscera may be involved. The average duration from diagnosis to extraneural metastasis has been reported as 18 months, although in some cases many years have elapsed following initial diagnosis before metastasis is identified (4,14,28,29,53). Bone scans usually demonstrate increased skeletal uptake but on occasion may be normal. The MRI of bone marrow metastasis tends to be a diffuse low-intensity signal on both T1-weighted and T2-weighted images, which may or may not enhance after administration of gadolinium (80).

CELL MARKERS

Identification of cell markers is adding to the current classification of medulloblastoma. In the past, classification schemes were based on microscopy, immunohistochemistry, and ultrastructural features. One school of thought suggests that a medulloblastoma represents a primitive, undifferentiated cell and that differentiation within the tumor suggests the presumed fate of the transformed malignant cell. Another scheme suggests that differentiation occurs any time in the life of the cell and that malignant transformation may occur independent of the stage of cytogenesis in committed as well as uncommitted cells. These views confound the ability of the neuropathologist to prognosticate on the basis of light microscopy and ultrastructural features. On the other hand, increasing knowledge of oncogene expression and monoclonal antibodies directed toward neuronal or glial elements are being used to classify and potentially stage tumors. For the most part, medulloblastomas do not react to glial antigens such as GFAP. Studies based on use of antibodies suggest that medulloblastomas may contain both neuronal and astrocytic differentiation, at times reflecting dual differentiation in the same cell, neuronal differentiation alone, astrocytic differentiation alone, or no evidence of differentiation (41,43,95). Monoclonal antibodies to a variety of markers have affirmed the observations by classical histopathologists that a complex pattern of differentiation must exist in medulloblastomas and suggests significant phenotypic heterogeneity from tumor to tumor (95).

Flow cytometry data have suggested that desmoplastic tumors are a homogeneous group of neoplasms on the basis of morphology, immunocytopathology, and DNA distribution. Unlike the more classical medulloblastoma, desmoplastic lesions are apt to be GFAP-positive, have a near diploid number and a monomodal DNA distribution, suggesting homogeneity with differentiation without evidence of heterogeneity or cycling cells. This implies that this variety of tumor is apt to have a better prognosis, although clinical experience, at best, only minimally supports these observations (47,104).

Unlike desmoplastic medulloblastomas, classical medulloblastomas are a more heterogeneous group that show a variable degree of differentiation. These tumors tend to be GFAP-negative and stain for neuronal antibodies. Flow cytometry indicates that this group of tumors may be tetraploid, triploid, or aneuploid. This, plus bimodal histograms, suggests that more cells may be cycling with DNA content somewhere between G_1 and G_2. These findings imply that diploidy and low proliferative index correlate with favorable clinical outcome, whereas features of aneuploidy or triploidy and tetraploidy suggest more aggressive behavior and a larger mitotic index (104). Conversely, Yasue et al. (119) have suggested that aneuploidy (greater than 5% change in DNA content) rather than diploidy imparts the most favorable prognosis.

Goldberg-Stern et al. (48), looking at histologic and immunohistochemical properties of 53 medulloblastomas, attempted to correlate clinical features and survival. They were unable to correlate histologic features such as mitosis, hemorrhage, necrosis, endothelial proliferation, desmoplasia, calcification, rosettes or glomerular arrangement, or oligodendroglial cells with survival. Of interest, however, 82% of their patients whose tumors stained positively for glial fibrillary acidic protein survived more than 5 years, whereas survival was 30% in those patients who were GFAP-negative.

Overexpression or amplification of n-myc, c-myc, and $erbB_1$ as well as chromosomal abnormalities such as isochromosome 17_q have been identified in medulloblastoma (24,96,116). These chromosomal abnormalities and findings of oncogene expression are of interest but unfortunately have not been consistent and have not correlated with prognosis (44). The finding of an i(17q) chromosome has led to the observation that the P53 found on the short arm of chromosome 17 may be deleted (103). This gene has also been implicated in the etiology of the Li-Fraumeni syndrome. Of some interest is the observation that the c-myc oncogene is associated with a low level of

GFAP expression, suggesting that this oncogene may in some manner be instrumental in limiting cell differentiation (7,34,43,69).

The group from Duke University has published the characteristics of several medulloblastoma cell lines that have been used to define karyotype, oncogene expression, and monoclonal antibodies directed to specific cell markers. Attempts have also been made to correlate findings in cell lines with histopathologic features of differentiation and desmoplasia. At present, the world library of published medulloblastoma lines is no more than seven, five of which have been defined at Duke University. For the most part, these lines do not express class 1 or class 2 HLA antigens, GFAP, lymphoid-associated antigens, or nerve growth factor receptors. On the other hand, they do express synaptophysin and neural filament proteins of high, low, and middle molecular weight. These characteristics are not common to all identified cell lines, as at least one reported lineage has been found to be positive for monoclonal antibodies to glial and associated antigens and HLA class 1 antigens (41–43).

Unfortunately, despite the ever increasing sophistication of monoclonal technology and the ability to map DNA content and apply molecular genetic techniques to this tumor system, little unambiguous information has been gathered. These techniques, to date, have provided a confusing and often uninterpretable array of data.

DIAGNOSTIC STUDIES

Before the advent of computerized tomography (CT), confirmation of clinical findings required invasive techniques such as air ventriculography and angiography. CT with contrast enhancement and now MRI with gadolinium have replaced all other diagnostic modalities (122) (Fig. 9-3). The MRI of medulloblastomas is characterized by low to intermediate signal on short TE. The signal is increased relative to muscle and decreased relative to white matter. On T2-weighted images with a long TR and TE, these tumors are of intermediate to moderately high signal. Signal heterogeneity may occur as a result of intratumoral cysts, small blood vessels, or calcifications. Gadolinium enhancement tends to be variable. Nonenhancing studies with gadolinium have been reported (75,93). Unlike cerebellar astrocytomas, cysts are uncommon, and unlike ependymomas, calcification is seen in less than 10% of cases. Before operation, neurosurgeons may still require angiography to obtain information concerning the blood supply to the tumor.

Polyamines have been used to assess the possible recurrence of medulloblastomas. The polyamines putrescine, spermidine, and spermine are elevated in biologic tissue characterized by high growth rate and rapid turnover. A correlation between putrescine levels and the recurrence of medulloblastomas has been described. The existence of these compounds in the cerebral

A 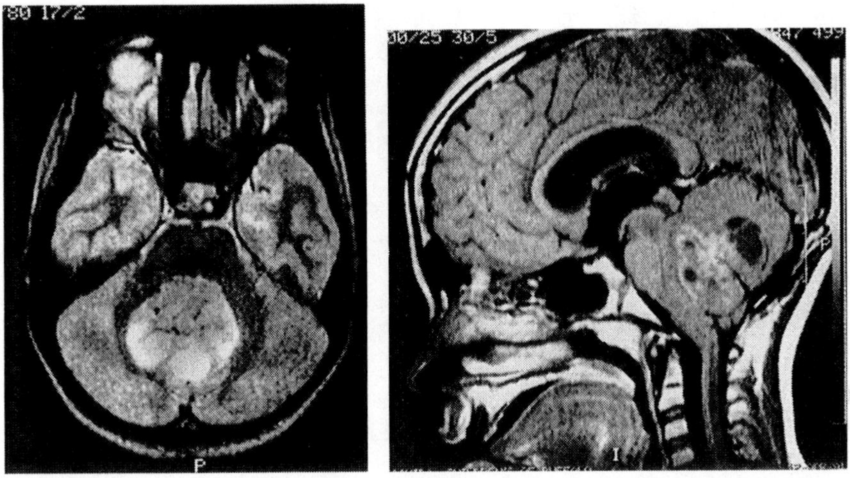 B

FIG. 9-3. Axial and sagittal MRI demonstrating large posterior fossa mass. Compatible with the pathologic diagnosis of a medulloblastoma.

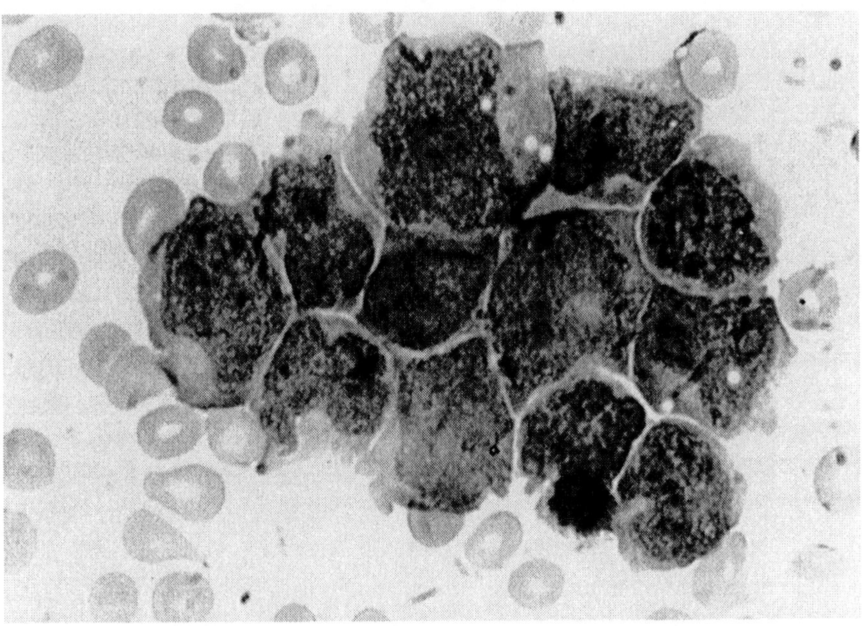

FIG. 9-4. CSF cytology of a patient with metastatic medulloblastoma. Note the large clumped cells, prominent nucleoli, and limited cytoplasm.

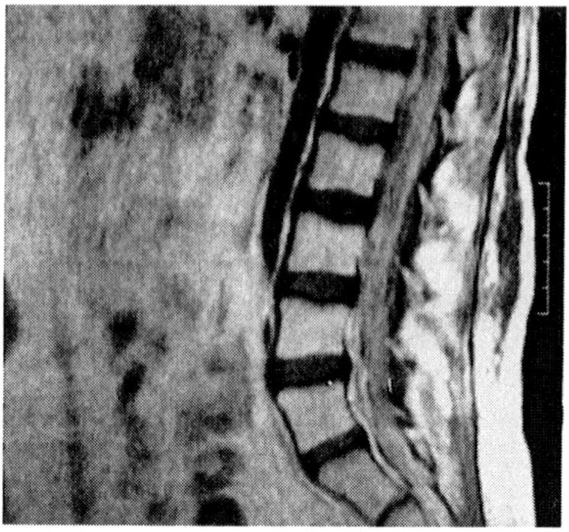

FIG. 9-5. T1-weighted MRI scan in the sagittal plane showing the entire spinal canal occluded by metastatic tumor (Chang Stage M_3).

spinal fluid (CSF) raised the possibility of making the diagnosis of recurrence prior to clinical or CT evidence of tumor (71,72). Although touted as a prognostic measurement, CSF polyamines have not proved to be an effective means of monitoring patients for tumor recurrence.

Because medulloblastomas are well known to disseminate throughout the subarachnoid space, cytologic examination of the CSF may yield malignant cells (Fig. 9-4). Unfortunately, although at times cytolopy has been positive, the low yield limits the diagnostic value of this method. In addition, the findings of malignant cells have not correlated with the extent of metastases. The most accurate means of assessing recurrence in the posterior fossa is the MRI scan with and without gadolinium enhancement. For tumor in the spinal cord, MRI with gadolinium can be exceptionally helpful and is rapidly replacing CT myelography as the procedure of choice (Fig. 9-5) (26–28).

STAGING OF TUMORS

Upon diagnosis and as a prelude to planning treatment, the tumor should be staged and the extent of local and distal involvement ascertained. Staging defines the extent of tumor spread and provides a criterion on which to base prognosis and most recently has influenced therapeutic selection.

Several studies have emphasized the need to establish the presence or absence of subarachnoid spread (28,37). Deutsch's studies (25–27) have suggested that subarachnoid dissemination at diagnosis is greatest in those under 5 years of age. Deutsch et al. and Dorwart et al. (28) have reported an incidence of 36 to 43% of tumor found on myelography but not suspected clinically. The small number of patients studied in these and other reports may

TABLE 9-1. *Chang staging of medulloblastoma as modified by Langston*

T_1	Tumor less than 3 cm in diameter
T_2	Tumor greater than or equal to 3 cm in diameter
T_{3a}	Tumor greater than 3 cm in diameter with extension into the aqueduct of Sylvius and/or into foramen of Luschka
T_{3b}	Tumor greater than 3 cm in diameter with unequivocal extension into the brain stem
T_4	Tumor greater than 3 cm in diameter with extension up past the aqueduct of Sylvius and/or down past the foramen magnum
No consideration is given to the number of structures invaded or the presence of hydrocephalus	
T_{3b} can be defined by intraoperative demonstration of tumor extension into the brain stem in the absence of radiographic evidence	
M_0	No evidence of gross subarachnoid or hematogenous metastasis
M_1	Microscopic tumor cells found in cerebrospinal fluid
M_2	Gross nodular seedings demonstrating in the cerebellar, cerebral subarachnoid space, or in the third or lateral ventricles
M_3	Gross nodular seeding in spinal subarachnoid space
M_4	Metastasis outside the cerebrospinal axis

account for the apparent high percentage of positive myelograms. The true incidence of CSF seeding may be substantially smaller.

The clinical classification by Harisiadis and Chang (49), based on the extent of tumor and the degree of metastasis in conjunction with current diagnostic methods, may provide a valuable prognostic index for predicting survival (see Table 9-1). In Chang's report, children classified as T_1, i.e., a tumor less than 3 cm and limited to the vermis, had 5- and 10-year survival rates of 75%. In those tumors classified as T_4, i.e., tumors with local extension spreading through the aqueduct, third ventricle, or midbrain, the 5-year survival rate was 0%. Where staging has been utilized, T_1 through T_{3a} and M_0 carry the best prognosis and are considered standard risk. High-risk patients are those with T_{3b} or greater tumor and M stage of one or more. Berry et al. (6), in their analysis of the Toronto experiences, found this staging system to be of limited prognostic value. Survival rates were more directly related to extent of surgical removal than to extent of tumor. Survivals of 64% are quoted for total removal, 56% for subtotal, and 33% for biopsy alone. Preliminary reports from the Children's Cancer Study Group show results similar to those by Berry et al. A report by Norris et al. (79) suggests that staging after operation may be more predictive. Staging is based on the extent of the tumor remaining postoperatively. The medulloblastoma protocol committee of the Pediatric Oncology Group has considered using a postoperative staging system. Stage I refers to a totally excised tumor with either an equivocal or negative CT scan. Stage II refers to a partially excised tumor with posterior fossa extension. Patients with Stage III tumors have extension outside the posterior fossa, but within the central nervous system. Stage IV tumors refer to extraneural metastasis (61). Because the most common site of extraneural metastases is the bone and bone marrow, appropriate staging prior to initiating therapy should also, at a minimum, include a radionuclide bone scan.

Because the validity of any staging criteria has yet to be substantiated, additional verification with more patients is necessary. Currently at our institution and at member institutions of the Pediatric Oncology Group, we are recommending assessment of spinal fluid and CT or MRI myelography 1 to 3 weeks after surgery and prior to starting radiotherapy. This should allow for more accurate staging and may provide more reliable prognostic information.

SURGERY

The treatment of medulloblastomas begins with as complete as possible operative removal of the tumor (1). The consistency of the tumor at surgery may give some clues about resectability. Cushing was one of the earliest to use the term "suckable" in describing the consistency of a medulloblastoma. He indicated that these tumors can be easily drawn into the tube of a suction apparatus, which is not true of the more rubbery astrocytomas or desmoplastic medulloblastomas. Aggressive surgery without compromising neural function not only provides definitive pathologic diagnosis and establishes CSF integrity but also should eliminate in most cases the need for intraoperative shunting, thus closing a possible portal for extraneural surgical metastasis. Although the literature suggests substantially higher operative mortality, modern techniques should permit mortality figures of less than 5%. Table 9-2 illustrates the downward trend in operative mortality since Cushing's time.

Bulk removal of the tumor is considered the first line of defense in any comprehensive therapeutic treatment program. Cushing (23) recognized the value of aggressive surgery when he stated in 1930 that "radical surgery has greatly augmented the operative mortality rate but . . . in survivors has notably prolonged the subsequent symptom free period." Because both radiation and chemotherapy destroy tissue by a log kill hypothesis, bulk re-

TABLE 9-2. *Tabulation of deaths within 1 month of surgery*

Author	Year	Deaths	Percent
Cushing (18)	1930	20/61	32
Newton et al. (77)	1968	11/35	31
Aron (2)	1971	3/20	15
Mealey and Hall (74)	1977	4/37	11
McIntosh (67)	1979	11/85	13
Mazza et al. (70)	1981	4/36	11

Note the declining mortality since Cushing's report in 1930.

moval is absolutely essential to the success of other treatment modalities. The smaller the amount of tumor left after surgery, the more likely is adjuvant therapy to be helpful.

In comparing radical removal (apparent gross total resection), subtotal removal (80% of the tumor), and partial removal and biopsy of the tumor, Raimondi and Tomita (92) found significantly different survival rates. Those patients treated with radical resection had 1-year survival rates of 92% and 5-year survival rates of 42%. Survival rates for subtotal or partial resection and/or biopsy did not differ among themselves, but were significantly lower than the survival rate for total resection, i.e., 65% survival for 1 year and 30% survival for 5 years. Understandably, depending on subsequent treatment, survival after initial surgery is apt to decline precipitously after 1 year. The influence of degree of surgical resection was supported in a study program from Toronto, Canada (6), in which a group of patients received modern radiotherapy after surgery. Five-year survivals of 64% after total resection contrasted with 5-year survivals of 56% for subtotal resection and 33% for biopsy despite similar radiotherapy. Although the need for gross total resection of medulloblastoma remains controversial, with some reports supporting and others refuting survival advantage for total resection, it is universally agreed that there is a decreased survival for patients treated with biopsy alone. Increasingly, more recent studies underscore the need for aggressive surgery (10,35). The surgical goal should be as complete a resection as possible without neurologic compromise (43,85). Postoperative mutism, pseudobulbar palsy, pseudomeningocele, and communicating hydrocephalus are all unwanted but not unexpected operative complications. Because these complications are, for the most part, self-limited and resolve, their potential occurrence should not deter aggressive debulking surgery.

RADIOTHERAPY

Assuredly, many factors influence the changing prognosis of medulloblastomas (13,66). Among others, these include aggressive surgery with attempts at total removal, better anesthesia, and the addition of chemotherapy. Despite these advances, there is an overwhelming worldwide consensus attesting to the major role of radiotherapy in extending survival rates. The switch to high-energy sources and the increased doses of radiation to the posterior fossa and neuraxis areas account for the major changes in survival. Today, virtually all authorities agree that after bulk removal, craniospinal radiation should be undertaken.

Why medulloblastomas are radiosensitive is not clear. In an effort to assess the radiosensitivity of these tumors, Weichselbaum et al. (117) reported on the radiobiology of in vitro medulloblastoma cells. Tumor tissue was explanted in monolayer cultures, characterized histologically by light and electron microscopy, and then irradiated with a 220-kV machine. Cultures were then analyzed for survival of cells. The doubling time for each of the four cell lines studied varied from 39 to 59 hours. Despite the elegance of these experiments, there was no difference between the survival curves of the medulloblastoma cells and skin fibroblasts. In addition, there were no differences in survival parameters of these cells as compared with cells from glioblastomas. These studies suggest that the radiation sensitivity of medulloblastomas may relate to in vivo factors such as tissue oxygenation and growth kinetics rather than to an inherent radiosensitivity of the neoplastic cells.

As in much of clinical medicine, the theoretical basis for a given theory may lag many years behind its application. As early as 1953, Paterson and Farr (2,86), using orthovoltage equipment, showed that radiation of the entire neuraxis might be associated with a cure of this tumor. They reported the results of treatment for 27 patients with medulloblastomas in Manchester, England, between 1941 and 1951. The brain and spinal cord were irradiated through a single posterior directed portal, which led to dose inequality. Despite this, only 8 of 22 patients had a recurrence, and 11 of 17 were alive after 3 years. This was the first report to suggest that radiation of the entire neuraxis should be undertaken in medulloblastomas. Since that time there has been a substantial change in radiation technology as well as philosophy regarding optimum dosage. Before 1965, radiation was administered by 250-kV equipment. The late 1960s and the decade of the 1970s saw a significant change in the quality of equipment. Today, radiation is delivered in megavolt quantity, with either ^{60}Co or accelerator beams with a nominal energy of no less than 4 MeV.

In 1969, Jenkin (52) compared partial and whole CNS radiation and documented the value of prophylactic craniospinal irradiation for medulloblastomas. He was the first to show that survival for those treated with whole CNS irradiation was significantly better than for those in whom the CNS was partially irradiated. Survival patterns suggest a clear reduction in recurrences for those who have had craniospinal irradiation.

Radiation dosages and schedules have altered with changes in technology. In the late 1960s, less than 4,000 cGy was considered adequate radiation to the posterior fossa, and 3,000 cGy was considered adequate to the spinal cord. Currently, recommended radiation doses are 5,000 to 5,500 cGy to the posterior fossa and 3,500 to 4,500 cGy to the neuroaxis (51). Five-year survival rates close to 80% have been reported with radiation doses of 5,000 cGy (59,65,109,112). Treatment failures and local recurrences have been related in part to local dosage schedules of less than 5,000 cGy (20). In planning radiation ports, care should be taken to include underdosed areas of the neuroaxis such as the retro-orbital and subfrontal regions, and to avoid overlap areas in the spinal cord and base of the brain.

Attention to these details has measurably increased 5-year survivals and limits to some extent the possibility of radiation necrosis (6). Five-year survivals of 20% reported in the 1960s stand in marked contrast to the 5-year survivals of 50 to 70% reported during the 1970s (56). The 1969 report by Bloom et al. (10) indicated that 40% of their patients completing therapy survived 5 years and 30% survived for 10 years. Most deaths took place in the 3 years immediately after diagnosis. As in Bloom's report, more recent studies detailing radiotherapy results are encouraging. The best results are reported in those series in which surgery has been the most extensive and radiation therapy has been completed (10,21,66). Today, even the conservative view accepts that radiation after surgery is curative in one-third of patients completing a full course of postoperative irradiation. Table 9-3 compares the 5-year and 10-year survival rates in children with medulloblastomas who completed radiotherapy. Because the concept of total craniospinal radiation with a posterior fossa boost is relatively recent, 10-year survival statistics are limited.

The medulloblastoma protocol committee of the Pediatric Oncology Group in the United States recommends the following approach to radiation. The entire CNS is to be irradiated. Treatment volume is in three parts: the brain, spinal contents, and the posterior fossa. The field for the whole brain extends anteriorly to include the frontal lobes and region of the cribriform plate, but does not include the orbit. The inferior border extends to 0.5 cm below the base of the skull. Spinal treatment volume should extend laterally on both sides so that a 1.0-cm margin exists on either side of the vertebral body. The lower border extends to the second sacral segment or the termination of the filum terminale. The inferior border of the posterior fossa boost is described as the C1–C2 interspace. The apex of the tentorium is considered to be one-half the distance from the foramen magnum to the vertex. Thus, the superior border of the posterior fossa boost is defined as 1.0 cm above the apex of the tentorium. Because the tentorium-cerebelli extends to the posterior clinoids, the anterior limit of the posterior fossa should extend to this anatomic reference point. Although an attempt is made to shield the pituitary fossa, the posterior medial half of the hypothalamus remains within the radiation points. The radiation dose to the whole brain is 4,000 cGy, with a boost of approximately 1,500 cGy to the posterior fossa. Irradiation to the spine is 3,500 cGy. The dose per fraction is not to exceed 200 cGy, and most treatment schedules are between 150 and 180 cGy per fraction. Although dosage schedules are modified for children under 2 years of age, radiation is not recommended as the initial postoperative treatment for children in this age group (see Chapter 20).

The need for doses as high as 3,600 cGy to the neuroaxis has been recently established. In the past, several reports have described tumor control in those patients with the lower Chang stages despite reduction in neuroaxis radiation to 2,400 to 2,500 cGy (64,113). However, a recent joint Pediatric

TABLE 9-3. *Five- and 10-year survival in children with medulloblastomas (after radiotherap*

Author	Year	Number of patients	% 5-year survival	% 10-ye survivа
Packer et al. (81)	1983–1988	26	96% at two years	
Bloom et al. (9)	1975–1979	286	56% CT ÷ RT 42% RT alone	
Evans et al. (35)	1975–1981	233	65	
Tarbell et al. (110)	1970–1983	50	55	
	1984–1991	39	72	
Hughes et al. (51)	1968–1984	60	68	44
Raimondi and Tomita (92)	1966–1979	51	34.5	
Tokars et al. (112)	1966–1984	9	73	
Garton et al. (45)	1965–1984	58	50	33
McIntosh (67)	1965–1969	33	3	
	1970–1974	23	48	
Chin and Maruyama (20)	1964–1976	10	80	
>5,000 rads				
<5,000 rads		9	11	
Harisiadis and Chang (49)	1963–1975	58	40	
	(T_1)[a]	5	75	31
	(T_2)	20	51	75
	(T_3)	29	32	44
	(T_4)	4	0	13
Bloom et al. (9,10)	1962–1970		18	
	1971–1974		27	
	1975–1977		38	
Mazza et al. (70)	1960–1978	37	27	
Belza et al. (5)	1959–1986	79	55	44
Berry et al. (6)	1958–1978	119	56	
	<1966	30	47	
	>1966	89	64	43
Brown et al. (13) (composite series; 3–5-year survivals)	1957–1972	34	67	
Mealey and Hall (74)	1953–1973	32	41	28
Hope-Stone (50)	1950–1962	13	77	
Aron (2)	1946–1968	14	46	
Cushing (23) (operative results)	1930	61		1.5% a yr

[a] T, tumor staging.

Oncology Group and Children's Cancer Study Group protocol randomized patients with low-risk medulloblastoma to one group receiving 24 Gy and another receiving 36 Gy neuroaxis radiation. The study was closed prematurely due to the presence of a statistically significant increase in leptomeningeal failures among those children treated with lower doses of radiation.

CHEMOTHERAPY

Although 5-year survival rates have improved dramatically, 10-year survival rates remain limited, and recurrence of medulloblastoma is invariably followed by death of the patient. It is unlikely that increasing radiation doses will improve survival. The present radiation doses are at the limits of tolerance of both the brain and the spinal cord (11,97,113). As such, the use of chemotherapy as primary adjuvant therapy or as treatment for recurrent disease is a logical consideration (70). Chemotherapeutic cures are known for several solid tumors, i.e., neuroblastoma, choriocarcinoma, Wilms' tumor, and Burkitt's lymphoma. In addition, combined treatment modalities have been highly effective in preventing, and at times eliminating, seeding of the CNS with acute lymphoblastic leukemia (22,33,111,118). Chemotherapy may be given before, after, or when radiation is used, as a radiosensitizer.

With this as background, reports began to appear in the 1960s suggesting a role for chemotherapy in the treatment of CNS neoplasia. Medulloblastomas are theoretically well suited for treatment with chemotherapy. Rapid growth rate, high mitotic index, location, and close proximity to the ventricular cavity and subarachnoid space make these tumors ideal candidates for a chemotherapeutic approach. In addition, chemotherapy has a role in the treatment of either overt or occult extraneural metastases. Reports (60,77,78,98,99,102,107) in limited numbers of patients touting the effects of intrathecal (IT) methotrexate and intravenous (IV) vincristine appeared in the mid-1960s. Since the 1970s, the alkylating agents have been an integral part of most protocols used in the treatment of CNS tumors (37,106,115,118). These drugs have a technical advantage because of their physical characteristics of low molecular weight, high lipid solubility, and lack of ionization at physiologic pH. This allows this class of agents readily to cross cell membranes, including the blood–brain barrier (108). In a 1981 Italian report (70), results of primary adjuvant chemotherapy with 1-(2-chlorethyl)3-cyclohexyl-1-nitrosourea (CCNU) alone was compared with the results of radiotherapy without adjuvant chemotherapy. Of 10 patients treated in the former group, 80% were alive after 1 year, 60% after 3 years, and 30% after 5 years. This was compared with 62%, 37%, and 25% survivals at 1, 3, and 5 years in 17 patients treated with radiotherapy alone. Although these results are substantially worse than the best series with radiotherapy, the results nonetheless suggest a positive chemotherapeutic effect. Other single agents that have been used in a limited way are actinomycin, adriamycin, cyclophosphamide, procarbazine, and VM-26 (18,39,74,97,114). Many of these have been used in the treatment of extraneural metastases and exist as case reports in one or two patients (76).

Results of combination chemotherapy regimens have been reported as early as the late 1960s. Our results (33) reported in 1979 suggested good results from a combination of IT/IV methotrexate, vincristine, BCNU, and prednisone. Because of the potential to develop leukoencephalopathy from the combination of IT/IV methotrexate and radiation, this drug combination has been abandoned. The eight-drug-in-one regimen (methylprednisone, vincristine, CCNU, procarbazine, hydroxyurea, cis-platinum, cytosine, arabinoside, and cyclophosphamide) used in a large CCSG trial showed a 50% response rate (89).

In a recent study (81,82) from the Children's Hospital of Philadelphia, 26 "high-risk" patients were treated with cis-platinum, CCNU, and vincristine. The treatment group included children less than 5 years of age at the time of diagnosis; those with partially resected or biopsied tumors; children whose tumors were disseminated at the time of diagnosis; and those who had evidence of cellular differentiation. Radiation was reduced in children between the ages of 15 months and 3 years in an effort to decrease known side effects. Ninety-five percent of these patients who are on study were alive and free of disease at a median of 24 months from the time of diagnosis. Five-year and 10-year survivals are yet to be reported.

A chemotherapy post-operative preradiation study (58) of patients with high-risk medulloblastoma was recently published. Induction therapy consisted of a 9-week course of cis-platin and vincristine followed by radiation. For those under 2 years, MOPP therapy (nitrogen mustard, vincristine, and procarbazine) was given until age 2, at which time they were referred for radiotherapy. Five of 13 with measurable disease following surgery had a definite response, and another 5 had a measurable response. Another POG pilot study (57) from St. Jude's evaluated preradiation chemotherapy using cis-platinum and VP16 in patients with newly diagnosed medulloblastomas, pineoblastomas, and cerebral neuroblastomas. All the children with medulloblastomas responded. None showed signs of progression between 8 and 48 months following diagnosis (57). Pilot studies using high-dose chemotherapy with autologous bone marrow rescue have been reported. Unfortunately, to date, there has been no selective advantage to this treatment, and toxicity has been high (38).

The largest studies evaluating the results of treatment in patients with medulloblastomas were reported in 1990 from England by the group from the Royal Marsden Hospital, the International Society of Pediatric Oncology, and the Childrens Cancer Study Group (CCSG) (10,34). Surgery and radiotherapy alone were compared with surgery, radiotherapy, and chemotherapy. The chemotherapy used in the SIOP trial was vincristine and CCNU and for the CCSG trial was CCNU, vincristine, and prednisone. Variables such as staging, age of the patient, and site of recurrence all influenced outcome. The Royal Marsden group analyzed their results in medulloblastomas from 1950 to 1981. Those completing radiotherapy had 5-year survival rates of 42%, 10-year survivals of 33%, and 15-year survivals of 29%. Total excision in 19 patients resulted in a 5-year survival of 62% compared to 41% for patients who had subtotal resection. From 1970 to 1981 38 of 53 patients had adjuvant chemotherapy. Their results were compared with the 105 patients extending over the entire length of the study who did not receive chemotherapy. Five- and 10-year survivals for the chemotherapy treated group were 65 and 56%, respectively. These results, when compared to historical controls, should be viewed circumspectly because improvements over time in surgery and radiation may bias results.

The SIOP trial was conducted between 1975 and 1979 and consisted of 286 children in 44 centers in 15 countries. CT scanning was not routinely used. Patients were not uniformly staged, and extent of resection was based on operative observations. Some centers reported their results independently. For instance, the study included an Italian report (46) in which 30 patients were evaluated for the effects of chemotherapy, 28 of 30 of whom had an actuarial survival of 28 months with a range of 13 to 56 months. Three had evidence of local recurrence. The authors did not compare their patients with the radiotherapy group, and although they suggest useful effects from the chemotherapy, the follow-up was too short for reliable assessment. Similarly, the Swiss Oncology Group (106) compared their results for 20 patients treated with CCNU, vincristine, and prednisone with the results reported by SIOP and CCSG. These results compared a group of patients receiving chemotherapy with those not receiving chemotherapy and suggested that the chemotherapy did not measurably prolong survival. When the entire International Society of Pediatric Oncology trials were analyzed as a whole, the disease-free 5-year survival was 58% for the chemotherapy arm and 48% for those receiving radiotherapy alone. This difference was not found to be statistically significant. However, in the subset containing children under 2 years of age, those undergoing subtotal or partial excision, and those with brain stem involvement, there was a significant advantage to chemotherapy. This study looked only at T staging and did not examine the effect of chemotherapy on metastatic disease (M staging).

The American Medulloblastoma trial sponsored by the Childrens Cancer Study Group and Radiation Therapy Oncology Group involved 230 children treated from June, 1975, to June, 1981. The 5-year event-free survival was 59% for children treated with radiation and chemotherapy compared with 50% for patients treated only with radiation. As in the SIOP trial, there was no statistical advantage for those treated with chemotherapy except in certain subgroups. Patients with advanced Chang staging had significantly better event-free survivals with chemotherapy. Chemotherapy toxicity was significant in that high numbers of patients developed bacterial meningitis and other infections. At times, hematologic toxicity resulted in interruption in the radiation schedules. These studies, as well as those from single institutions, demonstrate that children with low-risk medulloblastoma, i.e., those with T_1 Chang classification, do not benefit from the addition of chemotherapy. However, high-risk patients appear to benefit. Primary postoperative chemotherapy is the current recommendation for children less than 3 years old with medulloblastoma because of the severe neurotoxicity associated with radiation of the young child's nervous system as well as the poor survival with standard radiation treatment (see Chapter 20).

SUMMARY

In conclusion, although the beneficial role of chemotherapy in the treatment of medulloblastomas has yet to be firmly established, there is sufficient evidence to warrant a continued search for the appropriate drug combinations and routes of administration. Because the dosage of radiotherapy appears to be at the upper limits of tolerance, it appears unlikely that continued increase in survival will result from newer radiotherapy technology. Chemotherapy, moreover, will continue to play a role in the treatment of extraneural metastases as well as local recurrences. Unfortunately, improving survivals have been associated with increasing concerns over quality of life (Chapter 23). The rationale for the development of new and different methods of chemotherapy is the hope that radiation doses can be reduced and, in turn, the side effects on intellect and endocrine function can be diminished.

The ideal chemotherapy regimen has yet to be defined. Increasingly, stratification of patients to high- and low-risk groups will influence treatment options. The more potentially toxic therapies by design will be restricted to those patients stratified to high-risk groups, while those strategies with a wider risk:benefit ratio will be recommended for patients considered to be of low-risk. The cancer consortiums in the United States and elsewhere are continually turning to increasing dose intensity schedules, preradiation chemotherapy followed by postradiation chemotherapy, and the exploration of biologic response modifiers. Novel strategies are presently being explored by both children's cancer consortiums in the United States and other groups abroad. Future treatment options for patients with low-risk disease (i.e., T_1-T_{3a}, M_0) will likely include reduced dosage of neuroaxis radiation, possibly coupled with adjuvant chemotherapy. These concepts, in fact, are being tested in newly opened phase II and III medulloblastoma protocols in the United States. Radiation sensitizers, hyperthermia, and heavy particle-beam radiation, although having the potential of more tumor destruction, are not accompanied by increasing margins of safety. Thus, the search for effective combinations of chemotherapy with other treatment modalities of treatment must continue.

Despite the above, of all malignant brain tumors, results continue to be the most encouraging with medulloblastomas. Today, the child over 3 years of age treated with aggressive surgery, newer techniques of radiotherapy, and combination multiagent chemotherapy can reasonably expect 5-year survival rates in the 50 to 70% range. Unfortunately, 10-year survivals continue to hover between 30 and 55%. Since enough time has not elapsed to evaluate confidently the more recent studies, predictions about 10-year survivals continue to reflect results obtained from older treatment protocols.

REFERENCES

1. Albright AL, Wisoff JH, Zeltzer PM, Deutsch M, Finlay J, Hammond D. Current neurosurgical treatment of medulloblastomas in children: a report from the Children's Cancer Study Group. *Pediatr Neurosci* 1989;15:276–282.
2. Aron BS. Medulloblastoma in children: twenty-two years experience with radiation therapy. *Am J Dis Child* 1971;121:314–317.
3. Bailey P, Cushing H. Medulloblastoma cerebelli: a common type of mid-cerebellar glioma of childhood. *Arch Neur Psychiatr* 1925;14:192–224.
4. Banna M, Lassman LP, Pearce GW. Radiological study of skeletal metastases from cerebellar medulloblastoma. *Br J Radiol* 1970;43:173–179.
5. Belza MG, Donaldson SS, Steinberg GK, Cox RS, Cogen PH. Medulloblastoma: freedom from relapse longer than 8 years—a therapeutic cure? *J Neurosurg* 1991;75:575–582.
6. Berry MP, Jenkin RD, Colin MB, Keen W, Nair BD, Simpson WJ. Radiation treatment for medulloblastoma: a 21-year review. *J Neurosurg* 1981;55:43–51.
7. Bigner SH, Friedman HS, Vogelstein B, Oakes WJ, Bigner DD. Amplification of the c-myc gene in human medulloblastoma cell lines and xenografts. *Cancer Res* 1990;50: 2347–2350.
8. Bloom HJG. Intracranial tumors: response and resistance to therapeutic endeavors. *Int J Radiat Oncol Biol Phys* 1982;8:1083–1113.
9. Bloom HJG, Glees J, Bell J. The treatment and long-term prognosis of children with intracranial tumors: a study of 610 cases, 1950–1981. *Int J Radiat Oncol Biol Phys* 1990; 18:773–745.
10. Bloom, HJG, Wallace ENK, Henk JM. The treatment and prognosis of medulloblastoma in children: a study of 82 verified cases. *AJR* 1969;105:43–62.
11. Boden G. Radiation myelitis of the cervical spinal cord. *Br J Radiol* 1948;21:464–469.
12. Boyett JM, Viehi TJ. Role of clinical trials and cooperative group studies in children. *Cancer* 1985;56:1984–1986.
13. Brown RC, Gunderson L, Plenk HP. Medulloblastoma, a review of the LDS hospital experience. *Cancer* 1977;40:56–60.
14. Brutschin P, Culver GJL. Extracranial metastasis from medulloblastoma. *Radiology* 1973; 107:359–362.
15. Burger PC, Fuller GN. Pathology: trends and pitfalls in histologic diagnosis, immunopathology, and applications of oncogene research. In: Cohen ME, Duffner PK, eds. *Neurologic clinics: brain tumors in children*. Philadelphia: WB Saunders, May 1991;9(2):249–271.
16. Burger PC, Grahmann FC, Bleistle A, Kleihues P. Differentiation in the medulloblastoma: a histologic and immunologic study. *Acta Neuropathol* 1987;73:115–123.
17. Caputy AJ, McCullough DC, Manz HJ, et al. A review of the factors influencing the prognosis of medulloblastoma: the importance of cell differentiation. *J Neurosurg* 1987; 66:80–87.
18. Castro-Vita H, Salazar OM, Cova M. Cerebellar medulloblastoma: spread and failure patterns following irradiation. *Int J Radiat Oncol Biol Phys Suppl* 1979;2[Suppl]:211–212.

19. Chatty EM, Earle KM. Medulloblastoma: a report of 201 cases with emphasis on the relationship of histologic variants to survival. *Cancer* 1971;28:977–983.
20. Chin HW, Maruyama Y. Results of radiation treatment of cerebellar medulloblastoma. *Int J Radiat Oncol Biol Phys* 1981;7:737–742.
21. Collins VP. Wilms' tumor: its behavior and prognosis. *J La State Med Soc* 1955;197: 474–480.
22. Crist WM, Ragab AH, Vietti TJ, Ducos R, Chu JY. Chemotherapy of childhood medulloblastoma. *Am J Dis Child* 1976;130(6):639–642.
23. Cushing H. Experiences with cerebellar medulloblastoma: a critial review. *Acta Pathol Microbiol Scand* 1930;7:1–86.
24. Cusimano MD. An update on the cellular and molecular biology of brain tumors. *Can J Neurol Sci* 1989;16:22–27.
25. Deutsch M, Reigel DH. Myelography and cytology in the treatment of medulloblastoma. *Int J Radiat Oncol Biol Phys* 1981;7:721–725.
26. Deutsch M. Medulloblastoma: staging and treatment outcome. *Int J Radiat Oncol Biol Phys* 1988;14:1103–1107.
27. Deutsch M, Reigel DH. The value of myelography in the management of childhood medulloblastoma. *Cancer* 1980;45:2194–2197.
28. Dorwart RH, Wara WM, Norman D, Levin VA. Complete myelographic evaluation of spinal metastases from medulloblastoma. *Radiology* 1981;139:403–408.
29. Drachman DA, Winters TS III, Karon M. Medulloblastoma with extracranial metastases. *Arch Neurol* 1963;9:518–530.
30. Duffner PK, Cohen ME. Extraneural metastases in childhood brain tumors. *Ann Neurol* 1981;10:261–265.
31. Duffner PK, Cohen ME, Flannery JT. Referral patterns of childhood brain tumors in the state of Connecticut. *Cancer* 1982;50:1636–1640.
32. Duffner PK, Cohen ME, Myers MH, Heise HW. Survival of children with brain tumors: SEER Program, 1973–1980. *Neurology* 1986;36:597–601.
33. Duffner PK, Cohen ME, Thomas PRM, Sinks LF, Freeman AI. Combination chemotherapy in recurrent medulloblastoma. *Cancer* 1979;43:41–45.
34. Engelhard III HH, Butler AB, Bauer KD. Quantification of the c-myc oncoprotein in human glioblastoma cells and tumor tissue. *J Neurosurg* 1989;71:224–232.
35. Evans AE, Jenkin RDT, Sposto R, et al. The treatment of medulloblastoma. *J Neurosurg* 1990;72:572–582.
36. Farwell JR, Dohrman GJ, Flannery JT. Central nervous system tumors in children. *Cancer* 1977;40:3123–3132.
37. Fewer D, Wilson CB, Baldrey E, Enab KJ, Powell MR. The chemotherapy of brain tumors: clinical experience with BCNU and vincristine. *JAMA* 1972;222:549–552.
38. Finlay JL. High-dose chemotherapy followed by bone marrow rescue for recurrent brain tumors. In: Packer RJ, Bleyer WA, Pochedly C, eds. *Pediatric neurooncology*. Philadelphia: Hardwood Academic Publishers; 1992:278–297.
39. Flannery AM, Tomita T, Radkowski M, McLone DG. Medulloblastomas in childhood: postsurgical evaluation with myelography and cerebrospinal fluid cytology. *J Neurooncol* 1990;8:149–151.
40. Friedman HS, Burger PC, Bigner SH, et al. Establishment and characterization of the human medulloblastoma cell line and transplantable xenograft D283 MED. *J Neuropathol Exp Neurol* 1985;44:592–605.
41. Friedman HS, Oakes WJ. Recurrent brain tumors in children. *Pediatr Neurosci* 1987;13: 233–241.
42. Friedman HS, Burger PC, Bigner SH, et al. Phenotypic and genotypic analysis of human medulloblastoma cell line and transplantable xenograft (D341 MED) demonstrating amplifications of c-myc. *Am J Pathol* 1988;130:472–484.
43. Friedman HS, Oakes WJ, Bigner SH, Wikstrand CJ, Bigner DD. Medulloblastoma: tumor biological and clinical perspectives. *J Neurooncol* 1991;11:1–15.
44. Fujimoto M, Sheridan PJ, Sharp D, et al. Proto-oncogene analyses in brain tumors. *J Neurosurg* 1989;70:910–915.
45. Garton GR, Schomberg PJ, Scheithauer BW, et al. Medulloblastoma—prognostic factors and outcome of treatment: review of the Mayo Clinic experience. *Mayo Clin Proc* 1990; 65:1077–1086.

46. Gerosa MS, di Stefano E, Olivi A, Carteri A. Multidisciplinary treatment of medulloblastoma: a 5-year experience with the SIOP trial. *Childs Brain* 1981;8:107–118.
47. Giangaspero F, Chieco P, Ceccarelli C, et al. "Desmoplastic" versus "classic" medulloblastoma: comparison of DNA content, histopathology, and differentiation. *Virchows Archiv [A]* 1991;418:207–214.
48. Goldberg-Stern H, Gadoth N, Stern S, Cohen IJ, Zaizov R, Sandbank U. The prognostic significance of glial fibrillary acidic protein staining in medulloblastoma. *Cancer* 1991;68: 568–573.
49. Harisiadis L, Chang CH. Medulloblastoma in children: a correlation between staging and results of treatment. *Int J Radiat Oncol Biol Phys* 1977;2:833–841.
50. Hope-Stone HF. Results of treatment of medulloblastomas. *J Neurosurg* 1970;32:83–88.
51. Hughes EN, Shillito J, Sallan SE, Loeffler JS, Cassady JR, Tarbell NJ. Medulloblastoma at the Joint Center for Radiation Therapy between 1968 and 1984. *Cancer* 1988;61:1992–1998.
52. Jenkin RDT. Medulloblastoma in childhood: radiation therapy. *Can Med Assoc J* 1969; 100:51–53.
53. Jereb B, Sundaresan N, Horten B, Reid A, Galicich JH. Supratentorial recurrences in medulloblastoma. *Cancer* 1981;47:806–809.
54. Kleihues P, Burger PC, Scheithauer RW. In: Sobin L, ed. *Histologic typing of tumors of the central nervous system.* New York: Springer-Verlag; 1992.
55. Kleinman GM, Hochberg FH, Richardson EP. Systemic metastasis from medulloblastoma: report of two cases and review of the literature. *Cancer* 1981 48:2296–2309.
56. Kopelson G, Linggood RM, Kleinman GM. Medulloblastoma in adults: improved survival with supervoltage radiation therapy. *Cancer* 1982;49:1334–1337.
57. Kovnar EH, Kellie SJ, Horowitz ME, et al. Preirradiation cisplatin and etoposide in the treatment of high-risk medulloblastoma and other malignant embryonal tumors of the central nervous system: a phase II study. *J Clin Oncol* 1990;8:330–336.
58. Kretschmar CS, Tarbell NJ, Kupsky W, et al. Pre-irradiation chemotherapy for infants and children with medulloblastoma: a preliminary report. *J Neurosurg* 1989;71:820–825.
59. Landberg TG, Lindgren ML, Cavallin-Stahl EK, et al. Improvements in the radiotherapy of medulloblastoma 1946–1975. *Cancer* 1980;45:670–678.
60. Lassman LP, Pearce GW, Gang J. Sensitivity of intracranial gliomas to vincristine sulfate. *Lancet* 1965;1:296–297.
61. Laurent JP, Chang CM, Cohen ME. A classification system for primitive neuroectodermal tumors (medulloblastoma of the posterior fossa). *Cancer* 1985;56:1807–1809.
62. Lefkowitz IB, Packer RJ, Ryan SG, et al. Late recurrence of primitive neuroectodermal tumor/medulloblastoma. *Cancer* 1988;62:826–830.
63. Lefkowitz IB, Packer RJ, Siegel KR, Sutton LN, Schut L, Evans AE. Results of treatment of children with recurrent medulloblastoma/primitive neuroectodermal tumors with lomustine, cisplatin, and vincristine. *Cancer* 1990;65:412–417.
64. Levin VA, Rodriguez LA, Edwards MSB, et al. Treatment of medulloblastoma with procarbazine, hydroxyurea, and reduced radiation doses to whole brain and spine. *J Neurosurg* 1988;68:383–387.
65. Lowery GS, Ferree CR, Raben M. Medulloblastoma: treatment results with radiation therapy. *South Med J* 1981;74:1047–1049.
66. McFarland DR, Horwitz H, Saenger EL, Bahr G. Medulloblastoma: a review of prognosis and survival. *Br J Radiol* 1969;42:198–214.
67. McIntosh N. Medulloblastoma:. a changing prognosis. *Arch Dis Child* 1979;54:200–203.
68. McLendon RE, Burger PC. The primitive neuroectodermal tumor: a cautionary view. *J Pediatr Neurosci* 1987;3:1–8.
69. MacGregor DN, Ziff, EB. Elevated c-myc expression in childhood medulloblastomas. *Pediatr Res* 1990;28:63–68.
70. Mazza C, Pasqualin A, DaPian R, Donati E. Treatment of medulloblastoma in children: long term results following surgery, radiotherapy and chemotherapy. *Acta Neurochir* 1981; 57:163–175.
71. Marton LS, Edwards MS, Levin MA, Lubich WP, Wilson CB. CSF polyamine: a new and important means of monitoring medulloblastoma. *Cancer* 1981;47:757–760.
72. Marton LS, Edwards MS, Levin VA, Lubich WP, Wilson CB. Predictive value of cerebral spinal fluid polyamines in medulloblastoma. *Cancer Res* 1979;39:993–997.

73. Matsumoto T, Tani E, Kaba K, et al. Amplification and expression of a multidrug resistance gene in human glioma cell lines. *J Neurosurg* 1990;72:96–101.
74. Mealey J, Hall PV. Medulloblastoma in children. *J Neurosurg* 1977;46:56–64.
75. Meyers SP, Kemp SS, Tarr RW. MR imaging features of medulloblastomas. *AJR* 1992; 158:859–865.
76. Nathanson L, Kovacs SG. Chemotherapeutic response in metastatic medulloblastoma: report of two cases and a review of literature. *Med Pediatr Oncol* 1978;4:105–110.
77. Newton WA, Sayers MP, Samuels LD. Intrathecal methotrexate therapy for brain tumors in children. *Cancer Chemother Rep* 1968;52:257–261.
78. Norrell H, Wilson CB. Brain tumor chemotherapy with methotrexate given intrathecally. *JAMA* 1967;201:15–17.
79. Norris DG, Bruce DA, Byrd RL, et al. Improved relapse-free survival in medulloblastoma utilizing modern techniques. *Neurosurgery* 1981;9:661–664.
80. Olson EM, Tien RD, Chamberlain MC. Osseous metastasis in medulloblastoma: MRI findings in an unusual case. *Clin Imaging* 1991;15:286–289.
81. Packer RJ, Siegel KR, Sutton LN, et al. Efficacy of adjuvant chemotherapy for patients with poor-risk medulloblastoma: a preliminary report. *Ann Neurol* 1988;24;503–508.
82. Packer RJ, Sutton LN, D'Angio G, et al. Management of children with primitive neuroectodermal tumors of the posterior fossa/medulloblastoma. *Pediatr Neurosci* 1986;12: 272–282.
83. Packer RJ, Sutton LN, Rorke LB, et al: Prognostic importance of cellular differentiation in medulloblastoma of childhood. *J Neurosurg* 1984;61:296–301.
84. Palmer JO, Kasselberg AG, Netsky MG. Differentiation of medulloblastoma: studies including immunohistochemical localization of flial fibrillary acidic protein. *J Neurosurg* 1981;55:161–169.
85. Parks TS, Hoffman JN, Hendrich EB, et al. Medulloblastoma, clinical presentation and management; experience at the Hospital for Sick Children, Toronto, 1950–1980. *J Neurosurg* 1983;58:543–552.
86. Paterson R, Farr RF. Cerebellar medulloblastoma: treatment by irradiation of the whole central nervous system. *Acta Radiol* 1953;39:323–336.
87. Pearl GS, Takei Y. Cerebellar "neuroblastoma:" nosology as it relates to medulloblastoma. *Cancer* 1981;47:772–779.
88. Pearson ADJ, Craft AW, Ratcliffe JM, et al. Two families with the Li-Fraumeni cancer family syndrome. *J Med Genet* 1982;19:362–365.
89. Pendergrass TW, Milstein JM, Geyer JE, et al. Eight-drugs-in-one-day chemotherapy for brain tumors; experience in 107 children and rationale for preradiation chemotherapy. *J Clin Oncol* 1987;5:1221–1231.
90. Quest DO, Brisman R, Antunes JL, Housepian EM. Period of risk for recurrence in medulloblastoma. *J Neurosurg* 1978;48:159–163.
91. Raimondi AJ, Mullan S, Evans JP. Human brain tumors: an electron microscopic study. *J Neurosurg* 1962;19:731–753.
92. Raimondi AJ, Tomita T. Medulloblastoma in childhood. *Acta Neurochir* 1979;50:127–138.
93. Rollins N, Mendelsohn D, Mulne A, et al. Recurrent medulloblastoma: frequency of tumor enhancement on Gd-DTPA MR imaging. *AJNR* 1990;11:583–587.
94. Rorke LB. The cerebellar medulloblastoma and its relationship to primitive neuroectodermal tumors. *J Neuropathol Exp Neurol* 1983;42:1–15.
95. Rorke LB, Molenaar WM, Trojanowski JQ. Advances in diagnosis and basic science. I: The impact of monoclonal antibody studies on changing nosology and biological concepts of brain tumors. In: Packer RJ, Bleyer WA, Pochedly C, eds. *Pediatric neuro-oncology: new trends in clinical research.* vol 3. Philadelphia: Harwood Academic Publishers; 1992: 8–32.
96. Rouah E, Wilson DR, Armstrong DL, Darlington GJ. N-myc amplification and neuronal differentiation in human primitive neuroectodermal tumors of the central nervous system. *Cancer Res* 1989;49:1797–1801.
97. Rubin P, Casarett GU, eds. Central nervous system. In: *Clinical radiation pathology.* vol 2. Philadelphia: WB Saunders, 1968;609–661.
98. Rubin R, Owens E, Rall D. Transport of methotrexate by the choroid plexus. *Cancer Res* 1968;28:689–694.

99. Rubinstein LJ, Herman MM, Hanbery JW. The relationship between differentiating medulloblastoma and dedifferentiating diffuse cerebellar astrocytoma: light electron microscopic tissue and organ culture observations. *Cancer* 1974;33:675–690.
100. Rubinstein LJ. *Tumors of the central nervous system*. Washington, DC: Armed Forces Institute of Pathology; 1972:127–153.
101. Rubinstein LJ, Northfield DWC. The medulloblastoma and the so-called arachnoid cerebellar sarcoma: a clinical re-examination of a nosological problem. *Brain* 1964;87:379–412.
102. Sayers MD, Newton WA Jr, Samuels LD. Intrathecal methotrexate of brain tumors in childhood. *Ann NY Acad Sci* 1969;159:608–613.
103. Saylors RL III, Sidranski D. Friedman HS, et al. Infrequent p53 gene mutations in medulloblastomas. *Cancer Res* 1991;51:4721–4723.
104. Schofield DE, Yunis EJ, Geyer JR, Albright AL, Berger MS, Taylor SR. DNA content and other prognostic features in childhood medulloblastoma: proposal of a scoring system. *Cancer* 1992;69:1307–1314.
105. Shuster J, Hart Z, Stimson CW, et al. Ataxia telangiectasia with cerebellar tumor. *Pediatrics* 1966;37:776–786.
106. Seiler RW, Bernasconi S, Berchtold W, et al. Adjuvant chemotherapy with procarbazine, vincristine and prednisone for medulloblastomas. *Helv Paediatr Acta* 1981;36:249–254.
107. Selawry OS, Hananian J. Vincristine treatment of cancer in children. *JAMA* 1963;183: 741–746.
108. Shapiro WR. Chemotherapy of primary malignant brain tumors in children. *Cancer* 1975; 35:965–972.
109. Smith CE, Long DM, Jones TK, Levitt SH. Medulloblastoma: an analysis of time–dose relationships and recurrence patterns. *Cancer* 1973;32:722–728.
110. Tarbell NJ, Loeffler JS, Silver B, et al. The change in patterns of relapse in medulloblastoma. *Cancer* 1991;68:1600–1604.
111. Thomas P, Duffner PK, Cohen ME, Sinks LF, Tebbi C, Freeman AI. Multimodality therapy for medulloblastoma. *Cancer* 1980;45:666–669.
112. Tokars RP, Sutton HG, Griem ML. Cerebellar medulloblastoma: results of a new method of radiation treatment. *Cancer* 1979;43:129–136.
113. Verity GL. Tissue tolerance: central nervous system. *Radiology* 1968;91:1221–1225.
114. Walker RW, Allen JC. Cisplatin in the treatment of recurrent childhood primary brain tumors. *J Clin Oncol* 1988;6:62–66.
115. Ward HWC. CCNU in treatment of recurrent medulloblastoma. *Br Med J* 1974;1:642.
116. Wasson JC, Saylors RL III, Zeltzer P, et al. Oncogene amplification in pediatric brain tumors. *Cancer Res* 1990;50:2987–2990.
117. Weichselbaum RR, Liszczak TM, Phillips JP, Little JB, Epstein J, Kornblith PL. Characterization and radiobiologic parameters of medulloblastoma in vitro. *Cancer* 1977;40: 1087–1096.
118. Wilson CB. Medulloblastomas: current views regarding the tumor and its treatment. *Oncology* 1970;24:273–290.
119. Yasue M, Tomita T, Englehardt H, et al. Prognostic importance of DNA ploidy in medulloblastoma of childhood. *J Neurosurg* 1989;70:385–391.
120. Yates PO. Tumors of the central nervous system in children. *J Clin Pathol* 1964;17: 418–423.
121. Young JL, Miller W. Incidence of malignant tumors in U.S. children. *J Pediatr* 1975;86: 254–258.
122. Zimmerman RA, Bilaniuk L, Pahlajanl H. Spectrum of medulloblastoma demonstrated by computed tomography. *Radiology* 1978;126:137–141.

10

Cerebellar Astrocytomas

Cerebellar astrocytomas represent approximately 11% of brain tumors in children less than 18 years of age (43). They are the second most common tumor of the cerebellum in children and comprise approximately one-third of childhood posterior fossa tumors (18,31,43). Their peak incidence is in the latter half of the first decade, with a second peak in the first half of the second decade. There is no clear sex preference.

As early as 1926, Bailey and Cushing (4) recognized that patients with astrocytomas of the cerebellum had a longer postoperative survival than patients with astrocytomas in other locations. In 1931, Cushing (14) reported on his experience with 76 cases of cerebellar astrocytomas. As in early reports, he differentiated them from cerebral astrocytomas and stressed their favorable postoperative prognosis. However, he did not discuss microscopic differences from astrocytomas located in the cerebrum. Bergstrand (46), in 1937, reported detailed microscopic anatomy of these tumors, and named them "gliocytoma embryonale" because of his impression that the cerebellar astrocytoma was a congenital malformation of the cerebellar leptomeninges. Later pathologists have not supported Bergstrand's concept of a congenital malformation and have considered the cerebellar astrocytoma a true neoplasm.

Cerebellar astrocytomas may occur anywhere in the cerebellum, and may involve the vermis, the hemispheres, or both regions simultaneously. Occasionally they may be present largely within the cavity of the fourth ventricle. Although Cushing stressed their primarily midline location in the cerebellum, many of his cases had a midline mural nodule, with a large cyst extending into one lateral hemisphere (14). Similarly, 50% of the tumors in the series by Ringertz and Nordenstam (46) were purely midline, whereas 17.2% were lateral, and 32.1% were hemispheric as well as midline. Other authors have found that approximately 50% of cerebellar astrocytomas are predominantly hemispheric in location (7,16,45). Thus, the popular concept that cerebellar astrocytomas are primarily hemispheric tumors is not valid.

Overall, approximately 80% of cerebellar astrocytomas are cystic (29). Several authors have found that hemispheric tumors are more often cystic, whereas solid tumors are more commonly located in the vermis (8,24,46). As tumors of the vermis have been reported to have a higher operative

Brain Tumors in Children: Principles of Diagnosis and Treatment, 2/e, edited by M.E. Cohen and P.K. Duffner, Raven Press, Ltd., New York, 1994.

mortality, location in some series has influenced prognosis (29). However, if postoperative deaths are excluded, at least one series suggests that midline cerebellar astrocytomas have the best results (16).

PATHOLOGY

Cerebellar astrocytomas are generally well circumscribed, demarcated from surrounding tissue, and noninvasive. They may consist of a large cyst with a solid mural nodule or may be largely solid with smaller cysts throughout the substance of the tumor (Fig. 10-1). The wall of the cyst may be poorly cellular, contain reactive nonneoplastic tissue, or have an ependymal ventricular lining. Occasionally, the cyst may be fringed by tumor growth (28). The cyst cavity contains yellow or brown fluid, which is highly coagulable and has a high protein content. In one study, 78.6% of 111 tumors contained large cysts. Of these, 51% had the appearance of a large cyst with a solid mural nodule (46). It was Cushing who showed that the mural nodule represents the only neoplastic element in these tumors. Cerebellar astrocytomas are generally avascular, although at times the mural nodule may be hemorrhagic. Gross calcification has been reported in as many as 25% of the cases. Twenty percent of cerebellar astrocytomas are mainly solid on

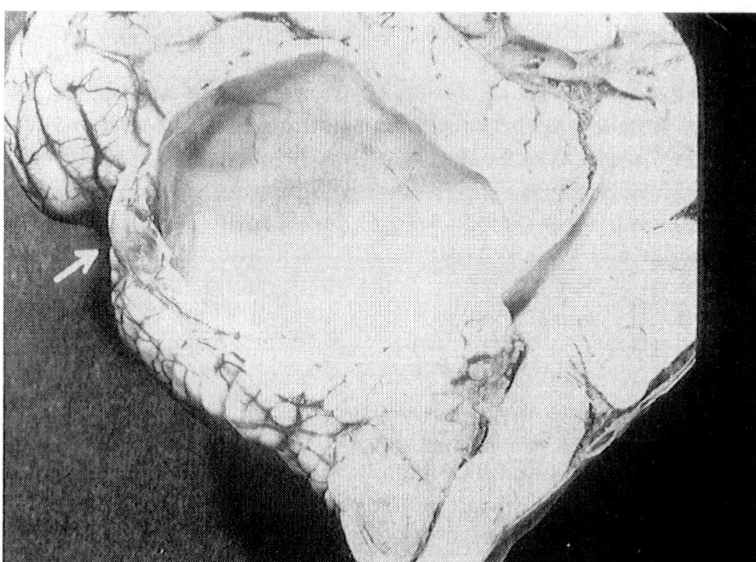

FIG. 10-1. Gross pathology of a large hemispheric cystic cerebellar astrocytoma. The *arrow* points to the mural nodule.

inspection of gross pathology and are similar to those found in the cerebral hemispheres.

Russell and Rubinstein (48) describe two distinct histologic types of cerebellar astrocytomas. The most common form consists of areas of compact, strongly fibrillated cells, which are often fusiform or polar in appearance, alternating with areas that are loose, spongy, and composed largely of microcysts. At times, the microcysts can coalesce into larger cysts. Compact areas are generally devoid of microcysts but contain an abundance of Rosenthal fibers. Rosenthal fibers are eosinophilic, beaded, or cigar-shaped swellings of astrocytes and are thought to represent a benign degenerative change. The spongy areas consist of sparse nonfibrillated stellate astrocytes often arranged around small cavities (47). It is in these areas that microcystic degeneration is frequently encountered (Fig. 10-2). The second, less frequent type, found in approximately 15 to 20% of the total, is the diffuse form of cerebellar astrocytoma (48). This tumor is identical with its counterpart in the cerebral hemispheres. The tumor consists of fibrillated stellate or piloid cells, and microcysts are rare.

Oligodendroglial cells may be found in both types of cerebellar astrocytomas. Microscopic calcification is present in 13 to 26% of cases, and is more common in cerebellar astrocytomas than in medulloblastomas (42,48). The most common microscopic pattern of calcification is characterized by small

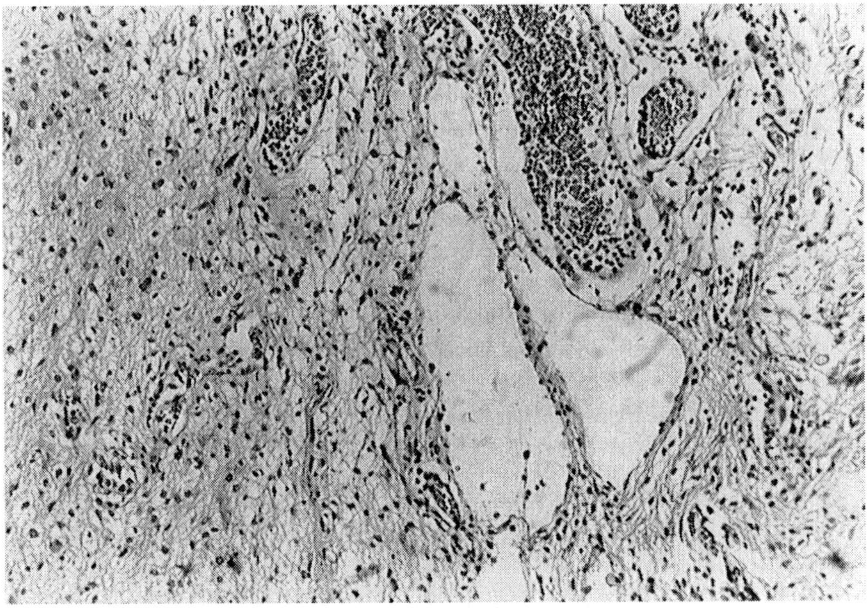

FIG. 10-2. Microscopic appearance of cystic cerebellar astrocytoma. Note the loose stroma and multiple microcysts. Anaplastic features are lacking.

globules or calcospherites within the adventitia or media of smaller vessels and within the endothelium of the capillaries (42). Ultimately, the vessels may become entirely calcified. The presence of calcification has no correlation with survival.

Invasion of the leptomeninges with tumor is common and has been reported in 55% of one series. Vascular endothelial hyperplasia may be present in as many as 15% of cases. Of importance, Rubinstein (47) has pointed out that the presence of multinucleated giant cells, nuclear hyperchromasia, and vascular endothelial proliferation does not impart a malignant potential to the tumors. However, mitoses are conspicuously absent, and when present malignancy should be suspected.

Attempts have been made to correlate the microscopic appearance of cerebellar astrocytomas with prognosis. In 1978, Gjerris and Klinken (27) reviewed 44 children with cerebellar astrocytomas. They divided the patients into two groups on the basis of microscopic anatomy: (a) the classic juvenile cerebellar astrocytoma, as described by Russell and Rubinstein, and (b) the diffuse astrocytoma. The juvenile cerebellar astrocytoma consists of compact areas of strongly fibrillated fusiform cells alternating with loose areas of nonfibrillated stellate astrocytes with microcysts. The "diffuse" type has equal distribution of glial fibrils, uniform cells, and small, evenly dispersed cavities. Seventy percent of their patients had "juvenile astrocytomas," and 30% were found to be "diffuse." The diffuse form was found more often in the older age group, i.e., 10 to 14 years of age, whereas the juvenile form was found in 88% of children with cerebellar astrocytomas less than 10 years of age. Children with the juvenile type had a 25-year cumulative survival of 94% compared with 38% for the diffuse type. Of interest, the macroscopic appearance of the tumor (cystic versus solid) had no correlation with survivals.

Gilles et al. (22,26,39) have also studied cerebellar gliomas in an attempt to define prognostic microscopic features. Their studies do not restrict themselves to traditional cerebellar astrocytomas, but rather include any glioma of the cerebellum. Therefore, ependymomas, glioblastomas, and other gliomas of the cerebellum are included in their categorization. (It should be emphasized that medulloblastomas are not included in this grouping.) Various factors have been identified which distinguish good from poor prognosis (59). Glioma A tumors contain any of the following four microscopic findings: (a) microcysts, (b) leptomeningeal deposits, (c) Rosenthal fibers, or (d) oligodendroglia (cluster A). The 10-year survival of patients with these pathologic findings is 94%. Glioma B tumors contain (a) perivascular pseudorosettes; (b) one or more of the following features: high cell density, necrosis, mitosis; or (c) calcification (cluster B). The 10-year survival for this group is 29%. The prognostic significance of the individual factors varies in these clusters. For example, patients with perivascular pseudorosettes, or at least two other factors of cluster B, will have a high mortality. If they have only one factor from cluster B, then mortality is lower. Cysts were found in 69.6% of glioma A and 23% of glioma B. Ten-year survivals for patients with cysts were 85%, suggesting a good prognosis. These findings are in contrast to those of Gjerris and Klinken, who found that the presence of cysts had no prognostic value for survival. Similar to the findings of Russell and Rubinstein, pleomorphism, endothelial proliferation, and hypervascularity did not influence survival.

The influence of histology on prognosis was analyzed at the Medical College of Wisconsin. Conway et al. (13,59), using the Gilles classification of glioma type A and B, found that patients with glioma type A had 5-year survivals of 100% compared with patients in the glioma type B category, in whom the 5-year survival was 41%. Progression-free survival was also different, as children with glioma type A had progression-free survivals of 66% compared with glioma type B, in which there was a 0% progression-free survival. Patients with glioma type B tumors had both a higher incidence of disease progression and also accounted for all deaths in the study. Recent articles have opted for the Gjerris and Klinken classification of the juvenile versus the diffuse astrocytoma rather than the Gilles categories of glioma type A and B. Gjerris and Klinken objected to the Gilles classification because patients were not followed long enough to identify late recurrences. Indeed, Gjerris and Klinken suggest that their classification of juvenile and diffuse astrocytoma falls into the subtype of type A gliomas. Ten-year survivals for type A gliomas are 94%, for juvenile astrocytomas 98%, and for diffuse astrocytomas 78%. By 15 years, the diffuse astrocytoma has a 70% survival, but by 25 years there is only a 38% survival, whereas the juvenile astrocytomas remain relatively recurrence-free. It appears that the juvenile pattern of astrocytoma in the absence of high cell density, necrosis, and mitosis is associated with the best long-term prognosis. Alternatively, type B gliomas and the diffuse type of cerebellar astrocytoma are associated with the highest recurrence rate (Table 10-1).

Whereas there has been debate regarding the prognostic significance of histology and macroscopic appearance, there is uniformity of opinion that patients with brain stem invasion and age less than 4 to 5 years are associated with early recurrence and poor survival (23,55,57). Of interest, early recurrence relates to both the degree of surgical resection and diffuse type of pathology, but late recurrence does not appear to have any relationship to either histologic grouping or extent of initial surgery (15).

True glioblastoma multiforme of the cerebellum is unusual in any age group and distinctly so in children. As of 1988, there were only 21 reports of primary malignant astrocytomas of the cerebellum in children less than 15 years of age, including 13 glioblastoma, one gliosarcoma, and seven malignant astrocytomas (25). The mean age is approximately 8 years, and there is no sex predominance. The majority of primary malignant astrocytomas are located in the cerebellar hemispheres, in contrast to benign cerebellar astrocytomas in which midline location can be found in as many as 50% of cases. The histopathology

TABLE 10-1. *Prognostic indicators in cerebellar astrocytomas*

	Glioma A	Glioma B	Juvenile	Diffuse
Criteria for diagnosis	All cerebellar tumors have one or more of the following: (1) Microcysts (2) Rosenthal fibers (3) Leptomeningeal deposits (4) Focus of olidodendroglia	All cerebellar tumors with either: (1) One or more perivascular pseudorosettes (2) Two or more of the following: (a) Necrosis (b) High cell density (c) Mitosis (3) Calcification in the absence of any glioma A features	Compact area of fibrillated fusiform cells alternated with loose areas	Equal distribution of glial fibrils, uniform cells
Initial surgery (GTR)[a]	80%	27%	94%	77%
Macrocysts	69.6%	23.3%	81%	69%
Age diagnosis	5 years (median)	3 years (median)	0–4 yr 35% 5–9 yr 39% 10–14 yr 26%	0–4 yr 15% 5–9 yr 8% 10–14 yr 77%
10-year survival	94%	29%	98%	78%
25-year survival	—	—	94%	38%

Glioma A and glioma B from Gilles et al. (26).
Juvenile and diffuse from Gjerris and Klinken (27).
[a] GTR, gross total resection.

of glioblastoma multiforme is the same regardless of location (21,40,56). Malignancy may be difficult to judge because endothelial hyperplasia, nuclear atypia, and giant cells, when found in cerebellar tumors, do not necessarily connote malignancy. Frequent mitoses, necrosis, and dense cellularity are necessary for the diagnosis of a malignant astrocytoma in the cerebellum.

Rarely, benign cerebellar astrocytomas may dedifferentiate into a more malignant variety. There have been eight reports to date of malignant transformation of well differentiated or pilocytic astrocytomas. The interval from initial diagnosis to malignant recurrence ranges from 7 to 48 years, with most occurring after 20 years (1,5,9,35,52,58). In all but one reported case, patients had been treated with postoperative radiation. Whether this evolution from benign to malignant pathology was due to dedifferentiation of the initial tumor or secondary to radiation-induced oncogenesis cannot be determined. The interval from radiation to malignant transformation fits quite well with other reported cases of second tumors following cranial irradiation. The third possibility, i.e., the development of a second tumor unrelated to either the primary neoplasm or radiation therapy, appears least likely.

SIGNS AND SYMPTOMS

The clinical presentation of the child with a cerebellar astrocytoma was well described by Cushing in 1931 (14):

> A child apparently normal in all respects begins toward the end of the first decade, possibly after a fall or an attack of whooping cough to have early morning headaches and vomiting. Nothing much is made of this by the family doctor, should he be called in, for the child subsequently feels perfectly well, has had breakfast, and wants to go out and play. This daily performance may continue for a considerable time, the child even going to school meanwhile. There may then be a remission of weeks, or perhaps months, and the episode be forgotten. On their re-occurrence, the symptoms are likely to be more pronounced and are apt to be ascribed to some gastrointestinal disturbance. This appears the more probable since the child finds that straining at stool brings on a headache and there is a tendency to become constipated. What is more, a mild daily laxative usually serves to completely mask the symptoms.
>
> This sort of thing continues off and on until it becomes evident that the child is a little clumsy at play and is knocked over easily. Very possibly, before this, the periodic headache and vomiting will have ceased completely or at least to have occurred at much longer intervals; and if parents are observant, they may notice that the child's head in the interim has increased in size more rapidly than it should. This, however, is usually discounted for the child meanwhile has become free from complaints and in all respects appears alert and well. Matters may run in this way for an indefinite time, possibly with some increase in clumsiness of movement or in some instances with no noticeable change whatever until it suddenly becomes apparent, perhaps at school, that the child's sight is poor. To counteract this, glasses are usually prescribed; but even should ophthalmoscope be resorted to, the child's retina is less easily examined than that of an adult, and, because of the decompressive effects of the enlarging head, the optic papillae often show no measurable swelling and the fact of their being pale and with margins blurred may easily pass unrecognized.
>
> Due to the insidious nature of the symptomatic onset, it is in this preamaurotic stage of the process that even today the victims of these midcerebellar astrocytomas unfortunately continue to be admitted to hospitals.

The major complaints of children with cerebellar astrocytomas are caused by increased intracranial pressure. Headache and vomiting are the most common initial presenting symptoms (24,42). Vomiting associated with a cerebellar tumor generally occurs in the morning and may be unassociated with nausea (43). Because the symptom is intermittent, the child may undergo gastrointestinal evaluation before the correct diagnosis is made. Non-focal symptoms are followed in frequency by gait disturbances. Presenting symptoms may predict the location of the tumor. The child with the more midline tumor will present with truncal ataxia, whereas children with tumors located in the cerebellar hemispheres will have appendicular signs (29). Patients may be apathetic, irritable, and complain of stiffness or pain in the neck. Attacks of unconsciousness, so-called "cerebellar fits," were present in 11% in one series (28). Rarely, patients may present with subarachnoid hemorrhage (20).

The duration of symptoms may vary from days to years. Eighty percent of the children have symptoms for 2 years or less (46). Children with midcerebellar tumors have a slightly shorter mean duration of symptoms than those with hemispheric tumors (15.8 months versus 18 months) (29). In comparison, children with medulloblastomas have a mean duration of symptoms before diagnosis of only 5 months. There is a longer duration of symptoms before diagnosis in adolescents and young adults, whereas the history is shorter in younger children.

Papilledema, gait ataxia with or without arm drift, and dysmetria are the most common presenting physical signs. The correlation of tumor location with lateralization of dysmetria on finger-to-nose and heel-to-shin maneuvers is usually high (24). Coarse nystagmus to the side of the lesion is of localizing value and must be distinguished from vestibular nystagmus, which is directed to the contralateral side of involvement (28). Head tilt away from the lesion is rare, but when present, correlates well with the side of the lesion (29). The presence of a sixth nerve palsy may be a false localizing sign indicative of increased intracranial pressure or may suggest invasion of the brain stem by tumor. In general, hyperreflexia and Babinski responses suggest tumor extension into the brain stem.

It should be stressed that some patients present with few or no complaints and on examination may have evidence of only papilledema. Sometimes their healthy appearance belies a massive cerebellar tumor. Cushing (14) described them as children who are "apt to be well nourished, placid, friendly, cooperative children who quickly become ward pets."

DIAGNOSIS

The presence of a cystic cerebellar astrocytoma is easily demonstrated on CT scan (Figs. 10-3 and 10-4). Tumor cysts have a high protein content and thus may be differentiated from arachnoid cysts and postoperative defects. MRI is also able to differentiate CSF from abnormal cyst fluid because the protein content is apt to be significantly elevated in the tumor cyst, imparting to the MRI different signal characteristics than CSF (41). The sagittal view readily depicts the anatomical location of the tumor. Contrast enhancement on CT may be present in those cystic lesions that are lined with tumor. This is of important clinical significance because there is no enhancement in cysts lined with nonneoplastic tissue. Mural tumor nodules have been shown in some series to have marked contrast enhancement. In solid cerebellar astrocytomas, the CT scan will demonstrate slightly decreased density and uniform enhancement. Medulloblastomas, on the other hand, will enhance uniformly but will have increased density. Ependymomas are of variable density and enhancement and may contain calcium. Thus the presence of a low-density mass, typically in the cerebellar hemispheres often with a cystic component, is suggestive of a cerebellar astrocytoma. Furthermore, the presence of an enhancing nodule adjacent to a cyst is compelling evidence of a cystic astrocytoma (34). Although the presence of calcification on CT scan is not pathognomonic of cerebellar astrocytomas, it is present in approximately 10% of cases (34).

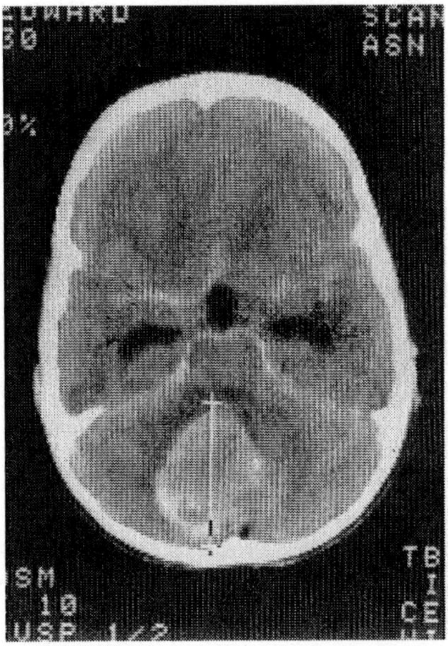

FIG. 10-3. Axial CT scan of a 5-year-old child with a diffuse cerebellar astrocytoma.

CT scans are also of value in identifying recurrent tumors. Because cyst fluid has increased density relative to CSF in a postoperative defect, differentiation of a cystic lesion from a CSF collection is possible. Alterations in the anatomy of the cerebellar pontine angle, perimesencephalic cisterns, and fourth ventricle may signify recurrent tumor (60). Schneider (51) has reported that contrast enhancement at the edge of the resection may develop on CT scan after an interval of approximately 5 months. The significance of this delayed enhancement is unclear. None of the children described in his study

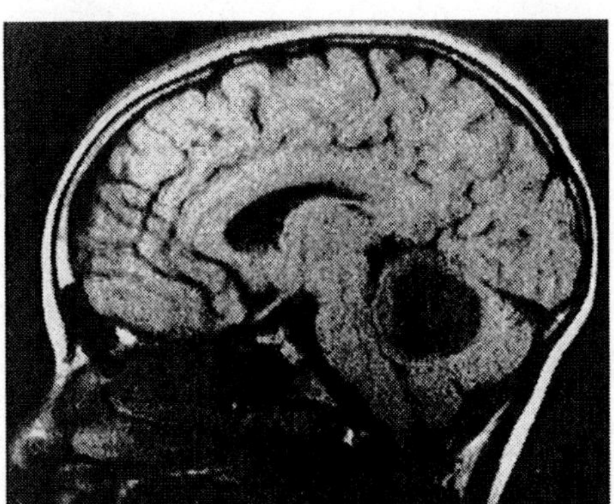

FIG. 10-4. Sagittal MRI of a 13-year-old boy with a history of ataxia and vomiting. The scan reveals a 4-cm primarily cystic mass occupying the superior cerebellar vermis and extending into the cerebellar hemisphere. Brain stem is displaced anteriorly and the aqueduct is compressed.

went on to develop tumor recurrence (mean follow-up, 5 years). In three patients, the enhancement eventually disappeared. Recurrence, therefore, should be identified only when the initial area of enhancement increases on serial scans (15).

TREATMENT

Surgery

> Not all gliomas are highly malignant, many are slow growing and favorable for surgical removal. (Harvey Cushing, 1930)

Cushing (14) operated on 76 cerebellar astrocytomas before 1931. During his first 15 years of surgical experience with these tumors, the goal was removal of the large cyst. Cushing initially did not recognize that the mural nodule represented the neoplastic elements of the tumor, and without removal of the nodule, the cyst would recur. Once the neoplastic nature of the nodule was identified, Cushing's results improved dramatically. Early surgical mortality was high. However today, with improved surgical techniques, less than a 5% operative mortality can be expected. Preoperative shunting is controversial. Some neurosurgeons (32) believe the shunt will stabilize the patient and decompress the ventricles, relax the brain, and permit surgery under the most optimal conditions. Others (17), however, believe the risk of upward herniation after ventricular shunting outweighs this advantage.

The goal of surgery is complete removal of the tumor. If achieved, gross total resection, without further therapy, will offer a nearly 100% 5-year survival (19,30,32,38,54). Although several series documented recurrence following total resection, most of these reports relied on the surgeon's opinion that a total resection had been achieved. Schneider et al. (51) studied patients with a "gross total resection" with CT scans, with and without contrast, within 3 days following surgery. They found that the surgeon was a poor predictor of the degree of surgical resection. Thus it is probable that many cases of recurrence following "gross total resection" occurred in patients who had only been subtotally resected. Another factor that may account for recurrence in the face of a gross total resection has been failure to excise the cyst wall. Although removal of the mural nodule is usually sufficient, Burger and others (3) have suggested that in those tumors in which there is an enhancing cyst wall, the wall of the cyst as well as the nodule must be removed. At the very least, the cyst wall should be biopsied to determine whether it is lined by neoplastic tissue and, if present, should be removed in toto (51). The most important factor limiting gross total resection of tumor is brain stem invasion. It is recommended that a scan be done within 3 to 4 days following surgery to confirm the degree of surgical resection. If residual tumor is present, other than in the brain stem, reoperation should be considered.

Recurrence is much more common after subtotal resection. Since the pathology of the local recurrence is typically identical to the histology of the original tumor, repeat surgery may offer a cure. In some cases, subtotal resection without further treatment has been associated with prolonged survivals (23). It has been theorized that in these cases, cell loss may equal or exceed cell production (3). Aggressive surgical intervention may not be associated with major morbidity, as removal of the cerebellar cortex rarely gives rise to serious cerebellar dysfunction. Only when the central cerebellar nuclei, the efferent tracts in the superior cerebellar peduncle, or the afferent cerebellar pathways in the brain stem are damaged is cerebellar dysfunction significant (7).

Radiotherapy

The role of radiotherapy in the treatment of cerebellar astrocytomas has been questioned. Since cure can be achieved in most cases with surgery alone, patients with gross total resection do not require radiation therapy. However, it is clear that children with subtotal resections have significantly worse progression-free survivals than children who have had gross total resections. Cushing reported a 29% progression-free survival at 5 years in subtotally resected patients; and, more recently, Griffin (30) reported a 36% progression-free survival in a similar group of children. Overall survivals are still good in the subtotally resected patients but are less than those achieved with gross total resection. Analysis of the role of radiation in subtotally resected tumors is limited by the lack of prospective studies. For example, a retrospective review of children who had received radiation following subtotal resection was reported by Garcia (23). Although his conclusion was that patients did not benefit from postoperative radiation, the studies extended from 1928 to 1980, thus severely limiting meaningful interpretation of the efficacy of modern-day radiation therapy. Even in this study, although radiation did not significantly increase survival of children with subtotal resection, progression-free survival was longer with postoperative radiation. Griffin (30) also evaluated the role of radiation therapy in children with cystic cerebellar astrocytomas who had undergone a subtotal resection. The relapse-free survival was 36% compared with those who had received postoperative radiation for both primary and recurrent disease, who had a relapse-free survival of 83%. These encouraging results were muted by Austin's (3) review of three radiation series. He found no statistically significant difference in the incidence of either early or late recurrence in children who had received postoperative radiation. The Pediatric Oncology Group and the

Children's Cancer Group, in response to these radiation questions, have mounted a two-arm study in which children greater than 5 years of age with subtotally resected cerebellar astrocytomas are given either local radiation or supportive care. The investigators hope to determine both the efficacy and neurotoxicity of radiation for this population of patients.

Results of the Pediatric Oncology Group/Children's Cancer Group study will not be forthcoming for several years. In the meantime, the currently accepted approach to children with cerebellar astrocytomas, both juvenile and diffuse, is the following. A gross total resection, when possible, should be sought. In such patients, further treatment is unnecessary. Patients should be followed closely for the first 3 to 4 years because this is the highest period of risk of recurrence. Although late recurrences occur in only 4% of patients, long-term follow-up is necessary. In those children with a subtotal or partial resection, repeat surgery is recommended if it can be performed without causing irreparable neurologic dysfunction. In those patients in whom there are contraindications to repeat surgery or in whom brain stem invasion is present, the patient can either be followed longitudinally or committed to radiation treatment. If children have evidence of recurrence, reoperation to achieve gross total resection is recommended. If this is not possible, repeat surgery should be followed by radiation consisting of 5,000 to 6,000 cGy to the tumor volume with a margin of 2 to 3 cm (37). In infants and very young children, however, radiation is not recommended as the first line of treatment at recurrence. In those patients in whom repeat surgery is not possible, chemotherapy may be an alternative approach. Although the literature on chemotherapy in cerebellar astrocytomas is extremely limited, information will be forthcoming in the future: the new Pediatric Oncology Group infant brain tumor study (vincristine, Cytoxan, cis-platinum, VP16) includes children with recurrent low-grade astrocytomas. Although less aggressive chemotherapy, as has been used in the optic glioma trial (carboplatinum), is an appealing approach, there is currently no information regarding efficacy in cerebellar astrocytomas.

Earlier literature suggested that cerebellar astrocytomas do not seed the CSF pathways. More recently, seeding through the CSF with metastatic implants has been reported even in histologically benign tumors. In one study of three cases, the tumors were in the vermis or paraventricular portion of the cerebellum and thus had access to the CSF. Although metastatic, the implants behaved in an indolent manner and appeared to respond to aggressive surgical intervention (53). Auer et al. (2) reported a histologically benign cerebellar astrocytoma with massive craniospinal leptomeningeal spread before surgical intervention. The tumor encased the brain and spinal cord at the time of autopsy. These cases, however, are sufficiently unusual so that routine spinal irradiation is not recommended. Extraneural metastases have also been reported. Brust et al. (6) reported one child with a malignant astrocytoma of the vermis who had extraneural metastases to the pleura and lymph nodes. Another author (33) reported local recurrence of a benign tumor with invasion of the musculature, soft tissues, and lymph nodes of the neck.

Children with glioblastoma of the cerebellum are at far greater risk for early death than children with low-grade cerebellar astrocytomas. Consequently, therapy will differ. Although radiotherapy is universally recommended after surgical removal, the volume of radiation has been debated. Salazar and Rubin (50) reported 13 children with glioblastomas of the cerebellum. Six children were treated with cranial irradiation alone and had a median survival of 10 months. In contrast, 7 patients were treated with craniospinal irradiation and had a median survival of 48 months. By 3 years, the survivals were significantly different, $p < 0.005$. The dose of radiation employed was 5,000 to 5,500 cGy to the cranium and 3,000 to 3,600 cGy to the spinal cord. Although the main pattern of failure was local recurrence, Salazar and Rubin stressed the development of spinal subarachnoid seeding in 5 of 6 patients treated only with cranial irradiation. None of those patients treated with craniospinal irradiation developed spinal metastases. Furthermore, 2 of 4 patients treated with local radiotherapy to the tumor bed alone developed supratentorial spread. Consequently, these authors (49) recommend full craniospinal irradiation for children and adults with glioblastomas of the cerebellum. Kopelson (36) agrees that local regional invasion, with involvement of the brain stem, adjacent leptomeninges, and soft tissues of the operative site and upper cervical spinal cord is common with glioblastomas of the cerebellum. However, in his study of 8 patients, none demonstrated evidence of subarachnoid spread. Thus Kopelson recommends only local regional radiation to the posterior fossa and adjacent areas. Chamberlain et al. (12) reported failures at the primary site concurrent with leptomeningeal and supratentorial metastases in 28% of cases. Since failure either occurred simultaneously at both the primary site and the leptomeninges or failure could be attributed to inadequate local radiation, they, like Kopelson, use high-dose limited-field irradiation to the primary tumor. Because glioblastoma of the cerebellum is an unusual tumor, especially in children, resolution of the value of craniospinal versus local radiation has not been forthcoming.

Although there is limited experience in the use of chemotherapy for this tumor type, it is now generally accepted that children less than 3 or 4 years of age with progressive disease should receive chemotherapy rather than be commited to the toxic effects of cranial irradiation (37).

SUMMARY

Cerebellar astrocytomas have the best prognosis of any intracranial tumor in childhood. Patients present with signs of increased intracranial pressure and, depending on location, have a midline cerebellar syndrome or more lateralized cerebellar dysfunction. The tumors develop in a slightly older age group than medulloblastomas and occur with approximately equal frequency. Children with cerebellar astrocytomas have a longer duration of symptoms before diagnosis than children with medulloblastomas. The majority of cerebellar astrocytomas have either a large cyst with a solid mural nodule or multiple smaller cysts. Overall, 18 to 20% of the tumors will be solid in nature. Microscopic pathology suggests that the juvenile type of cerebellar astrocytoma carries a better prognosis for long-term survival than the diffuse type. The preferred treatment for cerebellar astrocytomas is complete surgical removal of the tumor. Although removal of the cyst will prolong survival, cure only occurs on removal of the mural nodule. In cases of partial resection, reoperation is recommended. If complete surgical removal is impossible due to invasion of the brain stem or postoperative complications, radiation to the tumor bed should be considered. The necessity for postoperative radiation in partially resected tumors awaits future cooperative group studies.

REFERENCES

1. Alpers CE, Davis RL, Wilson CB. Persistence and late malignant transformation of childhood cerebellar astrocytoma. *J Neurosurg* 1982;57:548–551.
2. Auer RN, Rice GPA, Hinton GG, Amacher AL, Gilbert JJ. Cerebellar astrocytoma with benign histology and malignant clinical course. *J Neurosurg* 1981; 54:128–132.
3. Austin EJ, Alvord EC Jr. Recurrences of cerebellar astrocytomas: a violation of Collins' law. *J Neurosurg* 1988;68:41–47.
4. Bailey P, Cushing H. *A classification of the tumors of the glioma group*. Philadelphia: Lippincott, 1926.
5. Bernell WR, Kepes JJ, Seitz EP. Late malignant recurrence of childhood cerebellar astrocytoma: report of two cases. *J Neurosurg* 1972;37:470–474.
6. Brust JCM, Moiel RH, Rosenberg, RN. Glial tumor metastases through a ventriculo-pleural shunt: resultant massive pleural effusion. *Arch Neurol* 1968;18:649–653.
7. Bucy PC, Gustafson WA. Structure, nature, and classification of cerebellar astrocytomas. *Am J Cancer* 1939;35:327–353.
8. Bucy PC, Thieman PW. Astrocytomas of the cerebellum: a study of a series of patients operated upon over 28 years ago. *Arch Neurol* 1968;18:14–19.
9. Budka H. Partially resected and irradiated cerebellar astrocytoma of childhood: malignant evolution after 28 years. *Acta Neurochir* 1975;32:139–146.
10. Butler AR, Horii SC, Kricheff II, Shannon MB, Budzilovich GN. Computed tomography in astrocytomas. *Radiology* 1978;129:433–439.
11. Carmel PW. Cerebellar tumors in childhood. *Dev Med Child Neurol* 1972;14:809–811.
12. Chamberlain MC, Silver P, Levin VA. Poorly differentiated gliomas of the cerebellum: a study of 18 patients. *Cancer* 1990;65:337–340.
13. Conway PD, Oechler HW, Kun LE, Murray KJ. Importance of histologic condition and treatment of pediatric cerebellar astrocytoma. *Cancer* 1991;67:2772–2775.
14. Cushing H. Experiences with the cerebellar astrocytomas: a critical review of seventy-six cases. *Surg Gynecol Obstet* 1931;52:129–191.
15. Davis CH, Joglekar VM. Cerebellar astrocytomas in children and young adults. *J Neurol Neurosurg Psychiatr* 1981;44:820–828.
16. Elvidge AR. Long-term survival in the astrocytoma series. *J Neurosurg* 1968;28:399–404.
17. Epstein F, Murali R. Pediatric posterior fossa tumors: hazards of the preoperative shunt. *Neurosurgery* 1978;3:348–350.

18. Farwell JR, Dohrmann GJ, Flannery JT. Central nervous system tumors in children. *Cancer* 1977;40:3123–3132.
19. Fazekas JT. Treatment of grades I and II brain astrocytomas: the role of radiotherapy. *Int J Radiat Oncol Biol Phys* 1977;2:661–666.
20. Fogelson MH, Oppenheim RE, McLaurin RL. Childhood cerebellar astrocytomas presenting with hemorrhage. *Neurology* 1980;30:669–670.
21. Fresh CB, Takei Y, O'Brien MS. Cerebellar glioblastoma in childhood: a case report. *J Neurosurg* 1976;45:705–708.
22. Fulchiero A, Winston K, Leviton A, Gilles FH. Secular trends of cerebellar gliomas in children. *J Natl Cancer Inst* 1977;58:839–843.
23. Garcia DM, Latifi HR, Simpson JR, Picker S. Astrocytomas of the cerebellum in children. *J Neurosurg* 1989;71:661–664.
24. Geissinger JD, Bucy PC. Astrocytomas of the cerebellum in children: long term study. *Arch Neurol* 1971;24:125–135.
25. Georges PM, Noterman J, Flament-Durand J. Glioblastoma of the cerebellum in children and adolescents: case report and review of the literature. *J Neurooncol* 1983;1:275–278.
26. Gilles FH, Winston J, Fulchiero A, Leviton A. Histologic features and observational variation in cerebellar gliomas in children. *J Natl Cancer Inst* 1977;58:175–181.
27. Gjerris F, Klinken L. Long-term prognosis in children with benign cerebellar astrocytoma. *J Neurosurg* 1978;49:179–184.
28. Gol A. Cerebellar astrocytomas in children. *Am J Dis Child* 1963;106:21–24.
29. Gol A, McKissock W. The cerebellar astrocytomas: a report on 98 verified cases. *J Neurosurg* 1959;16:287–296.
30. Griffin TW, Beaufait D, Blasko JC. Cystic cerebellar astrocytomas in childhood. *Cancer* 1979;44:276–280.
31. Heiskanen O. Intracranial tumors of children. *Childs Brain* 1977;3:69–78.
32. Hendrick EB, Hoffman HJ, Humphreys RP. Treatment of infratentorial gliomas in childhood. *Recent Results Cancer Res* 1975;51:102–106.
33. Kepes JJ, Lewis RC, Vergara GG. Cerebellar astrocytoma invading the musculature and soft tissues of the neck: case report. *J Neurosurg* 1980;52:414–418.
34. Kendall BE. The CT scanner in posterior fossa tumors of childhood. *Br J Radiol* 1979;52:769–776.
35. Kleinman GM, Schoene WC, Walshe TM III, Richardson EP. Malignant transformation in benign cerebellar astrocytoma. *J Neurosurg* 1978;49:111–118.
36. Kopelson G. Cerebellar glioblastoma. *Cancer* 1982;50:308–311.
37. Larson DA, Wara WM, Edwards MSB. Management of childhood cerebellar astrocytoma. *Int J Radiat Oncol Biol Phys* 1989;18:971–973.
38. Leibel SA, Sheline GE, Wara WM, Boldrey EB, Nielsen SL. The role of radiation therapy in the treatment of astrocytomas. *Cancer* 1975;35:1551–1557.
39. Leviton A, Fulchiero A, Gilles FH, Winston K. Survival states of children with cerebellar gliomas. *J Neurosurg* 1978;48:29–33.
40. Luccarelli G. Glioblastoma multiforme of the cerebellum: description of 3 cases. *Acta Neurochir* 1980;53:107–116.
41. Maravilla KR, Sory WC. Magnetic resonance imaging of brain tumors. *Semin Neurol* 1986;6:33–42.
42. Martin F, Lemmen LJ. Calcification in intracranial neoplasm. *Am J Pathol* 1952;28:1107–1118.
43. Matson DD: Cerebellar astrocytoma in childhood. *Pediatrics* 1956;18:150–158.
44. Mervis B, Lotz J, Handler LC, Wright M. Computed tomography of infratentorial masses in children. *S Afr Med J* 1979;56:47–49.
45. Obrador S, Blazquez MG. Benign cystic tumors of the cerebellum. *Acta Neurochir* 1975;32:55–68.
46. Ringertz N, Nordenstam H. Cerebellar astrocytoma. *J Neuropathol Exp Neurol* 1951;10:343–367.
47. Rubinstein LJ. In Firminger HI, ed. *Tumors of the central nervous system*. Washington, DC: Armed Forces Institute of Pathology; 1972:32–34.
48. Russell DS, Rubinstein LJ. *Pathology of tumors of the nervous system*. Baltimore: Williams and Wilkins; 1989:152–157.

49. Salazar OM. Primary malignant cerebellar astrocytomas in children: a signal for postoperative craniospinal irradiation. *Int J Radiat Oncol Biol Phys* 1981;7:1661–1665.
50. Salazar OM, Rubin P. The spread of glioblastoma multiforme as a determining factor in the radiation treated volume. *Int J Radiat Oncol Biol Phys* 1976;1:627–637.
51. Schneider JH, Raffel C, McComb JG. Benign cerebellar astrocytomas of childhood. *Neurosurgery* 1992;30:58–63.
52. Schwartz AM, Ghatak NR. Malignant transformation of benign cerebellar astrocytoma. *Cancer* 1990;65:333–336.
53. Shapiro K, Shulman J. Spinal cord seeding from cerebellar astrocytomas. *Childs Brain* 1976;2:177–186.
54. Shin KH, Webster JG. Astrocytoma in children. *J Can Assoc Radiol* 1979;30:167–169.
55. Szenasy J, Slowik F. Prognosis of benign cerebellar astrocytomas in children. *Childs Brain* 1983;10:39–47.
56. Tibbs PA, Mortara RH. Primary glioblastoma multiforme of the cerebellum: a case report. *Acta Neurochir* 1980;52:13–18.
57. Undjian S, Marinov M, Georgiev K. Long-term follow-up after surgical treatment of cerebellar astrocytomas in 100 children. *Childs Nerv Syst* 1989;5:99–101.
58. Ushio Y, Arita N, Yoshimine T, Ikeda T, Mogami H. Malignant recurrence of childhood cerebellar astrocytoma: case report. *Neurosurgery* 1987;21:251–255.
59. Winston J, Gilles FH, Fulchiero A. Cerebellar gliomas in children. *J Natl Cancer Inst* 1987; 58:833–838.
60. Zimmerman RA, Bilaniuk LT, Bruno L, Rosenstock J. Computed tomography of cerebellar astrocytoma. *AJR* 1978;130:929–933.

11
Ependymomas

The pathologic entity of ependymoma was first described by Bailey (1) in 1924. He critically reviewed previous reports of "ependymal gliomas" and divided the tumors into ependymomas and ependymoblastomas on the basis of the degree of differentiation of the tumor cells. In 1937 Kernohan and Fletcher-Kernohan (28) further subdivided ependymomas on the basis of cytologic architecture into epithelial, myxopapillary, and cellular types. However, because this histologic variability did not predict biologic behavior, ependymomas were later subdivided on the basis of degree of anaplasia. In this classification, the grade of malignancy was correlated with postoperative survival time (38).

Ependymomas constitute approximately 6% of all intracranial tumors in children and adults (46). In the SEER registry series of 1,200 children aged 0 to 18 years, with brain tumors, 10% were diagnosed as having ependymomas. The mean age of diagnosis is 5 to 6 years, with approximately 60% less than 5 years of age, and only 4% greater than 15 years of age at the time of diagnosis (11). The mean age of children with fourth ventricular ependymomas tends to be younger than the age of children with ependymomas in other locations (2,66). The overall ratio of males to females is nearly 1, although a male predominance has been suggested with supratentorial ependymomas (1.4:1) (11) (also see Chapter 21).

LOCATION

Intracranial ependymomas may arise in relation to any part of the ventricular system. Of 455 intracranial ependymal tumors reported in a combined series, 151 (33%) were supratentorial, and 304 (67%) were infratentorial (2,11, 29,32,44,58,66). One study (11) in children suggested that malignant ependymomas were more frequently supratentorial (81% versus 19%), whereas low-grade ependymomas were more likely to be found in the posterior fossa (61% versus 39%).

Infratentorial tumors arise from the roof, floor, or lateral recesses of the fourth ventricle. The tumor may occlude the ventricle and extend cephalad to the aqueduct, caudad through the foramen magnum into the upper cervical spinal cord, or through the foramina around the brain stem and into the

Brain Tumors in Children: Principles of Diagnosis and Treatment, 2/e, edited by M.E. Cohen and P.K. Duffner, Raven Press, Ltd., New York, 1994.

cerebellar pontine angle. In the last location, the tumor may fill the posterior fossa without actually encroaching upon the lumen of the fourth ventricle.

Supratentorial ependymomas are presumed to arise from the ependymal lining of the lateral and third ventricles, and may be either entirely intraventricular or partially intraventricular and partially extraventricular. However, they may be found anywhere within the cerebral hemispheres and may be entirely extraventricular. In such cases, they are presumed to arise from ependymal cell rests, possibly the result of a malformation in the infolding of the neural tube (71). The tumors have a predilection for the frontal, temporal, and parietal lobes, and the third ventricle (71).

PATHOLOGY

Macroscopic

Ependymomas are usually well-defined and homogeneous. The tumors may be extensively cystic (71). One study (10) reported the presence of large cysts in supratentorial tumors, whereas small multiple cysts were present in infratentorial tumors. Cysts may be present in all grades of tumor, and solid tumor may occasionally line the cyst wall. Gross calcification may be found in ependymomas, regardless of location or degree of malignancy (71). Tumors of the fourth ventricle tend to extend dorsally and laterally and surround the medulla and upper cervical spinal cord (56).

Microscopic

In the nonneoplastic state, ependymal cells may assume various morphologic formations. Rosettes, cells grouped about a central lumen, will form if the ependymal cells are dislocated and no longer able to form surface epithelium. Alternatively, the cells may form solid clusters. These formations may be seen posteriorly in the occipital horns or near the atrium of the ventricles. Cilia and blepharoplasts are normally found along the free edges of the ependymal cell when it coats the surface of the ventricle. If these cells are no longer on the surface of the ventricle, then cilia are lost and blepharoplasts cluster near the nucleus.

Low-grade ependymomas are cellular tumors with a regular histologic pattern. Nuclei are regular, round, or slightly ovoid, and cell bodies are polygonal or fusiform. Cilia may be present. Blepharoplasts, the basal bodies of cilia, are found along the free borders of the ependymal cells and may be demonstrated by phosphotungstic acid hematoxylin (PTAH) stains (11). Tumor cells may be fibrillated. Ependymal rosettes are diagnostic and consist of tumor cells lined around a small central lumen (Fig. 11-1). Perivascular pseudorosettes are seen even more commonly than ependymal rosettes.

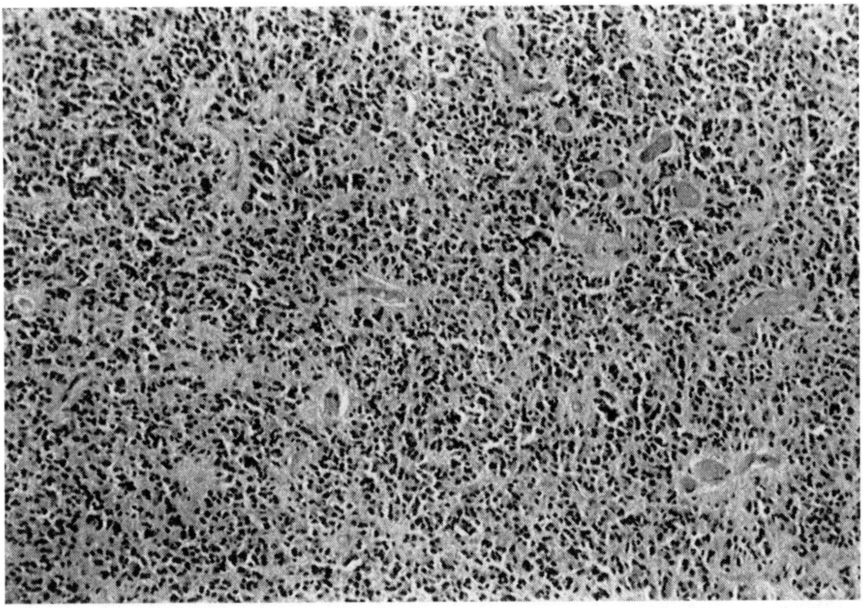

FIG. 11-1. Cellular tumor composed of neoplastic ependymal cells which typically form perivascular rosettes. Neoplastic elements are arranged around blood vessels, leaving a nuclear-free zone adjacent to the vascular channel (H & E).

Pseudorosettes consist of radiating, tapering processes of tumor cells oriented toward the blood vessel wall, with the nucleated body of the cell remote from the vessel (56). Rarer microscopic findings are the presence of papillary structures in which the cells form papillae and tubules. Cartilage may be present in some tumors of the fourth ventricle (55). Cells indistinguishable from oligodendroglia may be found in 39% of ependymomas. Indeed, some sections of the tumor may be more characteristic of oligodendrogliomas than ependymomas (60). Likewise, areas resembling astrocytomas are often seen (33,34).

Ependymomas have been grouped according to microscopic criteria into the cellular, epithelial, and myxopapillary or papillary groups (28). The cellular group of ependymomas describes tumors in which the bulk consists of compact masses of ependymal cells; processes are few but large. Although pseudorosettes are frequently found, neuroglial fibrils are not present. The epithelial group of ependymomas is characterized by cells growing side by side similar to cuboidal or columnar epithelium. Pseudorosettes and true rosettes are common in this type. The cells are not ciliated but may contain broad processes, and neurofibrils are not present. The third type is the myxopapillary or papillary group of ependymomas typically found in the cauda equina. Ependymal cells are cuboidal in type with a process attached to the papilla. Mucus is formed as the core of the papilla undergoes varying degrees of degeneration. This tumor has a much better prognosis than the other histologic types.

A four-grade classification was developed by Mabon et al. (38) in 1949 in an effort to judge malignancy. In this classification, grade I tumors reveal no evidence of anaplasia as characterized by pleomorphism, hyperchromatism, or mitotic figures. In grade II tumors, although the majority of the cells appear to be normal ependymocytes, the remaining cells have early anaplastic transformation. However, mitotic figures are not present. Grade III tumors are characterized by a fragmentary architectural pattern. Approximately half the cells show evidence of pleomorphism of the cytoplasm and nuclei. Mitotic figures and hyperchromatism of nuclei are also present. Grade IV tumors are generally disorganized and have few normal-appearing ependymal cells. The cells show evidence of pleomorphic cytoplasm and nuclei, hyperchromatic nuclei, and abundant mitotic figures.

Today, most neuropathologists recognize two grades rather than four, i.e., the benign or differentiated ependymoma and the malignant or anaplastic ependymoma. Malignant, high-grade, or anaplastic ependymomas have typical features of ependymomas but in addition have pleomorphism, necrosis, increased cellularity, mitoses, multinucleation, and giant cells. Histologically, the tumor appears to be dedifferentiating toward glioblastoma multiforme. High-grade neoplasms of the type described above are more commonly located in the supratentorial regions. Not all studies have identified the anaplastic variants as having a worse prognosis than the differentiated variety (53). This discrepancy may relate in part to disagreements among pathologists about the definitions of the various grades of this lesion. Schiffer et al. (61) attempted to correlate histologic characteristics of ependymomas with prognosis. Endothelial hyperplasia, vessel glomeruli, and necrosis were not meaningful for the diagnosis of anaplasia. The two most important histologic factors associated with prognosis in supratentorial ependymomas were increased cell density and increased number of mitoses (61). Several cooperative group studies are underway using strict histologic criteria to determine the effect of histology on prognosis in children with ependymomas.

There has been a great deal of confusion in the literature over the use of the term "ependymoblastoma," because the designation has been used interchangeably with "malignant ependymoma" by some authors. Although malignant, the ependymoblastoma (unlike the malignant ependymoma) is an extremely unusual tumor of primitive origin with characteristic microscopic features (54). Thus, "malignant ependymoma" and "ependymoblastoma" are not the same tumor, and these terms should not be used synonymously. Rather, ependymoblastomas are considered part of the wider category of embryonal tumors and will not be addressed specifically in this chapter (see Chapter 19).

The value of immunohistological phenotypes is being explored. Although generally considered a marker for astrocytes, GFAP may be present in ependymomas. Preliminary results suggest that the presence of GFAP is associated with a good prognosis, whereas vimentin is seen in more anaplastic lesions. Thus, a high GFAP: vimentin ratio is considered to carry a good prognosis (16).

SUBEPENDYMOMA

The subependymoma is a variant of the ependymoma in which the fibrillary subependymal astrocyte is the dominant cell. The tumors may arise in the fourth ventricle, septum pellucidum, and cervical cord. They appear as a sparsely cellular astrocytoma intermixed with ependymal cells. Blepharoplasts may be present. The tumors are usually incidental findings at the time of autopsy, and only rarely do they assume clinical significance. However, Scheithauer (60) reported a series of 21 tumors with clinical symptomatology secondary to obstructive hydrocephalus. The tumors were found arising in the septum pellucidum, the floor of the fourth ventricle, and the lateral ventricular walls. The large tumors were found to have cysts, microcalcification, and vessel degeneration with hemorrhage. A subgroup was composed of an admixture of classic subependymoma and features of a cellu-

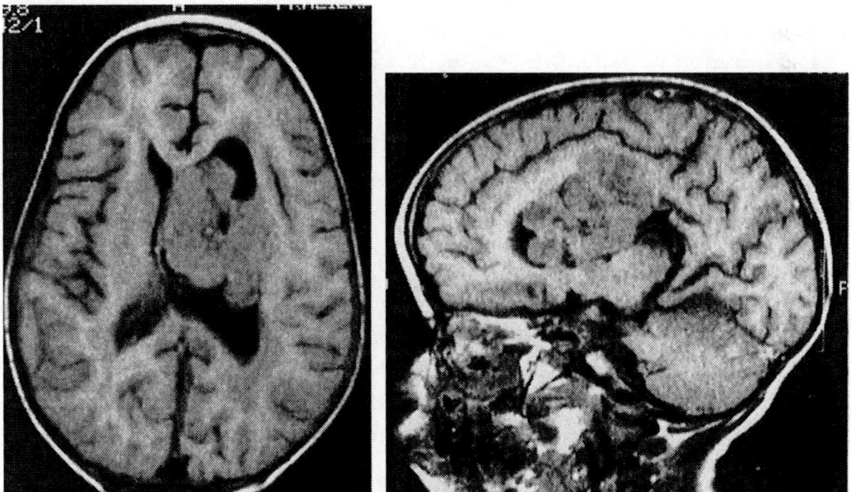

A B

FIG. 11-2. **(A)** Axial and **(B)** sagittal T1-weighted MRI of 2-year-old who presented with herniation syndrome. Heterogeneous mass involving the region of the body of the left lateral ventricle with involvement of third ventricle and region of hypothalamus. Mass measures 6 × 5 × 4 cm. The mass did not enhance with gadolinium. Diagnosis, subependymoma.

lar ependymoma. One-half of this mixed group of tumors occurred in children within the first decade of life, and all were found within the fourth ventricle. Mortality, as opposed to the usually good prognosis of subependymomas, was 80% (Fig. 11-2).

SIGNS AND SYMPTOMS

The symptoms of children with ependymomas vary with the location of the tumor. Nausea, vomiting, and headaches are relatively nonspecific, and are the most common presenting symptoms in both supratentorial and infratentorial tumors. In general, posterior fossa tumors present with symptoms of increased intracranial pressure (e.g., vomiting and headaches) as well as unsteady gait. Supratentorial tumors more commonly present with focal motor weakness, visual disturbances including field abnormalities, and seizures. Seizures may be present in 25% of the children with supratentorial ependymomas. Neck pain and stiffness are common with posterior fossa location, presumably related to encroachment of the tumor on the upper cervical nerve roots (42).

The most common physical finding in patients with ependymomas of any location is papilledema. Other signs vary with tumor location. Thus, nystagmus, meningismus, and dysmetria are frequently seen with posterior fossa lesions, whereas hemiparesis, hyperreflexia, and visual field abnormalities are more common with supratentorial tumors. Ataxia is present in both supratentorial and infratentorial cases (11).

The duration of symptoms varies, but in one series (12), the duration of symptoms before diagnosis varied between 1½ and 36 months, with the majority present for about 12 months. Duration of symptoms before diagnosis varies with location and grade. Supratentorial tumors have an average duration of symptoms before diagnosis of 7 months (2 weeks to 3 years), whereas posterior fossa tumors have an average duration of 9 months (2 weeks to 2 years) (32,75). In general, benign lesions have a longer history before diagnosis than malignant tumors (10). Grossly invasive posterior fossa tumors have symptoms for an average of 5.4 months, whereas tumors that are not grossly invasive have an average duration of symptoms of 11 months. Duration of symptoms before diagnosis is significantly longer in patients with calcified versus noncalcified supratentorial ependymomas. However, there is no such difference in duration of symptoms in calcified versus noncalcified posterior fossa tumors (41).

NEURORADIOLOGIC DIAGNOSIS

On CT scan, the posterior fossa ependymoma appears as a midline mass, often filling the fourth ventricle, and is associated with hydrocephalus.

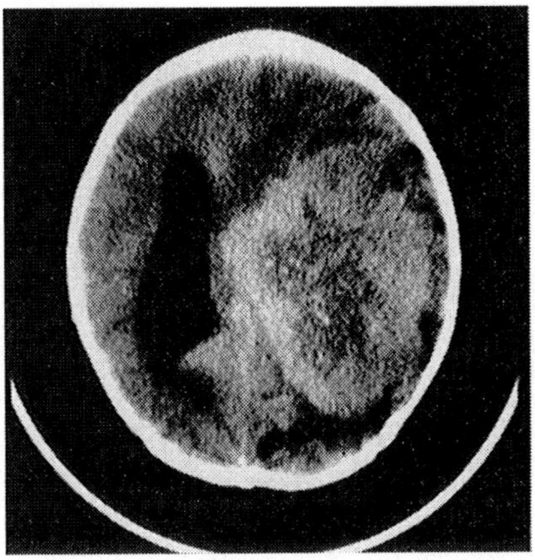

FIG. 11-3. Contrast enhanced CT scan in the axial plane showing a large supratentorial ependymoma with associated hydrocephalus. By the time of presentation, tumor had eroded through the child's skull.

Tumor density is usually increased relative to the brain. Those lesions which have decreased density or are isodense are less likely to be ependymomas (30). Cyst formation is common in ependymomas and is readily identified on CT scan. Calcification is present in as many as 44% of cases and may be either diffuse or coarsely nodular. Supratentorial ependymomas are hyperintense on CT with mixed attenuation and, at times, cystic structures (33) (Fig. 11-3). Tumor enhancement is typically present (25).

The signal intensity on MRI does not distinguish ependymomas from other intracranial gliomas. However, location and gross morphology can be defined extremely well on MRI (particularly on the sagittal view for posterior fossa lesions) and are very characteristic of ependymomas (Fig. 11-4). The MRI will demonstrate extension of the tumor from the fourth ventricle into the cerebellar pontine angle via the lateral recesses of the fourth ventricle and the foramen of Lushka. The downward extension of the tumor into the

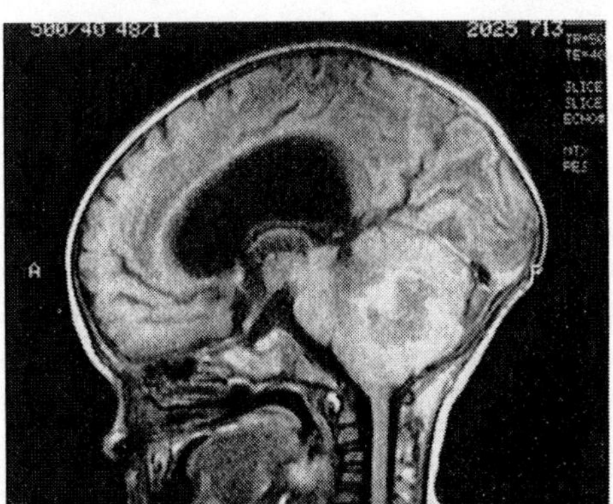

FIG. 11-4. MRI scan of 1-year-old with fourth ventricular ependymoma. Child had presented with vomiting, failure to thrive, and enlarged head circumference. Tumor completely fills the fourth ventricle.

cisterna magna and the cervical spinal canal through the foramen of Magendie is also readily appreciated by MRI. This presentation accounts for the description of ependymomas as "oozing out of the foramen." The ability to define accurately the caudal extent of tumor has an important influence on radiation treatment planning. The radiation tolerance of the cervical cord is close to that necessary for tumor control in the posterior fossa and, as such, restricting radiation volumes as much as possible is important to reduce neurotoxicity (24).

Solid ependymomas reveal heterogeneity of signal on MRI, which likely represents hemosiderin, necrosis, calcification, and vascularity (69). The cystic neoplasms are sharply defined with round or oval margins. They have a uniform signal intensity that is either equivalent to or slightly hyperintense relative to spinal fluid. Since as many as 50% of ependymomas typically calcify, the lack of reliable imaging of calcium on MRI limits its usefulness in this tumor type. Although gadolinium can distinguish enhancing tumor from nonenhancing edema, it is not specific for ependymomas. Overall, MRI is superior to CT in delineating tumor size and extent, especially in posterior fossa lesions. CT, however, is superior for demonstrating calcification (25).

Local recurrence, subarachnoid spread, and ventricular metastasis may be readily recognized on CT well before the presence of clinical signs (15). Indirect signs of recurrence are obliteration of the basal cisterns, protrusion of brain tissue, and displacement or obliteration of the fourth ventricle. Enhancement of the tentorium suggests subarachnoid spread of the tumor (7). At times, a cast of the ventricles is recognized (Fig. 11-5).

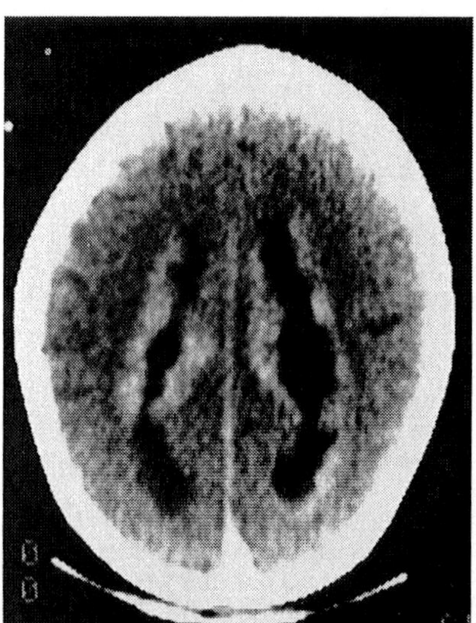

FIG. 11-5. A 4-year-old child with a fourth ventricular ependymoma. The tumor was disseminated throughout the subarachnoid space and ventricular system. The CT scan reveals seeding of the lateral ventricles, producing a "cast-like" appearance.

SPINAL CORD SEEDING

Ependymomas are well known to seed the CSF pathways. However, the incidence of subarachnoid seeding and its relationship to tumor grade and location are not well delineated. We combined the results of 21 series of children and adults with intracranial ependymomas. Of 703 intracranial ependymomas identified, 66 (9%) were associated with seeding of the spinal subarachnoid space, at either diagnosis, recurrence, or on autopsy (Table 11-1). Reports of clinical seeding tend to underestimate the true incidence of this phenomenon because routine myelograms were not done in most series. A recent analysis of clinically evident spinal seeding in patients with posterior fossa ependymomas revealed a 6% incidence compared to 15% noted in Table 11-1 (36).

The incidence of subarachnoid seeding varies with location. Patients with supratentorial tumors had an 8% incidence of spinal subarachnoid seeding, whereas those patients with posterior fossa tumors had a 15% incidence

TABLE 11-1. *Spinal seeding cord from intracranial ependymomas*

	Overall		Supratentorial		Posterior fossa		High grade		Low grade	
Author	No. seeded	%	No. seeded	%	No. seeded	%	No. seeded	%	No. seeded	%
Tarlov and Davidoff (1946)	3/8	38								
Svien et al. (1953)	6/19	32			6/12	50				
Bouchard and Peirce (1960)	0/12	0								
Kricheff et al. (1964)	1/69	1								
Phillips et al. (1964)	2/42	5								
Sagerman et al. (1965)	5/11	45	2/4	50	3/7	43				
Barone and Elvidge (1970)	0/47	0								
Salazar et al. (1975)	1/28	4	0/11	0	1/17	6	0/12	0	1/16	6
Shuman et al. (1975)	3/68	4	0/18	0	3/50	6				
Kim and Fayos (1977)	11/32	34	1/11	9	10/21	48	6/21	29	1/11	9
Bloom (1978)	6/35	17			5/24	21	5/19	26		
Renaudin et al. (1979)	4/19	21	2/10	20	2/9	22	3/9	33	1/10	10
Marks and Adler (1982)	5/46	11	1/20	5	4/26	15				
Salazar (1983)[a]	5/51	10								
Wallner (1986)	1/20	5			1/12	8	0/8	0	1/8	12.5
Tomita (1988)	1/22	4.5							1/22	4.5
Goldwein (1990)	6/36	16.6								
Nazar (1990)	1/32	3			1/32	3				
Healey (1991)	2/33	6								
Kovnar (1991)[b]	2/43	4.6								
Total	66/703	9	6/74	8	36/240	15	14/69	20	5/67	9

[a] Excluding direct tumor extension.
[b] Seeding at initial diagnosis.

of seeding. There was also a difference in drop metastases depending on pathologic grade. Thus, 20% of high-grade tumors seeded the spinal subarachnoid space, whereas low-grade tumors seeded the spinal cord in only 9% of cases. In general, high-grade tumors are more likely to metastasize in the spinal subarachnoid space than low-grade tumors. In addition, infratentorial tumors have a higher incidence of seeding than supratentorial tumors. Unfortunately, the relative importance of these risk factors has not been determined. Thus, the risk of subarachnoid seeding for tumors that are classified as high risk because of pathologic grade but low risk because of location, for example, is not known.

The likelihood of leptomeningeal failure impacts directly on decisions regarding volume of radiation. Although CSF seeding identified at autopsy is relatively common, prospective neuraxis staging prior to radiation has revealed a surprisingly low incidence of dissemination except in young children. The Pediatric Oncology Group (31) has recently completed a prospective ependymoma study. None of 43 children had either positive myelograms or spine MRIs prior to radiation. Two had positive cytology (one a well differentiated ependymoma and the other an anaplastic ependymoma). A somewhat higher incidence of seeding at diagnosis was found in the Philadelphia study (23), in which 3 of 17 patients evaluated prospectively for dissemination were found to have leptomeningeal disease at diagnosis: 1 had positive CSF cytology, 1 had an abnormal myelogram, and 1 had a tumor deposit in the lateral ventricle remote from the primary site. Clearly those patients in whom CSF dissemination is recognized at diagnosis will require craniospinal radiation. The question remains as to the risk of isolated failure outside the primary site. In the Pediatric Oncology Group study there were no cases of isolated subarachnoid failure regardless of histology, location, or extent of resection. Concurrent local and subarachnoid failure, however, did occur in 3 of the 43 patients (31). Healy et al. (25) reported isolated subarachnoid relapse in only 1 of 16 failures. An additional child had simultaneous failure in the CSF as well as in the primary site. Thus, in most cases leptomeningeal dissemination occurs concurrently with failure at the primary site with approximately a 3% likelihood of an isolated neuraxis relapse (62).

TREATMENT

The treatment of patients with ependymomas has been controversial, in part due to limited numbers and the differences in prognosis depending on pathologic grade and location. Unlike cerebellar astrocytomas, surgery is rarely curative (68). Surgical morbidity has been high, approaching 20 to 36% in some modern series (10,74). This high degree of morbidity associated with the surgical removal of posterior fossa ependymomas is due to their frequent attachment to the floor of the fourth ventricle. There has been some controversy in the literature as to the influence of gross total resection on prognosis. This may relate in part to the fact that determination of gross total resection can be based on either the surgeon's report or postoperative scan. If only the postoperative CT or MRI is utilized, highly significant differences in survival relative to degree of resection have been found (i.e., 75% PFS for children without residual disease vs. 0% in those with residual disease) (25). These improved survivals following gross total resection are found in infants as well, assuming the absence of leptomeningeal disease (13). Thus, despite higher surgical morbidity, an attempt at gross total resection is currently recommended (45).

Although radiation is clearly indicated for ependymomas, controversies have arisen concerning the volume of radiation to be administered to the brain, spinal cord, and tumor bed. Gadolinium-enhanced MRI of the spine and evaluation of CSF cytology should be performed at diagnosis in all children with ependymomas, regardless of grade or location. Those patients with evidence of disseminated disease will require craniospinal radiation. Less clear is the need for large-volume radiation in those children without documented CSF dissemination at diagnosis. Table 11-2 compares several radiotherapy treatment plans. Low-grade supratentorial ependymomas, which are at a low risk for subarachnoid seeding because of both favorable location and grade, are treated by most radiotherapists with local radiation to the tumor bed (5,33,34,42,53,54,56). Conversely, high-grade posterior fossa tumors, which are at a high risk for drop metastases because of unfavorable location and grade, usually receive full craniospinal radiation (4,39,40,57,58, 63,64,66).

The major radiotherapy controversies regard tumors with conflicting risk

TABLE 11-2. *Radiotherapy*

Author	High-grade supratentorial*	Low-grade supratentorial*	High-grade posterior fossa*	Low-grade posterior fossa*
Bloom (5,6)	CS	Local (wide)	CS	CS
Salazar et al. (58)	CS	WB	CS	WB to C5
Sheline (63)	WB	Local	CS	Local
Marsa et al. (40)	CS	Local	CS	Local
Marks and Adler (39)	Local (wide)	Local (wide)	CS	Local (wide)
Phillips et al. (49)	Local	Local	Local	Local
Sheline (64) (14 respondents)	CS (13/14)	Local (11/14)	CS (13/14)	Local (11/14)
Shuman et al. (66)	CS	Local (wide)	CS	Local (wide)
Sagerman et al. (57)	CS	CS	CS	CS
Kun (personal com)	Local	Local	Local	Local
Wallner (76)	CS	Local (wide)	CS	Local (wide)
Healey (25)	CS	Local (2-cm margin)	CS	Local (2-cm margin)
Goldwein (23)	CS	Local	CS	Local

Abbreviations: CS, craniospinal; WB, whole brain; wide, wide margins.
* Patients with no evidence of leptomeningeal disease.

factors. The low-grade posterior fossa ependymoma carries a high risk for seeding by location but a low risk by pathologic grade. Most radiotherapists, when confronted with this dilemma, use local radiation to the tumor bed but employ wide margins (39,40,63,64,66). Some radiotherapists extend the field down to C5. Although it is recognized that posterior fossa ependymomas may seed, it has also become clear that the vast majority of patients who fail do so in the primary site. Therefore, it is increasingly recommended to give only local radiation so long as a neuraxis evaluation reveals no evidence of metastatic disease (25,32,36,62,76).

Another controversy concerns high-grade supratentorial tumors, which are at high risk for seeding because of pathologic grade but low risk because of location. Those radiotherapists who place more emphasis on the high risk of seeding associated with malignant pathology tend to give these patients full craniospinal irradiation (6,39,40,49,57,58,63,66). Other respected radiotherapists emphasize the low risk of seeding associated with tumors in this favorable location, and either treat the whole brain or in some cases only the tumor bed, without delivering spinal irradiation.

The appropriate volume of radiation is being studied in a Pediatric Oncology Group protocol, which was based on results of a previous POG study (31). Detailed surveillance screening was performed at diagnosis in 43 children with ependymomas. There was only a 5% (2/43) incidence of CSF seeding at diagnosis. More important, there was no case of isolated neuraxis relapse regardless of histology or location. Concurrent failure at the primary site and the subarachnoid space occurred in 3 of the 13 failures. Since all patients failed initially at the primary site, the current protocol treats all children with posterior fossa ependymomas who have negative surveillance testing (regardless of histology) with local hyperfractionated radiation to the posterior fossa and upper cervical cord using a total dose of 69.6 Gy. If the second study confirms that failure occurs first in the primary site, craniospinal radiation may no longer be recommended in the future in those children with posterior fossa ependymomas who have negative surveillance testing.

The dose of radiation also influences survival. Several retrospective studies have demonstrated improved survivals, i.e., 46 to 70% versus 10 to 30% in those patients receiving ≥45 Gy – 55 Gy versus <45 Gy.

Chemotherapy

Although many centers have used single and combination chemotherapy in patients with ependymomas, the overall number of patients in each of these studies is small. Results with nitrosoureas have been variable. Three out of 3 patients failed to respond to 1-(chlorethyl)3-cyclohexyl-1-nitrosourea (CCNU) in one study, but in another study 1 patient responded for 11 months (52,78). Three out of 6 patients reported by Wilson et al. (78) responded to

1,3Bis(2-chlorethyl)-1-nitrosourea (BCNU). However, only 1 of 4 patients responded to BCNU in a study reported by Edwards et al. (14). Cis-platinum appears to be the most active agent studied to date, with 10 of 29 children with recurrent ependymomas having partial or complete responses in one study (18). In another study (3), 4 of 7 patients treated with cis-platinum had either a partial or a complete response. Carboplatinum, with its putative lower ototoxicity, also has produced partial responses in 2 of 14 children with recurrent ependymomas. Better response rates were found in those not having been previously treated with cis-platinum, i.e., 40% response rate (19).

Bloom (6) treated children with ependymomas with the same chemotherapy regimen employed in medulloblastomas, i.e.,CCNU and VCR. There was a 70% 5-year survival in chemotherapy-treated patients compared with a 44% 5-year survival for historical controls treated with surgery and radiation. However, after 6 to 7 years, the lines converged and there was no difference. CCNU, vincristine, and cis-platinum were used in combination with radiation therapy in 17 newly diagnosed children in another study (22). No difference in outcome was found when compared with children not treated with chemotherapy. The same group treated children with recurrent ependymal tumors with a variety of chemotherapeutic regimens. Cis-platinum appeared to be the most active agent, with 4 of 10 children demonstrating stable disease. Survival following recurrence in the cis-platinum-treated patients was 60% at 2 years compared to only 30% for those who received chemotherapy but no cis-platinum.

The International Society of Pediatric Oncology (6) treated 37 children with high-grade ependymomas in a randomized study of surgery plus radiation versus surgery plus radiation plus chemotherapy from 1975 to 1979. There was no demonstrated difference in the two treatment groups. More recently, a chemotherapy regimen consisting of cyclophosphamide and vincristine for children less than 3 years of age with malignant tumors revealed a 48% response rate in those children with ependymomas (13).

Although results of chemotherapy are available in only a limited number of patients, there is the suggestion that this tumor may be chemosensitive, particularly to cis-platinum and a combination of cyclophosphamide and vincristine. Future trials through the national cooperative groups will need to test whether adjuvant chemotherapy will increase progression-free and overall survivals.

EXTRANEURAL METASTASES

Extraneural metastases are far less common than seeding through the cerebrospinal fluid axis (9,12,20,37,47,48,65,67,77). Of interest, 90% of these

TABLE 11-3. *Extraneural metastases from intracranial ependymomas*

Author	Age of patient at diagnosis	Primary location of tumor	Metastatic spread	Survival
Perry (48)	39 years	Parietal	Liver, bone marrow	5.8 years
Sherbaniuk and Shnitka (65)	16 years	Parietal–occipital	Scalp, lungs	13.0 years
Maass (37)	27 years	Occipital	Lymph nodes	2.5 years
Duffner and Cohen (12)	9 years	Parietal–occipital	Lungs, lymph nodes, bone, diaphragm	4.0 years
Smith et al. (67)	31 years	Parietal	Lungs, lymph nodes	8.0 years
Breslich (9)	13 years	Occipital	Pleura, lungs, lymph nodes	2.0 years
Perrin (47)	2 years/9 months	Cerebellum	Lungs, mediastinum	6 months
Perrin (47)	4 years/8 months	Thalamus	Bone	14 months
Wen and Barrows (77)	9 years	Frontal	Lungs, lymph nodes, scalp	17 months
Glasauer and Yuan (20)	2 years/6 months	Parietal–Occipital	Lungs, lymph nodes	14 months
Salazar (59)	9 years	Supratentorial	Ribs, long bones	21 months
	6 years	Supratentorial	Scalp, neck nodes	6 months
	9 years	Supratentorial	Orbit	86+ months
Tomita (73)	5 years		Bone	26+ months

metastases occurred with supratentorial tumors. The most common site of spread is to the lymph nodes and lungs; these sites were found in 8 of 10 reported cases. Other areas of metastatic spread include liver, bone marrow, scalp, and diaphragm. Perry (48) commented that several reported cases had in common multiple operations, postoperative radiation, and prolonged survivals. Survivals have ranged from 6 months to 13 years, with 6 of 10 patients surviving 2 years or greater and only 3 patients surviving greater than 5 years (Table 11-3) (also see Chapter 21).

Prognosis

Although some authors claim a good prognosis for ependymomas, this unfortunately is not the usual scenario. Much of the literature is confounded by combining adult and pediatric cases. Survivals in those series consisting of children alone are much lower. Furthermore, some of the series either include or exclude postoperative deaths, which impacts on survival statistics. This not only influences overall 5-year survivals but is important in calculating risk by location. For example, most series that include postoperative deaths report that posterior fossa tumors have a worse prognosis than supratentorial tumors, with 20% 5-year survivals (74). Mork and Loken (44), who excluded postoperative deaths, found a better survival with posterior fossa tumors. Thus, these reports must be interpreted carefully (Table 11-4).

Prognostic factors vary from series to series. Virtually all series agree that very young age at diagnosis, i.e., less than 2 to 3 years, is associated with a significantly worse prognosis. For example in one study (25), there was a 0% 10-year survival for children less than 24 months of age at diagnosis compared to a 62% survival for older patients. The poor survivals in very young children were not related to radiation dose, because they had received similar amounts of radiation as the older children, i.e., a median tumor dose of 5,233 cGy compared to that for older patients of 5,400 cGy. In another study (23), children less than 4 years of age at diagnosis had a 2-year actuarial survival of 20%, compared to a rate of 83% for older children. Another potentially important prognostic factor is degree of surgical resection. Most, but not all, studies have shown either a trend toward better survival (35) or significantly improved survival (25,32,45) with gross total resection. In contrast, Goldwein (23) did not find that degree of resection impacted on survival. There is also controversy as to the influence of histologic grade of tumor on prognosis. Thus, whereas Shaw (62) has suggested that the difference between survivals in children with ependymomas versus anaplastic ependymomas is 74% versus 29%, others (31) have found evidence that histologic grade does not influence overall survival. As noted above, this discrepancy may relate to differences in pathologic interpretation, but at present histologic malignancy remains a questionable prognostic factor. It is likely that recurrence is related in part to the dose of radiation. Goldwein (23), for example, demonstrated that a dose of greater than 4,500 cGy was associated with a 51% survival compared with an 18% survival in children receiving less than 4,500 cGy. Finally, evidence of brain stem invasion of the tumor on the basis of either neuroimaging or neurologic signs that suggest cranial nerve involvement is associated with a poor prognosis (45).

Most pediatric series (23,74) report 5-year survivals of 27 to 58%. These numbers change quite dramatically if the study includes only very young children. For example, Lyons (36) found only a 14% 5-year survival in children less than 5 years of age. Most patients suffer a recurrance fairly quickly, with a median time to failure of 18 months. There is a somewhat longer time to recurrence in patients who have had gross total resection, where recurrence may not occur for 2 to 3 years (73). Several studies have suggested that Collins' rule is valid in the very young child; i.e., if a child survives more than 9 months plus the age at which the tumor was diagnosed, a cure may be anticipated. Unfortunately, this has not been the case in the POG infant brain tumor study, in which late failures have occurred.

TABLE 11-4. *Five-year survival of children with ependymomas*

Author	S	RT	Overall	Supra-tentorial	Infra-tentorial	High-grade	Low-grade
Kricheff (32), 1964							
(INC) $T = 36$	+	+	25% (3 yr)				
Phillips (49), 1964							
(INC) $T = 7$							
<5 years of age	+	+	0%				
Barone and Elvidge (2), 1970							
(INC) $T = 47$							
<15 years of age	+	+			25%		
Hendrick (27), 1975							
(INC) $T = 23$	+	+		25%			
Onoyama (46), 1975							
(EX) $T = 13$	+	+	44.4%				
Sheline (64), 1975							
(EX) $T = 14$	+	+			29%	78%	
Shuman (66), 1975							
$T = 28$	+	+	3%				
(EX) $T = 15$	+	+ ≤3,600	0%				
$T = 17$	+	+ ≥4,500	47%				
Dohrmann (11), 1976							
$T = 19$	+	+	25%	29%	17%	14%	33%
(INC) $T = 22$	+	−	15%	21%	10%	15%	21%
Coulon and Till (10), 1977						0% (SUPRA)	9.9% (SUPRA)
(INC) $T = 39$	+	+	12.5%	10%	13.7%	0% (PF)	22% (PF)
Farwell (16), 1977							
(INC) $T = 44$	+	+	18%	26%	19%		
Heiskanen (26), 1977							
(EX) $T = 16$	+	+	27%				

Bloom (5), 1982 (EX) $T = 30$	+	+	47%			40%	
Salazar (59), 1983 (EX) $T = 51$	+	+	69%[b]				
Wallner (76), 1986 (EX) $T = 20$	+	+	67%				
Shaw (62), 1987 (EX) $T = 18$	+	+	51%				
Bloom (4), 1989 (EX) $T = 47$	+	+	53%			21%	47%
Goldwein (23), 1990 $T = 51$	+	+	46%	35%	50%	42%	
Nazar (45), 1990 $T = 35$	+	+	44.6%			12.1%	70.5%
Undjian (74), 1990 (INC) $T = 60$	+	+	20%	26.1%	16.2%	19.6%	20.6%
Ernestus (15), 1991 $T = 29$	+	+ –	58%	58%	—	31%	75%
Healey (25), 1991 (EX) $T = 29$	+	+	62%				
Lyons (36), 1991[a] (INC) $T = 7$	+	+	14%		14%		

INC, including postoperative deaths; EX, excluding postoperative deaths; PF, posterior fossa; SUPRA, supratentorial.

[a] All patients less than 5 years.

[b] 10-year survival.

SUMMARY

Ependymomas represent 8 to 10% of intracranial tumors in childhood, with a mean age at diagnosis of 5 to 6 years. The tumors may arise in relation to any part of the ventricular system, although they occur twice as frequently in the posterior fossa as in the supratentorial regions. The signs and symptoms on presentation vary with location of the tumor. In general, longer duration of symptoms before diagnosis is associated with low pathologic grade and location in the posterior fossa.

Spinal cord seeding is found in approximately 9% of intracranial ependymomas at some time in their course, although less common at diagnosis (5%). The incidence of seeding varies with location and grade. Up to 20% of high-grade tumors are associated with spinal cord metastases, compared with only 8% of low-grade tumors. Location also influences the incidence of seeding; 15% of posterior fossa tumors, compared with 8% of supratentorial tumors, are associated with seeding of the spinal subarachnoid space. The highest incidence of seeding is associated with malignant ependymomas located in the posterior fossa.

Treatment approaches reflect this tendency of the tumor to seed the CSF pathways. Surgery is the initial approach to ependymomas but is not curative. Radiation controversies continue regarding the volume of radiation to be administered to brain, spinal cord, and tumor bed. Most radiotherapists treat low-grade ependymomas regardless of location with local radiation, whereas anaplastic ependymomas have typically been treated with craniospinal radiation. Staging procedures must be done prior to initiating radiation, as those patients with positive cytology and/or positive myelograms (even if pathology of the primary tumor is of low grade) will require radiation to the craniospinal axis. Studies are now underway to determine whether progression-free survivals will differ based on volume of radiation. If most patients fail first at the primary site, craniospinal radiation may not be recommended in the future. Chemotherapy has been used in a limited fashion. Excellent response rates have been seen with cis-platinum and cyclophosphamide/vincristine combination.

The overall 5-year survival in children with intracranial ependymomas ranges from 28 to 60%, although most series tend toward the lower number. The worst prognostic factor is young age at the time of diagnosis. Other prognostic factors associated with poor prognosis are incomplete surgical resection, metastases at diagnosis, parenchymal and brain stem invasion with concomitant brain stem signs, and radiation dosages less than 4,500 cGy. Overall, although some patients with ependymomas may have prolonged survivals, the majority fail between 18 and 24 months following diagnosis. Salvage therapy is rarely successful. Future studies will include more aggressive adjuvant chemotherapy as well as hyperfractionation in order to maximize radiation and limit neurotoxicity.

REFERENCES

1. Bailey P. Tumors arising from ependymal cells. *Arch Neurol Psychiatr* 1924;11:1–27.
2. Barone B, Elvidge A. Ependymomas: a clinical survey. *J Neurosurg* 1970;33:428–438.
3. Bertolone SJ, Baum ES, Krivit W, Hammond GD. A phase II study of cisplatin therapy in recurrent childhood brain tumors. *J Neurooncol* 1989;7:5–11.
4. Bloom HJG. The role of adjuvant chemotherapy in the primary treatment of medulloblastoma and ependymoma. In: Pochedly C, ed. *Controversies in pediatric and adolescent hematology and oncology*. St. Louis: CV Mosby; 1989.
5. Bloom HJG. Intracranial tumors: response and resistance in therapeutic endeavors 1970–1980. *Int J Radiat Oncol Biol Phys* 1982;8:1083–1113.
6. Bloom HJG. Management of some extracranial tumors in children and adults. *Prog Clin Biol Res* 1978;25:56–84.
7. Bock WJ, Clar HE, Weichert HC, Gerhard L. Follow-up studies in the posterior fossa in children using computerized tomography. *Neurochirugia* 1981;24:2–5.
8. Bouchard J, Peirce CB. Radiation therapy in the management of neoplasm of the central nervous system, with a special note in regard to children: twenty years' experience, 1939–1958. *AJR* 1960;84:610–628.
9. Breslich PJ. Ependymoma of the right occipital lobe with death from extracranial metastases. *Lancet* 1957;77:99–103.
10. Coulon RA, Till K. Intracranial ependymomas in children: a review of 43 cases. *Childs Brain* 1977;3:154–168.
11. Dohrmann GJ, Farwell JR, Flannery JT. Ependymomas and ependymoblastomas in children. *J Neurosurg* 1976;45:273–283.
12. Duffner PK, Cohen ME. Extraneural metastases in childhood brain tumors. *Ann Neurol* 1981;10:261–265.
13. Duffner PK, Howowitz ME, Krischer JP, et al. Postoperative chemotherapy and delayed radiation in children less than 3 years of age with malignant brain tumors. *N Engl J Med* 1993;328:1725–1731.
14. Edwards MS, Levin VA, Wilson CB. Chemotherapy of pediatric posterior fossa tumors. *Childs Brain* 1980;7:252–260.
15. Ernestus RI, Wilcked O, Schroder R. Supratentorial ependymomas in childhood: clinicopathological findings and prognosis. *Acta Neurochir* 1991;111:96–102.
16. Farwell JR, Dohrmann GJ, Flannery JT. Central nervous system tumors in children. *Cancer* 1977;40:3123–3132.
17. Figarella-Branger D, Gambarelli D, Dollo C, et al. Infratentorial ependymomas of childhood: correlation between histological features, immunohistological phenotype, silver nucleolar organizer region staining values and post-operative survival in 16 cases. *Acta Neuropathol* 1991;82:208–216.
18. Friedman SH, Oakes WJ. The chemotherapy of posterior fossa tumors in childhood. *J Neurooncol* 1987;5:217–229.
19. Gaynon PS, Ettinger LJ, Baum ES, Siegel SE, Krailo MD, Hominid GD. Carboplatin in childhood brain tumors. *Cancer* 1990;66:2465–2469.
20. Glasauer FE, Yuan RHP. Intracranial tumors with extracranial metastases: case report and review of the literature. *J Neurosurg* 1963;20:474–493.
21. Goldwein JW, Corn BW, Finlay JL, Packer RJ, Rorke LB, Schut L. Is craniospinal irradiation required to cure children with malignant (anaplastic) intracranial ependymomas? *Cancer* 1991;67:2766–2772.
22. Goldwein JR, Galser TA, Packer RJ, et al. Recurrent intracranial ependymomas in children. *Cancer* 1990;66:557–563.
23. Goldwein JW, Leahy JM, Packer RJ, et al. Intracranial ependymomas in children. *Int J Radiat Oncol Biol Phys* 1990;19:1497–1502.
24. Griffin BR, Shuman WP, Wisbeck W, Berger M, Spence A. Improved localization of infratentorial ependymomas by magnetic resonance imaging: implications for radiation treatment planning. *J Neurooncol* 1988;6:147–155.
25. Healey EA, Barnes PD, Kupsky WJ, Scott RM, Sallan SE, Black PM, Tarbell NJ. The prognostic significance of postoperative residual tumor in ependymoma. *Neurosurgery* 1991;28:666–671.

26. Heiskanen O. Intracranial tumors of children. *Childs Brain* 1977;3:69–78.
27. Hendrick EB, Hoffman HJ, Humphreys RP. Treatment of infratentorial gliomas in childhood. *Recent Results Cancer Res* 1975;51:102–106.
28. Kernohan JW, Fletcher-Kenohan EM. Ependymomas: a study of 109 cases. *Pub Assoc Res Nerv Ment Dis* 1937;16:182–209.
29. Kim YH, Fayos JV. Intracranial ependymomas. *Radiology* 1977;124:805–808.
30. Kingsley DPE, Kendall BE. The CT scanner in posterior fossa tumors of childhood. *Br J Radiol* 1979;52:769–776.
31. Kovnar E, Kun L, Krischer J. Patterns of dissemination and recurrence in childhood ependymoma: preliminary results of Pediatric Oncology Group protocol #8532. *Ann Neurol* 1991;30:457.
32. Kricheff II, Becker M, Schneck SA, et al. Intracranial ependymomas: a study of survival in 65 cases treated by surgery and irradiation. *AJR* 1964;91:167–175.
33. Kun LE, Kovnar EH, Sanford RA. Ependymomas in children. *Pediatr Neurosci* 1988;14: 57–63.
34. Liu HM, Boggs J, Kidd J. Ependymomas of childhood. 1: Histological survey and clinicopathological correlation. *Childs Brain* 1976;2:92–110.
35. Lorentzen M, Hagerstrand I. Congenital ependymoblastoma. *Acta Neuropathol* 1980;49: 71–74.
36. Lyons MK, Kelly PJ. Posterior fossa ependymomas: report of 30 cases and review of the literature. *Neurosurgery* 1991;28:659–665.
37. Maass L. Occipital ependymoma with extracranial metastases. *J Neurosurg* 1954;11: 413–421.
38. Mabon RF, Svien NJ, Kernohan JW, Craig WM. Symposium on a new and simplified concept of gliomas: ependymomas. *Proc Staff Meet Mayo Clin* 1949;24:65–71.
39. Marks JE, Adler SJ. A comparative study of ependymomas by site of origin. *Int J Radiol Oncol Biol Phys* 1982;8:37–43.
40. Marsa GW, Goffinet DR, Rubinstein LJ, Bagshaw MA. Megavoltage irradiation in the treatment of gliomas of the brain and spinal cord. *Cancer* 1975;36:1681–1689.
41. Martin F, Lemmen LJ. Calcification in intracranial neoplasm. *Am J Pathol* 1952;28: 1107–1131.
42. Matson DD. *Neurosurgery of infancy and childhood*. Springfield, IL: Charles C Thomas; 1969.
43. Mervis B, Lotz J, Handler LC, Wright M. Computed tomography of infratentorial masses in children. *S Afr Med J* 1979;56:47–49.
44. Mork SJ, Loken AC. Ependymoma: a follow-up study of 101 cases. *Cancer* 1977;40: 907–915.
45. Nazar GB, Hoffman HJ, Becker LE, Jenkin D, Humphreys RP, Hendrick B. Infratentorial ependymomas in childhood: prognostic factors and treatment. *J Neurosurg* 1990;72: 408–417.
46. Onoyama Y, Abe M, Takahashi M, Yabumoto E, Sakamoto T. Radiation therapy of brain tumors in children. *Radiology* 1975;115:687–693.
47. Perrin EV. Extracranial metastases from intracranial gliomata: report of 2 cases in children. *Am J Clin Pathol* 1958;30:244–251.
48. Perry RE. Extracranial metastasis in a case of intracranial ependymoma. *Arch Pathol* 1957; 64:337–341.
49. Phillips TL, Sheline GE, Boldrey E. Therapeutic consideration in tumors affecting the central nervous system: ependymomas. *Radiology* 1964;83:98–105.
50. Renaudin JR, DiTullio MV, Brown WJ. Seeding of infratentorial ependymomas in children. *Childs Brain* 1979;5:408–412.
51. Ringertz N, Reymond A. Ependymomas and choroid plexus papillomas. *J Neuropathol Exp Neurol* 1949:8:355–390.
52. Rosenblum ML, Reynolds AF, Smith KA, Rumack BH, Walker MC. Chloroethyl-cyclohexyl-nitrosourea (CCNU) in the treatment of malignant brain tumors. *J Neurosurg* 1973; 39:306–314.
53. Ross GW, Rubinstein LJ. Lack of histopathological correlation of malignant ependymomas with postoperative survival. *J Neurosurg* 1989;70:31–36.
54. Rubinstein LJ. The definition of the ependymoblastoma. *Arch Pathol* 1970;90:35–45.

55. Rubinstein LJ. *Tumors of the central nervous system*. Washington, DC: Armed Forces Institute of Pathology; 1972:104–124.
56. Russell DS, Rubinstein LJ. *Pathology of tumours of the nervous system*. Baltimore: Williams & Wilkins; 1989.
57. Sagerman RH, Bagshaw MA, Hanbery J. Considerations in the treatment of ependymoma. *Radiology* 1965;84:401–408.
58. Salazar O, Rubin P, Bassano D, Marcial VS. Improved survival of patients with intracranial ependymomas by irradiation: dose selection and field extension. *Cancer* 1975;35:1563–1573.
59. Salazar OM, Castro-Vita H, VanHoutte P, Rubin P, Aygun C. Improved survival in cases of intracranial ependymoma after radiation therapy. *J Neurosurg* 1983;59:652–659.
60. Scheithauer BW. Symptomatic subependymoma. *J Neurosurg* 1978;49:689–696.
61. Schiffer D, Chio A, Giordana MT. Histologic prognostic factors in ependymoma. *Childs Nerv Syst* 1991;7:177–182.
62. Shaw EG, Evans RG, Scheithauer BW, Ilstrup DM, et al. Postoperative radiotherapy of intracranial ependymoma in pediatric and adult patients. *Int J Radiat Oncol Biol Phys* 1987; 13:1457–1462.
63. Sheline GE. Radiation therapy of brain tumors. *Cancer* 1977;39:873–881.
64. Sheline G. Conventional radiation therapy of gliomas. *Recent Results Cancer Res* 1975: 125–133.
65. Sherbaniuk RW, Shnitka TJ. Metastasizing intracranial ependymomas. *Am J Pathol* 1956; 32:53–65.
66. Shuman RM, Alvord EC, Leech RW. The biology of childhood ependymomas. *Arch Neurol* 1975;32:731–739.
67. Smith DR, Hardman JM, Earle KM. Metastasizing neuroectodermal tumors of the central nervous system. *J Neurosurg* 1969;31:50–58.
68. Smith WA, Fincher EF. Intracranial tumors in children: preliminary study of 100 cases. *South Med J* 1942;35:547–554.
69. Spoto GP, Press GA, Hesselink JR, Solomon M. Intracranial ependymoma and subependymoma: MR manifestations. *AJNR* 1990;11:83–91.
70. Sutton LN, Goldwein J, Perilongo G, Lang B, Schut L, Rorke L, Packer R. Prognostic factors in childhood ependymomas. *Pediatr Neurosurg* 1990–91;16:57–65.
71. Svien H, Mabon RF, Kernohan JW, Craig WM. Ependymoma of the brain: pathologic aspects. *Neurology* 1953;3:1–15.
72. Tarlov IM, Davidoff LM. Subarachnoid and ventricular implants in ependymal and other gliomas. *J Neuropathol Exp Neurol* 1946;5:213–224.
73. Tomita T, McLone DG, Dasl D, Brand WN. Benign ependymomas of the posterior fossa in childhood. *Pediatr Neurosci* 1988;14:277–285.
74. Undjian S, Marinov M. Intracranial ependymomas in children. *Childs Nerv Syst* 1990;6: 131–134.
75. Vincent FM. Intracranial ependymomas: report of a case and literature review. *Minn Med* 1975;58:877–881.
76. Wallner KE, Wara WM, Sheline GE, Davis RL. Intracranial ependymomas: results of treatment with partial or whole brain irradiation without spinal irradiation. *J Radiat Biol Phys* 1986;12:1937–1941.
77. Wen HL, Barrows LJ. Ependymoma with extracranial metastases. *J Neuropathol Exp Neurol* 1957;16:112.
78. Wilson CB, Gutin P, Boldrey EB, Crafts D, Levin V, Enot JG. Single agent chemotherapy of brain tumors: a five year review. *Arch Neurol* 1976;33:739–744.

12

Brain Stem Tumors

Approximately 10 to 20% of brain tumors in the pediatric age group are found in the brain stem (21). Brain stem tumors, by definition, occupy the region of the brain traversed by the aqueduct of Sylvius and the fourth ventricle. Tumors that are found cephalad in the diencephalon or caudally below the medulla generally are not considered brain stem tumors. Neoplasms of the brain stem have been identified in children under 1 year of age as well as in adults in their third to fourth decade. However, most tumors of this region are seen in children in the second half of the first decade of life, with a slight male preponderance.

As a group, the prognosis and presentation of these tumors varies significantly from those for tumors in the spinal cord or in the diencephalon. Tumors of the brain stem usually follow a relentlessly progressive course resulting in death of the patient. Five-year survivals rarely exceed 30% and in most reports vary from 5 to 30% (5). Despite this, examination of actuarial survival curves suggests there may be two populations of patients. The majority of these are short-term survivors who die within 1 to 2 years of diagnosis. However, there is a smaller group of long-term survivors who have an extended course. Thus, even within this group of highly malignant tumors there may be a subcategory of patients who may survive long-term. Neuroimaging, duration of signs and symptoms prior to diagnosis, and to some extent histopathology have been used in an effort to further define prognosis (15). Several studies (67) have suggested that children with signs and symptoms of less than six months duration, with multiple brain stem signs and diffuse lesions on neuroimaging within the pons, have the poorest prognosis. Conversely, those brain stem tumors that present in an exophytic manner, are focal in nature, originate in anatomic structures adjacent to the cerebellar peduncle or cervical medullary junction, or are associated with cysts that may be amenable to surgery have a better prognosis. Similarly, there is evidence (47,56) that brain stem gliomas in patients with neurofibromatosis, regardless of imaging characteristics, have a different biology and a better prognosis than those in patients without neurofibromatosis. There has also been some suggestion that the pathology of the tumor may relate to prognosis (i.e., the more neoplastic tumors having the most truncated course). Others suggest that tumors of the brain stem, in reality, are mixed gliomas and that

Brain Tumors in Children: Principles of Diagnosis and Treatment, 2/e, edited by M.E. Cohen and P.K. Duffner, Raven Press, Ltd., New York, 1994.

with any given tumor, malignant features of anaplasia as well as features associated with a more benign pathology can be identified, depending on the area of tumor sampled. All these observations must be taken into consideration when treatment decisions are made.

PATHOLOGY

The pathology of brain stem tumors is quite variable. Most are either fibrillary or pilocytic astrocytomas, or the more malignant glioblastoma multiforme (10). In the past, spongioblastoma polare was considered as a separate grouping but is currently believed to be the same as the fibrillary astrocytoma. Cysts may be found in either the malignant or the slowly growing tumors. Cysts associated with glioblastomas are generally hemorrhagic and necrotic. Distortion in the structure of the normal architecture with hemorrhage and necrosis characterize the glioblastoma multiforme (Fig. 12-1). In contrast, slowly growing astrocytomas, rather than destroying tissue, tend to be insinuated between or adjacent to normal nerve fascicles. Unlike the more malignant gliomas, low-grade astrocytomas push and compress normal tissue rather than destroy it. The tendency for an astrocytoma to extend both cephalad and caudad produces diffuse enlargement of the pons, ac-

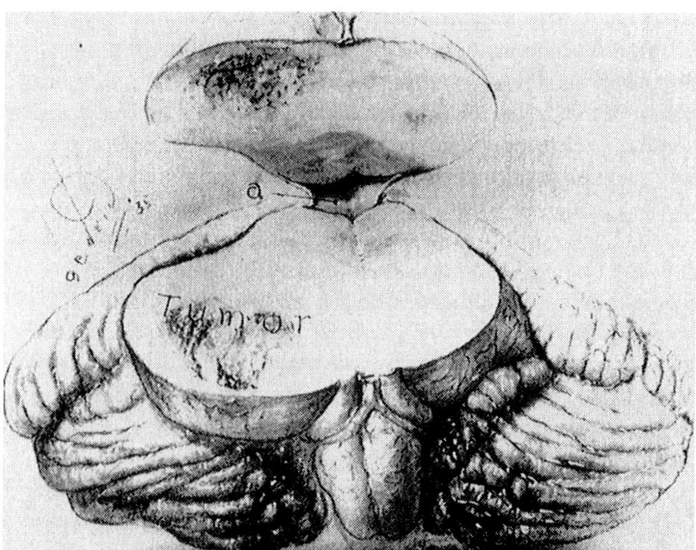

FIG. 12-1. Artist's rendition of a glioma of the pons demonstrating necrosis and pontine enlargement.

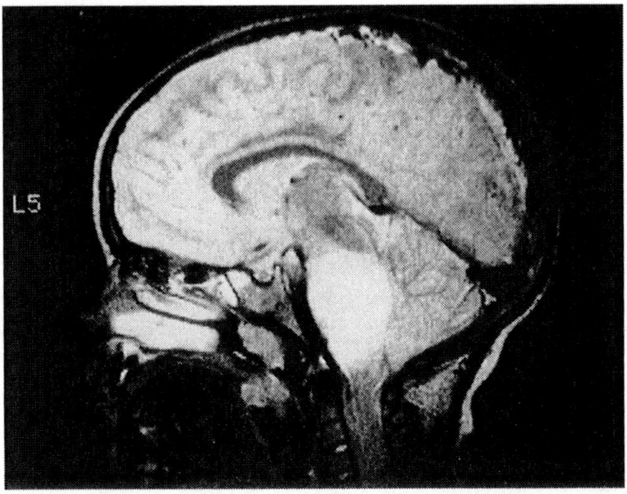

FIG. 12-2. T1-weighted MRI in sagittal plane showing diffuse pontine hypertrophy.

counting for the terminology "pontine hypertrophy" (Fig. 12-2). The growth of tumor between nerve fiber tracts may produce a pilocytic rather than a fibrillary appearance to the astrocytes. Hence, the pilocytic nature of the tumor is, in all probability, an epiphenomenon resulting from specific patterns of growth (5,65).

Although most tumors of this area are intrinsic to the brain stem, there is a small group of slowly growing tumors that have an exophytic presentation. These tumors may be found on the floor of the fourth ventricle, occupying the cerebellar pontine angles, or extending into the lateral recesses. Unlike intrinsic tumors of the brain stem, the fungating presentation of this tumor is surgically accessible and potentially treatable (34).

There has been some suggestion that low-grade astrocytomas are more likely to be found in the upper pons and midbrain, whereas glioblastomas are more commonly found in the lower pons and medulla. The location of the tumor as well as the histology and manner of presentation, both independently and in combination, relate to the overall prognosis.

In an autopsy study (45) of 25 patients with brain stem gliomas, tumor spread was found to be dependent on the site of origin and the histologic grade of malignancy. Tumors occurring in the pons tend to invade adjacent structures more readily than those occurring in the midbrain or the medulla. In this study, 48% of the tumors analyzed were glioblastoma multiforme. Distal tumor implants involving the cauda equina are seen with the more malignant tumors (76). As has been the observation of others, the more histologically aggressive tumors are apt to be found in the pons and medulla. In addition, when compared with tumors arising in the upper brain stem, the more aggressive tumors of the pons and medulla are noted to have the greatest cephalad and caudal involvement (10).

SIGNS AND SYMPTOMS

Consideration of a brain stem tumor begins with a triad of clinical findings consisting of long-tract signs, cranial neuropathies, and ataxia. Signs and symptoms consist of motor abnormalities (63), gait disturbances, vomiting, headaches, dysarthria, facial paresis, dysphasia, drowsiness, head tilt, and hearing loss. The most commonly involved cranial nerves are IX, X, V, VI, XII, VIII, VII, and III (29). Involvement of the third and fourth cranial nerves resulting in either diplopia, oculomotor paresis, or nystagmus suggests a mesencephalic component to the tumor.

Many varieties of nystagmus have been identified in patients with brain stem lesions. Nystagmus may suggest either an end-organ abnormality or intrinsic disease of the stem. Vertical nystagmus on upward gaze, bilateral nystagmus on lateral gaze, primary position nystagmus on horizontal gaze, and nonfatigable positional nystagmus are all considered intrinsic abnormalities of the brain stem. Primary position upbeat nystagmus has been associated with tumors presenting at the pontine–mesencephalic junction (80). Downbeating, small amplitude, primary position nystagmus, and ocular myoclonus suggest a medullary location (13). Localization to the midbrain is suggested by a median longitudinal fasciculus syndrome or convergence retraction nystagmus. Seesaw nystagmus localizes the pathology to the region of the diencephalon. In addition, oculomotor gaze disorders have been described (54,86).

Bulbar signs, including swallowing and feeding abnormalities, reflect medullary involvement. Because the descending tract of V has a long intracranial course from the point of entrance into the brain stem to as far caudal as the upper cervical cord, sensory loss over the face may suggest involvement of the brain stem at any point from a midpontine level to the medulla. Asymmetry of the palate, absent gag reflex, atrophy of the tongue, and nasal regurgitation of food all reflect medullary involvement. Ataxia, both limb and appendicular, suggests either direct involvement of the cerebellum or, more likely, compromise of pathways of the cerebellum passing through any of the three cerebellar peduncles. Motor difficulties relate in equal proportion to abnormalities of the cerebellum and corticospinal tracts.

Ventricular dilatation has been noted in approximately two-thirds of cases (57). Papilledema is seen in approximately one-third of patients at some time in the course of the illness. The findings of ventricular dilatation in the absence of papilledema suggest that obstruction of spinal fluid is slow in development. Thus, presenting signs, rather than those of increased intracranial pressure, are more likely to represent specific dysfunction of the brain stem.

Tumors of the stem are usually considered to be relentlessly progressive with an inexorable course to death. However, duration of symptoms until diagnosis may vary as long as several weeks to several years. There are limited reports (68) of neoplasms of the brain stem characterized by a remitting and exacerbating course. Presentation in this manner may lead the unwary physician to consider demyelinating disease and/or a parainfectious etiology. Presumably, remission relates to the resolution of edema or necrosis in the area of the tumor. Likewise, evacuation of a cyst may be associated with clearing of symptoms only to be followed by a recurrence of the symptomatology several months later. In addition, because the brain stem is located in a relatively narrow space, resolution of a tamponade effect secondary to edema or hemorrhage may be associated with improvement in symptoms or signs.

The differential of failure to thrive in infancy should include a pontine tumor. The finding of an emaciated infant with facial paresis, absent cough response during suctioning, depressed gag reflex, and respiratory irregularity, should lead to consideration of an intrinsic lesion of the stem (74).

Even in Cushing's time, it was recognized that pontine tumors may be associated with mental symptoms. Most authors have commented on personality changes in patients with brain stem tumors. These changes consist of apathy, withdrawn behavior, emotional lability, and decline in school performance. Several reports suggest that these youngsters may become agitated and aggressive, physically abusive, and have deterioration of handwriting and speech. As might be expected with abnormalities of the brain stem, dysarthria is often present.

DIAGNOSTIC STUDIES

The clinical suspicion of a pontine mass is further confirmed by additional diagnostic studies. Before the advent of computed tomography, air encephalography via the lumbar route was the diagnostic procedure of choice. Demonstration of an enlarged pons, particularly in the sagittal view, lead to the inferential diagnosis of pontine hypertrophy and, by extension, a pontine glioma. Pneumoencephalographic signs consisted of obliteration of the prepontine cisterns and distortion with upward and backward extension of the fourth ventricle. Findings of dilation of the third and lateral ventricles suggested obstructive hydrocephalus and a pontomesencephalic location of the tumor. The above is of interest only as a historical descriptor. Modern neuroimaging has replaced this approach.

Detailed descriptions of the arteriographic features of brain stem tumors were given in the late 1960s and early 1970s. The most readily recognized angiographic features are anterior displacement of the basilar artery and terminal portion of the vertebral artery against the clivus with obliteration of the prepontine cistern. Unfortunately, anatomical alteration of the basilar artery is not invariably found; enclosure of the vessel by tumor may prevent anterior displacement of this vessel. Furthermore, changes in the larger vessels do not allow differentiation of an extraaxial from an intraaxial mass. However, close attention to the distribution of the branches and segments of the superior, middle, and inferior cerebellar arteries allows characterization of the location and extent of the brain stem mass. Attention to the arteriovenous phase of the angiogram permits localization of the mass in multiple planes. For the surgeon, examination of detailed vascular anatomy continues to be necessary to delineate the vascular supply of the tumor and to rule out the infrequent arteriovenous malformation of the brain stem (37). Currently, MRI angiography has the potential of replacing more conventional methods.

CT and MRI scanning have virtually replaced all other diagnostic modalities (6,41,46,77). CT readily identifies calcification and displacement or distortion of the ventricular system. MRI is superior to CT because of the superior resolution of the anatomy, which can be visualized in all anatomic planes, i.e., coronal, sagittal, and axial (13). The ability to identify brain stem tumors accurately by CT and MRI is greater than 90%. The lowest portion of the brain stem is the most difficult to evaluate by CT, and it is best evaluated with MRI in both the coronal and axial planes. Several groups have emphasized the need to compare the normal distance from the dorsum sella to the anterior fourth ventricle. The sagittal plane is the most effective in identifying pontine hypertrophy (11).

CT features of brain stem tumors are quite variable. In an English report (40), the CT scans of 25 patients with brain stem tumors were analyzed. Thirty percent were found to have isodense lesions, 49% showed high density lesions, 52% were of low density, and 8% were of mixed density. Calcification was seen in 12%, hydrocephalus in 28%, and periventricular lucencies in 12%. Cystic changes were noted in 12%. Contrast enhancement occurred in over 50% of patients. Of those enhancing, 12% were diffuse, 42% were patchy, 14% showed even-ring enhancement, 25% showed uneven-ring enhancement, and 33% showed nodular enhancement (Fig. 12-3). Also, because many of the tumors are isodense on noncontrast films and are nonenhancing with contrast, CT diagnosis, like air, depends on recognition of altered anatomy (5,6).

For the most part, the MRI of tumors of the brain stem is characterized by decreased signal on T1-weighted images and increased signal on T2-weighted images. Ring-enhancement patterns with gadolinium have been described. The MRI, more than the CT scan, is helpful in identifying the extent of anatomical involvement and leptomeningeal seeding. MRI has suggested that tumor is rarely confined to the pons and that an exophytic pattern of growth is quite common. Because of this, MRI is rapidly becoming the procedure of choice in staging patients for treatment approaches (4) (Fig. 12-4). In those patients who have received high-dose hyperfractionated radiation, intrale-

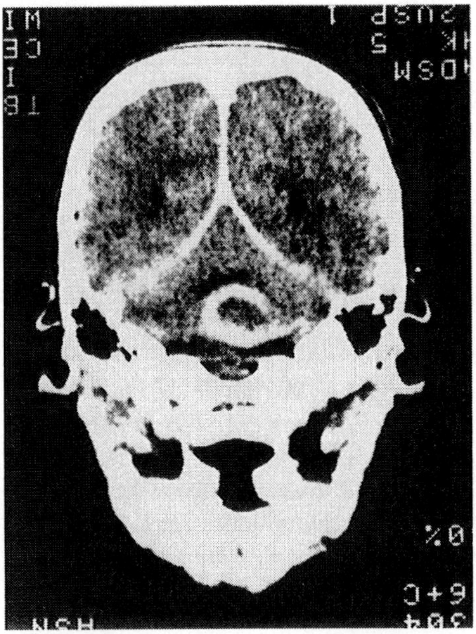

FIG. 12-3. CT scan with contrast in coronal plane showing ring enhancement of a necrotic tumor.

sional necrosis, not correlated with clinical symptomatology, is more frequently identified on MRI than on CT scanning.

Epstein (18,19) has identified four categories of brain stem tumors on the basis of anatomic location. These include tumors that are diffuse, focal, or cystic, or that are found at the cervical medullary junction. The diffuse tumor is the most common and has the worst prognosis. These tumors are characterized by areas of hypodensity throughout the pons and may extend into

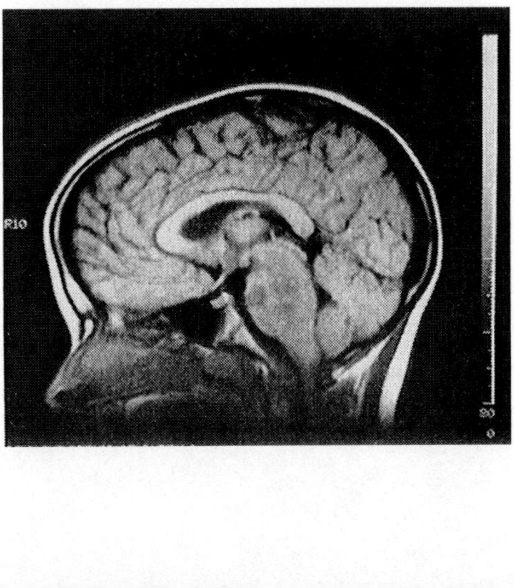

FIG. 12-4. T1-weighted MRI in sagittal plane demonstrating enlargement of the pons. Decreased T1 signal in the mass suggests tumor heterogeneity.

the midbrain or the medulla. On sagittal view they are identified as marked enlargement of the pons and correlate with the pathologic description of "diffuse pontine hypertrophy." These tumors may or may not enhance with contrast agents. On MRI, the tumor may appear more extensive than on CT, especially when T2-weighted paradigms of imaging are used. This, in all likelihood, is secondary to the marked edema associated with the tumor.

Focal tumors are characterized by areas of contrast enhancement on CT and absence of hypodensity. The MRI may either corroborate the findings of a focal tumor or suggest a more diffuse nature to the tumor and hence a more malignant potential.

Cystic brain stem tumors have the same limited potential for growth and the same imaging characteristics as cerebellar astrocytomas. On neuroimaging, whether by CT or MRI, an enhancing mural nodule with contrast may be identified associated with the cyst. These tumors may be found in the pons and extend laterally into the cerebellar peduncle. A more limited group of brain stem gliomas may present at the cervical medullary junction extending from the medulla caudally into the cervical cord. These tumors rarely extend above the pontomedullary junction and are readily identified on sagittal MRI.

Auditory brain stem evoked responses have also been used to assess brain stem function. The auditory response is a time-locked response to an auditory signal, either mixed or pure tone. Background noise from an EEG is averaged by computer so that the time-locked response may be readily identified. Five to seven wave forms are reproducibly elicited at a sensation level 40 dB above threshold. Each wave form is thought to represent neurogenerators at varying anatomical locations in the auditory pathway. Wave I is putatively representative of the eighth cranial nerve; wave II, the cochlear nucleus; wave III, the superior olivary complex; wave IV, the nucleus of the lateral lemniscus; wave V, the inferior colliculus; wave VI, the medial geniculate body; and wave VII, the cortical radiations (Fig. 12-5).

Multiple criteria have been used to suggest abnormalities. These include increased latency of the fifth wave, decreased amplitude, alterations in wave form, the lack of response stability (i.e., the ability to reproduce the same response), absence of different peaks, and intrapeak latency differences. Intrapeak latency differences are obtained by stimulation of both ears and comparing the latency of the fifth wave between ears. In a study (50) of seven children with brain stem tumors, six of seven had at least four abnormalities on auditory-evoked response. The remaining patients had two out of seven abnormalities. Others (37) have suggested that evoked responses in combination with impedance, pure tone, and speech audiometry are necessary to differentiate a peripheral from a central origin. There are also reports that the configuration of far-field generators may be altered in tumors of the brain stem. These findings imply that the recording of the spatial distribution

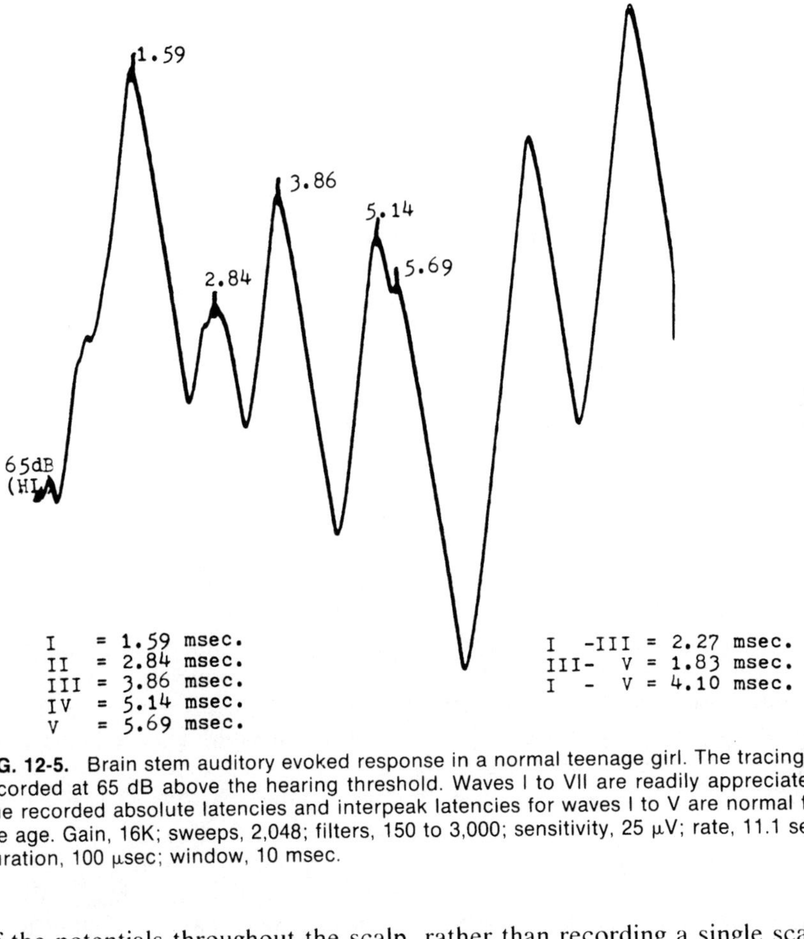

FIG. 12-5. Brain stem auditory evoked response in a normal teenage girl. The tracing is recorded at 65 dB above the hearing threshold. Waves I to VII are readily appreciated. The recorded absolute latencies and interpeak latencies for waves I to V are normal for the age. Gain, 16K; sweeps, 2,048; filters, 150 to 3,000; sensitivity, 25 μV; rate, 11.1 sec; duration, 100 μsec; window, 10 msec.

of the potentials throughout the scalp, rather than recording a single scalp potential, may have some diagnostic significance (33).

The above audiologic measures, although of interest, have little to add to the diagnosis or treatment of brain stem tumors. In most instances, audiologic testing is considered when more definitive signs of brain stem dysfunction are apparent. It is the unusual situation in which these tests, independent of other modalities, have diagnosed an intrinsic lesion of the brain stem. Rather, they are best used to assess loss of integrity of the auditory complex resulting from either chemotherapy, radiotherapy, or surgery.

SURGERY

Traditionally surgery, followed by pathologic assessment, confirms the clinical suspicion of a brain tumor. Unfortunately, fears of brain stem swelling, irreparable neurologic damage, and the inability to approach the brain stem without causing significant residual have hampered the ability to obtain an accurate pathologic diagnosis and in the past has limited the role of surgery. The finding of a low-grade neoplasm on stereotactic biopsy cannot be viewed as definitive, as sampling error may miss the presence of malignant dedifferentiation in parts of the tumor not sampled. This consideration has led many to reject the need for pathologic confirmation and to suggest that treatment should be instituted on the basis of clinical features of brain stem localization and imaging characteristics of a brain stem tumor. Others (52), however, suggest that because most patients have pilocytic tumors, there tends to be a uniformity in structure with little regional variation. As early as 1979, Reigel (57) addressed the value of the surgical approach to brain stem tumors. He reported on his surgical experience with 26 patients, the average age of whom was 7.3 years. All these patients had a biopsy of the brain stem for a putative tumor. Sixty-two percent of these patients had significant hydrocephalus requiring a shunting procedure. The majority of patients requiring shunts had tumors in the upper brain stem and mesencephalon. Pathologically, these were found to be low-grade astrocytomas. Glioblastomas were more likely to be found in the lower brain stem and caudal pons. Of the 26 patients biopsied, 13 had astrocytomas, 6 glioblastomas, and 2 ependymomas. No tumor was identified in the remaining 5. There were no operative deaths. Operative mortality consisted primarily of cranial nerve deficits. Five children required tracheostomy after the operation, 3 of which were permanent. Survival times for those patients with glioblastoma treated with radiation alone averaged 5.9 months, whereas survival of those treated with radiation and chemotherapy using a Children's Cancer Study Group (CCSG) protocol averaged 7 to 9 months. Thirteen of the 14 patients with astrocytomas were alive 4 to 15 months after the operation.

More recent papers (31) have addressed the relationship of histopathology to therapy and outcome. A Japanese series (49) of 23 patients with histologically proven brain stem gliomas was recently reported. Eleven of these patients had glioblastomas, while the remaining were of low grade. The survival of those with malignant tumors was 15 months following diagnosis, suggesting a poor prognosis; those patients with low-grade tumors had a 5-year actuarial survival rate of 50%. The use of biopsy is further underscored in a paper (23) from Marseille in which 17% of 38 patients with putative brain stem tumors were found to harbor nonneoplastic lesions. Diagnoses included hemangiomas, hemorrhagic infarcts, arachnoid cysts, telangiectasia of the pons, cavernous hemangiomas, and hamartomas. This report and others (3) emphasize the value of pathologic confirmation before treatment is considered. Traditional fears regarding surgical morbidity may be a bit overstated. In the Marseille group, the mortality was 3%, temporary morbidity was 18%, and permanent morbidity was only 3%. On the basis of the above, it is our belief that, where feasible, surgical exploration may clarify the underlying neoplastic pathology and in the infrequent situation identify nonneoplastic pathology.

Attempts at debulking and curative surgery vary depending on anatomic location (38,79). Surgical treatment of tumors in each of these anatomical locations varies considerably. The laser and the ultrasonic surgical aspirator are used to debulk the tumor. Those that present as dorsally exophytic or as cysts with a mural nodule are amenable to surgery and have the best overall prognosis of all brain stem tumors. For some of these patients, radical surgery offers the best possibility of long-term remission and even cure. Surgery can be more radical in the upper cervical cord but must be approached with greater trepidation in the medulla because of the greater risk of injuring neurologically sensitive areas. Ultrasound is used to monitor the dissection in order to identify cysts that may be overlooked as surgery proceeds (18).

RADIOTHERAPY

For most patients, treatment with or without surgical confirmation has consisted of radiotherapy (8). In a few studies, 5-year survivals as high as 40 to 50% have been reported, but most statistics suggest 5-year survivals of 20 to 30% (4). Dose–response curves for radiation of the brain stem are not universally accepted because survival statistics do not vary appreciably with increasing doses of radiation (Table 12-1). The generally accepted dose of radiation is 5,000 to 5,500 cGy given directly to the tumor bed extending over 5 to 6 weeks. To avoid radiation necrosis, radiation should not exceed 180 cGy per day. Beyond this level, there is an increasing incidence of radiation damage to normal tissue. MRI with gadolinium, rather than CT, may be the best tool for identifying the extent of the brain stem tumor and thus the most useful modality for defining the volume of radiation (75). MRI permits identification of tumor that extends beyond the brain stem either superiorly into the hypothalamus or third ventricle, laterally into the cerebellar peduncle and basal cisterns, more inferiorly into the medulla and/or cervical cord, and dorsally into the fourth ventricle.

There are several large series in the literature assessing the value of radiotherapy. In general, the response to radiation occurs early in the course of treatment, followed by a plateau effect. Long-term survivals are well known and are generally seen in patients with a long history of symptoms before the diagnosis is made. As a generalization, long-term survivals are seen in patients with low-grade astrocytomas, and short-term survival is to be expected with more malignant glioblastomas.

In an earlier study by Panitch and Berg (53), the average survival of children radiated for brain stem tumors was 47.2 months, compared with 15.5 months for those not treated. Those patients who had an early response had

TABLE 12-1. *Survival rates in children with brain stem tumors after radiotherapy*

Author	No. patients	Radiation (cGy)	3-yr survival (%)	5-yr survival (%)	10-yr survival (%)
Bray et al. (9) (1958)	24	2,000–4,000	Mean survival 9 months		
Bouchard and Peirce (8) (1960)	41	5,000–6,000	44	37	24
Whyte et al. (72) (1969)	57	>4,000		45	
		<4,000		22	
Panitch and Berg (53) (1970)	31	3,600–5,000	30	23	
Stewart et al. (78) (1973)	144	Not stated		6	
Lee (43) (1975)	24	>5,000	45	14	14
		<5,000	0	0	
Villani et al. (70) (1975)	36	>5,000	45		
Sheline (73)(1977)	27	>5,000		41	33
Ryoo et al. (66) (1979)	20	4,000–5,200		30	
Kim et al. (39) (1980)	63	>5,000	40	35	28
		<5,000	29	0	
Littman et al. (44) (1980)	38	2,400–6,400		30	
Renier and Gabreels (58) (1980)	20	3,250–6,650	Mean survival 15 months		
Bloom (7) (1982)	57	>5,000		17	17
Freeman et al. (24) (1988)	34	6,600 (HFX)[a]	Mean survival 11 months		
Freeman et al. (25) (1991)	54	7,020 (HFX)	Mean survival 10 months		
Edwards et al. (17) (1989)	53	7,200 (HFX)	Mean survival 16 months		
Shibamoto et al. (75) (1989)	71	5,700–6,500		17	15
Packer et al. (51) (1990)	31	7,200 (HFX)		32% at 2 yr	
	17	6,480 (HFX)		20% at 2 yr	

[a] Hyperfractionation.

an average survival of 60.8 months, whereas those without an early response survived an average of 5.6 months. Survival of patients with low-grade astrocytomas was 32.4 months versus 6.4 months for those with glioblastomas. Radiation doses ranged from 3,600 to 5,000 cGy.

Radiation dose may influence survival. Kim et al. (39) reported on 63 patients treated with radiotherapy. Forty-five of these patients received over 4,000 cGy. Survival rates were somewhat better for those treated with greater than 5,000 cGy. A 40% survival rate was found after 3 years, a 35% survival after 5 years, and a 28% survival after 10 years. For those patients treated with less than 5,000 cGy, survival at 3 years was 29%, and 0% at 5 and 10 years. Those with high-grade malignancies did the poorest. These results were essentially no different than those reported by Bouchard and Peirce (8) 14 years earlier from the same institution. Lee (43) evaluated 24 patients treated with 3,000 to 5,000 cGy to the posterior fossa. Forty-five percent of those patients treated with greater than 5,000 cGy were alive after 3 years. None of those who had received less than 5,000 cGy survived 3 years. Similarly, Whyte et al. (84) reported on 57 patients who completed radiotherapy.

The 5-year survival for those who received more than 4,000 cGy was greater than 58%, compared with a 5-year survival of 22% for those receiving less than 4,000 cGy.

However, in a group of 20 patients studied by Renier and Gabreels (58), an 8.4% 5-year survival rate was reported, and neither radiation dose nor adjuvant chemotherapy had measurable effect on the results. Similarly, Littman et al. (44) reported on 38 patients treated in doses ranging from 2,400 to 6,400 cGy. Twenty-one of 58 patients were alive 3 months to 13 years after completion of the treatment. Forty-one patients died within 32 months, most within 2 years. Those patients with malignant glioblastomas, which were confirmed either at surgery or necropsy, died within 16 months of diagnosis. Those with well-differentiated tumors had a somewhat better survival rate. Overall, 5-year survival was 30%. The dose of radiation appeared to have no effect on long-term survival. Golden et al. (32) examined 13 patients who died soon after the diagnosis was made. The average life-span of children in this group was 4.3 months, and for adults, excluding a 26-month survivor, 6.3 months. At the time of autopsy these patients had either a glioblastoma multiforme or malignant astrocytoma. Radiation in this group was believed to have no influence on survival. In a group of 40 patients studied by Ryoo et al. (66), survival was correlated with anatomic location. Those patients treated for tumors in the thalamus and midbrain had a 43% survival rate, whereas those with tumors of the pons and medulla had a 30% 5-year survival rate. Death occurred within 3 years in those patients who did not show some sign of improvement within the first month.

Radiation, although rarely curative, does provide short-term improvement in neurologic status. In Sheline's (75) series of 27 patients there was a 41% 5-year survival rate and 33% 10-year survival rate post-therapy. Most patients were treated with 5,000 to 5,500 cGy to the tumor, regardless of the histologic pathology. The median survival of those who died was 6 months. Seventy-one percent showed early improvement after completion of the treatment, bearing out the repeated observation that improvement, if it happens, occurs early in the course of treatment. The results by Bray et al. (9) were similar in a group of 39 patients. Radiation doses ranged from 1,200 to 4,000 cGy. Twenty-four patients were followed until death. The average survival was 9 months. Of this group, 15 were judged to have responded favorably within the first 3 to 6 weeks of therapy. The average survival for those responding early was 11.25 months compared to an average survival of 4.75 months for those who did not have an early initial response. Eight children were alive 1 month to 13 years after completion of therapy. Three children were lost to follow-up. Villani et al. (81) treated 36 patients with radiotherapy in doses ranging from 5,000 to 6,000 cGy. Survival after 1 year was 45% and somewhat less at 3 years.

The above studies, when compared to survival rates in the older literature, suggest a limited, but nonetheless increasing, trend of improvement in survival. Although an optimal radiation dose has not been universally accepted, the experience of Bouchard and Peirce (8) in the older literature, as well as more recent data, suggest that 4,500 to 5,500 cGy directed to the tumor bed is the most effective. Response to radiotherapy depends on many variables. These include location, histology of the tumor, and early response to treatment.

The greatest change in treatment of brain stem tumors in the last decade has been an increasing emphasis on hyperfractionated radiation. Hyperfractionation allows for high doses of radiation to be given over a time similar to that used for standard radiation. Rather than 180 cGy of radiation given once a day for 5 to 6 weeks, radiation fractions of 110 to 120 cGy are given two times a day. This technique has allowed the total dose of radiation to be increased 10 to 20% over the standard radiation doses of 5,500 cGy. Theoretically, by decreasing the dose per fraction and increasing the total dose of delivered radiation, a greater tumoricidal effect may occur without increasing side effects.

The use of hyperfractionation rests on the concept that neoplastic cells are apt to be more sensitive to ionizing radiation while they are in the proliferating phase of the cell cycle. Radiation, for the most part, will affect proliferating cells and spare those cells in G_0 or in the resting phase of the cell cycle. As the tumor burden shrinks, more cells in the nonproliferating pool tend to enter the cell cycle. Theoretically, by delivering multiple fractions of radiation over a short period, cells moving form the G_0 to a proliferating phase of the cell cycle are more subject to cell kill. In addition, there is evidence to suggest that decreased dose per fraction given frequently is more effective in destroying radio-resistant hypoxic cells than standard dose schema.

On the basis of the above, many groups have explored phase II trials of hyperfractionated radiation. Beginning in the middle 1980s, several reports (17,24,25,51) appeared using sequentially increased doses of hyperfractionation ranging from 6,600 cGy to 7,800 cGy. All these studies have demonstrated the ability of normal tissue to tolerate increasing dose. Although the cell kill of 6,600 cGy given by hyperfractionation is probably the same as that of 5,500 cGy, larger doses of radiation have been associated with increasing progression-free survival. In a recent study of 34 patients treated with 7,200 cGy, the median time to progression was 44 weeks with a median survival of 64 weeks. Using 7,200 cGy, a 30% progression-free survival was noted at 20 months. The three Pediatric Oncology Group studies (24–26) that used escalating doses of hyperfractionation from 6,600 to 7,560 cGy have all demonstrated the ability of the nervous system to tolerate large doses of radiation given in a hyperfractionated manner. Although not statistically significant, there has been a tendency toward improved progression-free survival with increasing dose. Toxicities at the higher dose levels are a bit greater than those at the lower dose levels. In the Pediatric Oncology Group study, approximately 50% of patients remained on steroids for periods in excess of 3 months following the beginning of radiation. Steroid complications have included an increased incidence of opportunistic infections, decreased glucose tolerance, hypertension, osteoporosis, and mood swings. As might be expected at higher dose levels, cystic degeneration and intralesional necrosis were identified in a few patients. These complications can be managed conservatively, but surgical decompression, when necessary, may be required. In those patients in the POG study in whom decompression was undertaken, tissue removed from the necrotic lesions was benign in 3 out of 4 patients (Table 12-2).

The Pediatric Oncology Group studies have been influenced to some extent by selection criteria. Those patients chosen for hyperfractionation were those with an adverse set of prognostic criteria and consisted of children with a duration of symptoms and signs less than 6 months, tumors that infiltrated the brain stem proper, i.e., mesencephalon, pons, and medulla, and children who had evidence of two or three clinical signs, i.e., long-tract signs, cranial neuropathy, or cerebellar signs. Lesions that were focal or exophytic, or originated in the cerebellar peduncle or cervical medullary junction were by design excluded. In this group of patients, of those that were biopsied, the majority were found to have either glioblastoma or anaplastic astrocytoma.

TABLE 12-2. *Clinical and imaging characteristics of patients in POG study treated with hyperfractionation*

Variable	66 Gy	70.2 Gy	75.6 Gy	*p*
Evaluable pts	34	57	39	—
Male gender	56%	47%	54%	0.7
Median age	7.1 yr	6.5 yr	7.5 yr	0.4
Caucasian race	74%	68%	64%	0.7
Neurological findings				
Cranial nerve deficits				
midbrain (III, IV, V)	21%	11%	13%	0.4
pons (VI, VII)	74%	86%	92%	0.09
medulla (IX, X, XI, XII)	32%	21%	47%	0.03
Long tract signs	56%	60%	66%	0.7
Ataxia	73%	75%	84%	0.5
"Classical triad" of symptoms	36%	40%	53%	0.3
Imaging findings				
Pons only (CT or MR)	53%	16%	56%	<0.001
Diffuse involvement (CT or MR)	75%	92%	97%	0.008
Exophytic (CT or MR)	18%	67%	63%	<0.001
Hypodense, nonenhancing (CT)	38%	42%		0.8
Ring-like enhancement (CT or MR)	18%	9%	19%	0.2
Hydrocephalus (CT or MR)	32%	29%	13%	0.1

From Freeman CR, Krischer JP, Sanford RA, et al. Final results of a study of escalating doses of hyperfractionated radiotherapy in brain stem tumors in children: a Pediatric Oncology Group study. *Int J Radiat Oncol Biol Phys* 1993; *in press.*

Results from CCSG studies (17,51) that used up to 7,800 cGy have, like the POG study, demonstrated good tolerance but limited beneficial effect.

Although most studies that used hyperfractionated radiation have accrued a large number of patients, demonstrated the feasibility and relative safety of this approach, and revealed a tendency toward increasing progression-free survival with increasing dose, overall survivals have not measurably changed. The major value of these studies has been the observation that CNS toxicity is the limiting factor when escalation of doses of radiation is considered.

CHEMOTHERAPY

Assessing the results of chemotherapeutic trials in the treatment of brain stem tumors is even more difficult than assessing radiotherapy effects. Interpretation of chemotherapy benefits has been complicated by the multiplicity of drugs, varying dose schedules, short-term effects, multiple delivery systems, and total lack of uniformity in the approach to treatment. In addition, unlike those on radiotherapy, most series in which chemotherapy has been used have been distressingly small. Although positive responses are reported by most authors, results are invariably short-term or tempered by previous treatment with radiotherapy. Furthermore, treatment differences among single and varying combinations of drugs have yet to be established (42,64,69, 71,83,85). Reports from small groups of patients in whom either single agents or combination agents were used have generally been discouraging. Single-agent trials with procarbazine, vincristine, and methotrexate given either intrathecally (IT) or IV in high doses have been unsuccessful (22,48,62,72). Renier (58) found no effect in a series of children treated with either cyclophosphamide, methotrexate, 6-mercaptopurine, vincristine, or 1-(2-chlorethyl)3-cyclohexyl-1-nitrosourea (CCNU). Crafts and Wilson (12) in their review of a compiled composite analysis of 19 patients treated with 1,3 Bis (2-chlorethyl)-1-nitrosourea (BCNU) alone, reported only five possible responders. The doses of BCNU varied between 20 and 125 mg/m^2 per tumor dose. Increasing the dose did not seem to influence survival (83). CCNU has been used in doses varying from 125 to 150 mg/m^2 (61). Alternating dose schedules and increasing the dose does not influence survival. There is a single anecdotal report of a limited response to high-dose intravenous methotrexate (60). This result has not been substantiated, nor has administration of methotrexate by either the IV or the IT route been shown to affect outcome (48). In a small group of patients treated with vincristine, there was a suggestive response in 2 of 5 patients (62). More recently, chemotherapeutic protocols have been platinum-based. Unfortunately, as with other single agents, protocols using cis-platin, carboplatin (1,2,14,27,30,70,82,87), and iproplatin have been disappointing. As with single agents, multiagent chemotherapy has shown no benefit over radiation alone. The drugs chosen have been varying combinations of 5 FU, CCNU, hydroxyurea, misonidazole, procarbazine, cytoxan, cytarabrine, and nitrogen mustard (20,36,55,59). These agents have been available for more than a decade, and their ineffectiveness as single agents, or in combination, reflects the frustration that has accompanied the search for meaningful treatment of this tumor.

One of the largest reports on the chemotherapeutic treatment of children with brain stem tumors comes from the University of California at San Francisco (27). In this report of 45 patients, there was no difference in survival between patients treated with single drugs and those treated with combination therapies. Drug protocols using nitrosoureas showed no advantage over those using procarbazine. In the group of 25 patients treated with radiotherapy and chemotherapy, either at the time of diagnosis or at recurrence, the median time to progression was 23 weeks with a mean survival of 44 weeks. Thirty-two percent had a 1-year survival rate, and 8% had a 5-year survival rate. Thirty-three patients had histologic confirmation of their tumor either by biopsy or autopsy. Those with high-grade gliomas had substantially poorer survival rates than those with low-grade gliomas. There was a 25% 5-year survival rate for patients with low-grade gliomas and a 0% 5-year survival rate for those with glioblastomas. An earlier report (16) from the same group in California but with a smaller number of patients revealed similar findings. Survival was better in children whose tumors were located in the medulla or midbrain, and poorest in those children with tumors located in the pons. The tendency for the more anaplastic tumors to occur in the medulla, as well as the medullary location, presumably acted in combination to influence the outcome. More recently, the same group reported their results in 13 patients treated with a combination of 5-flourouracil, CCNU, hydroxyurea and 6-mercaptopurine. As with most chemotherapeutic reports, response has been measured in weeks rather than months. A few singular reports in the recent literature extol the virtues of one agent over the other. These have been anecdotal. No one treatment regimen or dosage schedule has been found to be superior.

SUMMARY

In conclusion, the treatment of tumors of the brain stem by either surgery, radiotherapy, chemotherapy alone, or in combination has been disappointingly poor. Of all the tumors of childhood, treatment has been least helpful in this group. Unfortunately, although brain stem tumors are bathed by spinal fluid, administration of chemotherapy, either via the lumbar route or systemically, has not had a measured benefit. As a result, in the last 10 years there has been a dearth of chemotherapy trials. Those that have been reported have been unsuccessful and in small groups of patients. Similarly, although

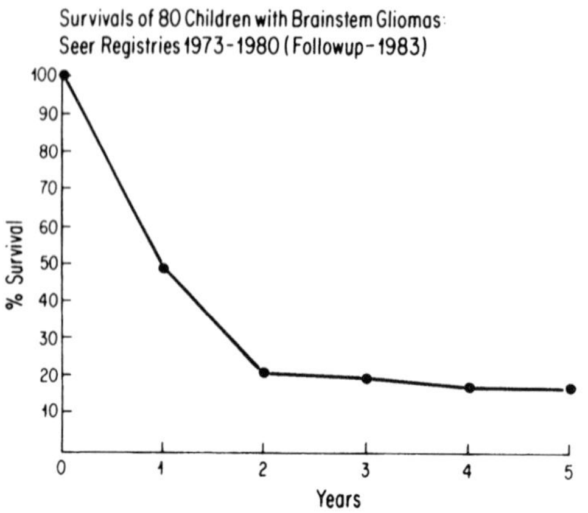

FIG. 12-6. Survival of children with brain stem glioma. Note the plateau at 2 years, suggesting two populations of patients: (A) a group in whom survival rate at 2 years is 20% and (B) a smaller group with long-term survival.

ample evidence suggests short-term benefits from radiotherapy, long-term results have been disappointingly poor. Radiation in many series is associated with an early response followed by a plateau effect. In select cases, radical surgery for dorsally exophytic tumors and those that present at the medullary cervical junction has produced long-term results and, at times, has been curative (19).

Survival may relate to the location as well as histopathology, rather than to the treatment. Thus, low-grade tumors occurring in the mesencephalon or in the medulla, those that present in an exophytic fashion, and those that are associated with neurofibromatosis have all been associated with long-term survival (Fig. 12-6).

The overall poor prognosis of brain stem tumors has led cooperative groups to consider protocols using increased doses of radiations, varying combinations of drugs, new drugs as single agents, or increasing dose intensity schema. Although well tolerated with limited side effects, hyperfractionation has had little impact on quality of life or survival. The Pediatric Oncology Group is now evaluating the effectiveness of nonchemosensitive doses of cis-platinum (100 mg/m^2) used as a radiosensitizer with increasing hyperfractionated doses. Novel approaches await the development of better drugs, different carrier systems, alternative methods of treatments such as immunotherapy and recombinant DNA, or more imaginative use of current treatment modalities.

REFERENCES

1. Allen JC, Hancock C, Walker R, Tan C. PCNU and recurrent childhood brain tumors. *J Neurooncol* 1987;5:241.
2. Allen JC, Walker R, Luke, et al. Carboplatin and recurrent childhood brain tumors. *J Clin Oncol* 1987;5:459–463.

3. Artigas J, Ferszt R, Brock M, Kazner E, Cervos-Navarro J. The relevance of pathological diagnosis for therapy and outcome of brain stem gliomas. *Acta Neurochir* 1988;42:166–169.
4. Barkovich AJ, Krischer J, Kun, et al. Brain stem gliomas: a classification system based on magnetic resonance imaging. *Pediatr Neurosurg* 1991;16:73–83.
5. Barnett HJ, Hyland HH. Tumors involving the brain stem: a study of 90 cases arising in the brain stem, IVth ventricle and pineal tissue. *Q J Med* 1952;83:265–284.
6. Bilaniuk LT, Zimmerman RA, Littman P, Gallo E, Rorke LB, Bruce DA, Schut L. Computed tomography of brain stem gliomas in children. *Radiology* 1980;134:89–95.
7. Bloom HJG. Intracranial tumors: response and resistance to therapeutic endeavors 1970–1980. *Int J Radiat Oncol Biol Phys* 1982;8:1083–1113.
8. Bouchard J, Peirce CB. Radiation therapy in the management of neoplasms of the central nervous system with a special note in regard to children: twenty years experience 1939–1958. *AJR* 1960;84:610–628.
9. Bray PF, Carter S, Taveras JM. Brain stem tumors in children. *Neurology* 1958;8:1–7.
10. Buckley RC. Pontine gliomas: a pathologic study and classification of twenty-five cases. *Arch Pathol* 1930;9:779–819.
11. Byrne JV, Kendall BE, Kingsley DPE, Moseley IF. Lesions of the brain stem: assessment by magnetic resonance imaging. *Neuroradiology* 1989;31:129–133.
12. Crafts DC, Wilson CB. Current status of pediatric brain tumor chemotherapy. In: O'Brien MS, ed. *Pediatric neurological surgery*. New York: Raven Press; 1978:87–100.
13. Curless RG. Acute vestibular dysfunction in childhood: central vs. peripheral. *Childs Brain* 1980;6:39–44.
14. Diez B, Monges J, Muriel FS. Evaluation of cisplatin in children with recurrent brain tumors. *Cancer Treat Rep* 1985;69:911–913.
15. Duffner PK, Klein DM, Cohen ME. Calcification in brain stem gliomas. *Neurology* 1978; 28:832–834.
16. Edwards MS, Levin VR, Wilson CB. Chemotherapy of pediatric posterior fossa tumors. *Childs Brain* 1980;7:252–260.
17. Edwards MSB, Wara WM, Urtasun RC, et al. Hyperfractionated radiation therapy for brain stem glioma: a phase I-II trial. *J Neurosurg* 1989;70:681–700.
18. Epstein F. Intra-axial tumors of the cervicomedullary junction in children. *Concepts Pediatr Neurosurg* 1987;7:117–133.
19. Epstein F, Wisoff JH. Intrinsic brain stem tumors in childhood: surgical indications. *J Neurooncol* 1988;6:309–317.
20. Ettinger LJ, Sinniah D, Siegel SE, et al. Combination chemotherapy with cyclophosphamide, vincristine, procarbazine, and prednisone (COPP) in children with brain tumors. *J Neurooncol* 1985;3:263.
21. Farwell JR, Dohrmann GJ, Flannery JT. Central nervous system tumors in children. *Cancer* 1977;40:3123–3132.
22. Fewer D, Wilson CB, Boldrey EB, Enot KJ. A phase II study of 1-2-chloroethyl-3-cyclohexyl-1-nitrosourea) (CCNU). *Cancer* 1972;56:421–427.
23. Frank F, Fabrizi AP, Frank-Ricci R, Gaist G, Sedan R, Peragut JC. Stereotactic biopsy and treatment of brain stem lesions: combined study of 33 cases (Bologna-Marseille). *Acta Neurochir* 1988;42:177–181.
24. Freeman CR, Krischer J, Sanford RA, Burger PC, Cohen M, Norris D. Hyperfractionated radiotherapy in brain stem tumors: results of a Pediatric Oncology Group study. *Int J Radiat Oncol Biol Phys* 1988;15:311–318.
25. Freeman CR, Krischer J, Sanford RA, Cohen ME, et al. Hyperfractionated radiation in brain stem tumors. *Cancer* 1991;68:474–481.
26. Freeman CR, Krischer JP, Sanford RA, et al. Final results of a study of escalating doses of hyperfractionated radiotherapy in brain stem tumors in children: a Pediatric Oncology Group study. *Int J Radiat Oncol Biol Phys*, 1993; *in press*.
27. Friedman HS, Kirscher JF, Burger P, et al. Treatment of children with progressive or recurrent brain tumors with carboplatin: a Pediatric Oncology randomized phase II study. *J Clin Oncol* 1992;10:249–256.
28. Fulton DS, Levin VA, Wara WM, Edwards MS, Wilson CB. Chemotherapy of pediatric brain stem tumors. *J Neurosurg* 1981;54:721–725.
29. Galbraith JG, Sahni P. Diagnosis of brain stem tumors. *Hosp Med* 1970;6:134–141.

30. Gayon PS, Ettinger LJ, Baum ES, et al. Carboplatin in childhood brain tumors. *Cancer* 1990;66:2465–2469.
31. Giunta F, Grasso G, Marini G, Zorzi F. Brain stem expanding lesions: stereotactic diagnosis and therapeutical approach. *Acta Neurochir* 1989;46:86–89.
32. Golden GS, Ghatak NR, Hirano A, French JH. Malignant glioma of the brain stem: a clinicopathological analysis of 13 cases. *J Neurol Neurosurg Psychiatr* 1972;35:732–738.
33. Hashimoto I, Ishiyama Y, Manaka S, Ebe M, Sano K. Spatial distribution of brain stem auditory evoked potentials and their alternations of the VIII nerve and brain stem. *Neurol Res* 1981;3:167–194.
34. Hoffman HJ, Becker L, Craven MA. A clinically and pathologically distinct group of benign brain stem gliomas. *Neurosurgery* 1980;7:243–248.
35. Huagn YP, Wolf BS. Angiographic features of brain stem tumors and differential diagnosis from fourth ventricle tumors. *AJR* 1970;110:1–30.
36. Jenkin RDT, Boesel C, Ertel I, et al. Brain stem tumors in childhood: a prospective randomized trial of irradition with and without adjuvant CCNU, VCR, and prednisone. *J Neurosurg* 1987;66:277–285.
37. Jerger J, Neely JG, Jerger S. Speech, impedance, and brain stem response audiometry in brain stem tumors. *Arch Otolaryngol* 1980;106:218–223.
38. Kelly PJ. Volumetric stereotactic surgical resection of intra-axial brain mass lesions. *Mayo Clin Proc* 1988;63:1186–1198.
39. Kim TH, Chin HW, Pollan S, Hazel JH, Webster JH. Radiotherapy of primary brain stem tumors. *Int J Radiat Oncol Biol Phys* 1980;6:51–57.
40. Kingsley DPE, Kendall BE. The CT scanner in posterior fossa tumors of childhood. *Br J Radiol* 1979;52:769–776.
41. Kirks DR, Harwood-Nash DCF. Computed tomography in pediatric radiology. *Pediatr Ann* 1980;9:66–76.
42. Kumar ARV, Renaudin J, Wilson CB, Boldrey E, Not K, Levin VS. Procarbazine hydrochloride in the treatment of brain tumors: phase 2 study. *J Neurosurg* 1974;40:365–371.
43. Lee F. Radiation of infratentorial and supratentorial brain stem tumors. *J Neurosurg* 1975; 43:65–68.
44. Littman P, Jarrett P, Bilaniuk LT, et al. Pediatric brain stem gliomas. *Cancer* 1980;45: 2787–2792.
45. Mantravadi RVP, Phatak R, Bellur S, Liebner EJ, Haas R. Brain stem glioma: an autopsy study of 25 cases. *Cancer* 1982;49:1294–1296.
46. Marks JE, Gado M. Serial computed tomography of primary brain tumors following surgery, irradiation and chemotherapy. *Radiology* 1977;125:119–125.
47. Milstein JM, Geyer JR, Berger MS, Bleyer WA. Favorable prognosis for brain stem gliomas in neurofibromatosis. *J Neurooncol* 1989;7:367–371.
48. Newton WA, Sayers MP, Samuels LD. Intrathecal methotrexate (NSC-740) therapy for brain tumors in children. *Cancer Chemother Rep* 1968;52:257–261.
49. Nishio S, Fukui M, Tateishi J. Brain stem gliomas: a clinicopathological analysis of 23 histologically proven cases. *J Neurooncol* 1988;6:245–250.
50. Nodar RH, Hahn J, Levine HL. Brain stem auditory evoked potentials in determining site of lesion of brain stem gliomas in children. *Laryngoscope* 1980;90:258–266.
51. Packer RJ, Allen JC, Goldwein JL, et al. Hyperfractionated radiotherapy for children with brain stem gliomas: a pilot study using 7,200 cGy. *Ann Neurol* 1990;27:167–173.
52. Packer RJ, Nicolson HS, Johnson DL, Vezura LG. Dilemmas in the management of childhood brain tumors: brain stem gliomas. *Pediatr Neurosurg* 1991;17:37–44.
53. Panitch ES, Berg BO. Brain stem tumors of childhood and adolescence. *Am J Dis Child* 1970;119:465–472.
54. Peiris JB, Wickremasinghe HR, Sivayoham ISS. An unusual brain stem astrocytoma producing complicated Parinaud's syndrome. *J Indian Med Assoc* 1975;64:340–341.
55. Pendergrass TW, Milstein JM, Geyer JR, et al. Eight drugs in 1 day chemotherapy for brain tumors: experience in 107 children and rationale for preirradiation chemotherapy. *J Clin Oncol* 1987;5:1221.
56. Raffel C, McComb JG, Bodner S, Gilles FE. Benign brain stem lesions in pediatric patients with neurofibromatosis: case reports. *Neurosurgery* 1989;25:959–964.

57. Reigel GH, Scarff TB, Woodford JE. Biopsy of pediatric brain stem tumors. *Childs Brain* 1979;5:329–340.
58. Renier WO, Gabreels FJM. Evaluation of diagnosis and nonsurgical therapy in 24 children with pontine tumors. *Neuropediatrics* 1980;11:262–273.
59. Rodriquez LA, Prados M, Fultond, et al. Treatment of recurrent brain stem tumors and other central nervous system tumors with 5-flouracil, CCNU, hydroxyurea, and 6-mercaptopurine. *Neurosurgery* 1988;22:691–693.
60. Rosen G. Ghavini F, Vanucci R, Deck M, Tan C, Murphy L. Pontine glioma: high-dose methotrexate and leucovorin rescue. *JAMA* 1974;230:1149–1152.
61. Rosenblum ML, Reynold AF, Smith KA, Rumack BH, Walker MD. Chloroethyl-cyclohexyl-nitrosourea (CCNU) in the treatment of malignant brain tumors. *J Neurosurg* 1973; 39:306–314.
62. Rosenstock JG, Evans AE, Schut L. Response to vincristine of recurrent brain tumors in children. *J Neurosurg* 1976;45:135–140.
63. Rothman SJ, Olanow CW. Brain stem glioma in childhood: acute hemiplegic onset. *J Can Sci Neurol* 1981:8:263–264.
64. Rubin RC, Ommaya AK, Henderson ES, Bering EA, Rall DP. Cerebrospinal fluid perfusion for central nervous system neoplasms. *Neurology* 1966;16:680–692.
65. Rubinstein LJ. In: *Tumors of the central nervous system*. Washington, DC: Armed Forces Institute of Pathology; 1972:19–50.
66. Ryoo MC, King GA, Chung CT, Sang YW, Sagerman RH. Irradiation of primary brain stem tumors. *Radiology* 1979;131:503–507.
67. Sanford RA, Freeman CR, Burger P, Cohen ME. Prognostic criteria for experimental protocols in pediatric brain stem gliomas. *Surg Neurol* 1988;30:276–280.
68. Sarkari NBS, Bickerstaff ER. Relapses and remissions in brain stem tumors. *Br Med J* 1969;2:21–23.
69. Sayers MP. Surgery and chemotherapy of brain tumors in children. *Prog Exp Tumor Res* 1972;17:414–422.
70. Sexauer CL, Khan A, Burger PC, et al. Cisplatin in recurrent pediatric brain tumors: POG phase II study. *Cancer* 1985;56:1497–1501.
71. Shapiro WR. Chemotherapy of primary malignant brain tumors in children. *Cancer* 1975; 35:965–972.
72. Shapiro WR, Chernik NL, Posner JB. Necrotizing encephalopathy following intraventricular instillation of methotrexate. *Arch Neurol* 1973;28:96–102.
73. Sheline GE. Radiation therapy of brain tumors. *Cancer* 1977;38:873–881.
74. Sieben RL, Nobuyoshi I. Brain stem glioma causing failure to thrive. *J Pediatr* 1971;47: 451–455.
75. Shibamoto Y, Takahashi M, Dokoh S, Tanabe M, Ishida T, Abe M. Radiation therapy for brain stem tumor with special reference to CT feature and prognosis correlations. *Int J Radiat Oncol Biol Phys* 1989;17:71–76.
76. Silbergold D, Berger M, Griffin B, et al. Brain stem glioma with multiple intraspinal metastases during life: case report and review of the literature. *Pediatr Neurosci* 1988;14:103–107.
77. Steele JR, Hoffman JC. Brain stem evaluation with CT cisternography. *Am J Radiol* 1981; 136:287–292.
78. Stewart AM, Lennox EL, Sanders BM. Group characteristics of children with cerebral and spinal cord tumors. *Br J Cancer* 1973;28:568–574.
79. Tomita T, McLone DG, Naidich TP. Brain stem gliomas in childhood. *J Neurooncol* 1984; 2:117–122.
80. Troost BT, Martinez J, Abel LA, Heros RC. Upbeat nystagmus and internuclear opthalmoplegia with brain stem glioma. *Arch Neurol* 1980;37:453–456.
81. Villani R, Gaini SM, Tomei G. Follow-up study of brain stem tumors in children. *Childs Brain* 1975;1:126–135.
82. Walker RW, Allen JC. Cisplatin in the treatment of recurrent childhood primary brain tumors. *J Clin Oncol* 1988;7:62–66.
83. Walker MD, Hurwitz BS. BCNU (1,3-Bis(2-chloroethyl)-1-nitrosourea: (NSC-409962) in the treatment of malignant brain tumor—a preliminary report. *Cancer Chemother Rep* 1970; 54:263–271.

84. Whyte TR, Colby MY, Layton DD. Radiation therapy of brain stem tumors. *Radiology* 1969;93:413–416.
85. Wilson CS, Gutin P, Boldrey E, Crafts D, Levin VA, Not J. Single agent chemotherapy of brain tumors. *Arch Neurol* 1976;33:739–744.
86. Zaret CR, Behrens MM, Eggers HM. Congenital ocular motor apraxia and brain stem tumor. *Arch Ophthalmol* 1980;98:438–330.
87. Zeltzer PM, Epport K, Nelson MD Jr, et al. Prolonged response to carboplatin in an infant with brain stem glioma. *Cancer* 1991;67:43–47.

13

Supratentorial Hemispheric Astrocytomas

The reported incidence of supratentorial tumors in childhood ranges from 34 to 55% (33,34,41,46,58,63). The majority of these tumors are astrocytomas, although other tumors, including oligodendrogliomas, ependymomas, and primitive neuroectodermal tumors, also arise in the cerebral hemispheres (25). Of 1,200 children with brain tumors reported to the Surveillance, Epidemiology, End Results (SEER) registries from 1968 to 1979, 32% had supratentorial astrocytomas (this series excluded craniopharyngiomas). Twenty percent of these tumors were classified as grades I and II, and 12% were grades III and IV, including glioblastoma multiforme. The incidence of glioblastoma multiforme in childhood varies from 2 to 10% (34). This variability in incidence figures may reflect series in which the inclusion criteria for children extends to 21 years.

The pathologic nosology of cerebral astrocytomas is complex. Some pathologists have subdivided the tumors according to cytologic architecture. Thus, Bailey and Cushing (3) referred to "protoplasmic" and "fibrillary" types of astrocytomas; Elvidge (22) subdivided the tumors into "diffuse," "protoplasmic," and "gemistocytic;" and Russell and Rubinstein (86) divided astrocytomas into "protoplasmic," "fibrillary" (diffuse or circumscribed), "pilocytic," "gemistocytic," and "anaplastic." Other pathologists have classified the tumors according to malignant potential. Thus, Kernohan et al. (47) graded astrocytomas I through IV according to increasing degree of anaplasia. In this classification, astrocytomas and glioblastomas represent different grades of malignancy of the same tumor. Grade I tumors, typically slow growing, are characterized by increased cellularity with most cells having normal characteristics, and few mitotic features. Endothelial proliferation is absent. Grade II tumors, previously designated "astroblastomas," are characterized by increased cellularity, polymorphic nuclei, and mitoses. There is no clear line of demarcation from normal tissue. Grade III tumors represent anaplastic astrocytomas characterized by increased cellularity, marked pleomorphism, and heightened mitotic index. Grade IV tumors represent the typical glioblastoma multiforme, characterized by cellular pleomorphism, endothelial proliferation, mitoses, necrosis, and multinucleated giant cells. Other authors have referred to grades I and II tumors as "low

Brain Tumors in Children: Principles of Diagnosis and Treatment, 2/e, edited by M.E. Cohen and P.K. Duffner, Raven Press, Ltd., New York, 1994.

grade'' and grades III and IV as ''high grade.'' Currently, a simplified system of three grades, i.e., astrocytoma, anaplastic astrocytoma, and glioblastoma multiforme, is in use by the Brain Tumor Study Group and the Pediatric Oncology Group (12) and will be used, where possible, in this discussion.

PATHOLOGY

Astrocytomas

Cerebral astrocytomas may appear diffuse and ill-defined with infiltration of central white matter, cortex, and basal ganglia. Others may be better defined and resemble the juvenile cystic cerebellar astrocytomas with a large cyst and mural nodule.

The most common microscopic pattern, according to Russell and Rubinstein (86), is the ''fibrillary'' astrocytoma. This pattern occurs most often in astrocytomas of the cerebellum, brain stem, and hypothalamus. The production of meningeal fibrils imparts a firm consistency to the tumor. Fine and coarse neuroglial fibrils occupy the matrix and form a criss-cross pattern among the cells. Cellular pleomorphism is not unusual. In parts of the tumor the cells may be small, and in others the cell borders are larger and more stellate. Mitoses are absent, and endothelial proliferation is not recognized.

A pure ''protoplasmic'' astrocytoma is rare. The tumor has poorly defined borders with cyst formation. Cells are evenly distributed and separated by an eosinophilic matrix. Tumor cells resemble protoplasmic astrocytes, but their cytoplasm is swollen, and their processes are fewer, shorter, and less branched than normal cells. They are usually devoid of neuroglial fibrils and often have a cobweb matrix, small microcysts, and microscopic degeneration. The superficial leptomeninges are frequently invaded by tumor.

''Pilocytic'' (hair-like) astrocytomas of the cerebrum, although usually in the midline, may also be located in the hemispheres. The cells are usually bipolar consisting of elongated, thin, and tapering process. They are often microcystic or may have a single large cyst with a tumor nodule resembling the cystic cerebellar astrocytoma. The latter form, although extremely rare in adults, is commonly seen in children and has been called a ''juvenile astrocytoma'' (37,85). Although vascular endothelial proliferation may be present in pilocytic astrocytomas of the cerebrum, it is not associated with malignant behavior.

''Gemistocytic'' astrocytomas develop in the cerebral hemispheres, rarely in a pure form. Eighty percent of these tumors subsequently evolve into glioblastoma multiforme. Grossly, the tumors are well circumscribed and may be cystic with tumor tissue surrounding the cystic cavity (22). On microscopic exam, cell bodies are seen to be globoid, with short fibrillated processes. Cytoplasm is homogeneous and lightly eosinophilic. The cells are

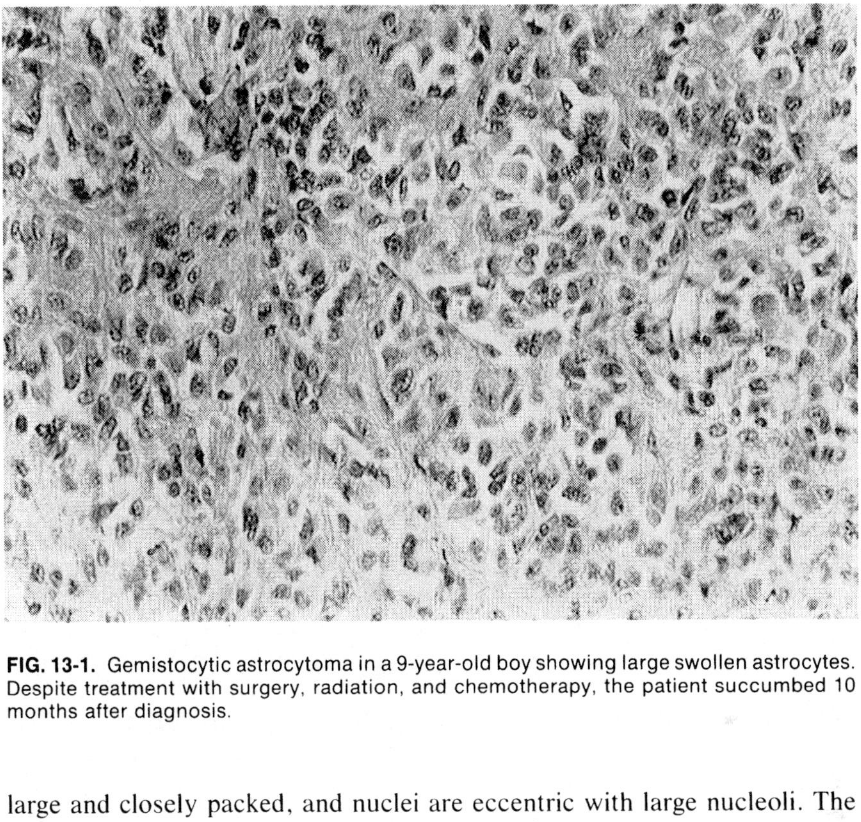

FIG. 13-1. Gemistocytic astrocytoma in a 9-year-old boy showing large swollen astrocytes. Despite treatment with surgery, radiation, and chemotherapy, the patient succumbed 10 months after diagnosis.

large and closely packed, and nuclei are eccentric with large nucleoli. The cells may form perivascular pseudorosettes (Fig. 13-1).

Anaplastic Astrocytomas

"Anaplastic" astrocytomas, according to the Russell and Rubinstein classification (86), are characterized by an admixture of features of both glioblastoma multiforme (i.e., increased cellularity, cellular pleomorphism, and mitoses) and features of typical astrocytomas. Histologically, these tumors appear to be dedifferentiating into glioblastoma multiforme. The nuclear–cytoplasmic ratio is increased compared to typical astrocytomas. Invasion of the cortex and extension into the subpial region is much more prominent than with astrocytomas (12).

Glioblastoma Multiforme

Glioblastoma multiforme appears either as a well-circumscribed globular mass or as a more diffuse mass lesion. The cut surface reveals necrosis, fatty degeneration, and hemorrhage. Necrosis may be found in 50% of glioblastomas. The tumors are most commonly solid, although cysts may be present. Rarely, the tumor consists of a solitary cyst and mural nodule (30).

The most commonly found microscopic features of glioblastoma multiforme are pleomorphism, endothelial proliferation, necrosis, and multinucleated giant cells. Mitoses are present in 70% and hemorrhages in 60%. Less frequent microscopic findings are overgrowth of vascular adventitia, pseudopalisading, and calcification (30).

SIGNS AND SYMPTOMS

The signs and symptoms of hemispheric supratentorial astrocytomas in children relate to the area of cortical involvement. Headaches and vomiting are the most common presenting symptoms (58,100). Although headache may be nonfocal, persistent focality of headaches correlates with true localization in 93% of cases (45). Seizures are a relatively common presenting symptom of hemispheric tumors. The incidence of seizures in patients with hemispheric tumors ranges from 30 to 60% (2,22,34,58,66) (Fig. 13-2). Tumors located in the sensory-motor regions of the brain and the temporal lobes tend to be the most epileptogenic (2). Seizures in general are related inversely to growth of the tumor. As such, seizures are more common with slow-growing astrocytomas than with rapidly evolving high-grade astrocytomas. Despite this, a study of glioblastoma multiforme (19) revealed 35% of

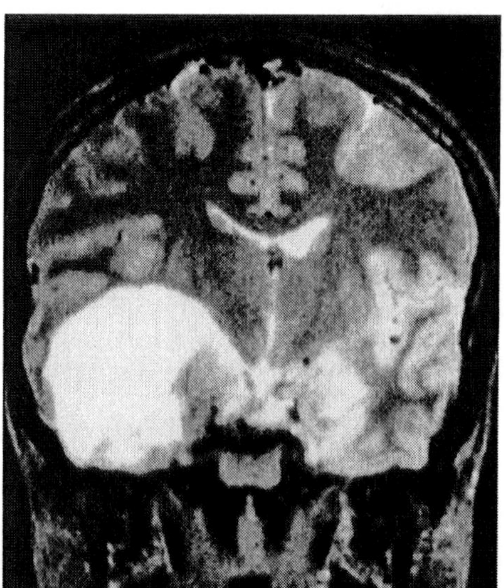

FIG. 13-2. T2-weighted MRI of 19-year-old boy who presented with a first tonic–clonic seizure. Despite the large size of the right temporal lobe tumor, his neurologic exam was normal.

the patients had seizures as presenting symptoms. Because of their inverse correlation with malignancy, seizures are considered a good prognostic sign. Seizures may be generalized, partial with complex symptomatology, or partial with elementary symptomatology with or without secondary generalization. Absence seizures are distinctly unusual as presenting symptoms of tumors, although some studies have reported the association of akinetic and myoclonic seizures with gliomas (58).

Although seizures are a common presenting symptom with hemispheric gliomas, the incidence of tumors in a population of childhood epileptics is quite low. Livingston (57) found only three tumors in a group of 1,518 children with seizures (0.2%). Page et al. (73) reviewed 10,450 children followed in the Boston Children's Hospital Seizure Unit and found 23 (0.2%) who had surgical verification of a supratentorial glioma. The age of onset of seizures ranged from 3 months to 8 years. Nineteen out of 23 patients had had seizures for at least half their lives before diagnosis of the tumor. Clues to the development of tumors in this population of epileptics were (a) change in personality and school performance, (b) change in pattern or frequency of seizures, (c) change in neurologic examination, (d) alterations in EEG, and (e) abnormalities on plain skull films (Fig. 13-3). The authors suggested that preexisting benign ectopias or hamartomas may evolve into malignancies. In their series of 23 patients, 11 had grades I and II astrocytomas.

Focal motor deficits with evidence of pyramidal dysfunction, visual field abnormalities, and papilledema are the most common physical signs of supra-

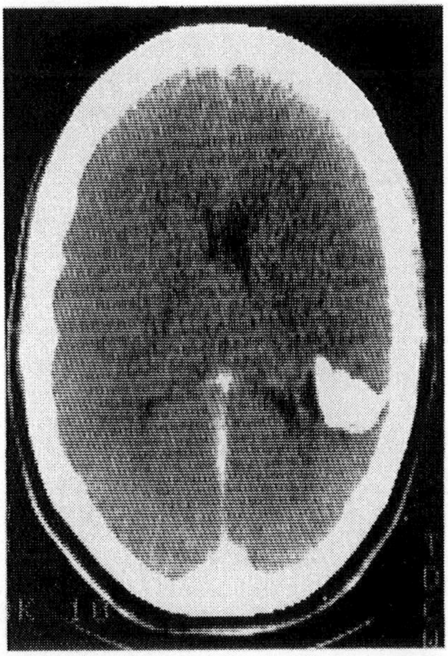

FIG. 13-3. CT scan of 15-year-old girl with a 5-year history of grand mal seizures who presented with new onset of partial complex seizures. CT revealed a calcified mass in the temporal lobe. Diagnosis, grade II astrocytoma.

tentorial gliomas (63). Of interest, ataxia may be present with tumors of the frontal lobes or thalamus, presumably related to impairment of frontopontine pathways (58). This clinical sign may at times lead the examiner mistakenly to suspect a posterior fossa tumor.

In general, duration of symptoms before diagnosis is longer with supratentorial astrocytomas than with infratentorial astrocytomas. Similarly, the mean duration of symptoms before diagnosis is longer with low-grade astrocytomas than with glioblastoma multiforme. Whereas children with low-grade gliomas may have symptoms for years before diagnosis, the average duration of symptoms before diagnosis for patients with glioblastoma is approximately 13 weeks (19). As would be expected, a long duration of symptoms before diagnosis correlates with a relatively longer survival than a short history of symptoms (71,112).

DIAGNOSTIC STUDIES

Computed tomography (CT) readily confirms the clinical diagnosis of a supratentorial mass lesion. Attempts have been made to correlate the pathologic grade of tumor with the CT findings of shape, density, mass effect, and contrast enhancement. Astrocytomas, in general, are well defined and regular in shape, whereas anaplastic astrocytomas and glioblastoma multiforme are often poorly defined, irregularly shaped lesions. Furthermore, glioblastoma multiforme is often associated with a finger-like configuration, which probably represents edema in subcortical white matter (56,108). The density pattern on CT of astrocytomas is homogeneous, whereas anaplastic astrocytomas are more heterogeneous. Glioblastoma are associated with mixed density lesions. Mass effect increases with the degree of malignancy (107). Approximately 50% of grade I astrocytomas, 93% of grades II and III astrocytomas, and 100% of grade IV astrocytomas will have CT characteristics of mass effect (114) (Fig. 13-4).

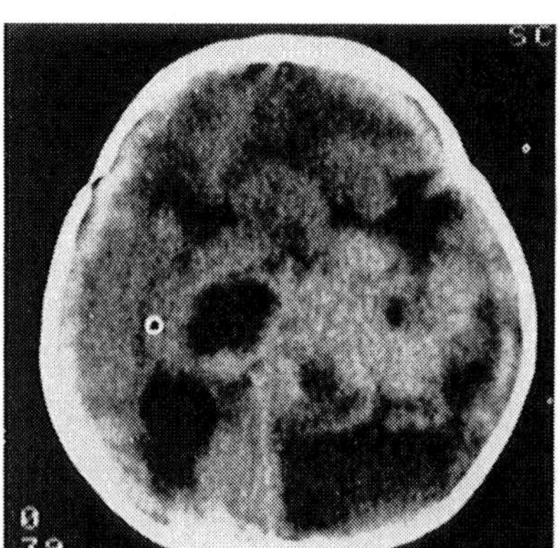

FIG. 13-4. Two-month-old baby who presented with increasing head circumference and bulging anterior fontanelle. Diagnosis, glioblastoma multiforme.

Contrast enhancement is believed to be related to alterations in the blood–brain barrier (14). Because of this, low-grade tumors might be expected to have an intact blood–brain barrier and not enhance, whereas high-grade tumors would be expected to have significant alterations in the blood–brain barrier. However, the correlation of contrast enhancement and degree of malignancy in tumors of childhood is not strong (101). Pedersen et al. (78) found contrast enhancement in 11 out of 11 grade I astrocytomas in childhood. Thus, although low-grade astrocytomas often do not enhance, the presence or absence of contrast enhancement in low-grade tumors is not a reliable prognostic sign.

Many reports have suggested that high-grade astrocytomas, especially glioblastoma multiforme, enhance in well over 90% of cases (108). Although glioblastoma multiformes predictably enhance, this is not always the case with malignant gliomas of lesser grade. Chamberlin (16) reported on 229 patients with supratentorial malignant gliomas. Contrast enhancement was not present in 4% of patients with glioblastoma multiforme, 30% with gemistrocytic astrocytomas, 31% with highly anaplastic astrocytomas, and 54% with moderately anaplastic astrocytomas.

The presence of enhancement on CT scan in a "ring-like" formation is characteristic of glioblastoma multiforme (105,108). Burger et al. (9) compared CT studies with pathologic studies of untreated patients with glioblastoma in order to correlate neuroimaging changes with pathology. The region of low density in the center of the ring lesion was necrosis; the enhancing ring was a cellular rim of viable neoplasm; and the perilesional low-density area was edema with tumor infiltration. In their initial study, all the tumor cells were either within the area of contrast enhancement or within the perilesional edema. None was farther than 3 cm from the periphery of the necrotic area. However, in a more recent comparison (11) of CT and pathology in patients with glioblastoma, Burger et al. (11) found that several patients had tumor infiltration beyond the outer limit of the peritumoral area of low density. The same author, using a similar scheme, also evaluated patients with recurrent glioblastoma. The highly cellular areas of the tumor corresponded to areas of contrast enhancement. Unlike the untreated lesions, however, malignant cells extended far beyond the areas of low density. Thus, those tumors that were diffusely infiltrating and of low cellularity were inadequately identified on CT scan. Furthermore, metastatic spread into the brain stem, identified histologically, was not identified on CT scan. Thus, in de novo lesions, the CT scan identifies most of the identifiable neoplasm, whereas in recurrent lesions, areas of low cell density that are metastatic from the primary lesion cannot be reliably identified in the cerebrum, cerebellum, or brain stem (9). The peritumoral area of low density on CT scan can either overestimate or underestimate the extent of the lesion. Furthermore, the contrast-enhancing area did not always define the full extent of the neoplasm (11).

In addition to shape, mass effect, density and contrast enhancement, tumor location can sometimes enable prediction of grade of tumor. Benign tumors tend to be midline, whereas malignant tumors are more lateral in location. The presence or absence of edema may also be predictive, as malignant tumors are typically surrounded by marked edema, whereas edema is unusual in low-grade astrocytomas (77).

MRI, like CT, has been used to suggest histologic type. Low-grade tumors on MRI are either isodense or barely perceptible on T1 images. In contrast, T2-weighted images are distinctly abnormal, with high signal extending well beyond the region of the tumor. Gadolinium permits assessment of breakdown of the blood–brain barrier and therefore helps to differentiate tumor from surrounding edema. However, as with CT scans, contrast enhancement may be present on MRI examinations in children with low-grade astrocytomas (104).

High-grade tumors tend to have an ill-defined heterogeneous area of low signal on T1. As with low-grade astrocytomas, T2-weighted signals are difficult to interpret because of surrounding edema. After administration of gadolinium, most high-grade tumors will markedly enhance, often demonstrating ring enhancement. It should be stressed that not all high-grade tumors enhance with gadolinium (104). As with CT scans, MRI is useful in identifying tumor but is not specific. One cannot reliably predict the grade of tumor on the basis of imaging characteristics.

EEGs may be localizing in as many as 61% of nonepileptic patients with supratentorial astrocytomas and are falsely negative in only 10%. Patients who have seizures and supratentorial astrocytomas are even more likely to have abnormal EEGs. In these patients, EEGs have been found to be of localizing value in 92% of cases (2). The abnormality on the EEG is most often polymorphic delta with maximum amplitude and longest duration of slow-wave abnormality directly over the tumor. Focal paroxysmal features such as spike and sharp wave as well as spike and slow wave patterns are present in as many as 69% of patients with gliomas (66).

TREATMENT

The literature specifically addressing the treatment of supratentorial astrocytomas occurring in childhood is limited. Therefore, much of the information in the following sections will incorporate the results of treatment in both adults and children. Review of the literature is confounded by multiple variables including age, pathologic grade, classification, and location of the tumor. Despite this, certain patterns are clear. Survival rates in children and adults with astrocytomas clearly correlate with the degree of anaplasia (35). Children with low-grade astrocytomas in two series (43,68) had 5-year survival rates ranging from 85 to 95%, although in a third study (25), low-grade astrocytomas had only a 58% 5-year survival. These results should be compared with a 4% 5-year survival in children with glioblastoma multiforme (25,69).

SURGERY

Surgical intervention is the first approach to any supratentorial hemispheric astrocytoma, regardless of grade. Complete surgical excision is difficult (38). An exception to this is the cystic hemispheric supratentorial astrocytoma. Total removal of the mural nodule is associated with the same excellent prognosis as in patients with cerebellar astrocytomas. In general, removal of the cyst wall does not appear to improve prognosis (74,75). However, since some cystic tumors of the hemispheres may actually be higher grade tumors, special attention should be paid to those cysts that enhance on CT scan. In those cases, biopsy and removal of the entire cyst wall is indicated. (59). Children with solid low-grade astrocytomas may also have a good prognosis following gross total resection alone. Hirsch et al. (43) reviewed a surgical series of 42 cases of benign astrocytic and oligodendrocytic tumors of the cerebral hemispheres in children. The progression-free survival at 5 years was 95%, even though only 2 of the 42 children had been treated with radiation.

The degree of surgical resection also influences survival in patients with glioblastomas. Jelsma and Bucy (45) reviewed their experience with 162 glioblastomas. Patients with extensive resection (>75%) had better survivals than patients treated with either partial resection or external decompression. Frankel and German (30) reviewed 219 cases of glioblastomas and compared survivals with the extent of operative procedure. The median survival for biopsied patients was 1 month, partial resection 2.5 months, and total resection 6 months. Relationships between gross total resection and improved survival and between subtotal or partial resection and survival were confirmed in a study of 285 adults with anaplastic gliomas (116). Although bulk removal offers an overall improved prognosis, surgery alone is not curative.

RADIATION THERAPY

Astrocytomas

The role of radiation therapy in low-grade astrocytomas in children is currently a subject of debate. Several studies (6,26) have shown significant differences in survival in patients who have received postoperative radiation compared to those who have not. The addition of radiation to partial resection in grade I astrocytomas increased the 5-year survival from 25 to 58% (98). Similarly, Leibel et al. (53) evaluated patients with grade I astrocytomas and found that those who received partial resection alone had a 25% 5-year survival versus a 58% survival in patients treated with postoperative radiation.

Most studies have reviewed grades I and II astrocytomas in combination. Thus, Leibel, et al. (53) compared children with grades I and II astrocytomas treated with surgery alone versus surgery and radiation. Five-year survivals in children treated with partial resection alone was 50% versus 81% in those treated with partial resection and postoperative radiation (these extremely good survivals may partly reflect the inclusion of cerebellar astrocytomas). Similarly, Fazekas (26) found a 13% 5-year survival in adults and children treated with surgery alone, compared with a 41% 5-year survival in patients treated with combination therapy.

Because few series solely address supratentorial hemispheric astrocytomas, accurate survival projections are difficult to ascertain. For example, Marsa et al. (62) reported a 72% 5-year survival in children treated with surgery and radiation for supratentorial astrocytomas. These statistics were biased by the inclusion of deep-seated midline tumors, which overall have a better prognosis. Similarly, although there was an 85% 5-year survival in 21 patients less then 20 years of age with astrocytomas treated with surgery and radiation, 15 of the children had cerebellar astrocytomas, which likely skewed the results toward longer survivals (96,97).

Another factor that influences interpretation of results is pathology. Even among low-grade astrocytomas, patients with pilocytic, "ordinary," and mixed oligoastrocytomas tend to fare differently. Patients with pilocytic tumors had 5- and 10-year survivals of 85% and 79%, respectively, compared to 51% and 23% for those with the other two tumor types. Radiation doses above 5300 cGy influenced survival in the "ordinary" astrocytomas and the oligoastrocytomas, but had no appreciable effect on the already good survivals of patients with pilocytic astrocytomas (95).

Although radiation treatment increases 5-year survivals of patients with partially resected tumors, 10-year survivals do not appear to be measurably influenced. Fazekas (26) found that 5-year survivals increased from 13 to 41% with radiation, but by 10 years there was a 26% survival in patients treated with radiation compared with a 32% survival in patients treated with surgery alone. It has therefore been suggested that radiation in low-grade astrocytomas is palliative rather than curative. As such, there has been increasing interest in delaying radiation in some patients until time of recurrence. Surgery alone, particularly gross total resection, has been associated with survival rates as good as those reported in patients in whom radiation follows surgical intervention (43) (Fig. 13-5). In addition, the long-term toxicities associated with radiation of the child's brain are sufficiently severe that a clear-cut risk/benefit ratio must be established before cranial irradiation can be routinely recommended in children with low-grade gliomas. To answer the question whether radiation is necessary at diagnosis, a combined Pediatric

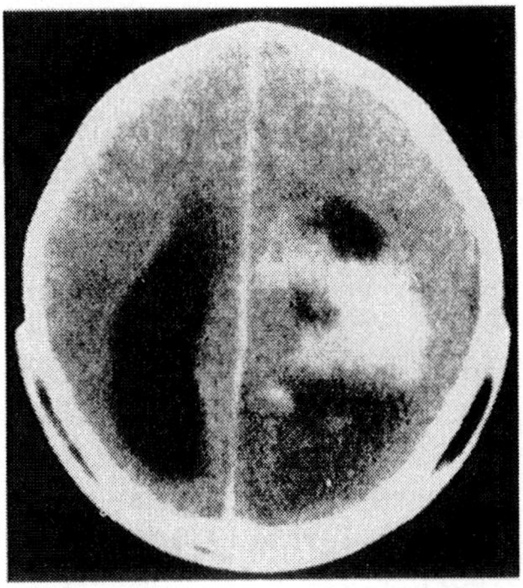

FIG. 13-5. Newborn infant diagnosed as having a low-grade astrocytoma. Tumor was totally resected and no further treatment was given. He remains free of disease 9 years later.

Oncology Group/Children's Cancer Study Group protocol has been established for children with low-grade supratentorial astrocytomas. Children with gross total resection will have no further therapy other than longitudinal follow-up. Patients with subtotal resections will be randomized to either local radiation or observation. Of interest, the European Organization for Research and Treatment of Cancer (EORTC), the Brain Tumor Cooperative Group, and the Radiation Therapy Oncology Group are studying low-grade astrocytomas and oligodendrogliomas in adults using similar guidelines (94). EORTC and the Mayo Clinic are also evaluating the appropriate dose of radiation to assess whether a lower dose provides protection equivalent that of high-dose radiation. The EORTC study is comparing the relative efficacy of 4,500 cGy versus 5,940 cGy localized brain radiation, and the Mayo Clinic is comparing results with 5,040 cGy versus 6,040 cGy. Thus, there is an increasingly conservative approach to the treatment of low-grade astrocytomas in both children and adults (15). The controversy regarding the need for postoperative radiation will be answered once the multi-institutional studies in both the United States and Europe are completed.

Anaplastic Astrocytoma and Glioblastoma Multiforme

Whereas it may be debatable as to whether children with low-grade astrocytomas require postoperative radiation, there is no question that some form of postoperative treatment must be given to children with anaplastic astrocytomas and glioblastoma multiforme. Several well-controlled studies (49,61,71, 87,88,98,109) have demonstrated that adults with anaplastic astrocytomas do significantly better with postoperative radiation. There is a 0 to 3% 5-year survival in adults treated with surgery alone compared with a 15 to 20% 5-year survival in patients treated with surgery and radiation. Five-year survivals range from 16 to 30% in adults with anaplastic astrocytomas, treated with either whole-brain or large-volume radiation in dosages of 3,500 to 6,500 cGy. Even better 5-year survivals are seen in children treated with high-dose radiation. Forty-five children with high-grade astrocytoma treated with postoperative radiation at the Royal Marsden had a 29% 5-year and 26% 10-year survival (5). In a study from Columbia Presbyterian Hospital (60), children with anaplastic astrocytomas who received 54 to 60 Gy had a 60% 5-year survival compared to 14% for those treated with doses of 35 to 50 Gy.

Unfortunately, these encouraging responses associated with cranial irradiation for patients with anaplastic astrocytomas have not been duplicated in patients with glioblastoma multiforme. Bloom (7) reviewed 450 patients with glioblastoma multiforme who had been treated with surgery alone, and 619 patients treated with surgery and radiation from 1952 to 1970. Two-year survivals were superior in the radiated group, but by 3 years, results were equally poor. Only 5 to 10% of these patients survived 5 years. Sheline (98) examined several series in the literature and found that combined treatment with surgery and radiation offered a 24% 1-year survival compared with an 8% 1-year survival with surgery alone. However, by 3 years after diagnosis, there was a 6% survival for patients treated with surgery and radiation versus a 9% survival for patients who received surgery alone. Thus, although glioblastomas initially respond better to surgery and radiation than to surgery alone, responses are only transient.

There is a significant dose–effect relationship between radiation dose and survival. Children with glioblastoma multiforme treated with radiation doses of 54 to 60Gy had a 9% 5-year survival compared with a 0% 5-year survival for children treated with 35 to 50 Gy (60). The Brain Tumor Study Group (111) compared survivals in patients with malignant glioma treated with less than 4,500, 5,000, and 6,000 cGy. Patients treated with 6,000 cGy had significantly better survival rates than patients treated with lower doses of radiation. However, doses of 7,000 to 8,000 cGy not only did not improve total survival but also were associated with a significant risk of radiation necrosis (88). Increasing the volume of radiation, i.e., whole brain versus limited volume, may not appreciably influence survival rates because failure almost always occurs either first at the primary site or simultaneously at both the primary and metastatic sites (31,99).

Fast neutron irradiation has been employed in patients with glioblastoma multiforme. Hypoxic cells are more resistant to conventional photon irradiation than to high linear energy transfer radiation such as fast neutrons. Since glioblastomas often have a component of hypoxic cells, use of fast neutrons has been considered a reasonable therapeutic approach. Unfortunately, improvement in length or quality of survival in fast neutron irradiated patients has not been seen. Autopsies of treated patients have shown coagulative necrosis of the tumor and a decreased amount of viable tumor, but there has also been evidence of radiation necrosis, diffuse gliosis, and demyelination of the cerebral, cerebellar, and brain stem white matter remote from the tumor (42,95).

Another treatment approach, developed to eliminate radioresistant hypoxic cells, has been the use of radiosensitizers. The nitroimidazole drugs appear to be selective in their effect on hypoxic tumor cells and have little effect on well-oxygenated tissue. The first controlled study of patients with glioblastomas treated with metronidazole and postoperative radiation transiently improved, but for only up to 12 months. Other studies have not found even these modest differences between misonidazole treated and control patients. The Royal Marsden Hospital (7) conducted a pilot study in children with cerebral malignant gliomas and brain stem gliomas using radiation and misonidazole. To date, there has been no evidence of improved survivals in these patients. Indeed, a review of the RTOG/ECOG studies (29) revealed that patients treated with misonidazole had a significantly worse prognosis than patients treated with radiation alone.

A third approach, primarily in patients with recurrent malignant gliomas, has been interstitial brachytherapy. The advent of CT and stereotaxy has made it possible to implant radioactive sources into the brain tumor without the need for open craniotomy. Patient selection is important. Potential candidates should have recurrent tumors that are less than 6 cm in size and located distant from the midline. In these selected cases, Leibel (52) reported a 36-month survival rate for patients with recurrent anaplastic astrocytomas of 28% and an 8% survival for those with glioblastoma multiforme. Prospective trials, which include both external beam radiation and brachytherapy with and without chemotherapy, should further elucidate the possible advantages of brachytherapy in high-grade localized gliomas (52).

CHEMOTHERAPY

In light of these poor results with surgery and radiation (particularly for patients with high-grade astrocytomas), chemotherapy has increasingly become a part of the treatment armamentarium. The information pertaining to patients with low-grade astrocytomas treated with chemotherapy is limited. We (106) reported a group of six children with recurrent low-grade astrocytoma treated with a combination of methotrexate, vincristine, 1,3 Bis(2-chlorethyl)-1-nitrosourea (BCNU), and dexamethasone. Although there were no cures, survivals after recurrence were longer than survivals before recurrence. Eight children with grades I and II astrocytomas were treated at the Royal Marsden Hospital with either 1-(-chlorethyl)3-cyclohexyl-1-nitrosourea (CCNU) or BCNU. Seventy-three percent of the patients showed an objective response to treatment (7). Since survivals are generally so good with low-grade astrocytomas, even with surgery alone, chemotherapy does not have much of a role other than at recurrence or for the very young child in whom radiation toxicity would be prohibitive.

Most of the experience with chemotherapy has been in the treatment of high-grade gliomas in adults. The nitrosoureas have been the agents most commonly used either singly or in combination (17,27,92). In 1980, Walker et al. (112) reviewed 467 adult patients from the Brain Tumor Study Group who had received additional therapy after surgery. The patients were randomly separated into four treatment groups, i.e. methyl-CCNU; radiation; BCNU and radiation; and methyl-CCNU and radiation. BCNU plus radiation was associated with the best survival, but this was not significantly better than either methyl-CCNU plus radiation or radiation alone. A similar study (82) using CCNU plus radiation showed no advantage over the use of radiation alone. At the Royal Marsden Hospital, patients with recurrent gliomas were treated with either CCNU or BCNU. Of 55 patients with either grade III or IV astrocytomas, there was only a 7% response rate (7). Although results with single-agent use of either BCNU or CCNU have been disappointing, the combination of CCNU with procarbazine and vincristine following radiation has shown promise in some studies (39,55). Encouraging results have also been reported (44) with a combination of surgery, radiation, and CCNU, procarbazine, vincristine, and methotrexate. This approach offered significantly better survival rates than postoperative treatment with either radiation or the same chemotherapy regimen used alone.

Another approach has been to deliver chemotherapy (VM-26 and CCNU) after surgery, and delay cranial radiation therapy for 6 months. Although this technique improved survivals over surgery and chemotherapy alone, neurotoxicity was significant. The authors (80,81) concluded that preradiation chemotherapy appeared to potentiate radiation CNS toxicity.

A variety of studies (18,33,50,92,115) have used drugs other than the nitrosoureas. Vincristine, procarbazine, cis-platinum, and methotrexate have all demonstrated temporary responses in patients with malignant gliomas, whereas bleomycin has not been effective following radiotherapy either alone or in combination.

High-grade gliomas in children appear to be more chemosensitive than those found in adults (84). The most intriguing results to date have come from a trial of the Children's Cancer Study Group (103) in which 58 children with high-grade astrocytomas were randomized to surgery plus radiation versus surgery, radiation, and CCNU, vincristine, and prednisone. The 5-year event-free survival was 46% for patients in the radiotherapy plus chemotherapy group and 18% for patients treated with radiation therapy alone. When the patients were categorized according to pathologic grade of tumor, i.e., anaplastic astrocytoma versus glioblastoma multiforme, differences were significant, with glioblastoma having a 3-year survival of less than 20% versus the anaplastic astrocytomas having a 3-year survival of approximately 60%. In another study from the University of California at San Francisco (79), children treated with postoperative radiation alone were compared with children treated with several different types of chemotherapeutic agents and radiation. Unlike the CCSG study, there was not a uniform approach to chemotherapy, but differences in survival between the two groups were still identified. Thus, the mean time to progression for children treated with radiation alone was 65 weeks, while the mean time for progression for patients treated with radiation plus chemotherapy was 3.5 years. Although differences have not reached statistical significance, the authors anticipate that with longer follow-up, statistical significance will be reached (79).

The newest chemotherapeutic approach to malignant gliomas of childhood is high-dose multiagent chemotherapy followed by bone marrow rescue. An objective response on neuroimaging of 60% (6 of 10) was reported on day 28 post-marrow infusion (28). The long-term results of this technique are as yet unknown.

Thus, the role of chemotherapy in high-grade astrocytomas is yet to be defined. The experience in adults has been relatively disappointing, but results in children with malignant gliomas have been encouraging. Whether the remarkable results from the CCSG trial will be sustained is unknown, but the data from several studies suggest that malignant gliomas in children react differently to chemotherapeutic agents than tumors with similar pathology in adults.

RECURRENCE

Supratentorial gliomas most commonly recur in their original site. Recurrences may consist of the same or more malignant pathology. Thus, of 72 grade I astrocytomas, 14% were unchanged at recurrence, 55.5% evolved into grade II, and 30.5% became glioblastomas. Of 65 grade II astrocytomas, 55.4% were unchanged at recurrence, and 44.6% became glioblastomas. Overall, approximately two-thirds of all supratentorial astrocytomas on recurrence will have evidence of increased malignancy (65). Recurrences may occur as long as 10 to 15 years after surgery (34). The time to recurrence depends on the nature of the primary tumor. Grade I tumors evolve into glioblastomas more slowly than do grade II astrocytomas. Most of the studies on astrocytoma dedifferentiation have been done in adult patients. However, a recent publication (20) has suggested that dedifferentiation may occur in children as well. Five cases of malignant gliomas arose in children at the sites of previously diagnosed low-grade tumors. Although these data are confounded by the fact that three patients had also received cranial irradiation (raising the specter of whether radiation was the causative factor), at least two cases occurred in the absence of radiation therapy.

CSF SEEDING

Children with high-grade gliomas tend to have a higher incidence of CSF seeding than adults. Although most cases of leptomeningeal dissemination have been identified on autopsy, there are increasing reports of patients who have been identified because of clinical symptomatology (20,21,23,51,71,72). In most series, those patients with clinical symptomatology tend to be younger, likely reflecting their better overall prognosis. Thus, the patients live long enough for their metastatic lesions to become symptomatic (71,110). Leptomeningeal dissemination may also rarely occur with low-grade gliomas. Ten children have been reported to date, but the tumors have been primarily in the cerebellum, spinal cord, or third ventricle (17). It has been suggested that those tumors with extensive CSF seeding are pathologically different than those tumors without extensive CSF dissemination. In one study, those patients who were GFAP negative tended to seed more often, but had less invasion at the primary site. In contrast, patients with very extensive parenchymal infiltration and who were GFAP positive had less evidence of CSF dissemination (71). As expected, the advent of leptomeningeal disease is associated with a poor prognosis. The mean survival between diagnosis of CSF metastases and death in one study was 2.8 months. The clinical response to radiation therapy was also extremely poor (110). We currently recommend neuraxis screening at diagnosis for children with anaplastic astrocytomas and glioblastoma multiforme. Routine craniospinal radiation is not recommended unless dissemination, as identified on MRI, myelography, or CSF cytology, is identified.

SUMMARY

Supratentorial hemispheric astrocytomas represent approximately 30 to 40% of brain tumors in children. Low-grade astrocytomas are more common than those of higher grade. The tumors with the best prognosis are cerebral cystic astrocytomas resembling their counterparts in the cerebellum which may be cured by total excision. Even in solid low-grade astrocytomas of childhood, 5-year survivals, in the absence of postoperative treatment, can range from 75–85%. Furthermore, freedom from recurrence following subtotal resection may extend for many years. At the present time, we suggest that children with totally resected low-grade astrocytomas be followed longitudinally rather than committed to radiation. In those children with subtotal resection, controversy exists between immediate radiation and "watchful waiting." It is anticipated that the results of ongoing studies will allow firm recommendations in the future. Children with high-grade astrocytomas have a far worse prognosis, with a 20–40% 5-year survival for anaplastic astrocytomas, and only a 4% 5-year survival for those with glioblastoma multiforme. Although radiation has significantly improved survivals in this population, responses are not long lasting. Those children with low-grade astrocytomas in whom radiation is recommended, should receive local radiation, whereas those with glioblastoma multiforme and anaplastic astrocytomas, should re-

TABLE 13-1. *Extraneural metastases in children from astrocytomas and glioblastomas*

Author	Age	Tumor	Location	Metastasis	Survival
Wolfe et al. (117)	14	Glio	Temp-occip	Lung, pleura, rib, vertebrae, sternum, mediastinum, lymph node	13 months
Schejbal (90)	9	Glio	Temp-occip	Cervical lymph node	
Smith et al. (102)	6	Glio + sarcoma	Temp	Lung	7 months
Komatsu et al. (48)	18	Glio	Thalamus	Cervical lymph node	7 months
Yao et al. (119)	18	Glio	Frontal-parietal	Lung, thyroid, neck, paratracheal mediastinal lymph nodes	19 months
Mosca and Baldini (64)	12	Astro	Pons	Lung and liver	
Russell and Rubinstein (86)	7	Glio	Temp	Liver, adrenal, hilar lymph node, pleura, vertebrae	
Russell and Rubinstein (86)	16	GC		Pleura, peritoneum, diaphragm	3 yr
Gyepes and D'Angio (40)	8	Glio	CPA Pons and midbrain	Bone, breast, lung, pleura	

Glio, glioblastoma multiforme; Astro, astrocytoma; GC, gliomatosis cerebri; Temp, temporal; Occip, occipital; CPA, cerebellopontine angle.

ceive either whole brain radiation or local radiation with wide margins. Chemotherapy may eventually play a major role in high-grade gliomas of childhood, if the early data which suggests adjuvant treatment significantly improves survivals, is confirmed in larger studies. Prognostic factors favoring prolonged survival include: seizures on presentation, young age (in adults), good performance status after surgery, low grade of tumor, longer duration of symptoms before diagnosis, postoperative tumor size on CT, and the presence of giant cells on pathologic exam (1,8,10,32,93,113,118). Extraneural metastases have been reported in both children and adults with astrocytomas and glioblastoma multiforme with extra-axial spread to the lung and lymph nodes (36,54,76,102) (Table 13-1). The small but significant incidence of CSF seeding will be of greater clinical importance once survivals of patients with high-grade gliomas are improved.

REFERENCES

1. Al-Mefty O, Nayef RF, Al-Rodhan MBBS, Phillips RL, El-Senossi M, Fox JL. Factors affecting survival of children with malignant gliomas. *Neurosurgery* 1987;20:416–420.
2. Backus RE, Millichap JG. The seizure as a manifestation of intracranial astrocytomas and oligodendrogliomas. *Pediatrics* 1962;29–978–984.
3. Bailey, Cushing H. *Classification of tumors of the glioma group on a histogenic basis with a correlated study of prognosis*. Philadelphia: JB Lippincott 1926.
4. Bloom HJG. Recent concepts in the conservative treatment of intracranial tumors in children. *Acta Neurochir* 1979;50:103–116.

5. Bloom HJG, Glees J, Bell J. The treatment and long-term prognosis of children with intracranial tumors: a study of 610 cases, 1950–1981. *Int J Radiat Oncol Biol Phys* 1990; 18:723–745.
6. Bloom HJG. Combined modality therapy for intracranial tumors. *Cancer* 1975;35:111–120.
7. Bloom HJG. Intracranial tumors: response and resistance to therapeutic endeavors, 1970–1980. *Int J Radiat Oncol Biol Phys* 1982;8:1083–1113.
8. Bouchard J, Peirce CB. Radiation therapy in the management of neoplasms of the central nervous system, with a special note in regard to children: twenty years' experience 1939–1958. *AJR* 1960;84:610–628.
9. Burger PC, Dubois PJ, Schold C, et al. Computerized tomographic and pathologic studies of the untreated, quiescent, and recurrent glioblastoma multiforme. *J Neurosurg* 1983;58: 159–169.
10. Burger PC, Green SB. Patient age, histologic features, and length of survival in patients with glioblastoma multiforme. *Cancer* 1987;59:1617–1625.
11. Burger PC, Heinz ER, Shibata T, Kleihues P. Topographic anatomy and CT correlations in the untreated glioblastoma multiforme. *J Neurosurg* 1988;68:698–704.
12. Burger PC, Vogel FS. *Surgical pathology of the nervous system and its coverings*. New York: John Wiley and Sons; 1982.
13. Burger PC, Vollmer RT. Histologic factors of prognostic significance in the glioblastoma multiforme. *Cancer* 1980;46:1170–1186.
14. Butler AR, Horii SC, Kricheff II, Shannon MG, Budzilovich GN. Computed tomography in astrocytomas: a statistical analysis of the parameters of malignancy and the positive contrast-enhanced CT scan. *Radiology* 1978;129:433–439.
15. Cairncross JG, Laperriere NJ. Low-grade glioma: to treat or not to treat? *Arch Neurol* 1989;46:1238–1239.
16. Chamberlain MC, Murovic JA, Levin VA. Absence of contrast enhancement on CT brain scans of patients with supratentorial malignant gliomas. *Neurology* 1988;38:1371–1374.
17. Civitello LA, Packer RJ, Rorke LB, et al. Leptomeningeal dissemination of low-grade gliomas in childhood. *Neurology* 1988;38:562–566.
18. Djerassi I, Kim JS, Shulman K. High dose methotrexate-citrovorum factor rescue in the management of brain tumors. *Cancer Treat Rep* 1977;61:691–694.
19. Dohrmann GJ, Farwell JR, Flannery JT. Glioblastoma multiforme in children. *J Neurosurg* 1976;44:442–448.
20. Dropcho EJ, Wisoff JH, Walker RW, Allen JC. Supratentorial malignant gliomas in childhood: a review of fifty cases. *Ann Neurol* 1987;22:355–364.
21. Eade OE, Urich H. Metastasizing gliomas in young subjects. *J Pathol* 1970;103:245–256.
22. Elvidge AR. Long-term survival in the astrocytoma series. *J Neurosurg* 1968;28:399–404.
23. Erlich SS, Davis RL. Spinal subarachnoid metastasis from primary intracranial glioblastoma multiforme. *Cancer* 1978;42:2854–2864.
24. European Organization for Research on Treatment of Cancer. Brain Tumor Group 1981: evaluation of CCNU, VM-26 plus CCNU and procarbazine in supratentorial brain gliomas. *J Neurosurg* 1981;55:27–31.
25. Farwell JR, Dohrmann GJ, Flannery JT. Central nervous system tumors in children. *Cancer* 1977;40:3123–3132.
26. Fazekas JT. Treatment of grades I and II brain astrocytomas: the role of radiotherapy. *Int J Radiat Oncol Biol Phys* 1977;2:661–666.
27. Fewer D. Wilson CB, Boldrey EB, Enot JK. Phase II study of 1-(2-chloroethyl)-3-cyclohexyl-1-nitrosourea (CCNU; NSC-79037J) in the treatment of brain tumors. *Cancer Chemother Rep* 1972;56:421–427.
28. Finlay JL, August C, Packer R, et al. High dose multi-agent chemotherapy followed by bone marrow "rescue" for malignant astrocytomas of childhood and adolescence. *J Neuro-oncol* 1990;9:239–248.
29. Fischbach AJ, Martz KL, Nelson JS, Griffin TW. Long-term survival in treated anaplastic astrocytomas. *Am J Clin Onc* 1991;14:365–370.
30. Frankel SA, German WJ. Glioblastoma multiforme: review of 219 cases with regard to natural history, pathology, diagnostic methods, and treatment. *J Neurosurg* 1958;15: 489–503.
31. Garden AS, Maor MH, Yung WKA, Bruner JM. Outcome and patterns of failure following limited-volume irradiation for malignant astrocytomas. *Radiother Oncol* 1991;20:99–110.

32. Gehan EA, Walker M. Prognostic factors for patients with brain tumors. *Natl Cancer Inst Monogr* 1977;46:189–195.
33. Gjerris F. Clinical aspects and long-term prognosis of intracranial tumors in infancy and childhood. *Dev Med Child Neurol* 1976;18:145–159.
34. Gjerris F. Clinical aspects and long-term prognosis of supratentorial tumors in infancy and childhood. *Acta Neurol Scand* 1978;57:445–470.
35. Gjerris F, Klee JG, Klinken L. Malignancy grade and long-term survival in brain tumors of infancy and childhood. *Acta Neurol Scand* 1976;53:61–71.
36. Glasauer FE, Yuan RHP. Intracranial tumors with extracranial metastases: case report and review of the literature. *J Neurosurg* 1963;20:474–493.
37. Gol A. Cerebral astrocytomas in childhood: a clinical study. *J Neurosurg* 1962;19:577–582.
38. Goldsmith MA, Carter SK. Glioblastoma multiforme: a review of therapy. *Cancer Treat Rev* 1974;1:153–165.
39. Gutin PH, Wilson CB, Kumar AR, et al. Phase II study of procarbazine, CCNU and vincristine combination chemotherapy in the treatment of malignant brain tumors. *Cancer* 1975;35:1398–1404.
40. Gyepes MT, D'Angio GJ. Extracranial metastases from central nervous tumors in children and adolescents. *Radiology* 1966;87:55–63.
41. Heiskanen O. Intracranial tumors of children. *Childs Brain* 1977;3:69–78.
42. Herskovic A, Ornitz RD, Shell M, Rogers CC. Treatment experience: glioblastoma multiforme treated with 15 MeV fast neutrons. *Cancer* 1982;49:2463–2465.
43. Hirsch JF, Rose CS, Kahn AP, Pfister A, Hoppe-Hirsch E. Benign astrocytic and oligodendrocytic tumors of the cerebral hemispheres in children. *J Neurosurg* 1989;70:568–572.
44. Jellinger K, Kothbauer P, Volc D, Vollmer R, Weib R. Combination chemotherapy (COMP Protocol) and radiotherapy of anaplastic supratentorial gliomas. *Acta Neurochir* 1979;51: 1–13.
45. Jelsma R, Bucy PC. The treatment of glioblastoma multiforme of the brain. *J Neurosurg* 1967;27:388–400.
46. Keith HM, Craig W, Kernohan JW. Brain tumors in children. *Pediatrics* 1949;3:839–844.
47. Kernohan JW, Mabon RF, Svien H, Adson AW. A simplified classification of the gliomas. *Mayo Clin Proc* 1949;24:71–75.
48. Komatsu K, Inaba Y, Hiratsuka H, Takahashi S, Kamisasa A. Widespread extracranial metastases of glioblastoma multiforme: report of a case and review of the cases in the literature. *Brain Nerve* 1972;24:339–351.
49. Kramer S. In: *Radiation therapy in the management of the malignant gliomas. Seventh National Cancer Conference Proceedings*. Philadelphia: JB Lippincott; 1973:823–826.
50. Kristiansen K, Hagen S, Kollevoid T, et al. Combined modality therapy of operated astrocytomas Grade III and IV: confirmation of the value of postoperative irradiation and lack of potentiation of bleomycin on survival time. *Cancer* 1981;47:649–652.
51. Kun LE, Kovnar E, Heideman R, et al. Malignant glioma in children: study of disease course and neuraxis dissemination. St. Jude Children's Research Hospital, Memphis TN. Presented to the Asilomar Conference, 1991.
52. Leibel SA, Gutin PH, Wara WM, Silver PS. Survival and quality of life after interstitial implantation of removable high-activity iodine-125 sources for the treatment of patients with recurrent malignant gliomas. *Int J Radiat Oncol Biol Phys* 1989;17:1129–1139.
53. Leibel SA, Sheline GE, Wara WM, Boldrey EB, Nielsen SL. The role of radiation therapy in the treatment of astrocytomas. *Cancer* 1975;35:1551–1557.
54. Leifer D, Moore T, Ukena T, et al. Multifocal glioblastoma with liver metastases in the absence of surgery. *J Neurosurg* 1989;71:772–776.
55. Levin VA, Silver P, Hannigan J, et al. Superiority of post-radiotherapy adjuvant chemotherapy with CCNU, procarbazine, and vincristine (PCV) over BCNU for anaplastic gliomas: NCOG 6G61 final report. *Int J Radiat Oncol Biol Phys* 1989;18:321–324.
56. Lewander R, Bergstrom M, Boethius J, Collins VP. Stereotactic computer tomography for biopsy of gliomas. *Acta Radiol [Diagn]* 1978;19:867–888.
57. Livingston S. *The diagnosis and treatment of convulsive disorders in children*. Springfield, IL: Charles C Thomas; 1954:24.
58. Low NL, Correll JW, Hammill JF. Tumors of the cerebral hemispheres in children. *Arch Neurol* 1965;13:547–554.

59. Maiuri F. Cysts with mural tumor nodules in the cerebral hemispheres. *Neurosurgery* 1988;22:703–706.
60. Marchese MJ, Chang CH. Malignant astrocytic gliomas in children. *Cancer* 1990;65: 2771–2778.
61. Marsa GW, Goffinet DR, Rubinstein LJ, Bagshaw MA. Megavoltage irradiation in the treatment of gliomas of the brain and spinal cord. *Cancer* 1975;36:1681–1689.
62. Marsa GW, Probert JC, Rubinstein LJ, Bagshaw MA. Radiation therapy in the treatment of childhood astrocytic gliomas. *Cancer* 1973;32:646–655.
63. Mercuri S, Russi A, Palma L. Hemispheric supratentorial astrocytomas in children: long term results in 29 cases. *J Neurosurg* 1981;55:170–173.
64. Mosca L, Baldini M. Early glial tumor metastases through a ventriculoatrial shunt. *Tumori* 1976;62:47–54.
65. Muller W, Afra D, Schroder R. Supratentorial recurrences of gliomas: morphological studies in relation to time intervals with astrocytomas. *Acta Neurochir* 1977;37:75–91.
66. Murphy JT, Gloor P, Yamamoto YL, Feindel W. A comparison of electroencephalography and brain scan in supratentorial tumors. *N Engl J Med* 1967;276:309–313.
67. Netsky MG, August B, Fowler W. The longevity of patients with glioblastoma multiforme. *J Neurosurg* 1950:7:261–269.
68. Nishio Sh, Takeshita I, Fujii K, Fukui M. Supratentorial astrocytic tumours of childhood: a clinicopathologic study of 41 cases. *Acta Neurochir* 1989;101:3–8.
69. Norbut AM, Mendelow H. Primary glioblastoma of the pineal region with leptomeningeal metastases: a case report. *Cancer* 1981;47:592–596.
70. Onda K, Tanaka R, Takahashi H, Takeda N, Ikuta F. Cerebral glioblastoma with cerebrospinal fluid dissemination: a clinicopathological study of 14 cases examined by complete autopsy. *Neurosurgery* 1989;4:533–540.
71. Onoyama Y, Abe M, Yabumoto E, Sakamoto T, Nishidai T, Suyama S. Radiation therapy in the treatment of glioblastoma. *AJR* 1976;126:481–492.
72. Packer RJ, Siegel KR, Sutton LN, Littman P, Bruce DA. Leptomeningeal dissemination of primary central nervous system tumors of childhood. *Ann Neurol* 1985;18:217–221.
73. Page LK, Lombroso CT, Matson DD. Childhood epilepsy with late detection of cerebral glioma. *J Neurosurg* 1969;31:253–261.
74. Palma L, Guidetti B. Cystic pilocytic astrocytomas of the cerebral hemispheres: surgical experience with 51 cases and long-term results. *J Neurosurg* 1985;62:811–815.
75. Palma L, Russo A, Mercuri S. Cystic-cerebral astrocytomas in infancy and childhood: long term results. *Childs Brain* 1983;10:79–91.
76. Pasquier B, Pasquier D, Golet AN, Panh MH, Coudere P. Extraneural metastases of astrocytomas and glioblastomas. *Cancer* 1980;45:112–125.
77. Pedersen H, Gjerris F, Klinken L. Malignancy criteria in computed tomography of primary supratentorial tumors in infancy and childhood. *Neuroradiology* 1989;31:24–28.
78. Pederson H, Gjerris F, Klinken C. Computed tomography of benign supratentorial astrocytomas of infancy and childhood. *Neuroradiology* 1981;21:87–91.
79. Phuphanich S, Edwards MSB, Levin VA, et al. Supratentorial malignant gliomas of childhood. *J Neurosurg* 1984;60:495–499.
80. Poisson M, Hauw JJ, Pouillart P, et al. Malignant gliomas treated after surgery by combination chemotherapy and delayed radiation. II: Tolerance to irradiation after chemotherapy. *Acta Neurochir* 1979;51:27–42.
81. Poisson M, Pouillart P, Bataini JR, Mashaly R, Pertuiset BF, Metzger J. Malignant gliomas treated after surgery by combination therapy and delayed irradiation. I: Analysis of results. *Acta Neurochir* 1979;51:15–25.
82. Reagan TJ, Bisel HF, Childs DS, et al. Controlled study of CCNU and radiation therapy in malignant astrocytoma. *J Neurosurg* 1976;44:186–190.
83. Rosenstock JG, Evans AE, Schut L. Response to vincristine of recurrent brain tumors in children. *J Neurosurg* 1976;45:135–140.
84. Rozenthal JM, Robins HI, Finlay J, Healey B. "Eight-drugs-in-one-day" chemotherapy administered before and after radiotherapy to adult patients with malignant gliomas. *Cancer* 1989;63:2475–2481.
85. Rubinstein LJ. Tumors of the central nervous system. Washington, DC: Armed Forces Institute of Pathology: 1972:19–84.

86. Russell DS, Rubinstein LJ. *Pathology of tumours of the nervous system*. Baltimore: Williams & Wilkins; 1989.
87. Rutten EHJM, Kazem I, Slooff JL, Walder-Alphons HD. Post operative radiation therapy in the management of brain astrocytoma: retrospective study of 142 patients. *Int J Radiat Oncol Biol Phys* 1981;7:191–195.
88. Salazar OM, Rubin P, Feldstein ML, Puzzutiello R. High dose radiation therapy in the treatment of malignant glioma: final report. *Int J Radiat Oncol Biol Phys* 1979;5:1733–1740.
89. Salazar OM, Rubin P. The spread of glioblastoma multiforme as a determining factor in the radiation treated volume. *Int J Radiat Oncol Biol Phys* 1976;1:627–637.
90. Schejbal V. Metastasizing glioma in childhood. *Neoplasma* 1962;9:585–592.
91. Seiler RM. Late results of multimodality therapy of high-grade supratentorial astrocytomas. *Surg Neurol* 1981;15:88–91.
92. Seiler RW, Greiner RH, Zimmerman A, Markwalder H. Radiotherapy combined with procarbazine, bleomycin, and CCNU in the treatment of high-grade supratentorial astrocytomas. *J Neurosurg* 1978;48:861–865.
93. Shapiro WR. Treatment of neuroectodermal brain tumors. *Ann Neurol* 1982;12:231–237.
94. Shaw EG, Daumas-Duport C, Scheithauer BW, Gilbertson DT. Radiation therapy in the management of low-grade supratentorial astrocytomas. *J Neurosurg* 1989;70:853–861.
95. Shaw CM, Sumi SM, Alvord EC, Gerdes AJ, Spence A, Parker RG. Fast-neutron irradiation of glioblastoma multiforme. *J Neurosurg* 1978;49:1–12.
96. Sheline GE. Conventional radiation therapy of gliomas. *Recent Results Cancer Res* 1975; 51:125–134.
97. Sheline GE. Radiation of primary tumors. *Semin Oncol* 1975;2:29–42.
98. Sheline GE. Radiation therapy of brain tumors. *Cancer* 1977;39:873–881.
99. Shibamoto Y, Yamashita J, Takahashi M, Yamasaki T, Kikuychi H, Mitsuyuki A. Supratentorial malignant glioma: an analysis of radiation therapy in 178 cases. *Radiother Oncol* 1990;18:9–17.
100. Shin KH, Webster JH. Astrocytoma in children: a review of 79 cases 1960–1976. *J Can Assoc Radiol* 1979;30:167–169.
101. Silverman C, Marks JE. Prognostic significance of contrast enhancement in low-grade astrocytomas of the adult cerebrum. *Radiology* 1981;139:211–213.
102. Smith DR, Hardman JM, Earle KM. Metastasizing neuroectodermal tumors of the central nervous system. *J Neurosurg* 1969;31:50–58.
103. Sposto R, Ertel IJ, Kenkin RDT, Boesel CP. The effectiveness of chemotherapy for treatment of high grade astrocytoma in children: results of a randomized trial. *J Neurooncol* 1989;7:165–177.
104. Stack JP, Antoun NM, Jenkins JPR, Metcalfe R, Isherwood I. Gadolinium-DTPA as a contrast agent in magnetic resonance imaging of the brain. *Neuroradiology* 1988;30: 145–154.
105. Steinhoff H, Grumme Th, Kazner E, et al. Axial transverse computerized tomography in 73 glioblastomas. *Acta Neurochir* 1978;42:45–56.
106. Sumer R, Freeman AI, Cohen ME, Bremer AM, Thomas PRM, Sinks L. Chemotherapy in recurrent non-cystic low grade astrocytomas of the cerebrum in children. *J Surg Oncol* 1978;10:45–54.
107. Tans J Th J, de Jongh IE. Computed tomography of supratentorial astrocytoma. *Clin Neurol Neurosurg* 1979;80:156–168.
108. Tchang S, Scotti G, Tergrugge K, et al. Computerized tomography as a possible aid to histologic grading of supratentorial gliomas. *J Neurosurg* 1977;46:735–739.
109. Uihlein A, Colby MY, Layton DD, Parsons WR, Carter TL. Comparison of surgery and surgery plus irradiation in the treatment of supratentorial gliomas. *Acta Radiol* 1966;5: 67–78.
110. Vertosick FT, Selker RG. Brain stem and spinal metastases of supratentorial glioblastoma multiforme: a clinical series. *Neurosurgery* 1990;27:516–522.
111. Walker MD, Strike TA, Sheling GE. An analysis of dose-effect relationship in the radiotherapy of malignant gliomas. *Int J Radiat Oncol Biol Phys* 1979;5:1725–1731.
112. Walker MD, Green SB, Byar DD, et al. Randomized comparisons of radiotherapy and nitrosoureas for the treatment of malignant glioma after surgery. *N Engl J Med* 1980;303: 1323–1329.

113. Weir B, Grace M. The relative significance of factors affecting postoperative survival in astrocytomas, grades one and two. *Can J Neurol Sci* 1976;3:47–58.
114. Weisberg LA. Cerebral computed tomography in the diagnosis of supratentorial astrocytoma. *Comput Tomogr* 1980;4:87–105.
115. Wilson CB, Gutin P, Boldrey EB, Crafts D. Single-agent chemotherapy of brain tumors: a five year review. *Arch Neurol* 1976;33:739–744.
116. Winger MJ, MacDonald DR, Cairncross JG. Supratentorial anaplastic gliomas in adults. *J Neurosurg* 1989;71:487–493.
117. Wolfe A, Cowen D, Stewart WB. Glioblastoma with extraneural metastasis by way of a ventriculopleural anastomosis. *Trans Am Neurol Assoc* 1954;79:140–142.
118. Wood JR, Green SB, Shapiro W. The prognostic importance of tumor size in malignant gliomas: a computed tomographic scan study by the brain tumor cooperative group. *J Clin Oncol* 1988;6:338–343.
119. Yao YT, Lin WSJ, Hung CC, Liu KN. A case of glioblastoma multiforme with extracranial metastasis. *J Formosan Med Assoc* 1975;74:220–228.

14

Craniopharyngiomas

Since the initial description by Erdheim in 1904, there has been universal acceptance that craniopharyngiomas arise from retained elements of Rathke's pouch, the embryologic forerunner of the anterior pituitary gland. It was not until 1932 that Cushing (19) named the tumor. In the same monograph he emphasized the complex surgical problems attendant with removal of the tumor as well as the resulting panhypopituitarism. Although the tumor is considered benign, its location, its slowly growing progressive nature, its tendency to encroach on surrounding tissue of functional importance, and its proclivity for recurrence make craniopharyngiomas a particularly vexing and challenging diagnostic problem (6).

This neoplasm is thought to result from embryonic squamous cell rests arising from the involuted tract of the hypophyseal pharyngeal duct. In 1838, Rathke commented on the presence of an irregular globular depression at the base of the skull in the roof of the primitive mouth of embryonic mammals. This depression, as he later learned, was to form the anlage of the anterior portion of the pituitary gland. Cell rests along the cranial pharyngeal duct, leading from the primitive stomodeum to Rathke's pouch, are considered to be the site of origin of craniopharyngiomas. As the embryo develops, the depressions forming Rathke's pouch and the cell rests associated with it tend to rotate from an inferior position at the base of the developing pituitary to a superior position above the gland. Subsequently, rests of squamous epithelial cells are found along the anterior surface of the pituitary infundibulum, presumably accounting for the suprasellar location of this tumor. Others (43) have suggested that these tumors, rather than resulting from embryonic rest cells, arise from metaplasia in cells of the adenohypophysis. Metaplasia of ectodermal cell rests tend to increase with increasing age.

Craniopharyngiomas account for 1.2 to 4% of all tumors in adults and from 6 to 10% of all tumors in children (53). Reflecting its embryonic origins, the tumor has been variously referred to as a Rathke pouch tumor, adamantinoma, ameloblastoma, or suprasellar epidermoid cyst. Diagnosis peaks in the second half of the first decade and the early part of the second decade. There is no clear-cut sexual preference. The tumor may be quite variable in location, size, texture, and adherence to surrounding structures. The majority of tumors are suprasellar in location, although on occasion they are found

Brain Tumors in Children: Principles of Diagnosis and Treatment, 2/e, edited by M.E. Cohen and P.K. Duffner, Raven Press, Ltd., New York, 1994.

in an intrasellar location (29). They may fill the cavity of the third ventricle or extend inferiorly and posteriorly along the dorsum sella and clivus, displacing structures at the base of the brain.

PATHOLOGY

Grossly, craniopharyngiomas are largely cystic or partially solid and cystic, with a firm capsule usually at the superior extent, at times blending imperceptibly into the surrounding tissue. The tumor is grayish-red in color, of varying size, with a smooth or finely nodular surface. It has a tenacious, gritty texture presumably secondary to foci of calcification. The cystic contents consist of thick, brownish yellow or green machine-oil-like fluid rich in cholesterol crystals. Cyst contents may be gelatinous rather than fluid. Suspended crystals of cholesterol impart a birefringent character to the fluid. A severe chemical arachnoiditis can result from spillage of cyst contents at the time of surgery (Fig. 14-1). Solid areas containing foci of calcification may also contain evidence of early bone formation.

Some authors (25,31,45) have emphasized that craniopharyngiomas are not encapsulated and are not separated by a leptomeningeal lining from the brain parenchyma. These authors have commented on the infiltrating nature of the tumor, which can permeate the brain, tuber cinereum, and hypothalamus, thus making total excision impractical. Others (27,44,62) have stated

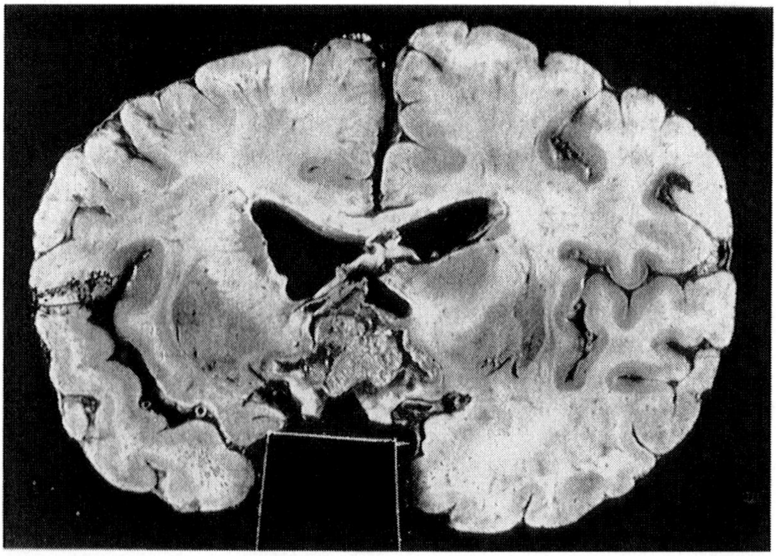

FIG. 14-1. Cystic craniopharyngioma identified at post mortem invading the third ventricle.

that cleavage planes between the tumor and parenchyma do exist but at times are so thin as to prohibit attempts at total excision. It is the adherent nature of the tumor that putatively relates to the postoperative endocrine and psychologic complications that accompany aggressive surgery.

Microscopically, the tumor presents as an epithelial microcystic tumor (53). Cells are found arranged in cords of angulated columnar cells resting on a collagen basement membrane. Keratin pearls may be among the areas of squamous epithelium. The keratin may become confluent and may undergo calcification and even bone formation. Nests of columnar elements are found embedded in a loose fibrillated stroma. Palisading of columnar cells is similar to that seen in embryonic dental and oral mucosa, and thus has been associated with adamantinomas found in the jaw. Degenerative changes and microcysts may be found in the adamantinomatous areas (Fig. 14-2). In adults, squamous epithelium without palisading is apt to predominate.

Three mechanisms thought to be responsible for the cyst formation are (a) degenerative changes in the adamantinomatous nest of cells, (b) degenerative changes in the stroma, and (c) sloughing of epithelial cells and maturation of the squamous epithelium (39). Both squamous cells and adamantinomatous areas are seen in the cystic and solid tumors. Small cystic areas may be found in the region of the tuber cinereum. Cystic cavities, lined by keratinizing squamous epithelium, are indistinguishable from epidermoid cysts (30,42,53). Carcinomatous changes have not been described, although small

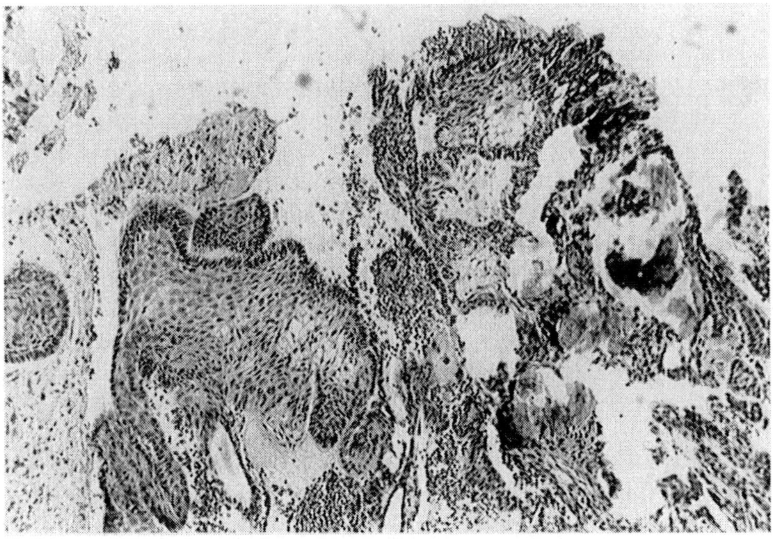

FIG. 14-2. Microscopic section of a craniopharyngioma. Sheets of columnar and squamous epithelial cells are easily recognized. Calcification, degenerative changes, and microcysts are seen throughout the section.

islands of cells separate from the main body of the tumor have been erroneously mistaken as carcinomatous invasion.

SIGNS AND SYMPTOMS

Clinical signs and symptoms depend on the extent of tumor and location. As in most intracranial tumors of childhood, complaints of headaches and vomiting are nonspecific signs of increased intracranial pressure or may reflect hydrocephalus secondary to obstruction of CSF pathways at the level of the foramen of Monro. Visual defects, depending on the location of the tumor below, above, or behind the visual axis, arise from compression of either the optic nerve, chiasm, or tract. Field defects are more likely to be asymmetric or unilateral, rather than that of a more classic bitemporal hemianopsia. Loss of a single field of vision suggests involvement of the optic tract, whereas unilateral loss with optic atrophy implies a tumor anterior and lateral to the chiasm. Unfortunately, because of the slowly progressive nature of the tumor, the patient is not apt to complain of visual loss. Involvement of the optic pathway is more likely to be suspected during a school visual examination or by findings of optic atrophy or papilledema during a routine funduscopic examination. Even in the absence of increased intracranial pressure, visual loss secondary to optic atrophy may accompany compression of the visual pathway. Seesaw or pendular nystagmus at presentation usually reflects visual loss rather than involvement of oculomotor pathways.

Endocrine abnormalities are quite variable (58). The severity of endocrinopathy has not been shown to have a relationship to the extent of the tumor or, for that matter, the anatomical location of the tumor. Unlike the less common presentation of an intrasellar mass, suprasellar craniopharyngiomas are associated with pituitary abnormalities late in their course or endocrine abnormalities at presentation may be absent altogether. In the perioperative period (i.e., before, during, and after surgery) skilled endocrine management is absolutely essential.

At presentation, the most likely endocrine abnormalities in children are apt to be deficits in stature, hypothyroidism, or diabetes insipidus. The children with growth retardation will present with delayed bone age and deceleration of linear growth. Growth retardation and decreased production of growth hormone may precede a clinical diagnosis of tumor by many years. Those with hypothyroidism will present with increased weight gain, easy fatigability, lethargy, and, possibly, declining school performance. Physical examination should reveal typical signs of decreased thyroid function. With involvement of the hypothalamus, diabetes insipidus may develop. Complaints of excessive thirst, frequent urination, and decreased urinary specific gravity raise the suspicion of diabetes insipidus. Less commonly, vegetative states, abnormalities of autonomic function, or disturbances in fluid or electrolyte balance may be seen as a result of a hypothalamic syndrome. Hypothalamic syndromes are more likely as an aftermath of surgery rather than as a presenting sign or symptom.

Other than visual abnormalities, neurologic findings are uncommon and when they do occur, suggest expansion of the tumor outside its usual location, either anteriorly, laterally, or inferiorly along the base of the brain. Loss of smell, with or without partial complex seizures, suggests extension of the tumor anteriorly to involve the olfactory tract, and laterally to involve the medial aspects of the temporal lobe. Impingement of the oculomotor nerves or the trigeminal nerves as they lie free in the subarachnoid space suggests backward and basilar extension of the tumor. Growth of the tumor along the base, in the unusual circumstance, may produce pyramidal and cerebellar signs.

Several studies (26,57) illustrate the difference between adults and children. Children, unlike adults, are more likely to present with symptoms of increased pressure secondary to hydrocephalus. Adults, rather than presenting with signs of pressure, are more apt to present with abnormalities of vision or endocrinopathies. Personality disorders, although unusual in children, may be found in upward of 25% of adults (5,7,16). Clinical features of 48 children seen at the Hospital for Sick Children in Toronto, Canada over a 25-year period serve to demonstrate the differences in children and adults (27). All the children but one had visual complaints. Papilledema was seen in 13, bitemporal hemianopsia in 25, unilateral temporal hemianopsia in 4, and homonymous hemianopsia in 4. In 17, visual acuity was unilaterally decreased, and it was bilaterally decreased in 11. Seesaw nystagmus was found in 3 patients. Over 50% had endocrine symptoms: 6 had diabetes insipidus, 7 were excessively obese, 9 were short, 2 had hypothyroidism, and 2 had evidence of deficient sex hormones. In a smaller series of 11 adults and children (27), 10 out of 11 presented with visual complaints. Endocrine findings of decreased libido, hypothyroidism, hypopituitarism, diabetes insipidus, amenorrhea, and galactorrhea were observed in isolated instances. In the series by Kramer et al. (42) of 26 adults and children, 20 out of 26 presented with visual loss, and 8 out of 26 presented with signs of increased intracranial pressure. Regardless of age, endocrinopathies were less common. Children more than adults were likely to present with increased intracranial pressure. In this series, although 8 out of 12 children presented with increased intracranial pressure, none of the 14 adults presented in this manner. A review from the Neurological Institute in New York City (60) of 109 patients seen over a 27-year period found that 39.5% of craniopharyngiomas were found in children under 15 years of age, with a peak incidence at age 6 to 10 years. Of these children 40% (i.e., 17 out of 43) presented with papilledema, 54% had visual complaints, 38% had short stature, 9% had diabetes insipidus, 7% had ataxia, and 1 had hemiparesis. Duration of symptoms ranged from 1 week to 2 years. Fifty percent of the children were symptomatic for less than 4 months. In comparison, 80% of the adults presented with visual loss. Only 8% had evidence of increased intracranial pressure, 40% had mixed endocrinopathy, 20% had mental disturbances, 8% had diabetes insipidus, and 5% had sixth-nerve palsies. Of the adults, 53% were symptomatic for more than 1 year. Fifty to 80% of children had evidence of calcification found either on plain x rays of the skull or by CT scan. Calcification was somewhat less common in adults.

Table 14-1 lists the common signs and symptoms of patients with craniopharyngiomas. Where indicated, incidence of symptomatology is differentiated between children and adults. As Table 14-1 shows, well over 50% of the patients will present with abnormalities of the visual axis. Visual abnormalities are either bilateral or unilateral, involve one or both fields of vision, and may or may not be associated with optic atrophy. All endocrinopathies are grouped together. Many patients have evidence of disturbances of one or more endocrine functions. At presentation, the most commonly documented abnormality is either a deceleration in growth or decrease in production of growth hormone. Approximately 50% of the patients can be expected to present with either vomiting, headaches, or papilledema. This triad of symp-

TABLE 14-1. *Usual signs and symptoms of craniopharyngiomas (%)*

Author	Patients	Abnormal vision	Headache	Papilledema	Endocrinopathy	Vomiting
Love and Marshall (42) (1950)	100	81[c]	88	28		
Kramer et al. (40) (1968)	26	50[a] 100[b]		70	42 7	
Matson and Crigler (44) (1968)	57	58[a]	81		39	
Svolos (61) (1969)	108	88[a]	88	28		41
Koos and Miller (38) (1971)		60[a]		28	38	74
Bartlett (8) (1971)	35	76[a] 74[b]		43 5	40 32	
Hoff and Patterson (26) (1972)	61	58[a] 80[b]	59 63	19	25 50	
Banna (5) (1973)	71	64[c]	66	31	41	50
Petito et al. (48) (1976)	190	71[c]	78		32	34
Hoffman et al. (27) (1977)	48	98[c]		28	50	
Sung et al. (60) (1981)	109	54[a] 80[b]		40 8	47	
Symon et al. (64) (1985)	20	75[c]		20		
Baskin et al. (9) (1986)	74	72[c]	50		88	
Adamson et al. (1) (1990)	25 26	84[a] 62[b]			52 (31 pts.[a]) 87 (40 pts.[b])	

[a] Children.
[b] Adults.
[c] Children and adults.

toms in general represents nonspecific signs of increased intracranial pressure.

DIAGNOSTIC STUDIES

Plain skull films may provide valuable diagnostic information. Calcification, either patchy, diffuse, or linear, may be seen in up to 80% of children with craniopharyngiomas. Intrasellar masses are suggested by downward displacement of the floor of the sella, erosion of the dorsum sella, and changes in the clinoid processes. Volumetric measurements and ballooning of the sella indicate enlargement of the cavity of the sella turcica. Suprasellar calcification, split sutures, changes in the shape of the dorsum sella, and elongation of the clinoid processes, without an increase in the depth or size of the sella, suggest an extrasellar mass.

With the advent of neuroimaging, there is limited need for plain films and virtually no need for air encephalography, other than to aid in delineating the extent of an intrasellar mass. The CT scan readily identifies the extent, location, and degree of calcification of a suprasellar mass. CT features characteristic of craniopharyngiomas are calcification, low density, cyst formation, and contrast enhancement. CT scanning has suggested a higher incidence of calcification than previously thought. Differentiation of a chiasmatic tumor from a hypothalamic mass by CT scan may be difficult (13).

Magnetic resonance imaging, even more than CT, has defined the anatomy of the tumor and its relationship to other structures within the calvarium (23,49) (Fig. 14-3). This includes the optic nerve, chiasm, hypothalamus, and

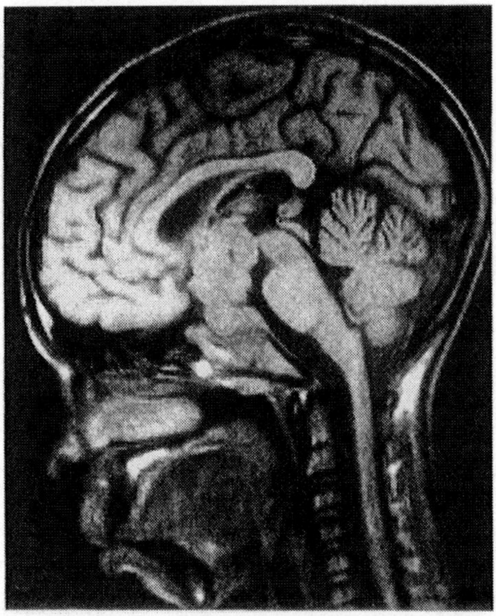

FIG. 14-3. Large suprasellar lobulated craniopharyngioma extending anteriorly and superiorly into the hypothalamus.

brain stem. MRI angiography helps to define the vasculature at the base of the brain. Because patients are apt to be on ventilators, postoperative MRI examinations are difficult to obtain. As such, preoperative CT scans continue to be necessary along with postoperative scanning in order to evaluate degree of surgical resection.

Preoperative knowledge of the vascular anatomy may be very helpful. The position of the carotid artery and the course of the anterior and middle cerebral arteries help to define the extent and location of the tumor and assist in operative planning. Unless the tumor is quite large, deviation of the supraclinoid portion of the internal carotid artery and elevation of the horizontal portion of the anterior cerebral artery may not be appreciated. Nonetheless, the circumfundibular plexus of small vessels will be elevated in most cases. There may be stretching of the posterior communicating artery and cisternal portion of the anterior cerebral arteries. Frontal extension of the tumor can be appreciated by elevation and posterior bowing of the horizontal portion of the anterior cerebral artery. Lateral extension is appreciated by stretching and bowing of the middle cerebral artery. As a result of an enlarged ventricle, the ventricular striate arteries may be stretched and lose their normal patterns. Diagnosis of the posterior extension of the tumor is suggested by alteration in the vertebral basilar arteries.

Before surgery, patients should have a complete endocrine and psychometric assessment. Evaluation should also include testing of visual fields and acuity. If not present preoperatively, postoperative endocrinopathies, primarily diabetes insipidus, are invariably present.

TREATMENT

Agreement is universal on the need for surgery, although the extent of surgery is controversial (14,61,64). Complete removal of craniopharyngiomas has been advocated by some, while others have suggested aspiration of cyst contents and partial removal followed by local irradiation (1,3,8,71). Virtually all authors agree that there is a high recurrence rate (9). With the advent of steroid replacement therapy preoperatively and postoperatively, operative mortality has dramatically declined (32). Skilled endocrine management has removed fears of intraoperative and postoperative hypopituitarism and, in turn, has led to more aggressive surgical management (4,36). The introduction of steroids has essentially eliminated intraoperative adrenal insufficiency. Initially, endocrinologists followed rigid replacement protocols during the operative and postoperative period. However, increased awareness of steroid biochemistry and greater understanding of the management of diabetes insipidus have greatly simplified the endocrine approach. In the 1950s and 1960s, Matson and Crigler (44) of the Harvard Medical School suggested that total radical excision of a craniopharyngiomas was possible in the context of preoperative and postoperative management of patients with high-dose steroids. Their approach, for the most part, reflects current endocrine management in the perioperative period.

Matson believed that craniopharyngiomas were more likely to recur in children and were apt to be more relentlessly aggressive. Furthermore, complications were more likely in those children requiring reoperation as opposed to those initially treated with surgical removal. Most of his cases were approached subfrontally with sparing of the optic nerve and chiasm. Complete removal was considered obtained in 46 of 57 patients. However, in reviewing Matson's cases, Katz (33) reported that only 34 were thought to have had total resection. Subsequently, 9 out of 34 were found to have evidence of recurrence of tumor, 6 within the first month postoperatively and 3 others within 3.5 to 4.5 years after surgery. At the time of Katz's report, 22 of 34 patients were alive without signs and symptoms of tumors. Three of the original series died as a result of endocrinopathy; autopsies failed to reveal tumor. Quality of life was rated good to excellent in 15 of the 22 survivors and fair in the remaining 7. Four patients had had total excision on reoperation, 2 of whom were considered to be doing well. Of 5 children with partial excision, 4 were doing well, and 1 was considered fair (i.e., dependent on others for some aspects of daily care). Eighty-seven percent of the patients in this series were hormone deficient. Despite the need for continuing hormone replacement, a good quality of life in the absence of tumor recurrence has been documented for well over a decade.

Hoffman et al. (27) have echoed the opinions of Matson and Crigler concerning total radical removal. They reported on 48 children seen in Toronto, Canada. Sixteen had aspiration of cyst contents, 15 had subtotal extirpation, and total removal was accomplished in 17. In all 16 patients treated by aspiration, tumors recurred. Of 15 with subtotal excision, 6 were irradiated because of tumor recurrence, 2 died, and the remaining 7 had no evidence of recurrence. Of the 13 survivors, the majority have had some form of endocrinopathy. Of the 17 patients who had total excision, 15 are alive with some degree of endocrinopathy but none with recurrent tumor. Fourteen had diabetes insipidus, 11 required steroids, 13 thyroid replacement, and 4 sex hormones. Overall, mortality was 62.4% for those surgically treated with aspiration, 13.3% for those treated with subtotal surgical excision, and 11.8% for those treated with total excision. In 8 patients in whom the operating microscope was used, morbidity and mortality was 0. Like Matson and Crigler, the Toronto group emphasized the relative ease of de novo tumor removal versus the increased difficulty of surgery for recurrent disease because of dense adhesions that prevent total removal of the tumor from the surrounding brain. Others have also reported good results following attempts at gross total resection. In several other series (52), successful total resection was reported in 74 to 90% of children with an operative mortality of 0 to 11%. For the

TABLE 14-2. *Survival rates of patients with craniopharyngiomas*

	Total surgical removal		Subtotal surgical removal		Radiotherapy surgery	
Author	No. of patients	(%)	No. of patients	(%)	No. of patients	(%)
Kramer et al. (40) (1968)					13[c]	65
					14[a]	79
Svolos (61) (1969)	25	36	53	13		
Bloom (10) (1975)					59[c]	76 (5 yr)[a]
					33[a]	61 (10 yr)
Katz (33) (1975)	34	88				
Urdaneta et al. (69)					9	55
Petito et al. (48) (1976) <1955					14	30 (5 yr)
>1955					17	55 (5 yr)
Hoffman et al. (27) (1977)	17	88			15	87
Humphreys et al. (29)	19	88	15	87		
Richmond and Wilson (51)	8	88 (5 yr)	4	51 (5 yr)	12	88 (5 yr)
(1980)	4	50 (10 yr)	4	50 (10 yr)	9	44 (10 yr)
Sung et al. (60) (1981)	C 14	100 (5 yr)	14	71 (5 yr)	14	93 (5 yr)
	14	100 (10 yr)	14	14 (10 yr)	14	80 (10 yr)
	A 23	59 (5 yr)	23	36 (5 yr)	18	81 (5 yr)
	23	24 (10 yr)	23	31 (10 yr)	18	73 (10 yr)
Baskin (9) (1986)			5	73	2	95
Yasargil et al. (71) (1990)	51	88	19	58		
Kahn et al. (32) (1973)		C	28	50		
		A	12	75		Overall[b]
Shapiro et al. (54) (1979)			60	38		Overall[b]
Mori et al. (45) (1980)		Steroid	34	50 (5 yr)		
			34	38 (10 yr)		
		Presteroid	41	51 (5 yr)		Overall[b]
			41	38		

[a] Where noted in literature survival in years is stated in parentheses.
[b] Overall refers to survival in all treatment groups; i.e., authors did not differentiate survival with various treatment modalities.
[c] A, adults; C, children.

most part, these reports fail to clarify the clinical outcome or degree of endocrinopathy (Tables 14-2, 14-3, and 14-4).

Others believe that although a total excision may be desired, this approach is impractical and potentially harmful. More often than not, these tumors either grossly invade the brain or there is absence of a surgical plane that permits total removal. In addition, in the series by Matson and Crigler, the long-term success rate for the total removal of a primary tumor, although impressive, is still only 55% and the long-term success rate for reoperation was only 17%. Of interest, a decade later, Shillito (55), commenting on his experience in Matson's clinic, favors a much more conservative approach. Shillito favored total excision only when tissue did not appear to invade the brain. For initial treatment he recommended subtotal resection with radiotherapy and for recurrence, radiation rather than reoperation. Surgical intervention, in his opinion, is indicated primarily to decompress the optic system. In addition, he recommends a tap of the recurrent cyst without craniotomy through an x-ray guide needle.

TABLE 14-3. *Recurrence rate of surviving patients with craniopharyngiomas*

Author	Total surgical removal		Subtotal surgical removal		Radiotherapy surgery	
	No. of patients	(%)	No. of patients	(%)	No. of patients	(%)
Hoff and Patterson (26) (1972)	0/4	0	13/18 16/18	72 (5 yr) 89 (10 yr)	9/22 12/19	41 (5 yr) 63 (10 yr)
Kahn et al. (31) (1973)					5/9	55
Katz (33) (1975)	9/31	29				
Hoffman et al. (27)	2/15	13	8/15	53		
Thompson et al. (66) (1978)					1/5	20
Richmond et al. (50) (1980)	3/8	38				
Rougerie (52) (1979)	4/32	12.5				
Humphreys et al. (29) (1979)	0/13	0	2/15	13		
Shapiro et al. (54) (1979)	5/22	23	7/9	78	11/22	50
Cabezudo et al. (14) (1981)	4/13	30	10/14	71	1/16	6
Sung et al. (60) (1981)						
C =	7/14	50	30/37	81	8/32	25
A =	11/23	48	(A and C)		(A and C)	

A, adults; C, children; number in parentheses, follow-up interval.

For most surgeons, subtotal resection appears to be the procedure of choice. This eliminates the pulling and tugging of the hypothalamus and the associated morbidity that accompanies aggressive surgery to the area of the hypothalamus (42,45,62,63). A review (47) of 155 cases indicated that the morbidity associated with total surgical extirpation was not warranted, and that palliative surgery followed by radiation was recommended. Despite the introduction of the operating microscope and recent advances in microscopic techniques, total surgical removal in many instances may lead to unacceptable hypothalamic damage. The microscopic presence of a tumor invading the brain makes total excision, even with the aid of a dissecting microscope, impossible. Ample surgical and pathologic evidence suggests that the lack of a glial capsule may not allow development of the surgical plane. The site of the tumor, its relationship to the visual apparatus, and preoperative endocrine function all influence the outcome and surgical approach.

A problem associated with total resection have been compromise of the

TABLE 14-4. *Quality of survival*

Author	Patients	Total excision (%)			Patients	Partial excision and radiotherapy (%)		
		Good	Fair	Poor		Good	Fair	Poor
Kahn et al. (31) (1973)	28	21						
Katz (33) (1975)	22	68	32	0				
Hoffman et al. (27) (1977)	15	33	60	7				
Richmond and Wilson (51) (1980)	6	100			14	100		
Thomsett et al. (67) (1980)	11	73	9	18	17	70	18	12
Sung et al. (60) (1981)	27	26	48	26	14	64	36	0
Yasargil et al. (71) (1990)	51	73	10	10	19	32	22	5

vascular supply to the visual apparatus resulting in postoperative visual deterioration. Furthermore, endocrine disturbances are apt to be more significant following aggressive surgery because of manipulation of the hypothalamus. In addition to diabetes insipidus, one needs to be concerned about possible postoperative Addison's disease and hypothyroidism. Abulia, associated with frontal lobe manipulations, may leave the patient mute with marked lack of motivation. In this group of patients, intelligence and memory quotients tend to be preserved.

A frequent complication of craniopharyngiomas is recurrence of the cystic portion of the tumor. In one of our patients who was thought to have a 95% subtotal resection, recurrence of a cyst resulted in compression of the optic chiasm, visual loss in one eye, and compromise of visual field in the remaining eye. In such situations, stereotactic intercyst injection of radioactive colloid has been tried with some success. If at the initial surgery decompression of the visual apparatus can be obtained by aspiration, then interstitial radiotherapy should be reserved for recurrent tumor.

RADIOTHERAPY

Radiation was first used in the treatment of craniopharyngiomas in 1937. Following Kramer's (39) observation in the early 1960s that these tumors arise from squamous epithelium and thus might be susceptible to high-dose radiation, an increasing number of reports have supported the value of radiation. Since then there has there been increasing acceptance of the use of radiotherapy in combination with subtotal excision for the treatment of craniopharyngioma (15). The recommended doses of local irradiation in children have been approximately 5,000 cGy, whereas those in adults have been as high as 7,000 cGy (38,41,42). Although radiation necrosis to the brain, visual apparatus, and parasellar structures has been reported, most authorities believe that these complications can be avoided if the dose per fraction does not exceed 150 to 180 cGy per day (18,25,66,69).

Results of radiation and subtotal surgical removal versus surgery alone suggest that recurrences are strikingly decreased in the radiation group (21). Even in those reports in which total excision has been advocated, the rate of recurrence approaches that of patients treated with radiotherapy. Furthermore, radiotherapy can be standardized from institution to institution. Hence, a good result need not be dependent on the skill of a specific individual, as it is with surgery.

Comparison of survival rates after surgery and irradiation are more difficult to document (70). Because many surgical reports include mortality in the immediate postoperative period, survival statistics are bound to favor radiotherapy. A review of the literature suggests that those patients with subtotal surgical removal followed by radiotherapy are apt to have better survival rates than those patients treated by biopsy and cyst aspiration after radiotherapy. Results of total excision compared to radiotherapy are more difficult to compare and are more nearly equal. On balance, most radiotherapists and neurosurgeons accept the concept of radiotherapy after a recurrence (10). Because recurrences in patients with total excision continue to be reported, a small but highly respected group of radiotherapists suggest radiation after attempts at total excision. As an alternative to x-ray therapy, there have been scattered reports of success with radioactive tracers delivered to the cystic cavity of craniopharyngiomas through an Ommaya device (24,65). This approach is limited to patients with large cystic cavities with or without recurrences (3,35,37). This is a striking departure from the philosophy of reoperation for recurrences, which represents the thinking of the 1960s and early 1970s (50,51).

Radiation complications include optic neuritis and pituitary hypothalamic damage and dementia (68) consisting of difficulties with memory, concentration, and intelligence. Arteritis is a reported but rare complication, as are radiation-induced second tumors (also see Chapter 23).

OUTCOME MEASURES

Tables 14-2 and 14-3 correlate the various treatment modalities with survival and recurrence. Survival of patients treated with radiation and partial excision appears to be as high as those treated with total excision. Radiotherapy and partial excision appear superior to partial excision alone. In many instances where total excision was considered present, recurrence rates approach those of patients treated with radiotherapy. In those patients treated with only aspiration, recurrence rates approached 100%. Similarly, recurrence was also high in a few series in which radiotherapy after aspiration was sorted out from radiotherapy with partial excision.

Quality of life is more difficult to judge, despite the abundant literature about treatment results (Table 14-4). Accurate assessment of patients is not discussed in a systematic way (59). On balance, there remains the suggestion that patients fare better when treated with partial excision and radiotherapy rather than by surgery alone. Morbidity after radiation and radical surgery is high in both groups. Survival may be poorer in adults than in children (27,29,45). Because of the location of this tumor, endocrinopathies are invariably found.

Attempts have been made to correlate functional results with treatment, pathologic features, and various roentgenographic features. The choice of treatment is the single most important factor influencing outcome. However, other variables cannot be excluded. Many authors have associated prognosis with the presence of calcification, size of the tumor, introduction of the operative microscope, and presence of endocrinopathies. Irregularities of the floor of the third ventricle and the presence of psychiatric symptoms have both been correlated with a poor prognosis, presumably because this represents an extension of the tumor into the hypothalamus. Absence of calcification, a tumor size smaller than 3 cm, negative cerebrospinal fluid findings, and diagnosis after 1955 have been associated with a favorable outcome (48,54).

Endocrinopathies, although not associated with mortality, do represent significant morbidity (1). Although deficits of hypothalamic pituitary function may not be present before diagnosis and treatment, they invariably occur after treatment. Delayed growth and/or decreased production of growth hormone, although not necessarily a symptom at presentation, may be present

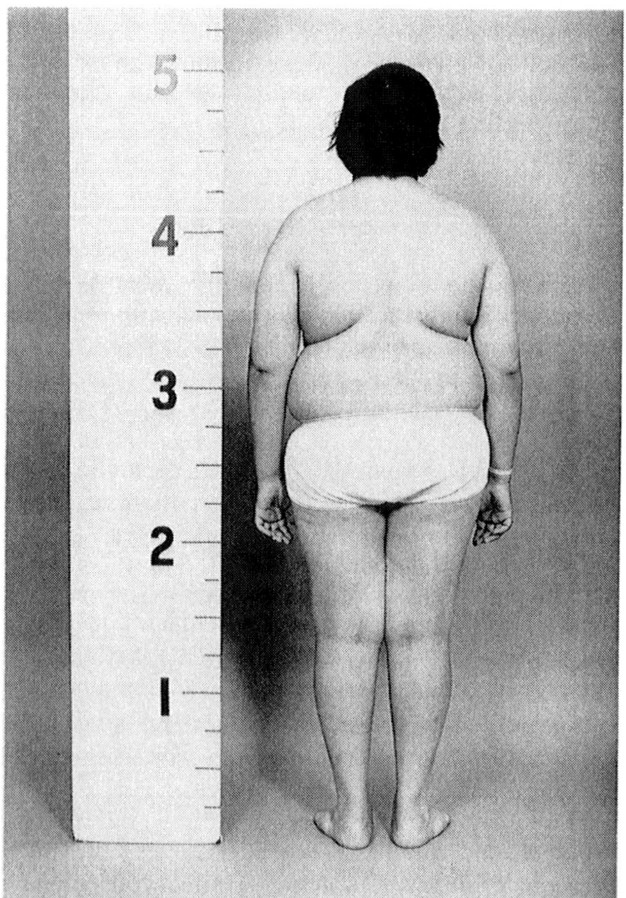

FIG. 14-4. Fourteen-year-old male with obesity and diabetes following surgical removal of a craniopharyngioma.

in over 50% of the cases (53). Most commonly reported endocrine abnormalities are decreased growth hormone, decreased ACTH, decreased TSH, decreased LH/FSH, decreased ADH, and decreased prolactin (58,67).

There have been several observations in the literature of normal growth after surgery and radiation despite deficiency of growth hormone (12,28,34). In fact, there is some evidence that normal modulation of growth occurs (56). Growth spurts above normal after surgery have been documented in several children (28). Why patients should have low growth hormone and catch-up growth after the removal of a craniopharyngioma has never been answered. Suggested possibilities relate to the level of somatomedin, insulin, and thyroid, and the effects of these hormones on promoting normal growth despite the absence of normal levels of growth hormone (17,20). Other explanations include hyperprolactinemia and normal 24-hour growth hormone production with low plasma growth hormone (22).

Hyperphagia with obesity is greatest immediately after surgery. Weight gain may or may not parallel gains in growth. Although appetite may decrease to preoperative levels, obesity is apt to remain a chronic problem (Fig. 14-4). Postoperatively, diabetes insipidus is likely to persist. Unlike the findings of decreased growth hormone production found preoperatively, diabetes insipidus is usually absent before surgery but invariably present postoperatively. Like thyroid deficiency, this complication responds well to replacement therapy. Overall, partial excision followed by radiotherapy has been associated with a better endocrinologic outcome than radical surgery alone.

SUMMARY

Craniopharyngiomas present with a complex set of medical and surgical problems. Successful total surgical removal with limited morbidity depends on the skill of the surgeon, the location of the tumor, the presence of a defined surgical plane, the size of the tumor, and occurrence in either a child or an adult. Both surgery and radiation are invariably associated with endocrine complications. Radiotherapy combined with partial excision has been associated with less immediate morbidity but with more long-term morbidity. Furthermore, as with surgery, radiotherapy is usually not curative. This consideration plus the observation that approximately 50% of patients treated surgically may have tumor recurrence suggests that radiotherapy should be considered at the time of recurrence rather than at the time of presentation. Long-term effects on intelligence, mood, behavior, and neurologic residuals, although commonly mentioned in the literature, have yet to be fully assessed. When possible, we continue to believe that attempts at total surgical excision may be the best approach. However, this view must be tempered by the observation that if a glial capsule is not identified at surgery, tugging and pulling at the hypothalamus may result in unacceptable morbidity and even death. Regrettably, total surgical excision is usually not possible, and subtotal excision should be, upon recurrence, followed by radiation. Whereas both approaches are associated with endocrinopathy, radiation has been more commonly associated with effects on intelligence. However, this approach may offer the best possibility for long-term survival and limited morbidity.

REFERENCES

1. Adamson TE, Wiestler OD, Kleihues P, Yasargil MG. Correlation of clinical and pathological features in surgically treated craniopharyngiomas. *J Neurosurg* 1990;73:12–17.
2. Ammirati M, Samii M, Sephernia A. Surgery of large retrochiasmatic craniopharyngiomas in children. *Childs Nerv Syst* 1990;6:13–17.
3. Anderson DR, Trobe JD, Taren JA, Gebarski SS. Visual outcome in cystic craniopharyngiomas treated with intracavitary phosphorus-32. *Ophthalmology* 1989;96:1786–1792.
4. Andler W, Roosen K, Clar HE. Pre- and post-operative evaluation of hypothalamo-pituitary function in children with craniopharyngiomas. *Acta Neurochir* 1979;45:287–299.
5. Banna M. Craniopharyngioma in adults. *Surg Neurol* 1973;1:202–204.
6. Banna M. Review article: craniopharyngioma: based on 160 cases. *Br J Radiol* 1976;49: 206–223.
7. Banna M, Hoare RD, Stanley P, Till K. Craniopharyngioma in children. *J Pediatr* 1973; 83:781–785.
8. Bartlett JR. Craniopharyngiomas: a summary of 85 cases. *J Neurol Neurosurg Psychiatr* 1971;34:37–41.
9. Baskin DS, Wilson CB. Surgical management of craniopharyngioma: a review of 74 cases. *J Neurosurg* 1986;65:22–27.
10. Bloom HJ. Combined modality therapy for intracranial tumors. *Cancer* 1975;35:111–120.
11. Burger PC, Vogel FS. *Surgical pathology of the nervous system and its coverings*. 2nd ed. New York: J Wiley & Sons; 1982:511–525.
12. Burns EC, Tanner JM, Preece MA, Cameron N. Growth hormone treatment in children with craniopharyngioma: final growth status. *Clin Endocrinol* 1981;14:587–595.
13. Cabezudo JM, Vaquero J, Garcia-de-Sola R, Leundo G, Nombela L, Bravo G. Computed tomography with craniopharyngioma: a review. *Surg Neurol* 1981;15:422–427.
14. Cabezudo JM, Vaquero J, Areitio E, Martinez R, Garcia-de-Sola R, Bravo G. Craniopharyngiomas: a critical approach to treatment. *J Neurosurg* 1981;55:371–375.
15. Carpenter RC, Chamberlin GW, Frazier CH. The treatment of hypophyseal stalk tumors by evacuation and irradiation. *AJR* 1937;38:162–177.
16. Clopper RR, Meyer WJ, Udvarhelyi GB, et al. Post-surgical IQ and behavioral data on twenty patients with a history of childhood craniopharyngioma. *Psychoneuroendocrinology* 1977;2:365–372.
17. Costin G, Kogut MD, Phillips LS, Daughaday WH. Craniopharyngioma: the role of insulin in promoting post-operative growth. *J Clin Endocrinol Metab* 1976;42:370–379.
18. Crompton MR, Layton DD. Delayed radionecrosis of the brain following therapeutic x-radiation of the pituitary. *Brain* 1961;84:85–101.
19. Cushing HW. Intracranial tumors: notes upon a series of two thousand verified cases with surgical-mortality percentages pertaining thereto. Springfield, IL: CC Thomas; 1932:97.
20. Finkelstein JW, Kream J, Ludan A, Hellman L. Sulfation factor (somatomedin): an explanation for continued growth in the absence of imunoassayable growth hormone in patients with hypothalamic tumors. *J Clin Endocrinol Metab* 1972;35:13–17.
21. Fischer EG, Welch K, Shillito J Jr, Winston KR, Tarbell NJ. Craniopharyngiomas in children: long-term effects of conservative surgical procedures combined with radiation therapy. *J Neurosurg* 1990;73:534–540.
22. Frasier SD, Smith FG. Return of normal growth following removal of a craniopharyngioma. *Am J Dis Child* 1968;116:311–314.
23. Fukushima T, Hirakawa K, Kimura M. Intraventricular craniopharyngioma: its characteris-

tics in magnetic resonance imaging and successful total removal. *Surg Neurol* 1990;33: 22–27.
24. Guevara JA, Bunge HJ, Heinrich JJ, et al. Cystic craniopharyngioma treated by Yttrium 90 silicated colloid. *Acta Neurochir [Suppl] (Wein)* 1988;42:109–112.
25. Harris JR, Levene MB. Visual complications following irradiation for pituitary adenomas and craniopharyngiomas. *Radiology* 1976;120:167–171.
26. Hoff JT, Patterson RH Jr. Craniopharyngiomas in children and adults. *J Neurosurg* 1972; 36:299–302.
27. Hoffman HJ, Hendrick EB, Humphreys RP, Buncic JR, Armstrong DL, Jenkin RDT. Management of craniopharyngioma in children. *J Neurosurg* 1977;47:218–227.
28. Holmes LB, Frantz AG, Rabkin MT, Soeldner JS, Crawford JD. Normal growth with subnormal growth hormone levels. *N Engl J Med* 1968;279:559–566.
29. Humphreys RP, Hoffman HJ, Hendrick EB. A long-term post-operative follow-up in craniopharyngioma. *Childs Brain* 1979;5:530–539.
30. Hunter IJ. Squamous metaplasia of cells of the anterior pituitary gland. *J Pathol Bacteriol* 1955;69:141–145.
31. Kahn EA, Gosch HH, Seeger JF, Hicks SP. Forty-five years experience with the craniopharyngiomas. *Surg Neurol* 1973;1:5–12.
32. Kang JK, Song JU. Results of the management of craniopharyngioma in children: an endocrinological approach to the treatment. *Childs Nerv Syst* 1988;4:135–138.
33. Katz EL. Late results of radical excision of craniopharyngiomas in children. *J Neurosurg* 1975;42:86–90.
34. Kenny FM, Iturzaeta NF, Mintz D, et al. Iatrogenic hypopituitarism in craniopharyngioma: unexplained catch-up growth in the three children. *J Pediatr* 1968;72:766–775.
35. Kobayashi T, Kageyama N, Ohara K. Internal irradiation for cystic craniopharyngioma. *J Neurosurg* 1981;55:896–903.
36. Kobayashi T, Kageyama N, Yoshida Y, Shibuya N, Yonezawa T. Pathological and clinical basis of the indications for treatment of craniopharyngiomas. *Neurol Med Chir (Tokyo)* 1981;21:39–47.
37. Kodama T, Matsukado Y, Uemura S. Intracapsular irradiation therapy of craiopharyngiomas with radioactive gold: indication and follow-up results. *Neurol Med Chir (Tokyo)* 1981; 21:49–58.
38. Koos W Th, Miller MH. Craniopharyngioma. In: *Intracranial tumors of infants and children*. St. Louis:CV Mosby; 1971:188–213.
39. Kramer S, McKissock W, Concannon JP. Craniopharyngiomas: treatment by combined surgery and radiation therapy. *J Neurosurg* 1961;17:217–226.
40. Kramer S, Southard M, Mansfield CM. Radiotherapy in the management of craniopharyngiomas: further experiences and late results. *AJR* 1968;103:44–52.
41. Kramer S. Craniopharyngioma: the best treatment is conservative surgery and postoperative radiation therapy. In: Morley TP, ed. *Current controversies in neurosurgery*. Philadelphia:WB Saunders; 1976:336–343.
42. Love JG, Marshall TM. Craniopharyngiomas (pituitary adamantinomas). *Surg Gynecol Obstet* 1950;90:591–601.
43. Luse SA, Kernohan JW. Squamous cell nests of the pituitary gland. *Cancer* 1955;8:623–628.
44. Matson DD, Crigler JF. Management of craniopharyngioma in childhood. *J Neurosurg* 1969;30:377–390.
45. Mori K, Handa H, Murata T, Takeuchi J, Miwa S, Osaka K. Results of treatment for craniopharyngioma. *Childs Brain* 1980;6:303–312.
46. Northfield DWC. *The surgery of the central nervous system*. Oxford: Blackwell Scientific; 1973:314–327.
47. Patterson RH Jr, Danylevich A. Surgical removal of craniopharyngiomas by a transcranial approach through the lamina terminalis and sphenoid sinus. *Neurosurgery* 1980;7:111–117.
48. Petito CK, DeGirolami U, Earle KM. Craniopharyngiomas, a clinical and pathological review. *Cancer* 1976;37:1944–1952.
49. Pusey E, Kortman KE, Flannigan BD, Tsuruda J, Bradley WG. MR of craniopharyngiomas: tumor delineation and characterization. *AJR* 1987;149:383–388.
50. Richmond IL, Wara WM, Wilson CB. Role of radiation therapy in the management of craniopharyngiomas in children. *Neurosurgery* 1980;6:513–517.

51. Richmond IL, Wilson CB. Parasellar tumors in children. II: Surgical management, radiation therapy and follow-up. *Childs Brain* 1980;7:85–94.
52. Rougerie J. What can be expected from the surgical treatment of craniopharyngiomas in children: report of 92 cases. *Childs Brain* 1979;5:433–449.
53. Rubinstein LJ. *Tumors of the central nervous system.* Washington, DC: Armed Forces Institute of Pathology; 1972:292–294.
54. Shapiro K, Till K, Grant N. Craniopharyngiomas in childhood: a rational approach to treatment. *J Neurosurg* 1979;50:617–623.
55. Shillito J. Craniopharyngiomas: the subfrontal approach or none at all? *Clin Neurosurg* 1980;27:188–205.
56. Sorva R. Children with craniopharyngioma: early growth failure and rapid postoperative weight gain. *Acta Paediatr Scand* 1988;77:587–592.
57. Sorva R, Jaaskinen J, Heiskanen O. Craniopharyngioma in children and adults: correlations between radiological and clinical manifestations. *Acta Neurochir (Wein)* 1987;89:1–3.
58. Sotos JF, Romshe CA. Pituitary tumors. In: Gardner LI, ed. *Endocrine and genetic disease of childhood and adolescence,* 2nd ed. Philadelphia: WB Saunders; 1975:187–219.
59. Stahnke N, Grubel G, Lagenstein I, et al. Long-term follow-up of children with craniopharyngioma. *Eur J Pediatr* 1984;142:179–185.
60. Sung DI, Chang CH, Harisiadis L, Carmel PW. Treatment results of craniopharyngiomas. *Cancer* 1981;47:847–852.
61. Svolos DG. Craniopharyngiomas: a study based on 108 verified cases. *Acta Chir Scand (Suppl)* 1969;403:1–44.
62. Sweet WH. Recurrent craniopharyngiomas: therapeutic alternatives. *Clin Neurosurg* 1980; 27:206–229.
63. Sweet WH. Radical surgical treatment of craniopharyngiomas. *Clin Neurosurg* 1976;23: 52–79.
64. Symon L, Sprich W. Radical excision of craniopharyngioma: results in 20 patients. *J Neurosurg* 1985;62:174–181.
65. Szeifert GT, Julow J, Slowik F, et al. Pathological changes in cystic craniopharyngiomas following intracavital Yttrium-90 treatment. *Acta Neurochir (Wein)* 1990;102:14–18.
66. Thompson IL, Griffin TW, Parker RG, Blasko JC. Craniopharyngioma: the role of radiation therapy. *Int J Rad Oncol Biol Phys* 1978;4:1059–1063.
67. Thomsett MJ, Conte FA, Kaplan SL, Grumbach MM. Endocrine and neurologic outcome in childhood craniopharyngioma: review of effect of treatment in 42 patients. *J Pediatr* 1980;97:728–735.
68. Tomita T. Management of craniopharyngiomas in children. *Pediatr Neurosci* 1988;14: 204–211.
69. Urdaneta N, Chessin H, Fisher J. Pituitary adenomas and craniopharyngiomas: analysis of 99 cases treated with radiation therapy. *Int J Radiat Oncol Biol Phys* 1976;1:895–902.
70. Wen BC, Hussey DH, Staples J, et al. A comparison of the roles of surgery and radiation therapy in the management of craniopharyngiomas. *Int J Radiat Oncol Biol Phys* 1989;16: 17–24.
71. Yasargil MG, Curcic M, Kis M, Siegenthaler G, Teddy PJ, Roth P. Total removal of craniopharyngiomas: approaches and long-term results in 144 patients. *J Neurosurg* 1990;73:3–11.

15

Tumors of the Diencephalon and Optic Pathway

Diencephalic tumors are those tumors that arise in the midline and are bordered anteriorly and inferiorly by the foramen of Monro and the intracranial portion of the optic nerves and optic chiasm; posteriorly by the aqueduct of Sylvius, pineal region, and the rostral portion of the midbrain; and laterally by the internal capsule and lateral ganglionic structures. Tumors of this region include thalamic, optic pathway, and hypothalamic neoplasms. They can occur at any age, but the age of onset is usually under 20 years.

THALAMIC TUMORS

Neoplasms of the thalamic region tend to be more aggressive and have a more truncated course than those found in the area of the hypothalamus, chiasm, or other portions of the optic pathway. Because a limited number of thalamic tumors are reported in the literature, an accurate appraisal of treatment effects and outcome is difficult. In many reports (6) thalamic tumors are included with those tumors occurring in the cerebral hemispheres. By and large, the duration of symptoms prior to diagnosis is less than 1 year. Infrequently, although commonly thought of as occurring in the pineal region or suprasellar region, germinomas have been reported in the lateral ganglionic area.

Signs and symptoms of a thalamic mass are surprisingly nonspecific and consist of headaches, papilledema, confusion, memory loss, and emotional lability. Increased intracranial pressure secondary to obstruction of the ventricular system is the most common presentation. Mental symptoms have been described with involvement of the medial thalamic nucleus and its projections to the frontal cortex. Abnormalities of speech production seen in thalamic tumors have been correlated with deficits in the ventrolateral thalamus (74). Lateralizing signs reflect involvement of the fibers, either leaving or entering the thalamus. An unusual case of ipsilateral hemiatrophy has been recorded with a thalamic tumor (58). Involvement of the cerebellorubrothalamic tracts may cause unilateral dysmetria, tremor, incoordination, or unsteady gait.

Brain Tumors in Children: Principles of Diagnosis and Treatment, 2/e, edited by M.E. Cohen and P.K. Duffner, Raven Press, Ltd., New York, 1994.

Motor abnormalities such as tremor and dysmetria may be mistakenly associated with cerebellar hemisphere lesions, whereas dystonic movements and unilateral chorea implicate abnormalities of the subthalamus or basal ganglia. These findings suggest either involvement of motor pathways projecting to the region of the thalamus or extension of the tumor outside the anatomic confines of the thalamus and the internal capsule.

Visual loss is secondary to either long standing increased intracranial pressure or involvement of the visual pathway. Hemianopsia may reflect involvement of the optic tract, geniculate bodies, or optic radiations. Pupillary inequality and conjugate gaze disturbances suggest extension of the tumor into the midbrain and quadrigeminal plate. Surprisingly, sensory findings in tumors of the region are not common and when present are mild in nature (87). The thalamic syndrome of Djerrine is virtually never encountered.

Clinical seizures are considered unusual, although a 30% incidence has been reported in at least one series (23,44,105). EEG abnormalities, unlike seizures, are quite common, and have been reported in 70 to 90% of patients (23,44). Nonspecific EEG findings, consisting of diffuse bursts of symmetrical high-voltage delta and theta waves occurring in the waking state, generally reflect increased intracranial pressure. More specific EEG correlations lateralize the findings to one hemisphere and consist of either ipsilateral depression of normal background rhythms, presence of lateralized polymorphic delta activity, or the findings of sleep spindles (i.e., sigma rhythms) during the waking state.

Thus, what emerges as characteristic of deep-seated cerebral tumors of the basal ganglia or thalamus is a clinical picture of nonspecific symptoms. The patients are usually under 20 years of age, with a duration of symptoms less than 1 year and evidence of increased intracranial pressure. Characteristically, lateralized motor signs with or without abnormality of movement or sensation complete the clinical picture. The signs and symptoms associated with thalamic masses suggest that functional derangement, not specifically related to the anatomic site of involvement, is the expected correlate of tumors of these areas (90).

Diagnostic Studies

Clinical suspicion of a thalamic mass is confirmed by appropriate diagnostic studies. CT scans obtained in both axial and coronal views show distortion and displacement of ventricular structures. The tumor mass is seen in the area of the thalamus or basal ganglia (Fig. 15-1). The density of the mass may be greater than, equal to, or less than that of surrounding tissue. Some degree of contrast enhancement is usual. As with CT, MRI provides exquisite definition of anatomy but adds little to the pathologic assessment.

Angiographic evidence of a deep-seated mass consists of displacement of

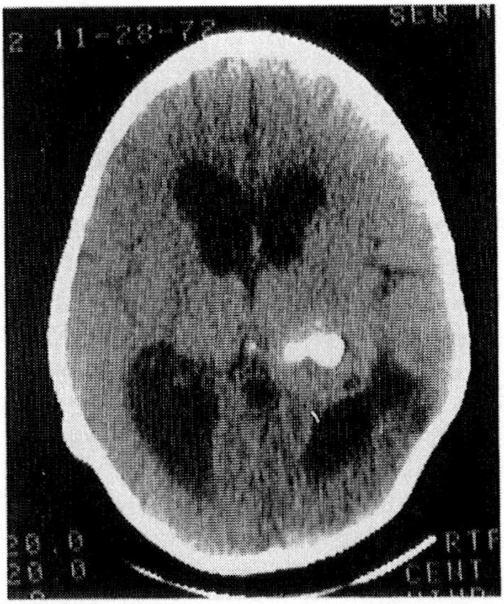

FIG. 15-1. CT showing calcified mass in the thalamus and basal ganglia.

the angiographic Sylvian point laterally with resultant straightening of the branches of the middle cerebral artery. There may be displacement of the lenticular striate vessels outward and inferiorly, and subtle changes in the course of the anterior and posterior choroidal vessels. In the venous phase, the venous angle is opened and the internal cerebral vein is displaced superiorly. Neovascularity and arteriovenous shunting are associated with increased malignancy of the tumor.

Treatment

Treatment of tumors of the thalamus, in general, has been unsatisfactory (7,44). Open craniotomy for biopsies and resection of thalamic gliomas has been associated with high morbidity and mortality. The infiltrative nature of the tumor rarely offers the hope of a surgical cure. Ventriculostomy and other surgical procedures are used to decompress the ventricle and relieve pressure. As with neoplasms in any region, it is axiomatic that proper treatment relies on histologic diagnosis. Kelly (54) reported on 72 patients from the Mayo Clinic who had histologically verified thalamic astrocytomas. Forty-four of these had stereotactic biopsy, 22 of whom had stereotactic resection of the tumor. Of 34 patients with a grade IV astrocytoma, the mean survival after surgery and radiation was somewhat greater than 21 weeks. Kelly emphasized that the computer-assisted volumetric stereotactic surgery produces several advantages over conventional surgery. The stereotactic approach allows the surgeon to maintain spatial orientation so that deep lesions may be located. It also permits the operator to stay within the boundaries of the lesion as defined by CT or MRI scan. Unlike open biopsy, stereotactic biopsies have been associated with low morbidity and mortality. Morbidity after biopsy was 6%, all of which occurred in the patients with high-grade tumors. In a small cadre of patients who have high-grade neoplasms, decompression of the ventricular system and debulking of the tumor mass in the lateral ganglionic regions followed by radiation may be associated with increased survival as compared to biopsy and radiation alone.

Overall results of radiotherapy are discouraging, with expected 5-year survivals of 20 to 30% and 10-year survivals of 17 to 30% (13,14). Survival is, for the most part, associated with degree of malignancy at the time of diagnosis. Because these tumors are infiltrative in nature, radiation has been given either in large volumes well beyond the confines of the tumor mass, or to the entire brain. Unlike malignant astrocytomas, low-grade tumors in this region may be associated with long-term survival (37). Because large series comparing treatment modalities are not available, it has been difficult to assess the role of adjuvant therapy. Compounding the difficulty in assessing treatment has been the practice of irradiating patients without the benefit of surgery or biopsy (13). As a generalization, this approach is to be avoided, and treatment decisions should be made only after an accurate pathologic diagnosis is obtained (12).

HYPOTHALAMIC TUMORS

Midline gliomas of childhood occupying the region of the third ventricle, hypothalamus, and optic chiasm generally have a different pathology and, by and large, a different biology than those occurring in the thalamus. Tumors arising in this region may blend imperceptibly into neoplasms originating in the optic chiasm, and thus distinction between these groups at times may be quite arbitrary. Pilocytic astrocytomas, hamartomas, gangliogliomas, germinomas, and craniopharyngiomas comprise the bulk of pathology seen in this area. Gliomas of this region, regardless of site, are apt to be classified as juvenile pilocytic astrocytomas. These tumors, unlike those found more laterally, are not histologically graded according to malignancy. Findings of necrosis and hemorrhage do not necessarily imply an aggressive nature. Rosenthal fibers and lack of vascular reaction are the usual histologic features. The surgical description is that of an avascular gelatinous mass (Fig. 15-2).

Signs and symptoms of hypothalamic masses depend on the location and extent of the tumor (93) (Fig. 15-3). A tumor may begin in the hypothalamus, invade the optic chiasm anteriorly, or extend inferiorly and posteriorly to invade the interpeduncular fossa and basal cisterns. Depending on location, presenting signs may be hypothalamic or visual. At times, differentiation

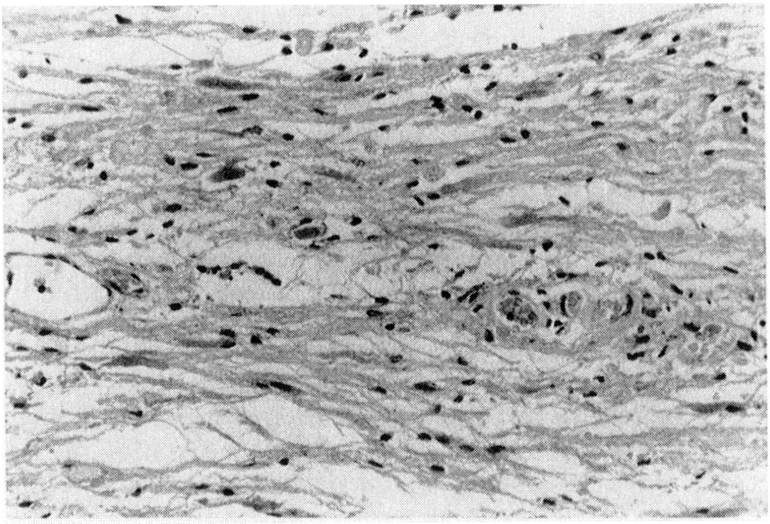

FIG. 15-2. Pilocytic astrocytoma. Many of the tumor cells are spindle-shaped (piloid). Rosenthal fibers are fusiform eosinophilic structures representing masses of astrocytic filaments.

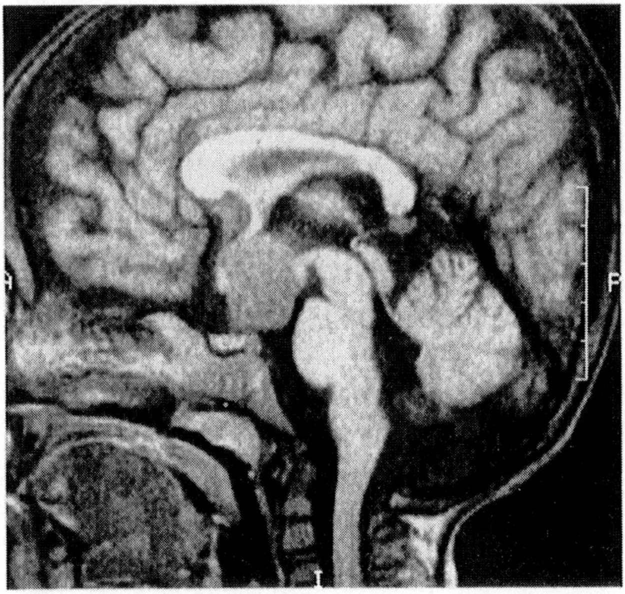

FIG. 15-3. MRI demonstrating large anterior hypothalamic mass in an 18-month-old presenting with a diencephalic syndrome.

prior to surgery from other parasellar masses, such as craniopharyngioma, may be impossible.

CT scan with contrast enhancement may show hydrocephalus with secondary occlusion of the foramen of Monro and obliteration of the interpeduncular cistern. CT features of pilocytic astrocytomas have been characterized as sharply demarcated tumors with smooth borders rarely associated with edema. Cyst formation can be observed, and tumor calcification is occasionally encountered. Calcifications on CT are rarely identified (59). MRI scan is characterized by either hypointense or isointense lesions on T1-weighted images and increased signal on T2-weighted images.

A spectrum of endocrine signs and symptoms characterizes hypothalamic tumors (93). Failure to thrive, emaciation, loss of subcutaneous fat, salt loss, hypoglycemia, and accelerated long bone growth suggest involvement of the anterior hypothalamus (103). Pendular searching nystagmus, with or without visual loss, in a young child with failure to thrive should suggest a tumor in the region of the optic chiasm with posterior extension into the anterior hypothalamus.

Since Russell's paper in 1951 (83), the diencephalic syndrome characterized by failure to thrive and inanition has been associated with astrocytomas of the anterior hypothalamus and optic chiasm (29,52,75,87,100). This syndrome is usually seen in young children between the ages of 18 months and 3.5 years (88). Why this syndrome does not occur in older children has never been adequately explained (39). The children present with a history of normal development followed by a period of profound inanition bordering on cachexia. Hypoglycemia may or may not be present. Anorexia or excessive appetite may be the predominant feature. Long bone growth continues or may even be accelerated. Emaciation with profound losses of subcutaneous tissue is regularly seen (3). Drop et al. (32) have discussed the varying endocrine theories that might account for increased lipolytic activity. These include excessive growth hormone, activation of pituitary peptides that contain lipolytic activity, and the possible presence of a lipid mobilizing factor. Normalization of growth hormone concentration has been reported after irradiation of the tumor (2). As a response to destruction of the preoptic areas, there may be a defective release of somatostatin.

Some authors have suggested that emaciation implies that the mass is limited to a small portion of the anterior hypothalamus. With subsequent tumor growth and extension into other portions of the hypothalamus, cachexia is replaced by obesity, vegetative signs, and delayed puberty. In fact, Bauer (10) has suggested that anorexia is an uncommon result of hypothalamic malfunction. Experimental animal work has shown that destruction of the lateral thalamic nuclei gives rise to cachexia, and destruction of the more midline hypothalamic nuclei is associated with obesity. Clinically, it has been postulated that the counterbalance of destructive lesions in both these areas of the hypothalamus may allow the production of seemingly paradoxical results, i.e., voracious appetite and emaciation (65). Despite a cachectic appearance, the children may maintain a surprising degree of equanimity and friendly behavior bordering on euphoria. Russell attributed the apparent paradoxical euphoria in the face of severe inanition to interruption of the frontothalamic-hypothalamic pathways.

The diencephalic syndrome is unusual and generally seen in children under 3 years of age (52,76) (Fig. 15-4). In a review of 51 neoplasms of the hypothalamus, obesity, diabetes insipidus, and hypogonadism were more common. Lethargy, rather than euphoria, was regularly described. As the tumor extends superiorly into the region of the foramen of Monro, obstructive hydrocephalus may develop as a result of increased intracranial pressure.

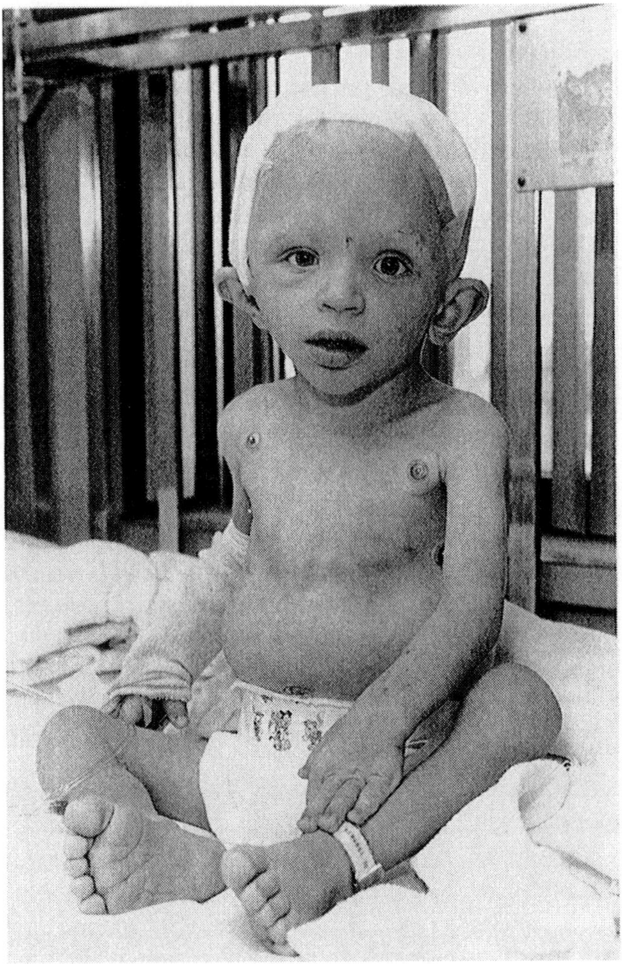

FIG. 15-4. 18-month-old with diencephalic syndrome. Note large head and emaciation.

Like the clinical features of the diencephalic syndrome, the findings of precocious puberty in a toddler can be dramatic and a certain sign of a hypothalamic mass. Hamartomas of the tuber cinereum, astrocytomas, ependymomas, ectopic pinealomas, suprasellar cysts, craniopharyngiomas, postinfectious states, neurofibromatosis, and hydrocephalus have all been associated with precocious puberty (8). Of interest are the comments commonly found in standard texts that the endocrine effects of tumors in this region are mechanical, as tumors of different histology presenting in the interpeduncular fossa and in the region of the tuber cinereum have nonselectively been associated with precocious puberty. There is, however, evidence that hamartomas may act as an accessory hypothalamus. Hochman et al. (45), using immunohistochemical techniques, have described luteinizing hormone releasing factor in at least one tumor and also electron microscopic evidence of neurosecretory tissue. In addition, findings of elevated gonadal steroids and gonadotropins have characterized the endocrinologically active hamartoma. At the time of surgery, hamartomas are generally small and found adherent to brain tissue in the region of the tuber cinereum and posterior hypothalamus. Other than endocrine abnormalities, because of the small size of the mass, neurologic signs may be minimal.

An uncommon location for neoplasms has been at the lateral ventricular wall. Tumors in this area have been variously described as astrocytomas, ependymomas, oligodendrogliomas, subependymomas, neurocytomas, and primitive neuroectodermal tumors. Tumor that arise from the ventricular wall, i.e., the groove and the head of the caudate and the submental plate, are thought to be related to cell rests arising from sites of the primitive germinal matrix. The cell rests are considered to be a source for the potential development of neoplasia along the lateral ventricular wall. Nishio et al. (71) described 19 such patients. Eight were diagnosed as intraventricular neurocytomas, e.g., tumors consisting of a uniform population with central round nuclei and clear eosinophilic cytoplasm. Burger (20) has described these tumors as cellular with nuclear uniformity and a rarity of mitosis. The tumors can resemble neuroblastomas or may have a histologic similarity to oligodendrogliomas. Tumors of this histology are not thought to be malignant. Long survivals and cures following surgery without additional therapy have been the rule. Treatment is dependent on histology rather than location.

Treatment

Prognosis of patients with hypothalamic tumors, unlike those with thalamic tumors, may be quite good. Treatment of hypothalamic tumors traditionally consists of surgical biopsy followed by either chemotherapy or radiotherapy. Some surgeons are now opting for debulking surgery followed by watchful waiting. A POG, CCSG combined protocol is now evaluating the efficacy of this approach. In centers where radiation is recommended, doses between 5,000 and 6,000 cGy have been given with reversal of symptoms and long-term cures. Five-year survival rates of 71% and 10-year survival rates of 56% have been documented (13,14,29). As with other tumors occurring in children under 3 to 5 years of age, radiation has been associated with significant morbidity. Results with chemotherapy have been inconclusive. There have been limited reports in the literature documenting the effectiveness of chemotherapy. A single report in the recent literature (22) suggested a beneficial response to multiagent therapy consisting of thioguanine, procarbazine, dibromoduleitol, CCNU, and vincristine. A pilot study of the Pediatric Oncology Group (35) published in 1992 demonstrating the effectiveness of carboplatin in low-grade tumors forms the basis of a group-wide protocol using this agent in optic pathway tumors in children less than 5 years of age. This report, plus those suggesting the effectiveness of chemotherapy in optic pathway tumors, underscores the rationale for considering chemotherapy in patients presenting with low-grade tumors in this region. More controversial, and not embraced by the North American community, are the reports from Europe using interstitial radiation. Iodine-125 and iridium-192 have been used in tumor volumes ranging between 2.5 and 3.5 cm^3. Survivals depended on the site, size, and histology of the tumor (33).

Because tumors of this region may behave in a benign fashion, the more conservative view endorses debulking surgery followed by observation. Adjuvant treatment is considered only on evidence of progression. A POG-CCSG combined study in the United States is now evaluating the wisdom of this approach. Because the natural history of tumors in this region has not been clarified, the appropriateness of either an aggressive or a conservative approach remains an open question.

TUMORS OF THE OPTIC PATHWAY

Optic gliomas, while not associated with complex endocrine features, are common neuroglial tumors found in the midline (30). These tumors represent approximately 3 to 5% of all childhood intracranial tumors. Because of their location either in the orbit or the cranium, their association with neurofibromatosis, a lack of information pertaining to accurate incidence figures and natural history, and a tendency for these tumors to remain indolent, there has been little consensus regarding how and when to treat neoplasms of this anatomic region. For the most part, tumors of the anterior visual pathway are histologically benign and are generally classified as pilocytic astrocytomas. Anaplastic tumors and glioblastomas are much less common.

Approximately 60 to 80% of optic pathway tumors will involve the optic nerves, chiasm, and tract with and without extension into the anterior third ventricle. The remaining 20 to 40% occur in the prechiasmatic portion of the optic pathway. Location, in part, refers to the anatomy of the visual pathway. The length of the optic nerve to the chiasm varies from 35 to 55 mm. The intraocular length is approximately 1 mm, and the orbital portion varies from 20 to 30 mm. That part of the optic nerve within the canal is 4 to 10 mm in length, and the intracranial portion of the optic nerve is approximately 16 mm. Thus, most tumors can be expected to involve either the intraorbital or intracranial portion of the optic pathway rather than the intraocular or canalicular part of the nerve (26,74).

The association of optic nerve tumors with neurofibromatosis has been recognized for many years. The incidence of optic gliomas in children 2 to 9 years old may be as high as 5 to 21%. Conversely, of children with optic gliomas, approximately 35 to 50% may have neurofibromatosis (48,63,94). Up to 15% of CT scans of children with NF-1 without visual or ocular abnormalities may reveal optic gliomas. Forty percent of children with NF-1 in one study had tumors which involved the chiasm and one or both optic nerves, 30% had isolated intraorbital tumors, and 30% had bilateral tumors. Mean age is 4.3 years with a range from 9 months to 21 years. It is noteworthy that patients with NF-2 may also have optic gliomas. The gene incidence of neurofibromatosis for NF-1 is 1 in 3,500, while that for NF-2 is 1 in 35,000. Because of the high incidence of optic gliomas in children with neurofibromatosis, the criteria for the diagnosis of NF-1 have been extended to include the presence of a bilateral intraorbital optic glioma. Although not confirmed in the literature, there is speculation that patients with optic pathway tumors who have NF are apt to be younger than those without neurofibromatosis. This putatively occurs because screening imaging results as a consequence of either finding cafe au lait spots, a family history of neurofibromatosis, or other manifestations of the syndrome (104). Conversely, patients without evidence of neurofibromatosis are apt to be identified only at the time of visual complaints. These dual observations, i.e, younger age and lack of symptoms, has prompted the observation that children with optic pathway tumors associated with neurofibromatosis are likely to have a more benign course. However, there are many exceptions to this rule.

Some authors have suggested a difference in biological behavior of optic gliomas with or without neurofibromatosis (95). A detailed pathologic report from Columbia University in New York City (94) describes the pathologic differences that may occur in those patients who do and do not have neurofibromatosis. A circumferential perineural growth pattern was described in patients with neurofibromatosis, whereas an expansile interneural growth pattern was correlated with those patients who did not have the syndrome. These observations failed to lead to histopathologic correlations with prognosis. Rather, the authors concluded that the pattern of growth seen in patients with neurofibromatosis more clearly resembled that growth pattern seen in true neoplasms rather than the growth pattern of hamartomas. The appropriateness of treatment, i.e., surgery and radiation versus limited treatment, is in some measure dependent on whether the mass is neoplastic or hamartomatous. Understandably, a hamartoma would be expected to have a better prognosis and be less invasive than a true neoplasm. Unfortunately, this controversy has not been resolved.

Gliomas of the optic pathway can be quite variable in presentation and may be limited to a single nerve, occur bilaterally, invade the optic chiasm anteriorly, or involve the entire chiasm (69). Fusiform enlargement of the nerve may be seen intraorbitally or limited to one side of the chiasm (1,34). The tumor may extend through the optic canal or can be partially intraorbital or partially intracranial. The usual behavior of intraorbital tumors is to remain within the orbit and not extend into the cranium. This appears particularly true for patients with neurofibromatosis (4). However, there are many exceptions to this rule. Intracranial tumors may arise in the optic chiasm, and they may extend anteriorly to involve the intracranial portion of the optic nerve or posteriorly to involve the anterior third ventricle. Conversely, particularly in patients with neurofibromatosis, growth in the orbit may extend intracranially along the optic pathway and even involve the optic radiations. This may not represent true neoplastic spread. High signal intensity on MRI involving the optic tract and geniculate bodies may reflect edema resulting from compression of white tracts by an extrinsic lesion rather than invasion by tumor. Unlike intraorbital tumors, the intracranial optic pathway tumor may involve the anterior hypothalamus and may be associated with obstruction of spinal fluid outflow tracts.

While the differential diagnosis of an intraorbital tumor is limited to an astrocytoma or less likely a meningioma, the differential diagnosis of tumors in the hypothalamic area includes suprasellar germinomas, craniopharyngiomas, gliomas, lymphomas, and histiocytosis X. If the tumor remains chiasmatic, is globular in nature, and does not extend beyond the anatomic confines of the visual axis, it is most likely a glioma of the optic pathway (26).

Signs and Symptoms

Diminished visual acuity is the most common presenting complaint. Because most children are unaware of gradual decrements in visual acuity, these signs may not be present until relatively late in the course of the disease. Decreased vision may be brought to the attention of an unsuspecting parent after a routine school eye evaluation. Irreducible and nonpulsatile proptosis suggests the presence of an intraorbital mass pushing the globe forward. Extraocular palsies are less common. Unlike proptosis, nystagmus suggests chiasmatic involvement (24). This form of nystagmus consists of a combination of constant short arcs and rapid oscillations with scanning or

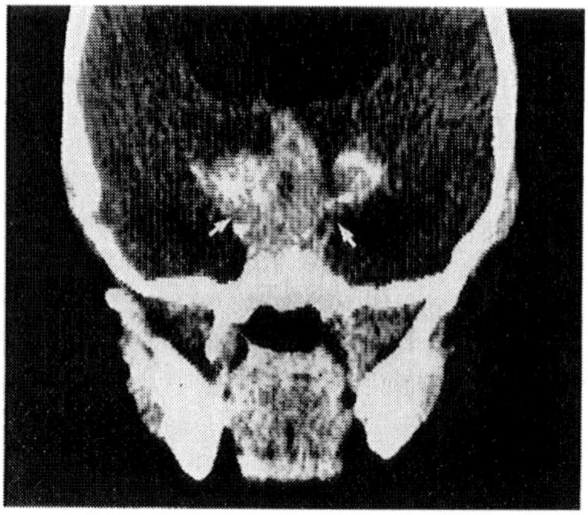

FIG. 15-5. Coronal CT showing a large glioma in an 18-month-old suspected of having congenital nystagmus.

searching, slow, wide arc movements. Spasmus nutans and congenital nystagmus have been incorrectly confused with tumors involving the visual pathway (5) (Fig. 15-5).

As might be expected with an infiltrative lesion, visual field defects are variable and consist of variations of central, central-cecal, and eccentric field cuts. Visual loss limited to one eye suggests unilateral involvement of the optic nerve. Although there are reports of monocular visual loss with chiasmatic tumors, bilateral field cuts (either congruous or incongruous) are more likely to suggest involvement of the optic chiasm or tract (24). Evidence of papilledema and signs of increased intracranial pressure suggest involvement of the anterior hypothalamus with obstruction of the foramen of Monro. Rather than suggesting chiasmatic extension, papillitis with blurring of the disc and loss of central vision suggests an intraorbital tumor.

Increased intracranial pressure results from the backward extension of a chiasmatic mass into the hypothalamus, or the findings of increased pressure with visual loss might imply origin in the hypothalamus with forward extension into the chiasm. To further confuse the clinical picture, the presence of optic atrophy with resultant thinning of the nerves may delay development of papilledema despite other evidence of increased intracranial pressure. As a generalization, the findings of blurred discs with visual loss suggest intraorbital involvement, whereas the finding of papilledema in the presence of visual loss with either a field cut or nystagmus suggests chiasmatic involvement. Sexual precocity in association with chiasmatic gliomas or signs of increased pressure suggests the backward extension of the tumor into the hypothalamus.

The findings in an asymptomatic child, aged 2 to 10 years, of axillary freckling, a large head, and cafe-au-lait spots, should raise the possibility of neurofibromatosis and initiate a search for an unsuspected optic glioma

(84,86). Furthermore, as neurofibromatosis is a dominant gene, the presence of an optic glioma and other stigmata of neurofibromatosis should prompt an investigation of all family members.

Pattern of Growth

Anatomically, the optic nerve is part of the central and not the peripheral system but differs from normal white matter in that it is partitioned by vascularized connective tissue septa derived from the dural sheath. Over 50 years ago, several histologic patterns were described. The first pattern consists of astrocytic or oligodendroglial proliferation. The second consists of a reticular pattern in which microcystic foci are found, containing mucous-like fluid. Spindle-shaped, fibrillated cells arranged in bundles characterize the third pattern. The third presentation is seen when the leptomeninges are invaded. Mitosis is usually not found. GFAP staining confirms the glial nature of the tumor. As in most low-grade tumors, Rosenthal fibers, i.e., degenerated glial processes, are seen in more prominent areas and interface with vascular connective tissue.

Rubinstein and Russell (84) have suggested that optic gliomas are mixed tumors consisting of both pilocytic and stellate astrocytes intermixed with oligodendroglia. This interpretation is compatible with findings in the optic pathway of a glial precursor cell (the O2A cell), which is thought to be capable of differentiating into either astrocytes or oligodendroglial lines. This precursor cell in the optic pathway was initially identified in tissue culture by Raff et al. (78) in 1982. Appropriate perturbations of the culture system with cytokines influenced the cultures to express features of astrocytes with the production of GFAP. Alternatively, the media could be induced to produce oligodendrogliocytes as characterized by monoclonals to galactocerebroside.

Course

For the most part, tumors of the optic pathway are characterized by slow growth and limited threat to life. Characteristically, there may be expansion of the leptomeningeal sheath with extension of the tumor into the subarachnoid space. This is probably a reactive response of the tumor rather than representing true neoplastic extension into the leptomeninges. The leptomeningeal proliferation may falsely give the appearance of enlargement of the nerve on neuroimaging. On the other hand, many papers describe an accelerated course and metastatic spread within the leptomeninges (19).

Many have suggested that tumors of the orbit are hamartomatous in nature; however, the majority view is that they are neoplastic with a well defined proliferative capability. Unfortunately, limited pathologic features can differentiate growth potential of tumors occurring in the intracranial portion of the optic nerve from those that arise in the intraorbital portion of the nerve. Malignant dedifferentiation when it occurs is apt to take the form of an anaplastic astrocytoma or a glioblastoma multiforme. Malignant dedifferentiation, for the most part, occurs in the older child or adult. The report of Bruggers (19) is an exception to this rule.

Alvord's (1) thoughtful analysis of 623 cases of optic gliomas provided actuarial information by which to assess the prognosis of patients with tumors of this region by age, site, treatment, extension into the hypothalamus, and presence of concomitant neurofibromatosis. He developed a mathematical model from which he concluded that low-grade astrocytomas in this area have a wide but continuous range of growth. Because the mitotic index is not high, the histologic, immunologic, and immunocytologic features used to measure proliferation are not helpful. Growth rate may be inferred by measuring the volume of mass at the time of diagnosis and at the point of progression. Alvord indicates there is a spectrum of growth consisting of a small number of tumors that have a rapidly progressive course to the larger, more usual, population that grow slowly and have a prolonged clinical course. As growth does not follow tumor kinetics, he suggests that deceleration in growth occurs at some point during the course of disease. The fact that optic gliomas do not follow cellular kinetics or predictable doubling times is explained by a multitude of factors. These include exfoliation of cells from the original bulk, intravening immunologic mechanisms, or a changing genetic makeup of the tumor, which alters its proliferative capacity. At the time of initial diagnosis, it remains a conundrum for the clinician to predict which tumor will progress and which, with a similar histology and location, will either decelerate in growth or not progress. Alvord was unable to define clearly if there was a difference in prognosis in those patients with intraorbital tumors with and without neurofibromatosis, although he suggests that patients without evidence of neurofibromatosis tend to do better than those with neurofibromatosis. There were no reported differences in prognosis of patients with chiasmatic gliomas.

Diagnostic Studies

Before the advent of CT scanning, roentgenographic evaluation was not carried out until the patient became symptomatic. Orbital roentgenograms of the skull in a patient with an intraorbital tumor demonstrate an enlarged optic foramen. Appropriate films of the optic canal reveal thinning of both anterior clinoids, an enlarged chiasmatic sulcus, flattening of the tuberculum sellae, and blunting of the posterior clinoids. Axial tomography of the canal demonstrates intracanalicular extension of the tumor. A difference of 1 mm between opposing canals or a canal diameter greater than 7 mm should be considered abnormal (34).

Presently, CT and MRI have all but eliminated other diagnostic modalities (77). This methodology allows direct visualization of the optic nerve within the orbit. The total anatomic extent of the tumor can readily be seen with CT. With the advent of high-resolution CT scans, the length and width of the optic nerve can readily be identified. Sections cut oblique to the horizontal and longitudinal axis allow detailed evaluation of the width and course of the nerve. Because optic nerve gliomas in general are isodense, intravenous contrast shows limited enhancement (21,99).

Enlargement of the optic nerve may be seen on CT examination as a result of papilledema (80). Furthermore, change in the size of an optic nerve or tortuosity in its course does not invariably imply an optic nerve tumor (21). To avoid misinterpretation of the findings of a tortuous intraorbital nerve, accurate CT assessment requires that the plane of the section be made parallel to the optic nerve. In the primary position of gaze, the optic nerve is most redundant. This tortuosity allows the freedom of action necessary to permit unrestricted movement of the eye through its range of motion. In order to ensure an artifact-free picture, the CT scan is best obtained with the nerve on stretch, that is, having the eye look straight, and either up or down (85). This approach is often not practical, because young children have difficulty in either cooperating or understanding the necessary directions. Fortunately, the newer scanning equipment eliminates the need for rigid positioning of the eye. As with intraorbital tumors, appropriate interpretation of the chiasmatic anatomy requires a uniform plane of the section. To view the chiasm optimally, 0.15- to 0.5-cm sections parallel and perpendicular to Reid's baseline (the canthomeatal line) are preferable (28).

MRI, unlike CT, allows mutiplanar visualization of the entire optic pathway and provides images in the axial, sagittal, coronal, and, when necessary, oblique planes (Fig. 15-6). Double-intensity tubular thickening suggesting perineural arachnoidal gliomatosis; elongation of the nerve, and kinking of the nerve in mid-orbit all suggest optic gliomas (50). In patients with neurofibromatosis, because of the high incidence of optic pathway tumors, we routinely screen the visual axis at the time of presentation. In patients with neurofibromatosis, MRI may reveal multicentric disease such as heterotopias, aqueductal stenosis, idiopathic macrocephaly, and increased T2-weighted signals on MRI scanning (Fig. 15-7). These features have made the MRI the procedure of choice. Furthermore, there is some suggestion that arachnoid gliomatosis in patients with neurofibromatosis can be recognized by T2-weighted scans. These consist of high signal intensity on T2 imaging within the tumor surrounding a demarcated central linear core of low signal intensity. MRI not only shows involvement of the optic nerve and chiasms but also is able to identify streaking along the visual pathway including the optic tracts, lateral geniculate, and optic radiations (18). It is not clear whether or not streaking along the pathway, specifically in patients with

A 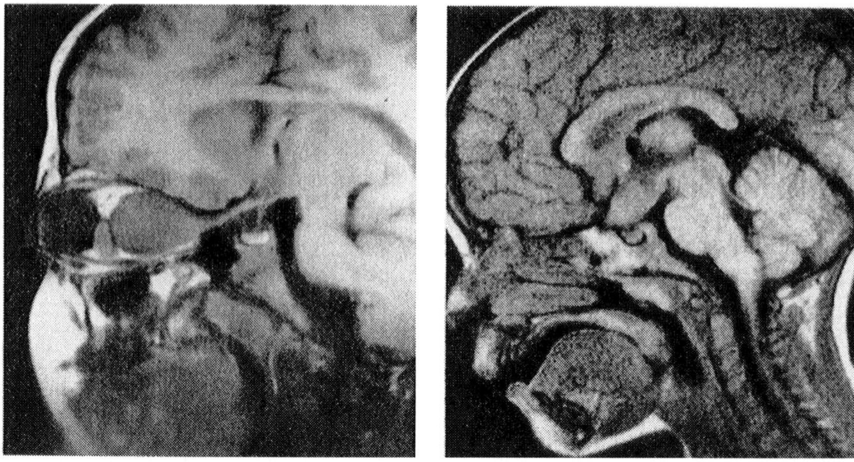 B

FIG. 15-6. A, T1-weighted MRI in sagittal plane showing large intraorbital tumor. **B,** T1-weighted MRI in sagittal plane showing large chiasmatic mass.

neurofibromatosis, represents neoplasm, edema, hamartomas, or some other pathology that may or may not precede the development of neoplasms.

In the asymptomatic patient, CT and MRI have demonstrated an unparalleled ability to identify the anatomy of the optic pathway but have provided little information regarding the functional integrity of the optic nerve. Visual evoked responses (VER) offer the possibility of identifying functional abnor-

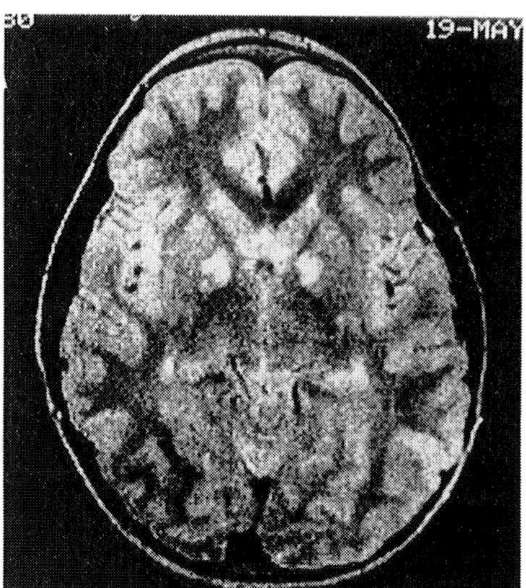

FIG. 15-7. T2-weighted MRI showing bilaterally symmetrical bright objects in the basal ganglia associated with neurofibromatosis. The pathology of these lesions is unknown.

malities in the optic pathway. Treatment remains controversial; therefore knowledge of the natural history of the tumor and its prognosis is increasingly important. Visual evoked responses are more apt to be abnormal in patients with chiasmatic gliomas than in those with tumors more anteriorly placed. We have evaluated several patients with well-defined anatomic abnormalities on neuroimaging with VER (25). Several of these patients were asymptomatic with normal visual acuity, and they were studied because of evidence of neurofibromatosis and neuroimaging evidence of an optic glioma. The criteria for functional involvement of the optic pathway were the finding of a normal electroretinogram (ERG) and either the complete absence of a VER or increased latency of the response (Fig. 15-8).

A VER is a time-locked response to a repetitive visual stimulus, using either a flashing light of known luminance (FVER) or an alternating checkerboard pattern subtending a known visual angle (PVER). These responses generally relate to stimulation of the foveal areas and primarily represent central vision. Latency of the P100 rather than amplitude is a more reliable indicator of visual involvement. Increased latency suggests decreased conduction along the visual pathway, while amplitude, although relating to visual function, is not well standardized. Although visual evoked responses theo-

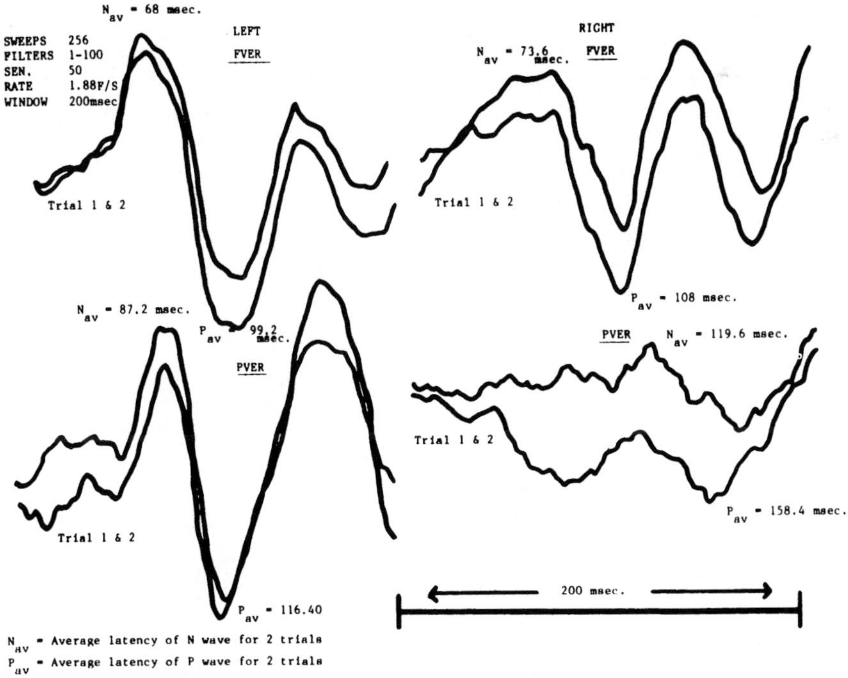

FIG. 15-8. VER in a patient with an intraorbital glioma on the right side. Note presence of the flash response and absence of pattern response.

retically provide reasonable physiologic information, this method has significant limitations when following patients with visual pathway tumors. Patients can unwittingly alter their evoked responses. It is recognized that attention to a task other than visual can cause the amplitude of the VER to decrease and the latency to decrease. Thus, visual evoked responses, although capable of indicating abnormality of the visual axis, are unable to determine the degree, extent, and progression of functional change.

Acuity and field loss remain the gold standard for measuring functional loss. Unfortunately, limitations regarding knowledge of the visual field in the very young reflect the inability to assess the field accurately rather than a lack of physiologic maturation. In nonverbal or illiterate children, the letters X, O, and E are substituted for the numbers on the Snellen chart. A simple hand-held E chart is used in which the child points in the direction of the lines. A behavior technique has been identified by which children are shown a series of 16 cards with varying sides. The child is encouraged to look to the right or left without preference being shown in either visual field. Using a staircase approach, one can then identify the patient's threshold and cycles per centimeter. Techniques using light-emitting diode perimeters and force field choices are being developed that may enable a more quantitative assessment of peripheral fields in the young. All these methods provide a less than satisfactory evaluation of the visual field and are complicated by the lack of knowledge of the size and nature of the visual fields of a young child. It is also important to be able to differentiate the amblyopia that accompanies strabismus from that associated with visual loss secondary to an intraorbital tumor. Color vision is a sensitive indicator of optic nerve function and is not altered by amblyopia. Thus, in those patients in whom the optic nerve is not compromised, but who have visual acuity of 20/200 or 20/400 from amblyopia, hyperopia, or astigmatism, color vision will remain normal.

Treatment

Descriptions of tumors of the optic pathway have existed for over 150 years. Despite the fact that many large series have been reported in the literature, there is no universal approach to treatment (11,42,51,55,64,68,92,108). Therapeutic considerations depend on many factors. Lessell (60) has articulated the quandary involved in arriving at a treatment decision. Those who advocate a laissez-faire approach are hampered by the lack of pathologic proof of a tumor to support their decision. Conversely, those who suggest surgical extirpation prevent the natural history of the tumor from expressing itself. The decision to surgically sacrifice a sighted eye when the tumor has not extended into the chiasm presumes that intraorbital tumors are malignant and if not treated will invariably progress. Pathologically, most of these neoplasms are pilocytic astrocytomas with a slow growth potential.

Compounding the above is the suggestion that those tumors associated with neurofibromatosis, rather than being true gliomas, are really hamartomas. However, the general consensus in the literature is that these are more likely to be neoplasms, rather than representing congenital rest cells.

A review of the literature suggests that approximately half of the patients followed will have a benign protracted course; unfortunately, it is difficult to know which half will behave in this fashion (53,62,79,106,107). There is a subset of patients whose tumor grows rapidly and who have a truncated course.

Robertson (81) has stated that although glial cells can be seen infiltrating neurons, mitosis is quite rare. Microscopic evidence suggests that the true tumor may be limited to a small portion of the nerve and that the bulk of the tumor, rather than consisting of neoplastic elements, may be composed of hyperplastic arachnoid cells (2,27,60,109). Furthermore, spontaneous improvement of vision and proptosis has been reported in the absence of treatment (36,61). For these reasons, controversy regarding treatment continues. To date, there are no long-term assessments of untreated patients with both radiographic evidence of enlargement of the optic nerves and normal visual acuity. Most series differentiate between tumors of the optic nerve and those of the chiasm. Tumors in the region of the chiasm may extend forward in the optic nerve or extend beyond the confines of the visual system into the hypothalamus. Thus, it may be difficult to know whether the tumor originated in the hypothalamus or optic pathway. These considerations usually cannot be resolved without surgical intervention.

Prognosis may be the most favorable in those patients with neurofibromatosis. In a group of patients studied at the Mayo Clinic, survival was better in those patients with chiasmatic gliomas who had neurofibromatosis than in those without neurofibromatosis. The British have had similar experiences (108). This observation has not been universal. Packer (73,83) reviewed his experience at the Children's Hospital of Philadelphia and compared the presence of optic pathway tumors in patients with and without neurofibromatosis. For the most part, those patients with neurofibromatosis had more extensive lesions and their course was more variable. Patients with neurofibromatosis with chiasmatic lesions were diagnosed on the presence of routine visual screening because of the known history of NF. These patients tended to have large lesions that streaked along the optic tract through the anterior visual pathway, and frequently extended into the optic radiations. Patients without NF, on the other hand, were apt to have more globular lesions isolated to the chiasm.

Surgery

Surgery, when considered, consists of either biopsy or excision of the nerve (31,79,87). Complete excision of the nerve should be flush with the optic chiasm. There are several reports in which excision has been associated with failure to remove the tumor extending into the chiasm. For this reason, some surgeons advocate total, rather than partial, amputation. A biopsy, unlike surgical extirpation, offers the advantages of histologic confirmation and the possibility of preserving vision. This approach permits correlation of histology with the choice of treatment and eventual outcome. Because a chiasmatic tumor may be associated with obstructive hydrocephalus, a shunt procedure may be necessary.

Radiation

Radiation is as controversial as surgery in the treatment of intraorbital or chiasmatic tumors (102). Although radiation may preserve vision, complications may be vascular necrosis, cataracts, and endocrinopathies. Some authors (48,76) have suggested that radiation has failed to show a treatment benefit. Others (47,70,76,96,101) unequivocally point to long-term benefits, and thus, confidently extol the virtues of radiation. Furthermore, since in isolated cases pilocytic tumors of the optic pathway undergo malignant transformation, a group of therapists (66,107) recommend radiation treatment at the time of diagnosis. Although low-grade astrocytomas are generally not considered responsive to radiotherapy, as with craniopharyngiomas, high-dose focal radiation may be quite effective. The dose of radiation varies between 4,000 and 6,000 cGy to the tumor bed given over 5 to 7 weeks (9,13,14). Unidentified bright objects seen on T2-weighted MRI scans in patients with neurofibromatosis are not considered neoplastic and should not be radiated. Rather, only those elements contiguous with the tumor should be considered neoplastic and included in the radiation port.

Radiation, unlike surgery, has the advantage of not compromising vision, although visual improvement is rarely seen. Abnormalities of the hypothalamic–pituitary axis are well documented following radiation (16). Proptosis has been known to resolve after radiotherapy. The effects of radiotherapy on chiasmatic lesions are less clear-cut, although long-term cures have been reported. A report published in 1990 (56) suggests 5-, 10-, and 15-year actuarial survivals of 94, 81, and 74%, respectively. Most chiasmatic tumors in patients over 20 years of age have a more malignant course than those in patients under 20 years and are generally found to be less responsive to either radiation or surgery (17,33,41). The prognosis is poorest in those individuals in whom hydrocephalus is present, and in whom the tumor extends into the posterior hypothalamus.

Chemotherapy

Unlike the literature on radiation therapy, the literature on chemotherapy for optic pathway tumors is very scanty (57). Several reports (73,82) examining a cohort of patients from the same center have advocated the use of vincristine and actinomycin. The Pediatric Oncology Group is presently evaluating single-agent, rather than multiple-agent, chemotherapy. This approach was chosen because of the indolent nature of these tumors and their limited threat to life. With this in mind, carboplatinum, a platinum derivative with limited ototoxicity and a good track record in low-grade astrocytomas, is currently undergoing clinical trials by the Pediatric Oncology Group.

SUMMARY

Regardless of whether the patient has neurofibromatosis, treatment, for the most part, is determined by whether the tumor is chiasmatic or intraorbital. Patients who present with intraorbital tumors without chiasmatic involvement may have decreased vision, proptosis, disc edema, optic atrophy, and a high incidence of neurofibromatosis. Patients with chiasmatic tumors tend to have optic disc pallor, decreased vision, nystagmus, strabismus, nausea, vomiting, hydrocephalus, and, possibly, endocrine symptoms. By and large, the prognosis in patients with tumors limited to the optic nerve is better than in those with chiasmatic extension.

Controversy exists as to the nature and extent of treatment (43,49,51, 55,91). Many favor radiotherapy, but morbidity may be quite significant, consisting of intracranial calcification, leukoencephalopathy, moya moya disease, dementia, and endocrinopathies (Chapters 22 and 23). As results of chemotherapy continue to be tentative, patients with chiasmatic extension of the tumor, with or without hydrocephalus or hypothalamic symptoms, should be considered for radiotherapy upon evidence of progression. In those patients under 5 years of age, in order to eliminate the unacceptable morbidity associated with radiation, treatment with chemotherapy may be the most prudent course.

For intraorbital tumors, surgical amputation of the optic nerve at the junction of the nerve and the chiasm is associated with a complete cure. However, this approach has the disadvantage of producing precipitous visual loss. Since the natural history of these tumors is not known, surgery, like radiation and/or chemotherapy, should be undertaken only when there is evidence of clear-cut progression or there is no useful vision.

We believe that continuous assessment of the patient with a suspected intraorbital glioma should include frequent evaluations, including CT or MRI, VER, visual acuity, and visual fields. CT and MRI allow long-term noninvasive evaluation of patients, particularly those with neurofibromatosis. This should allow documentation of progression of the lesion. In selected cases VER may identify abnormalities before the identification of a field defect on perimetry (38). If there is evidence of progression on visual

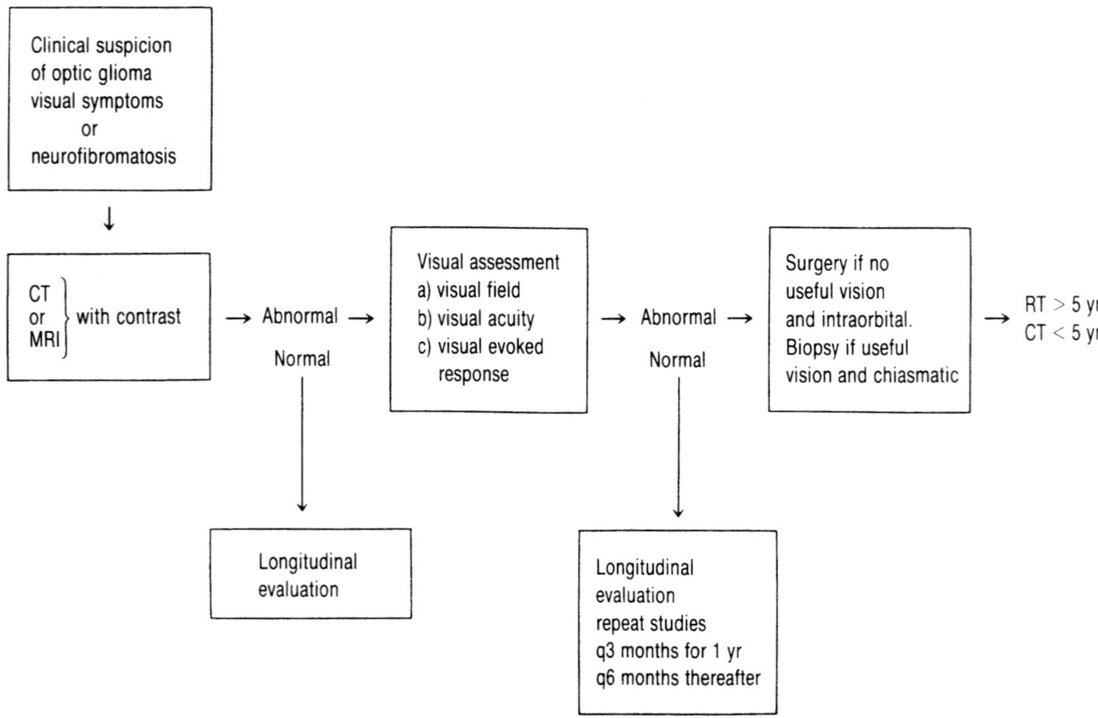

FIG. 15-9. The suggested approach for a child with an optic pathway tumor.

assessment, and the tumor has been shown to extend posteriorly into the optic canal, then we support amputation of the nerve at the junction of the nerve with the chiasm (Fig. 15-9).

REFERENCES

1. Alvord EC, Lofton S. Gliomas of the optic nerve or chiasm. *J Neurosurg* 1988;68:85–98.
2. Anderson DR, Spencer WH. Ultrastructural and histochemical observations of optic nerve gliomas. *Arch Ophthalmol* 1970;83:324–335.
3. Andler W, Stolecke H, Sirang H. Endocrine dysfunction in the diencephalic syndrome of emaciation in infancy. *Helv Paediatr Acta* 1978;33:393–400.
4. Tumor spread in unilateral optic glioma. Study Report No. 2. North America study group for optic glioma. ***Neurofibromatosis 1989;2:195–203.***
5. Antony JH, Ouvrier RA, Wise G. Spasmus nutans: a mistaken identity. *Arch Neurol* 1980; 37:373–375.
6. Arkhangelsky VN. Neoplasms of the optic nerve. *Ophthalmologica* 1966;151[Suppl]: 260–271.
7. Arseni C. Tumors of the basal ganglia: their surgical treatment. *Arch Neurol Psychiatr* 1958;80:18–24.
8. Balagura S, Shulman K, Sobel EH. Precocious puberty of cerebral origin. *Surg Neurol* 1979;11:315–326.
9. Bataini JP, Delanian S, Ponvert D. Chiasmal gliomas: results of irradiation management in 57 patients and review of literature. *Int J Radiat Oncol Biol Phys* 1991;21:615–623.
10. Bauer HG. Endocrine and other clinical manifestations of hypothalamic disease: survey of 60 cases with autopsies. *J Clin Endocrinol Metab* 1954;14:13–31.
11. Benes V, Julisova I, Julis I. Our treatment philosophy of gliomas of the anterior visual pathways. *Childs Nerv Syst* 1990;6:75–78.
12. Bernstein M, Hoffman HJ, Halliday WC, Hendrick EB, Humphreys RP. Thalamic tumors in children. *J Neurosurg* 1984;61:649–656.
13. Bloom HGJ. Recent concepts in the conservative treatment of intracranial tumors in children. *Acta Neurochir* 1979;50:103–116.
14. Bloom HJG. Intracranial tumors: response and resistance to therapeutic endeavors, 1970–1980. *Int J Radiat Oncol Biol Phys* 1982;8:1083–1113.
15. Brand WN, Hoover SV. Optic glioma in children. *Childs Brain* 1979;5:459–466.
16. Brauner R, Malandry F, Rappaport R, et al. Growth and endocrine disorders in optic glioma. *Eur J Pediatr* 1990;149:825–828.
17. Brooks WH, Packer JC, Young AB, Mortara RH. Malignant gliomas of the optic chiasm in adolescents. *Clin Pediatr* 1976;557–561.
18. Brown EW, Ricardi VM, Mawad M, Handel S, Goldman A, Bryan RN. MR imaging of optic pathways in patients with neurofibromatosis. *AJNR* 1987;1031–1036.
19. Bruggers CS, Friedman HS, Phillips PC, et al. Leptomeningeal dissemination of optic pathway gliomas in three children. *Am J Ophthalmol* 1991;111:719–723.
20. Burger PC, Fuller GN. Pathology: trends and pitfalls in histolgoic diagnosis, immunopathology, and application of oncogene research. In: Cohen ME, Duffner PK, eds. *Brain tumors in children, Neurologic Clinics*. Philadelphia: WB Saunders; 1991;9:249–271.
21. Cabanis EA, Salvolini U, Rodallee A, Menichelli F, Pasquini U, Bonnin P. Computed tomography of the optic nerve. II: Size and shape modifications in papilledema. *J Comput Assist Tomogr* 1978;2:150–155.
22. Chamberlain MC, Levin VA. Chemotherapeutic treatment of the diencephalic syndrome. *Cancer* 1989;63:1681–1684.
23. Cheek WR, Taveras JM. Thalamic tumors. *J Neurosurg* 1966;24:505–513.
24. Chutorian AM, Schwarts JF, Evans RA, Carter S. Optic glioma in children. *Neurology* 1964;14:83–95.
25. Cohen ME, Duffner PK. Visual-evoked responses in children with optic gliomas with and without neurofibromatosis. *Child's Brain* 1983;10:99–111.
26. Cohen ME, Duffner PK. Optic pathway tumors. *Neurol Clin* 1991;9:467–477.

27. Cooling RJ, Wright JE. Arachnoid hyperplasia in optic nerve glioma: confusion with orbital meningiomas. *Br J Ophthalmol* 1979;63:596–599.
28. Daniels DL, Haughton VM, William AL, Gager WF, Berns TF. Computed tomography of the optic chiasm. *Radiology* 1980;137:123–127.
29. DeSousa AL, Kaisbeck JE, Mealey J, Fitzgerald J. Diencephalic syndrome and its relation to opticochiasmatic glioma: review of twelve cases. *Neurosurgery* 1979;4:207–209.
30. Dodge AW, Love JG, McCraig W, et al. Gliomas of the optic nerves. *Arch Neurol Psychiatr* 1958;79:607–621.
31. Dosoretz DE, Blitzer PH, Wang CC, Linggood RM. Management of glioma of the optic nerve and/or chiasm: an analysis of 200 cases. *Cancer* 1980;45:1467–1471.
32. Drop SLS, Guyda JG, Colle E. Inappropriate growth hormone release in the diencephalic syndrome of childhood: case report and 4 year endocrinologic follow-up. *Clin Endocrinol* 1980;13:181–187.
33. Etou A, Mundinger F, Mohadjer M, Birg W. Stereotactic interstitial irradiation of diencephalic tumors with iridium 192 and iodine 125: 10 years follow-up and comparison with other treatments. *Childs Nerv Syst* 1989;5:140–143.
34. Fowler PD, Matson DD. Intraorbital glioma: case reports. *J Neurosurg* 1957;14:516–528.
35. Friedman HS, Krischer JP, Burger P, et al. Treatment of children with progressive or recurrent brain tumors with carboplatin or iproplatin; a Pediatric Oncology randomized phase II study. *J Clin Oncol* 1992;10:249–256.
36. Glaser JS, Hoyt WF, Corbett J. Visual morbidity with chiasmal glioma. *Arch Ophthalmol* 1971;85:3–12.
37. Grisby PW, Thomas PR, Schwartz HG, Fineberg BB. Multivariate analysis of prognostic factors in pediatric and adult thalamic and brainstem tumors. *Int J Radiat Oncol Biol Phys* 1989;16:649–655.
38. Halliday AM, Halliday E, Kriss A, McDonald WI, Mushin J. The pattern evoked potential in compression of the anterior visual pathway. *Brain* 1976;99:357–374.
39. Hamilton W. Diencephalic syndrome of infancy and childhood. *Dev Med Child Neurol* 1967;9:497–498.
40. Harper CG, Stewart-Wynne EG. Malignant optic gliomas in adults. *Arch Neurol* 1978;35: 731–735.
41. Harwood-Nash DC. Optic gliomas and pediatric neuroradiology. *Radiol Clin North Am* 1972;10:83–100.
42. Heiskanen O, Raitta C, Torsti R. Management and prognosis of gliomas of the optic pathways in children. *Mod Probl Pediatr* 1977;18:216–219.
43. Heiskanen O, Raitta C, Torsti R. The management and progress of glioma of the optic pathways in children. *Acta Neurochir* 1978;43:193–199.
44. Hirose G, Lomboso CT, Eisenberg H. Thalamic tumors in childhood. *Arch Neurol* 1975; 32:740–744.
45. Hochman HI, Judge DM, Reichlin S. Precocious puberty and hypothalamic hamartoma. *Pediatrics* 1981;67:236–243.
46. Hoffman HJ, Platt J, DeLima B, Soloniuk D, Humphreys RP, Drake JM, Becker L. Management of axial low-grade astrocytomas in childhood. *Int Pediatr* 1991;6:149–152.
47. Horwich A, Bloom HJG. Optic gliomas: radiation therapy and prognosis. *Int J Radiat Oncol Biol Phys* 1985;11:1067–1079.
48. Hoyt WF, Meshel LG, Lessell S, Schatz NJ, Suckling RD. Malignant optic glioma of adulthood. *Brain* 1973;96:121–132.
49. Imes RK, Hoyt WF. Childhood chiasmal gliomas: update on the fate of patients in the 1969 San Francisco study. *Br J Ophthalmol* 1986;70:179–182.
50. Imes RK, Hoyt WF. Magnetic resonance imaging signs of optic nerve gliomas in neurofibromatosis. *Am J Ophthalmol* 1991;111:729–734.
51. Iraci G, Gerosa M, Tomazzoli L, et al. Glioma of the optic nerve and chiasm: a clinical review. *Childs Brain* 1981;8:326–349.
52. Kagan H. Anorexia and severe inanition associated with a tumor involving the hypothalamus. *Arch Dis Child* 1958;33:257–260.
53. Kanter WR, Eldridge R, Fabricant R, Allen JC, Koerber T. Central neurofibromatosis with bilateral acoustic neuroma: genetic, clinical and biochemical distinction from peripheral neurofibromatosis. *Neurology* 1980;30:851–859.

54. Kelly PJ. Stereotactic biopsy and resection of thalamic astrocytomas. *Neurosurgery* 1989; 25:185–195.
55. Klug GL. Gliomas of the optic nerve and chiasm in children. *Aust N Z J Surg* 1977;47: 596–600.
56. Kovalic JJ, Grigsby PW, Shepard MJ, Fineberg BB, Thomas PR. Radiation therapy for gliomas of the optic nerve and chiasm. *Int J Radiat Oncol Biol Phys* 1990;18:927–932.
57. Kretschmar CS, Linggood RM. Chemotherapeutic treatment of extensive optic pathway tumors in infants. *J Neurooncol* 1991;10:263–270.
58. Kwak R, Saso S, Suzuki J. Ipsilateral cerebral atrophy with thalamic tumor of childhood. *J Neurosurg* 1978;48:443–449.
59. Lee Y, Van Tassel P, Bruner JM, Moser RP, Share JC. Juvenile pilocytic astrocytomas: CT and MR characteristics. *AJR* 1989;152:1263–1270.
60. Lessell S. Current concepts in ophthalmology. *N Engl J Med* 1978;299:533–536.
61. Liu GT, Lessell S. Spontaneous visual improvement in chiasmal gliomas. *Am J Ophthalmol* 1992;114:193–201.
62. Lowes M, Bojsen-Moller M, Vorre P, Hedegaard O. An evaluation of gliomas of the anterior visual pathways: a 10-year survey. *Acta Neurochir* 1978;43:201–216.
63. Lund AM, Skooby F. Optic gliomas in children with neurofibromatosis type I. *Eur J Pediatr* 1991;150:835–838.
64. MacCarty CS, Boyd AS, Childs DS. Tumors of the optic nerve and optic chiasm. *J Neurosurg* 1970;33:439–444.
65. Martin JB, Reichlin S, Brown GM. *Clinical neuroendocrinology*. Vol 19. Philadelphia: FA Davis; 1977:171–172.
66. Martuza RL, Kornblith PL, Liszczak TM. Characteristics of human optic gliomas in tissue culture. *J Neurosurg* 1977;46:78–84.
67. McKissock W, Paine JWE. Primary tumors of the thalamus. *Brain* 1958;81:41–63.
68. Miller NR, Iliff WJ, Green WR. Evaluation and management of gliomas of the anterior visual pathways. *Brain* 1974;97:743–754.
69. Mohadjer M, Etou A, Milios E, Baden R, Mundinger F. Chiasmatic optic glioma. *Neurochirurgia* 1991;34:90–93.
70. Montgomery AB, Griffin T, Parker RG, Gerdes AJ. Optic nerve glioma: the role of radiation therapy. *Cancer* 1977;40:2079–2080.
71. Nishio SN, Fujiwara S, Tashima T, Takeshita I, Fujii K, Fukui M. Tumors of the lateral ventricle wall, especially the septum pellucidum: clinical presentation and variations in pathological features. *Neurosurgery* 1990;27:224–230.
72. Ojemann GA, Ward AA. Speech representation in ventrolateral thalamus. *Brain* 1971;94: 669–680.
73. Packer RJ, Sutton LN, Bilaniuk LT, et al. Treatment of chiasmatic/hypothalamic gliomas of childhood with chemotherapy: an update. *Ann Neurol* 1988;23:79–85.
74. Pasztor E, Remenar L. Optic nerve gliomas. I: Clinical diagnosis and pathology. *Acta Neurochir* 1978;41:191–203.
75. Pelc S. The diencephalic syndrome in infants: a review in relation to optic nerve glioma. *Eur Neurol* 1972;7:321–334.
76. Pierce SM, Barnes PD, Loeffler JS, McGinn C, Tarbell NJ. Definitive radiation therapy in the management of symptomatic patients with optic glioma: Survival and long term effects. *Cancer* 1990;65:45–52.
77. Price HI, Danzinger A. The computerized tomographic findings in pediatric orbital tumors. *Clin Radiol* 1979;30:435–440.
78. Raff MC, Miller RH, Nobel M. A glial *progenitor* cell that develops in vitro into an astrocyte or an oligodendrocyte depending on culture medium. *Nature* 1983;303:390.
79. Redfern RM, Scholtz CL. Long term survival with optic nerve glioma. *Surg Neurol* 1980; 14:371–375.
80. Rekate HL, Ruch T, Nulsen FE, Roessmann U, Spence J. Needle biopsy of tumors in the region of the third ventricle. *J Neurosurg* 1981;54:338–341.
81. Robertson AG, Brewin TB. Optic nerve glioma. *Clin Radiol* 1980;31:471–474.
82. Rosenstock JG, Packer RJ, Bilaniuk L, et al. Chiasmatic optic glioma treated with chemotherapy. *J Neurosurg* 1985;63:862–866.
83. Russell A. A diencephalic syndrome of emaciation in infancy and childhood. *Arch Dis Child* 1980;26:274.

84. Rubinstein LJ, Russell DS. *Pathology of tumours of the nervous system*, 5th ed. Baltimore: Williams & Wilkins; 1989:370–376.
85. Salvolini U, Cabanis EA, Rodallec A, Menichell F, Pasquini U, Iba-Zizen MT. Computed tomography of the optic nerve. I: Normal results. *J Comput Assist Tomogr* 1978;2:141–149.
86. Savoiardo M, Harwood-Nash DC, Tadmor R, Scotti G, Musgrave MA. Gliomas of the intracranial anterior optic pathways in children. *Radiology* 1981;138:601–610.
87. Schuster H, Koos WT, Zaunbauer F. Results of microsurgical treatment of gliomas of the optic system and the hypothalamus in children. *Mod Prob Pediatr* 1977;18:211–215.
88. Scott EW, Mickle JP. Pediatric diencephalic gliomas: a review of 18 cases. *Pediatr Neurosci* 1987;13:225–232.
89. Smith KR, Weinburg WA, McAllister WH. Failure to thrive: the diencephalic syndrome of infancy and childhood—a case report. *J Neurosurg* 1965;23:348–351.
90. Smyth GE, Stern K. Tumors of the thalamus: a clinicopathologic study. *Brain* 1938;61: 339–374.
91. Spencer WH. Primary neoplasms of the optic nerve and its sheath: clinical features and current concepts of pathogenic mechanisms. *Trans Am Ophthalmol Soc* 1972;70:490–528.
92. Spoor TC, Kennerdell JS, Martinez AJ, Zorub D. Malignant gliomas of the optic nerve pathways. *Am J Ophthalmol* 1980;89:284–292.
93. Starceski PJ, Lee PA, Albright AL, Migeon CJ. Hypothalamic hamartomas and sexual precocity. *AJDC* 1990;144:225–228.
94. Stern J, DiGiacinto GV, Housepian EM. Neurofibromatosis and optic gliomas: clinical and morphologic correlations. *Neurosurgery* 1979;4:524–528.
95. Stern J, Jakoviec FA, Housepian EM. The architecture of optic nerve gliomas with and without neurofibromatosis. *Arch Ophthalmol* 1980;98:505–511.
96. Taveras J, Mount LA, Wood EH. The value of radiation therapy in the management of glioma of optic nerves and chiasm. *Radiology* 1956;66:518–528.
97. Tovi D, Schisano G, Liljeqvist B. Primary tumors of the region of the thalamus. *J Neurosurg* 1961;18:730–740.
98. Tym R. Piloid gliomas of the anterior optic pathways. *Br J Surg* 1961;49:322–331.
99. Usold R, Newton TH, Hoyt WF. CT examination technique of the optic nerve. *J Comput Assist Tomogr* 1980;5:560–563.
100. van den Berge JG, Blaauw G. Subdural cysts and diencephalic tumor. *Surg Neurol* 1980; 13:267–272.
101. Venes JL, Latack J, Kandt RS. Postoperative regression of opticochiasmatic astrocytoma: a case for expectant therapy. *Neurosurgery* 1984;15:421–423.
102. Weiss L, Sagerman RH, King GA, Chung CT, Dubowy RL. Controversy in the management of optic nerve glioma. *Cancer* 1987;59:1000–1004.
103. White PT, Ross AT. Inanition syndrome in infants with anterior hypothalamic neoplasms. *Neurology* 1963;13:974–981.
104. Whitehouse D. Diagnostic value of the cafe au lait spot in children. *Arch Dis Child* 1966; 41:316–319,
105. Williams D. The thalamus and epilepsy. *Brain* 1965;88:539–556.
106. Wilson WB, Feingod M, Hoyt WF, Nielsen SL. Malignant evolution of childhood chiasmal pilocytic astrocytoma. *Neurology* 1976;26:322–325.
107. Wright JE, McDonald WI, Call NB. Management of optic nerve gliomas. *Br J Ophthalmol* 1980;64:545–552.
108. Wright JE, McNab AA. Optic nerve glioma and the management of optic nerve tumors in the young. *Br J Ophthalmol* 1989;73:967–974.
109. Zimmerman LE. Arachnoid hyperplasia in optic glioma. *Br J Ophthalmol* 1980;64:638–639.

16

Pineal Region Tumors

Tumors arising in the region of the pineal are rare, representing 0.4 to 4.2% of all brain tumors. The variability in incidence is accounted for by the imprecision of the histology, the location of the tumors, and the differing rates of occurrence in Japan as opposed to Western countries including the United States. The incidence of germ-cell tumors and pineal area tumors is substantially higher in Japan than in the West, i.e., 2.6 to 6.5% in several Japanese reports versus 0.4 to 0.7% in the Western series (3,17,24,37,89). A recent survey reported that in Japan germinomas constitute 70 to 84% of all tumors in patients aged 15 to 35 years (58). Assessments of incidence figures are further confounded by the tendency to consider ectopic tumors of the pineal and suprasellar germinomas as misplaced pineal tumors. In addition, some authors (2), when reporting on the statistics of this area, distinguish between parenchymatous tumors of the pineal and teratomas. A widely accepted classification for tumors of the pineal region is that of Rubinstein (68) (Table 16-1). Edwards (22) has suggested that there are over 17 different histologic types that occur in the pineal region. The most common of these are germ-cell tumors. Germ-cell tumors have been divided into three groups: (a) the radiation-sensitive germinoma consisting of primordial germ cells infiltrated by lymphocytes, (b) nongerminoma germ-cell tumors that do not respond to radiation (i.e., embryonal carcinomas, yolk sac or endodermal sinus tumors, choriocarcinomas, and immature malignant teratomas, and (c) mature teratomas (81). Tumors of the pineal parenchyma, such as pineocytomas and pineoblastomas, are much less frequent (91).

The incidence of pineal area tumors peaks in the second half of the second decade of life, and these tumors are more common in boys than girls. Suprasellar germinomas, unlike those occurring in the region of the pineal, are apt to affect the sexes more equally or have a female preponderance (24,89).

PATHOLOGY

Krabbe (47) initially named tumors of this region *pinealomas*, reflecting his observation that the neoplasm represented a fetal pineal body. As the name implies, most of these neoplasms are found in the region of the pineal gland, but many are also recognized in the area of the third ventricle and

---

Brain Tumors in Children: Principles of Diagnosis and Treatment, 2/e, edited by M.E. Cohen and P.K. Duffner, Raven Press, Ltd., New York, 1994.

TABLE 16-1. *Classification of pineal region tumors*

I. Pineal area tumors
  A. Tumors of germ-cell origin
    Germinomas (pinealomas, atypical pineal teratomas, superasellar germinomas, or ectopic pinealomas)
  B. Teratomas
  C. Choriocarcinomas
  D. Embryonal carcinomas or endodermal sinus tumors
II. Tumors of the pineal parenchyma
  A. Pineocytomas
  B. Pineoblastomas
III. Other histologic types
  A. Gangliogliomas and ganglioneuromas, chemodectomas, pineal area cysts, gliomas, and meningiomas

suprasellar regions (93). The occurrence in the pineal area of tumors of varying histologic types reflects the diversity of anatomic sites from which the neoplasm may arise (73). These include the pineal, brain parenchyma, choroid plexus, and tentorial dura. Furthermore, the pineal contains at least two cell types that are capable of neoplastic growth. Midline rests of multipotential germinal cells allow for the occurrence of germinomas, embryonal cell carcinomas, and endodermal sinus carcinomas. The term "ectopic pinealoma" has been used for tumors present in the midline but not in the pineal area. Ectopic pinealomas may be found in the infundibulum, neurohypophysis, or mesencephalon (9). These tumors are either encapsulated or are less well-defined and infiltrative in nature. Ectopic pineals have also been reported outside a midline location in the basal ganglia and thalamus (45,84).

GERMINOMAS

Germinomas represent 50% of all tumors occurring in the pineal area (37). The morphologic similarity of tumors of this region to testicular seminomas was initially reported by Dorothy Russell. She felt that the tumor should more probably be called an atypical teratoma rather than a pineal gland tumor (16,69). Following this observation, Friedman (27) introduced the term "germinoma." This all-inclusive term refers not only to intracranial tumors of the pineal region but also to tumors found outside the central nervous system in the gonads, abdomen, and chest. Intracranial germinomas occurring in the suprasellar and pineal regions are considered as one group because of similar histology and the difficulty that arises in defining the site of origin (68). Those germinomas that occur in the pineal area are more commonly found in boys and are apt to be more radioresponsive than suprasellar germinomas. Tumors growing in the posterior region of the third ventricle may spread anteriorly to involve the cavity of the third ventricle, superiorly to involve the corpus callosum and roof of the third ventricle, and posteriorly to involve the cerebellar vermis or brain stem. At the time of surgery or necropsy, the tumor is rarely small and solely confined to the pineal. It is more likely to be extensive and infiltrating adjacent structures in all directions. Suprasellar germinomas may be multilobulated and encompass the region of the anterior third ventricle, pituitary stalk, or optic chiasm. Clinically, anterior third ventricle germinomas may easily be confused with gliomas or other intrasellar masses.

Microscopically, germinomas consist of two cell types, large vesicular cells and small cells resembling lymphocytes (Fig. 16-1). Transitional features are not seen. Mitosis is confined to the larger cell type. Occasionally, teratomatous features may be identified in mixed-cell tumors consisting of epithelial elements, mucous-secreting cells, cartilage, smooth muscle, and islands of squamous epithelium. The advancing edge of the tumor may be marked by neuroglial and microglial reactions. Granulomatous reactions characterized by multinucleated giant cells and inflammatory elements are similar to the pathology found in testicular and ovarian germinomas. Electron microscopy of the tumor reveals clear chromatin with a rope-like nucleolus and varying amounts of glycogen and annulated lamellae (32). Within the tumor bed, active phagocytosis and invasion of the tumor by T-lymphocytes has been recognized. The absence of a blood–brain barrier in the pineal region allows the bathing of this tumor with blood-borne elements, and presumably the development of an immune reaction.

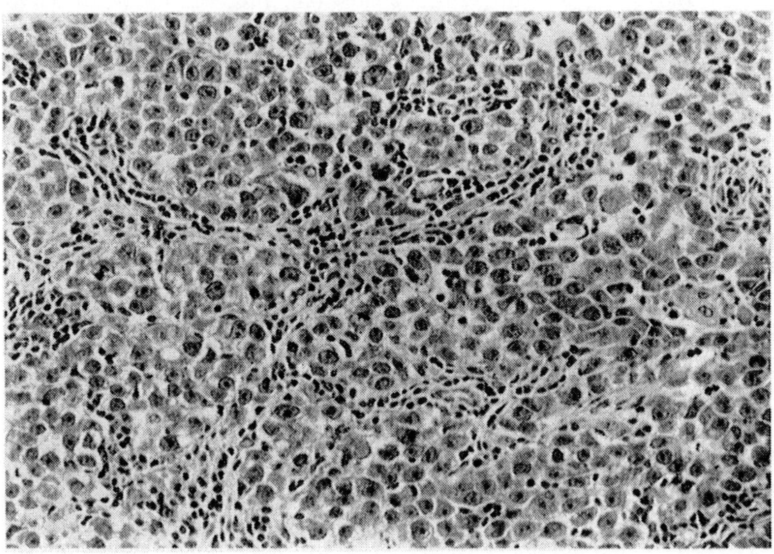

FIG. 16-1. H & E section of a germinoma. The tumor is composed of two populations of cells. The predominant cell is large and somewhat round with abundant cytoplasm. The nucleus is vesicular with a prominent nucleolus. The large cells are arranged in nests or clusters, separated by collections of small dark cells of lymphocytic origin.

NON-GERMINOMA GERM-CELL TUMORS: TERATOMAS, CHORIOCARCINOMAS, EMBRYONAL CARCINOMAS, YOLK SAC TUMORS

The findings of dermoids, teratomas, and epidermoids in the pineal region illustrate the potential of growth from the three primordial germ layers (ectoderm, mesoderm, and endoderm) (9). Teratomatous features without histologic elements of a germinoma characterize the benign teratoma. Grossly, these tumors may be lobulated with multicystic areas. Elements resembling all three germinal layers may be readily recognized on a cut section. The literature supports an uneasy separation of teratoma from germinoma, as both these tumors may have elements of the other. Up to 45 to 50% of recent series have reported mixed germ-cell tumors rather than tumors of a pure cell type (1). Unless the pathology is strictly limited to one cell type, prognosis on the basis of histology does not appear to be warranted (14).

Less common forms of tumors found in this area are choriocarcinomas and embryonal carcinomas. The choriocarcinoma is a highly malignant, rapidly growing tumor that is well known to metastasize extracranially. The embryonal carcinoma and endodermal sinus tumor or yolk sac tumors are rare, more primitive tumors than the germinoma. These tumors resemble those found in the testes and, like the testicular tumor, are highly malignant and invasive. As with choriocarcinomas, metastasis outside the central nervous system is well documented. Because embryonal tumors are rare, the taxonomy of this tumor remains incomplete.

PARENCHYMATOUS TUMORS OF THE PINEAL BODY

As the pineal gland develops from cells lining the roof of the embryonic prosencephalon, parenchymatous tumors may develop along glial or neuronal lines. This accounts for the occasional finding of ependymal glial tumors at this site. The pineal parenchymatous tumors are less common than germinomas and consist primarily of pineoblastomas and pineocytomas (7). These are not associated with cell markers, and there is no sex preference. Pineoblastomas develop in the younger patient and invariably are accompanied by signs of increased intracranial pressure. The tumor is characterized biologically by a short course, rapid growth, and seeding of the spinal fluid. Homer-Wright rosettes, few cytoplasmic processes, and giant cells characterize the histology. Response to radiation may be temporarily favorable. Biologically and histologically, these tumors resemble medulloblastomas, suggesting that the approach to treatment should be similar. Because the differentiation of pineoblastoma from medulloblastoma depends on location and age of presentation, separation of these tumor types may be difficult.

Medulloblastomas arising from the superior aspect of the cerebellar vermis are readily confused with pineoblastomas.

The pineocytomas, unlike pineoblastomas, arise in older children and adults. They are slower growing and occur as well-circumscribed, noninfiltrating masses. These tumors do not seed the cerebrospinal fluid, and in general have a much more protracted course than their more malignant counterpart. Histologically, the tumor is monotonous and monomorphic. Pineocytomatous rosettes characterize the tumor. The central zone of the rosette contains cell processes, whereas more peripheral areas contain the cell perikaryon. Unlike the solitary Homer-Wright rosettes, pineocytomatous rosettes are more confluent. Cell stains suggest a neuronal differentiation (33). Gangliogliomatous elements admixed with the pineocytomatous areas are features of the gangliogliomatous pineocytoma (67). An area suggesting a chemodectoma or paraganglioglioma completes the picture of the neuroectodermal elements that may be seen in association with pineocytomas. The presence of giant cells may be related to the occurrence of giant-cell formation in the normal pineal and therefore may not represent a malignant feature. Differentiating features of parenchymatous pinealomas can be seen in Table 16-2.

With the advent of neuroimaging, pineal cysts have been more readily recognized on routine scans of the head. The pineal cyst is characterized by decreased T1-weighted signal as compared to surrounding tissue and increased signal on T2-weighted images. Cysts can be small or large and may be associated with calcification along the walls. For the most part, patients do not develop signs and symptoms suggesting either involvement of the tectum or aqueductal compression. Other than longitudinal follow-up, no treatment is indicated. In a few cases, compression of the tectum may require surgical intervention. Of interest, although only recently recognized on imaging, cysts of the pineal gland have been reported (85) in 20 to 40% of patients coming to autopsy.

TABLE 16-2. *Characteristics of the parenchymatous pinealomas*

	Pineoblastoma	Pineocytoma
Age	Young	Adult
Tempo of progression	Fast	Slow
Length of illness	Short	Long
Expansion	Infiltration	Compression
Spread in CSF	Common	Rare
Cytoplasmic processes	Few	Many
Type of rosette	Homer-Wright	Pineocytomatous
Giant cells	Present	Present
Histologic variants	Subtle	Conspicuous

Modified from Borit A, Blackwood W, Mair WGP. The separation of pineocytoma from pineoblastoma. *Cancer* 1980;45:1408–1418.

METASTASES

Spinal seeding may occur in 2 to 15% of tumors (48). Seeding is more apt to occur with germinomas and pineoblastomas than with other histologic types. Extracranial metastases are much less common. Extracranial metastases, presumably secondary to hematogenous spread, have resulted in tumors in the lungs, lymph nodes, bone marrow, and pleura. Reports of germinomas metastasizing through a ventricular peritoneal shunt are well documented (31,48,65,94). More commonly, germinomas seed the ventricles and spread throughout the spinal subarachnoid space (52). Local extension and destruction at the base of the brain is well recognized (34).

Exfoliation of malignant cells into the spinal fluid may help aid in the differentiation of malignant from benign behavior and also in establishing the presence of recurrent tumor (44). The cytologic pattern in the cerebral spinal fluid is usually that of undifferentiated, large epithelial cells. The cells have an immature nucleus and a small to average amount of cytoplasm. Seminomatous areas are characterized by cells arranged singly or in groups with a fine chromatin pattern, vesicular nucleus, and finely textured cytoplasm (68,95). In summarizing their and other experiences, Fowler et al. (25) have documented 24 cases of cerebral spinal fluid seeding in 34 patients with germinomas.

CLINICAL PRESENTATION

Clinical presentation is variable and depends on the location of the tumor at the time of diagnosis (74). Signs of increased intracranial pressure and the presence of Parinaud's phenomenon, i.e., failure of upward gaze, lack of convergence, and failure of accommodation, suggest a pineal location. These classic signs refer to a lesion of the dorsal rostral midbrain and reflect compression from above. The syndrome results because the anatomic pathways serving these functions converge at the level of the midbrain. Vertical eye movements are controlled rostrally in the mesencephalon. Diminished pupillary light reflex results from damage to fibers coursing through the pretectal area to cells in the region of the Edinger-Westphal nucleus. Similar pathways cause pupillary constriction associated with accommodation. Thus, it is not surprising that compression of the dorsal midbrain affects pathways that are responsible for vertical gaze, pupillary light reflex, and movements underlying vergence. Visual loss, diabetes insipidus, precocious puberty, and emaciation imply involvement of the anterior hypothalamus either as a result of a tumor originating in this area or secondary to metastasis from the pineal area anteriorly into the third ventricle. Involvement of multiple cranial nerves as well as brain-stem syndromes suggests basilar and brain-stem extension of the tumor. Ataxia is thought to be secondary to involvement of the cerebellar thalamic tracts. Precocious puberty, when found, is almost exclusively seen in males. The true incidence of this phenomenon is probably small, because most of the patients with neoplasms of this region present after the onset of puberty. Conversely, an intracranial tumor may declare itself many years after the development of precocity or at the time of autopsy (90).

Headache, nausea, vomiting, lethargy, dementia, anorexia, secondary amenorrhea, growth failure, hiccups, and photophobia are all nonspecific signs. The nausea and vomiting, weight loss, and hiccups have been identified with tumors of the pineal gland, while growth failure, blurred vision, secondary amenorrhea, and obesity suggest hypothalamic and suprasellar involvement (16,24).

Classically, the suprasellar teratoma presents with a triad of symptoms consisting of visual loss, hypopituitarism, and diabetes insipidus. Involvement of the third ventricle in the area around the hypothalamus produces diabetes insipidus and other pituitary abnormalities. Infiltration of the optic nerves and chiasm can lead to visual defects, and obstruction at the level of the foramen of Monro may lead to hydrocephalus. Endocrinopathies, when seen, consist of growth retardation and either absence of secondary sex characteristics or precocious puberty. Thermal lability, somnolence, and alteration in consciousness suggest involvement of the hypothalamus (1).

Suprasellar germinomas may have a poorer prognosis than pineal region germinomas (40,42). It has been suggested that they metastasize more readily throughout the cerebral spinal fluid, are less responsive to radiotherapy, and have an overall poorer survival rate (9). However, a report by Legido et al. (49) suggests that the outcome in this group of patients may be similar to that in patients with tumors in the pineal region.

DIAGNOSTIC STUDIES

Pineal area tumors, by and large, derive their blood supply from the lateral and medial portions of the posterior choroidal arteries as well as from branches of the posterior cerebral and superior cerebellar arteries (78,86). Because tumors of this region are generally not very vascular, diagnostic angiography is usually not helpful. The diagnostic studies that yield the most information are plain skull films, CT scans with and without contrast, and MRI (17,23,66,83). The size, character, and position of calcification in tumors of the pineal have been characterized by Lin (51). In a series of 321 patients, Zimmerman et al. (97) found no pineal calcification in a group of children under 4 years of age. Calcification was found in 3% of 65 children 5 to 8 years of age, in 12% of 55 children 9 to 12 years of age, in 18.9% of 52 children 13 to 16 years of age, and in 43.3% of 67 children 17 to 20 years of age. Thus, this series, like others (10,52,53), suggests that pineal calcification rarely occurs in patients under 10 years of age.

More than 25 to 70% of patients with pineal area tumors may have evidence of calcification on skull films (10). Of interest, pineal calcification commonly occur in patients with germinoma and hence, when present may suggests a terminoma rather than a teratoma. In addition, teratomas may show evidence of fat, bone, or dental structures. Calcification is commonly seen in pineal parenchymatous tumors (51,88,97). There is some suggestion that calcification is more apt to be seen in patients under 20 with pineal tumors than in those over 20.

CT scans demonstrate the radiologic diversity seen in pineal tumors and suprasellar germinomas. Pineal region tumors present with a spectrum of isodense, noncalcified masses with irregular margins and nonhomogeneous contrast enhancement (17). Infiltration along the walls of the third ventricle suggests malignant behavior. CT scans of germinomas may also reveal tumors of high density that homogeneously enhance after IV contrast. Teratomas, on the other hand, may be heterogeneous and have fat density on CT. Lobulated hyperdense areas with focal calcification as well as multicystic lobulated tumors with patchy contrast enhancement have been described in teratomas (11).

MRI, like CT, readily identifies a tumor in the pineal region. As with CT, histologic diagnoses are difficult to infer by neuroimaging. In patients with germinomas, the lesions tend to be well defined and show homogeneous enhancement. Pineocytomas, on the other hand, tend to have a mixed signal on T1-weighted images, high signal intensity on T2-weighted images, and

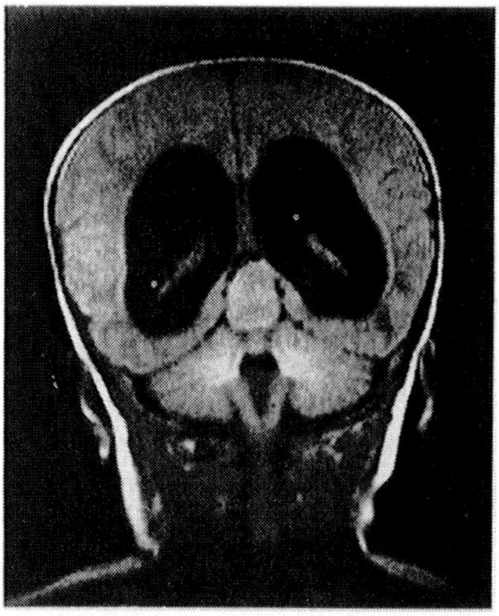

FIG. 16-2. T_1 weighted MRI of a 6-month-old demonstrating obstructive hydrocephalus secondary to a large tumor presenting in the pineal region. Patient subsequently was found to have a pineoblastoma.

variably enhance with gadolinium. Similar features are seen with pineoblastomas. With teratomas, there tends to be either a low signal intensity or isosignal on T1 and high signal on T2. In addition, a fatty component can sometimes be recognized. Gadolinium-enhanced images show cystic lesions with or without signal void suggesting calcium. Hemorrhage is uncommonly seen (6). Thus, MRI is exquisite in defining the location of the tumor and may be superior to CT in delineating subsequent intracranial extension or seeding throughout the cerebrospinal fluid axis. The advent of magnetic resonance angiography should also help define the vasculature of this area. As with all forms of neuroimaging, however, specific histology cannot be predicted with any degree of comfort (76,96) (Fig. 16-2).

TUMOR MARKERS

Oncofetal antigens have proven of limited value as markers used in estimating the presence of germ-cell tumors and in monitoring response to therapy (43,54). Two of these antigens, human chorionic gonadotrophin (HCG) and alpha-fetoprotein, have been of some use in assessing intracranial germinomas (55). HCG is normally synthesized by synctiotrophoblastic cells of the placenta. This marker is found to be abnormally elevated in the serum and spinal fluid of patients with embryonal carcinomas and choriocarcinomas (41). Two subunits have been recognized, alpha and beta. The alpha unit is identical to that found in luteinizing hormone (LH) and follicle-stimulating hormone (FSH). The beta subunit has been found to be elevated in patients with cranial germinomas and endodermal sinus tumors. Antisera to the beta subunit have minimal cross-reactivity with LH or FSH.

Alpha-fetoprotein is normally found in the serum of the fetus. Later in life, tumors arising from yolk-cell derivatives and liver may produce this protein. This marker is found to be elevated in patients with germ-cell tumors, although with less profusion than HCG. Its major use has been in monitoring patients with malignant teratomas (82). The finding of an increased serum alpha-fetoprotein in the presence of an avascular, cystic suprasellar, or pineal region tumor should therefore suggest a malignant teratoma rather than a germinoma.

CSF and serum levels of both the beta subunit of HCG and alpha-fetoprotein have correlated with the presence of intracranial embryonic carcinomas and choriocarcinomas (2). These tumors can produce high levels of these antigens. As with seminomas, HCG may be elevated in patients with intracranial germinomas. In these situations, HCG is only modestly elevated, being usually less than 100 mIU/ml. Levels higher than this suggests the presence of choriocarcinoma. Conversely, the presence of elevated alpha-fetoprotein should suggest the presence of a nongerminomatous tumor such as an endodermal sinus tumor or embryonal choriocarcinoma. Serum levels are usually lower than spinal fluid levels, and when the reverse is found systemic metastasis should be suspected (2,22).

TREATMENT

Surgery

To some extent, treatment of pineal region tumors depends on whether the tumor is of germ-cell origin or not (30,35,57,92). Operative approaches to these neoplasms are associated with high mortality and morbidity rates. Before 1970, operative mortality and morbidity for direct approaches to the area approached 60% (62,63). Operative mortality for subtotal resection and/or biopsy has been reported as high as 33 to 50% (18). Because of this, surgery, in the past, has consisted of shunting around the area of obstruction followed by radiotherapy. Ventricular cisternostomy is the most common diverting procedure for those patients in whom tumor occupies the cavity of the third ventricle. Continued growth of tumor and shunt obstruction may require frequent shunt procedures. Radiation following diversionary procedures carries an 8% morbidity with an average survival of 5 years, whereas in the past a 35 to 50% morbidity with biopsy or surgical removal without shunting could be anticipated (18).

In 1965, Davidoff's (15) comments regarding surgery were the order of the day. Writing in the bulletin of the *New York Academy of Medicine*, he stated:

> The radical surgical treatment of tumors originating in the pineal region, after 50 years more or less of bold, aggressive efforts on the part of several generations of neurosurgeons to extirpate them, is even to this day dismally unsuccessful. What the future may hold, when stereotactic methods are more skillfully used than they are today, is uncertain. I have grave doubts as to their applicability to these or, for that matter, to any other intracranial lesions that infiltrate neighboring brain structures. This would be particularly true in the region of the midbrain, where so many vital brain mechanisms are located. The reason for my skepticism is that destructive agents that can be delivered through a probe, whether it be supercold, superheat, or a radioisotope implant, are totally necrotizing. The margin between the zone of necrosis and the neighboring brain would have to be so exquisitely placed as to destroy all the tumor and yet spare all the surrounding brain. This, I submit, would be extremely difficult if not impossible to do. However, assuming even that it could be accomplished, it would be necessary either to carry the effect of the destructive agent deliberately into the neighboring brain tissues in cases of infiltrating tumors and thus destroy vital brain elements, or leave the infiltrating portions of the tumor behind, thus guaranteeing recurrence.

Direct approaches to the tumors of the pineal are difficult because of the large venous channels present in the area of the pineal. Lack of direct access to the tumor at times prevents surgical biopsy and does not allow debulking.

However, in the last decade the use of the operating microscope has permitted greater surgical access (5,12,36,48). Once adequate hemostatis is obtained and care is taken to avoid compromise of vascular channels, the tumor can be removed either by aspiration or by piecemeal dissection. Over the years, surgical approaches have varied. Poppen and Marino (62) have suggested an occipital-parietal approach, which requires manipulation of the deep venous system overlying and surrounding the tumor. This approach carries with it a high operative mortality. Stein (77,78), using the operative microscope and an infratentorial supracerebellar approach, claims limited surgical morbidity and mortality. The most often quoted series favoring the direct approach is that of Suzuki and Iwabuchi (80). The shortest length of hospital stay in this series was 37 days, and the longest was 5 months. Convulsions commonly occurred postoperatively, and many of their patients were left with significant motor weakness. Long-term follow-up of this series has been limited. Despite increasing advocacy of a direct approach, surgery of tumors of the pineal continues to be associated with a formidable morbidity.

Modern surgical techniques have reduced operative mortalities from 30 to 50% to 5 to 10%. Advances in medical/surgical techniques and improved anesthesia have led to more encouraging results (61). Several authors have pointed out that following the introduction of microsurgical techniques, pineal tumors operated on by either occipital, transtentorial, or suboccipital supracerebellar approaches carry the same degree of mortality and morbidity as that obtained with other intracranial tumors. In 30 patients reports by Edwards et al. (22) there were no operative deaths. He approached the pineal region through a suboccipital craniotomy. Stein (77), using a suboccipital supracerebellar microsurgical approach on 65 patients, had an operative mortality of 2% and a long-term morbidity rate of 2%. Increasingly, because of difficulties inherent in direct operative approaches, stereotactic techniques are being used to establish a diagnosis and treatment plan (20).

On the basis of the above and because treatment of tumors in this area is increasingly defined by histology, it is our opinion that attempts at biopsy or surgical removal should be considered in all patients with a pineal region tumor.

Adjuvant Treatment

The ultimate prognosis of tumors of this region relates to histology and presence of dissemination at the time at diagnosis (13,75). Benign teratomas and dermoids are associated with complete cure following gross total resection. Pure germinomas are more likely to be radiosensitive than the nongerminomatous malignant tumor. Ten-year survival for patients with germinomas receiving radiotherapy ranges from 60 to 80%. Nongerminomatous malignant germ-cell tumors are less radioresponsive and rarely curable with radiation therapy. For these tumors, high-dose collimated radiosurgery delivered to a small focal source has been recommended (19).

Because germinomas are radiosensitive, all contemporary authorities agree that following attempts at total excision, shunting, or biopsy, patients should be radiated (54,57,58,64,65). There is no universal agreement on the dose or volume of radiation, although most authors suggest 5,000 cGy to the tumor bed, 4,000 cGy to the head, and 3500 cGy to the spine (64). Five-year survival rates after radiation may be as high as 50 to 80% (7,13,16,23,39,43, 49,71). A 1978 series (39) of 52 patients irradiated at the Princess Margaret Hospital in Canada showed 5- and 10-year actuarial survival rates of 59 and 55%, respectively. In the 31 patients who did not have biopsy-proven disease, survival was strikingly age-dependent. Crude survival rates for those under 25 were 81%, compared to 37% for older patients. The radiation dose used by this group was 5,000 cGy to the tumor bed given over 5 to 6 weeks. Adjuvant cranial and craniospinal radiation varied between 2,000 and 4,000 cGy. A European report (29) has suggested that the cumulative risk of seeding of the spinal axis in unbiopsied patients with germinomas was approximately 6% following cranial radiotherapy.

Other groups (39,79) have reported a 1.7% incidence of spinal cord seeding in nonbiopsied patients as opposed to a 14% incidence in the biopsied patients. This raises the possibility that surgery may lead to increased spinal metastasis. The figure of 10 to 15% for meningeal seeding has been primarily based on autopsy rather than operative data (15,25,53,72,93). Jenkin reported a 5-year survival and relapse-free survival in 21 patients of 90 and 85%, respectively. Of those patients that did relapse, relapse occurred in the spinal axis and cerebral meninges. The relapsed patients had not received radiation to the spine. He reviewed 118 verified germinomas in the literature, 76% of which had good survivals. Thirty percent had received craniospinal radiation, and 70% had some form of local radiation without spinal cord irradiation. Spinal cord seeding was reported in 18% of the total group. His conclusion (38) after an extensive review of the literature was that uncomplicated patients with germinomas may respond to small-volume, low-dose radiation, and he suggested that this approach may be just as effective as craniospinal irradiation with a high-dose boost to the tumor burden following tumor resection. This hypothesis has not been tested, however.

Despite the above, most large series in the literature advocate high-dose radiation. For instance, the Royal Marsden experience (17) in England, reported in 1991, consisted of 34 histologically verified germinomas; 12 malignant teratomas, of which 4 had elevated spinal fluid AFP titers; and 21 patients with non-germ-cell tumors. As in most other series, the neoplasms were predominantly found in males and occurred in the second decade of life. Although treatment varied a bit over the three decades encompassed by this report, for the most part, patients were given 5,000 cGy to the tumor bed and 3,000 cGy to the craniospinal axis. The 5- and 10-year actuarial survival rates for germinomas were 82 and 70%, respectively. The survival for patients with malignant teratoma, as expected, was much less, with 5- and 10-year survivals of 18%. Those with non-germ-cell tumors had 5- and 10-year survivals of 64 and 47%, respectively. Of the 4 recurrences in the 34 cases with germinomas, 1 relapsed at the primary site and had widespread disease throughout the central nervous system and 2 others had recurrence outside the area of high-dose radiation. As in all other studies, this retrospective study (1962 to 1987) supported the excellent results obtained by radiotherapy for germinomas and the intermediate results obtained with this modality for other forms of pineal region tumors.

Although there has been some controversy over the dose of radiation recommended for germinomas, most authors have favored treating intracranial germinomas with high-dose radiation to 50 Gy. This recommendation has been increasingly supported in the literature, despite the observation that testicular seminoma may be eradicated with much smaller doses in the range of 20 to 35 Gy. Radiation volumes continue to be debated, but the more aggressive approach of radiating the tumor bed and the craniospinal axis is currently favored by most experts. Extensive intracranial disease, multiple foci of tumor, ventricular and meningeal seeding, extensive tumor spillage at surgery, and positive CSF cytology are all adverse risk factors supporting the need for full craniospinal irradiation (1).

Recurrence, when seen, may arise anywhere from 6 months to many years after the initial treatment. There is some suggestion that suprasellar germinomas are more apt to metastasize through the craniospinal subarachnoid space than pineal area germinomas. In the series by Sung et al. (79), 30% of the suprasellar tumors metastasized distally. Recurrence, when present, is likely to be in the spinal cord. This observation has in effect strengthened the argument for whole neuraxis radiation at the time of diagnosis.

Like radiation, adjuvant chemotherapy for pineal region germinomas is in a constant state of reexamination (70). For instance, the observation that chemotherapy may be effective treatment in extracranial germinomas raises the possibility of similar effects in CNS germinoma. Allen (1) has treated 11 patients with germinomas with two courses of cyclophosphamide prior to radiotherapy. Because there was no measurable disease in 10 following chemotherapy, radiotherapy was reduced by 33%. Nine of these 10 have remained in continuous remission for a median of 6 years posttreatment. Two patients died, one from recurrence outside the radiation field and another from a myelopathy secondary to an intramedullary hemorrhage. Another patient developed acute lymphoblastic leukemia, which was reported in remission. Okuno et al. (59) have reported encouraging results with cisplatin and VP16 in a patient with a germinoma refractory to radiation with extensive neuroaxis dissemination. Out of a total of 67 patients identified by the Royal Marsden Group between 1962 and 1987, 8 received chemotherapy, 6 of whom received platinum-based therapy. Most recurred following early responses (17). These results have supported the concept that adjuvant chemotherapy has the potential of reducing the dose of radiotherapy.

Unlike germinomas, which are highly chemosensitive and radiosensitive, nongerminomatous germ-cell tumors have an extremely poor response rate to conventional therapy. Although initial response to either radiotherapy or chemotherapy may be high, most cases relapse, and death within 1 year is the rule. Five-year survivals are exceptional. As with germinomas, chemotherapy has been platinum-based and has been included in protocols consisting of vincristine, VP16, bleomycin, and ifosfamide (2,33,46). Recently, Allen (1) has recommended neoadjuvant sandwich therapy consisting of 4 monthly cycles of platinum and VP16 followed by high-dose radiation to the primary tumor and 3,600 cGy to the craniospinal axis. Following completion of radiation, chemotherapy consists of vincristine, bleomycin, VP16, and carboplatinum. Carboplatinum replaces the cis-platinum in the induction therapy because of the concerns over ototoxicity. His preliminary report suggests objective responses in all patients studied. Others have used high-dose chemotherapy followed by autologous bone marrow rescue.

SUMMARY

In conclusion, the approach to pineal region tumors continues to be variable and depends, in large measure, on histology. Those with the best prognosis are patients with benign teratomas, dermoids, cysts, or pineocytomas, all of which can be operably cured. Because of their marked chemosensitivity and radiosensitivity, pure germinomas are associated with an 80% survival rate. Nongerminomatous tumors, i.e., choriocarcinomas, embryonal carcinomas, endodermal sinus tumors, and pineoblastomas, for the most part, are neither radiosensitive nor chemosensitive, and thus have a poor prognosis.

In the past, interpretation of radiotherapy data has been complicated by the absence of pathologic verification, and treatment has been decided on the basis of neuroimaging data. As ability to approach this area surgically has improved, many surgeons are now opting for debulking with cytoreduction in an effort to establish pathology and increase the effect of adjuvant therapy. Cytoreductive surgery has been facilitated by the operating microscope, cavitron, improved anesthesia, stereotactic approaches, and modern postoperative care. In germinomas, which are readily curable by radiotherapy, surgery has a limited role. For malignant teratomas, pineoblastomas, and the embryonal tumors, debulking surgery may enhance quality of survival if not prolong survival. Staging should include preoperative and postoperative MRIs with contrast evaluation of the entire spinal axis. Markers should be sought to help establish the presence of mixed-cell or nongerminomatous germ-cell tumors. The dose of radiation remains controversial, as does the recommended volume of radiation. Some authors have suggested local radiation will suffice for those tumors limited to the pineal region. For those tumors found in the suprasellar region, invading the ventricle, or associated with endocrinopathies or spinal fluid dissemination, whole brain and spinal radiation should be considered.

REFERENCES

1. Allen J, Kim J, Packer R. Neoadjuvant chemotherapy for newly diagnosed germ cell tumors of the central nervous system. *J Neurosurg* 1987;69:65–70.
2. Allen JC, Nisselbaum J, Epstein F, Rosen G, Schwartz MK. Alpha-fetoprotein and human chorionic gonadotropin determination in cerebrospinal fluid. *J Neurosurg* 1979;51:368–374.
3. Araki C, Matsumoto S. Statistical re-evaluation of pinealoma and related tumors in Japan. *J Neurosurg* 1969;320:146–149.
4. Arita N, Ushio Y, Abekura M, Koshino K, Hayakawa T. Embryonal carcinoma with teratomatous elements in the region of the pineal gland. *Surg Neurol* 1978;9:198–202.
5. Backlund E, Rahn T, Sarby B. Treatment of pinealomas by sterotaxic radiation surgery. *Acta Radiol* 1974;13:368–376.
6. Barkovich AJ, Edward MS. MR imaging of pineal tumors. *AJR* 1990;155:143–151.
7. Borit A, Blackwood W, Mair WGP. The separation of pineocytoma from pineoblastoma. *Cancer* 1980;45:1408–1418.
8. Bradfield JS, Perez CA. Pineal tumors and ectopic pinealomas. *Radiology* 1972;103: 399–406.
9. Camins MB, Mount LA. Primary suprasellar atypical teratoma. *Brain* 1974;97:447–456.
10. Chang CG, Kageyama N, Kobayashi T, Yoshida J, Negoro M. Pineal tumors: clinical diagnosis with special emphasis on the significance of pineal calcification. *Neurosurgery* 1981;8:656–668.
11. Chang T, Teng MMH, Guo WY, Sheng WC. CT of pineal tumors and intracranial germ cell tumors. *AJNR* 1989;10:1039–1044.
12. Chapman PH, Linggood RM. The management of pineal area tumors: a recent reappraisal. *Cancer* 1980;46:1253–1257.
13. Cummins FM, Taveras JM, Schlesinger EB. Treatment of gliomas of the third ventricle and pinealomas, with special references to the value of radiotherapy. *Neurology* 1960;10: 1031–1036.
14. Dattoli MJ, Newall J. Radiation therapy for intracranial germinoma: the case for limited volume treatment. *Am J Radiat Oncol Biol Phys* 1990;19:429–433.
15. Davidoff LM. Some considerations in the therapy of pineal tumors, Rudolf Virchow Lecture. *Bull NY Acad Med* 1967;43:537–561.
16. Dayan AD, Marshall AHE, Miner AA, Pick FJ, Rankin NE. Atypical teratomas of the pineal and hypothalamus. *J Pathol Bacteriol* 1966;92:1–28.
17. Dearnaley DP, A'Hern RP, Whittaker S, Bloom HJG. Pineal and CNS germ cell tumors: Royal Marsden Hospital experience 1962–1987. *Int J Radiat Oncol Biol Phys* 1990;18: 773–788.
18. DeGirolami U, Schmidek H. Clinicopathological study of 53 tumors of the pineal region. *J Neurosurg* 1973;39:455–462.
19. Dempsey PK, Kondziolka D, Lunsford LD. Stereotactic diagnosis and treatment of pineal region tumors and vascular malformations. *Acta Neurochir (Wien)* 1992;116:14–22.
20. Dempsey PK, Lunsford LD. Stereotactic radiosurgery for pineal region tumors. *Neurosurg Clin North Am* 1992;3(1):245–253.
21. Dupont MG, Gerard JM, Flament-Durand J, Baleriaux-Waha D, Mortelmans LL. Pathognomonic aspect of germinoma on CT scan. *Neuroradiology* 1977;14:209–211.
22. Edwards MSB, Hudgins RJ, Wilson CB, Levin VA, Wara WM. Pineal region tumors in children. *J Neurosurg* 1988;68:689–697.

23. El-Mahdi AM, Philips E, Lott S. The role of radiation therapy in pinealoma. *Radiology* 1972;103:407–412.
24. Farwell JR, Flannery JT. Pinealomas and germinomas in children. *J Neurooncol* 1989;7: 13–19.
25. Fowler FD, Alexander E Jr, Davis CH. Pinealoma with metastases in the central nervous system: a rationale of treatment. *J Neurosurg* 1956;13:271–288.
26. Friedman HS, Schold SC, Mahaley MS, et al. Phase II treatment of medulloblastoma and pineoblastoma with melphalan: clinical therapy based on experimental models of human medulloblastoma. *J Clin Oncol* 1989;7:904–911.
27. Friedman NB. Germinoma of pineal: its identity with germinoma (seminoma) of the testis. *Cancer Res* 1947;7:363–368.
28. Futrell NN, Osborn AG, Cheson BD. Pineal region tumors: computed tomographic-pathologic spectrum. *Am J Radiol* 1981;137:951–956.
29. Glanzmann C, Seelentag W. Radiotherapy for tumours of the pineal region and suprasellar germinomas. *Radiother Oncol* 1989;16:31–40.
30. Glasauer FE. An operative approach to pineal tumors. *Acta Neurochir* 1970;22:177–180.
31. Haimovic IC, Sharer L, Hyman R, Beresford HR. Metastasis of intracranial germinoma through a ventriculo-peritoneal shunt. *Cancer* 1981;48:1033–1036.
32. Hassoun J, Gambarelli D, Pellissier JF, Henin D, Toga M. Germinomas of the brain: light and electron microscopic study—a report of seven cases. *Acta Neuropathol* 1981;7: 105–108.
33. Herrick MK, Rubinstein LJ. The cytological differentiating potential of pineal parenchymal neoplasms (true pinealomas). *Brain* 1979;102:289–320.
34. Hertle RW, Robb RM. Pinealoblastoma metastatic to the optic nerve. *J Clin Neurol Ophthalmol* 1990;10:95–99.
35. Horrax G. Treatment of tumors of the pineal body: experience in a series of 22 cases. *Arch Neurol Psychiatr* 1950;64:227–242.
36. Jamieson KG. Excision of pineal tumors. *J Neurosurg* 1971;35:550–553.
37. Jellinger K. Primary intracranial germ cell tumors. *Acta Neuropathol* 1973;25:291–306.
38. Jenkin D, Berry M, Chan H, et al. Pineal region germinomas in childhood: treatment considerations. *Int J Radiat Oncol Biol Phys* 1989;18:541–545.
39. Jenkin RD, Simpson WJ, Keen CW. Pineal and suprasellar germinomas. *J Neurosurg* 1978; 48:99–107.
40. Jereb B, Zupancic N, Petric J. Intracranial germinomas: report of seven cases. *Pediatr Hematol Oncol* 1990;7:183–188.
41. Jordan RM, Kendall JW, McClung M, Kammer H. Concentration of human chorionic gonadotropin in the cerebrospinal fluid of patients with germinal cell hypothalamic tumors. *Pediatrics* 1980;65:121–124.
42. Kersh CR, Constable WC, Eisert DR, et al. Primary central nervous system germ cell tumors. *Cancer* 1988;2148–2152.
43. Klee GC, Go VLW. Serum tumor markers. *Mayo Clin Proc* 1982;57:129–132.
44. Kline T. Cytological examination of cerebrospinal fluid. *Cancer* 1962;15:591–597.
45. Kobayashi T, Kageyama N, Yoshihisa K, Yoshida J, Shibuya N, Okamura K. Unilateral germinomas involving the basal ganglia and thalamus. *J Neurosurg* 1981;55:55–62.
46. Kobayashi T, Yoshida J, Ishiyama J, Noda S, Kito A, Kida Y. Combination chemotherapy with cisplatin and etoposide for malignant intracranial germ-cell tumors. *J Neurosurg* 1989; 70:676–681.
47. Krabbe KH. The pineal gland, especially in relation to the problem on its supposed significance in sexual development. *Endocrinology* 1923;7:379–414.
48. Kun LE, Tang TT, Sty JR, Camitta BM. Primary cerebral germinoma and ventriculo-peritoneal shunt metastasis. *Cancer* 1981;48:213–216.
49. Legido A, Packer RJ, Sutton LN, et al. Suprasellar germinomas in childhood. *Cancer* 1989; 63:340–344.
50. Lewis I, Baxter DW, Stratford JG. Atypical teratomas of the pineal. *Can Med Assoc J* 1963;89:103–110.
51. Lin SR, Crane MD, Lin ZS, et al. Characteristics of calcification in tumors of the pineal gland. *Radiology* 1978;126:721–726.
52. Macpherson P, Matheson MS. Comparison of calcification of pineal, habenular commis-

sure, and choroid plexus on plain films and computed tomography. *Neuroradiology* 1979; 18:67–72.
53. Mincer F, Meltzer J, Botstein C. Pinealoma: a report of twelve irradiation cases. *Cancer* 1976;37:2713–2718.
54. Molenaar WM, Jansson DS, Gould VE. Molecular markers of primitive neuroectodermal tumors and other pediatric central nervous system tumors. *Lab Invest* 1989;61:635–643.
55. Neuwelt EA, Glasberg M, Frenkel E, Clark WK. Malignant pineal region tumors. *J Neurosurg* 1979;51:597–607.
56. Nichols C, Tricot G, Williams S, et al. Dose-intensive chemotherapy in refractory germ cell cancer: a phase I/II trial of high-dose carboplatin and etoposide with autologous bone marrow transplantation. *J Clin Oncol* 1989;7(7):932–939.
57. Obrador S, Soto M, Gutierrez-Diaz JA. Surgical management of tumours of the pineal region. *Acta Neurochir* 1976;34:159–171.
58. Oi S, Matsumoto S. Controversy pertaining to therapeutic modalities for tumors of the pineal region: a worldwide survey of different patient populations. *Childs Nerv Syst* 1992; 8(6):332–336.
59. Okuno S, Ishikawa J, Nozak K, Yamamoto K. Recurrent intracranial germinoma refractory to conventional irradiation: effective chemotherapy consisting of cisplatin and etoposide—case report. *Neurol Med Chir (Tokyo)* 1992;32:351–355.
60. Onoyama Y, Ono K, Nakajima T, Masahiro H, Mitsuyuki A. Radiation therapy of pineal tumors. *Radiology* 1979;130:757–760.
61. Pluchino F, Broggi G, Fornari M, Franzini CI, Solero CL, Allegranza A. Surgical approach to pineal tumors. *Acta Neurochir* 1989;96:26–31.
62. Poppen JL, Marino R Jr. Pinealomas and tumors of the posterior portion of the third ventricle. *J Neurosurg* 1968;28:357–364.
63. Rand RW, Lemmen LJ. Tumors of the posterior portion of the third ventricle. *J Neurosurg* 1953;10:1–18.
64. Rao YTR, Medini E, Haselow RE, Jones TK, Levitt SH. Pineal and ectopic pineal tumors: the role of radiation therapy. *Cancer* 1981;48:708–713.
65. Rosenfeld JV, Murphy MA, Chow CW. Implantation metastasis of pineoblastoma after stereotactic biopsy. *J Neurosurg* 1990;287–290.
66. Rubin P, Kramer S. Ectopic pinealoma: a radiocurable neuroendocrinologic entity. *Radiology* 1965;85:512–523.
67. Rubinstein LJ, Okazaki H. Gangliogliomatous differentiation in a pineocytoma. *J Pathol* 1970;102:27–32.
68. Rubinstein LJ. Tumors of the central nervous system. In: *Atlas of tumor pathology*. Washington, DC: Armed Forces Institute of Pathology; 1972:268–284.
69. Russell DS. The pinealoma: Its relationship to teratoma. *J Pathol Bacteriol* 1944;56: 145–150.
70. Sakoda K, Uozumi T, Kawamoto K. Responses of pineocytoma to radiation therapy and chemotherapy. *Neurol Med Chir (Tokyo)* 1989;29:825–829.
71. Sano K. Diagnosis and treatment of tumours in the pineal region. *Acta Neurochir* 1976;34: 153–157.
72. Sano K. Pinealoma in children. *Childs Brain* 1976;2:67–72.
73. Schmidbauer M, Budka H, Pilz P. Neuroepithelial and ectomesenchymal differentiation in a primitive pineal tumor ("pineal anlage tumor"). *Clin Neuropathol* 1989;8:610.
74. Scully RE, Mark EJ, McNeely BU. Case records of the Massachusetts General Hospital. *NEJM* 1981;9:542–549.
75. Sheline GE. Radiation therapy of tumors of the central nervous system in childhood. *Cancer* 1975;35:957–964.
76. Sprung C, Baerwald R, Henkes H, Schorner W. A comparative study of CT and MRI in midline tumors of childhood and adolescence. *Childs Nerv Syst* 1989;5:102–106.
77. Stein BM. The infratentorial supra-cerebellar approach to pineal lesions. *J Neurosurg* 1971; 35:197–202.
78. Stein BM. Surgical treatment of pineal tumors. *Clin Neurosurg* 1979;26:490–510.
79. Sung DK, Harisiadis L, Chang CH. Midline pineal tumors and suprasellar germinomas: highly curable by irradiation. *Radiology* 1978;745–751.
80. Suzuki J, Iwabuchi T. Surgical removal of pineal tumors (pinealomas and teratomas): experience in a series of 19 cases. *J Neurosurg* 1965;23:565–571.

81. Takei Y, Pearl GS. Ultrastructural study of intracranial yolk sac tumor. *Cancer* 1981;48: 2038–2046.
82. Takeuchi J, Handa H, Oda Y, Uchida Y. Alpha-fetoprotein in intracranial malignant teratoma. *Surg Neurol* 1979;12:400–404.
83. Takeuchi J, Handa H, Otsuka S, Takebe Y. Neuroradiological aspects of suprasellar germinoma. *Neuroradiology* 1979;17:153–159.
84. Tamaki N, Lin T, Shirataki K, et al. Germ cell tumors of the thalamus and the basal ganglia. *Childs Nerv Syst* 1990;6:3–7.
85. Tamaki N, Shirataki K, Lin T, Masumura M, Katayama S, Matsumoto S. Cysts of the pineal gland. *Childs Nerv Syst* 1989;5:172–176.
86. Tien RD, Barkovich AJ, Edwards MSB. MR imaging of pineal tumors. *AJNR* 1990;155: 143–151.
87. Tod PA, Porter AJ, Jamieson KG. Pineal tumors. *AJR* 1974;120:19–26.
88. Tucker WG, Leong ASY, McCulloch GAJ. Tumors of the pineal region: neuroradiologic aspects. *Australas Radiol* 1977;21:313–324.
89. Ueki K, Tanaka R. Treatments and prognosis of pineal tumors: experience of 110 cases. *Neurol Med Chir (Tokyo)* 1980;20:1–26.
90. van der Werff ten Bosh JJ. Isosexual precocity. In: Gardner LI, ed. *Endocrine and genetics diseases of childhood*. 2nd ed. Philadelphia: WB Saunders; 1969:616–639.
91. Vaquero J, Coca S, Martinez R, Escandon J. Papillary pineocytoma. *J Neurosurg* 1990; 73:135–137.
92. Vaquero J, Ramiro J, Martinez R, Coca S, Bravo G. Clinicopathological experience with pineocytomas: report of five surgically treated cases. *Neurosurgery* 1990;4:612–619.
93. Wara W, Jenkin RDT, Evans A, et al. Tumors of the pineal and suprasellar region: Children's Cancer Study Group treatment results 1960–1975. *Cancer* 1979;43:698–701.
94. Wood BP, Haller JO, Berdon WE, Lin SR. Shunt metastases of pineal tumors presenting as a pelvic mass. *Pediatr Radiol* 1979;8:108–109.
95. Zaharopoulos P, Wong JY. Cytology of common primary midline brain tumors. *Acta Cytol* 1980;24:384–390.
96. Zee C, Segall H, Apuzzo M, et al. MR imaging of pineal region neoplasms. *J Comput Assist Tomogr* 1991;15:56–61.
97. Zimmerman RA, Bilaniuk LT, Wood JH, Bruce DA, Schut L. Computed tomography of pineal, parapineal, and histologically related tumors. *Radiology* 1980;137:669–677.

17

Meningiomas

Meningiomas, although common in adults, are relatively rare in children. The reported incidence of primary tumors of the meninges in adults may be as high as 10 to 20% of all tumors, while that in children is something less than 2% (7,9,11,13,35,47). Most reported series in children are quite small, although there are notable exceptions (18). The literature, by and large, consists of a collation of reports from different institutions or an analysis of meningiomas over several decades in one institution. Meningiomas have no age predilection and have been described in infancy through senescence, with a tendency to increase with increasing age. The majority in children are found between 5 and 14 years of age (Table 17-1). In most series, there is a greater incidence in females than males (42). Before the age of 16, there is a slight preference for males, with a distinct male preponderance in infancy (46). As with adults, location is quite variable. The tumor has been found on the convexity of the brain, arising from the tentorium at the base of the brain, and in the lateral ventricles. A higher incidence of cyst formation, location in the lateral ventricle with absence of dural attachment, or origin in the posterior fossa characterizes the meningioma found in childhood (15,26, 41,48). The third ventricle is the least common ventricular location (43). The tumor is thought to originate from either the choroid plexus, velum interpositum, or tela choroidea. Some investigators suggest that there is a high incidence of sarcomatous meningiomas in childhood, with the proportion of cases being as high as 38% (14). Although these tumors have the shortest course, for the most part, pathologic type has not correlated well with prognosis. Long survival with good quality of life regardless of pathology has been reported.

PATHOLOGY

Grossly, meningiomas are large, globular, or multilobular tumors, or may be found growing en plaque in a "carpet-like" fashion. At surgery, the tumor is found either to be gray or red in appearance depending on its vascularity (28). Unlike tumors of glial origin, the meningioma is rarely infiltrative. The cut surface may be hard and gritty. Foci of calcification or even bone may be encountered. Multiple meningiomas have been associated with NF-2 and

Brain Tumors in Children: Principles of Diagnosis and Treatment, 2/e, edited by M.E. Cohen and P.K. Duffner, Raven Press, Ltd., New York, 1994.

TABLE 17-1. *Age distribution, rank order*

Age	
10–14	(~40–50% in most series)
5–9	(~30% in most series)
15–20	(~20% in most series)
1–4	(~10% in most series)
0–1	(rare in all series)

have been considered part of the oncogenic complications associated with this disease (17). Since Cushing and Eisenhardt's classical monograph (13) on meningiomas in 1938, trauma has been considered a possible etiology in the causation of these tumors. They suggested that a history of trauma is more likely to be found in meningiomas of children than those found in adults. Approximately 33% of 295 cases were found to have evidence of prior trauma, 24 of which were found to have a cicatrix or evidence of a fracture at the site of the tumor. In the Cavendish lecture of 1922, Cushing discussed the relationship of meningiomas to trauma. In discussing 85 verified cases of meningioma, he stated that in many of these, a tumor had been found at the exact location where a blow had been received to the skull years before. Cushing concluded that occlusion of arachnoid villi by either trauma or disease might lead to neoplastic deterioration. Decades after this observation, there has been little further substantiation supporting the development of a meningioma after either frank or surgical trauma to the meninges or dural sinuses (57).

The modern criteria for attributing a malignant growth to previous trauma were summarized by Auster (2) in 1961. He suggested that (a) the site of injury should be compared to the area in which the tumor developed; (b) trauma should be well authenticated; (c) there should be proof that neither metastatic nor primary disease was present before the injury; (d) the time between the injury and neoplasm must be significant; (e) there must be extension from the pathologic changes in the wounded area to the pathologic changes in the tumor; and (f) there must be microscopic evidence of a neoplasm. If these criteria are strictly followed, the case for a traumatic etiology for meningioma is considerably weakened (1,57).

Microscopic Pathology

Several different microscopic patterns of meningiomas have been described. In our view, Russell's (45) division of histologic types into five categories is the simplest and most workable grouping. The syncytial group is described as consisting of polygonal, poorly defined cells arranged in sheets. Fibroglial cells are generally absent. Elastic and collagen fibers are confined to the vascular trabeculae and give the appearance of dividing the tumor into islands or clusters of cells. In the transitional form, whorls are identified in which cells are wrapped around one another giving the appearance of a cut onion. The whorls may form psammoma bodies, which are defined as areas of concentric laminae of calcification deposited in degenerated areas (31). Rubinstein (44) has suggested that although psammomatous bodies may be the end result of concentric whorls seen in transitional meningiomas, their exact etiology has yet to be determined. In the fibroblastic type, the tumor is composed of spindle cells with prominent fibroglia. There may be a suggestion of palisading of nuclei and whorl formation. Between the individual cells, there is a dense development of reticulin and collagen fibers. The angioblastic type of meningioma is characterized by the presence of capillaries interspersed in the matrix of a cellular tumor. This imparts a spongy characteristic to the tumor. Mitotic figures may be readily identified, but this feature in itself does not imply malignant behavior. The differences between an angioblastic meningioma and a capillary hemangioblastoma may be quite difficult to define. The latter tend to be supratentorial, solid, and attached to the dura.

Sarcomatous meningiomas, more than the other forms detailed above, are more likely to be found in infants and young children. This variety of meningioma may be of leptomeningeal origin or arise from the tela choroidea of the choroid plexus. Those that arise in the brain parenchyma and do not reach the surface are theorized to arise from the pial covering of perforating blood vessels. Sarcomatous meningiomas have many mitotic features and a disorganized architecture. Other histologic variants seen with meningiomas but not considered to be distinct subtypes are the findings of melanin, foam cells containing sudanophilic lipid, giant cells, and myxomatous changes in bone and cartilage (44,45).

The incidence of the various histologic types of meningiomas was examined in 1,238 patients treated surgically, most of whom were adults (24). Of the total, endotheliomatous forms represented 63.3%, transitional 20.9%, fibroblastic 66%, angioblastic 8%, and atypical (malignant) meningiomas 1.2%. This series included both intracranial and spinal meningiomas. In one series of 178 meningiomas occurring in children under 16 years, there was a higher frequency of fibroblastic meningiomas in infants and a higher incidence of syncytial meningiomas in adolescence. In a paper by Davidson (14), a sclerosing type of meningioma has been characterized which appears to be peculiar to childhood. Histologically, these lesions consist of collagen with a sparse population of cells. In the cellular areas there are perinuclear halos. Cell membranes are poorly defined, and the architectural pattern is not visible. In these cases, the tumor was negative for GFAP and positive for vimentin. Although most cases show a fibroblastic pattern, a few have shown meningothelial whorling pattern. Invasion of the brain, at times, characterizes sclerosing meningiomas. This feature, coupled with the clear cells and focal areas of hypercellularity, suggests malignant behavior. However, for the most part, these tumors consist of primarily collagenous sclerosis with only small parts of the lesion appearing to have viable cells.

LOCATION

Although the convexity is a common location in both adults and children, (Fig. 17-1), posterior fossa meningiomas and intraventricular meningiomas are more readily found in the child than the adult (39,40,49). Unlike in adults, lack of dural attachment defines the meningioma occurring in childhood as does location on the convexity within the cerebral hemispheres or ventricular system and in the posterior fossa (Fig. 17-2). Table 17-2 compares the location of meningiomas in adults in several large series, and Table 17-3 indicates

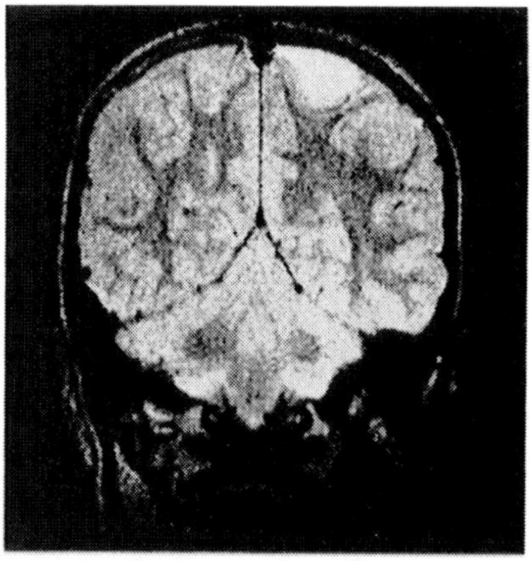

FIG. 17-1. T2-weighted coronal view of an 8-year-old with a convexity meningioma.

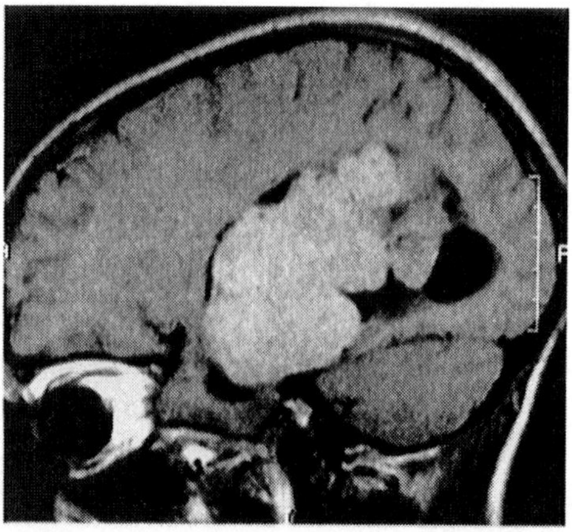

FIG. 17-2. T2-weighted sagittal view of a 6-year-old boy with a large intraventricular meningioma.

TABLE 17-2. *Common location of meningioma in adults*

Location	Simpson (50) (%)	Cushing and Eisenhardt (13) (%)	Olivecrona et al. (39) (%)	Glaholm et al. (20) (%)
Intraventricular	6/339 (2)	4/294 (1)	11/608 (3)	
Sphenoid	57/339 (17)	53/294 (19)	111/608 (18)	30/186 (16)
Parasagittal	107/339 (32)	77/294 (26)	143/608 (14)	18/186 (26)
Convexity	67/339 (20)	51/294 (18)	91/608 (15)	38/186 (20)
Parasellar	21/339 (6)	28/694 (10)	42/608 (7)	20/186 (15)
Other	81/339 (23)	75/294 (26)	203/608 (33)	50/186 (23)

the usual location of meningiomas in childhood. Meningiomas may also be found, on occasion, arising from the velum interpositum. It has been postulated that these tumors arise from the pia arachnoid of the roof of the third ventricle or from the connective tissue stroma of the pineal body (43). In childhood, meningiomas are apt to be cystic, and located over the convexity of the cerebral hemispheres The peritumoral cyst may be larger than the tumor itself, and in up to 50% there is no evidence of dural attachment. Although reported, congenital meningiomas are extremely rare and when found tend to occur on the convexities and to be extremely large.

An even rarer location for a meningioma in childhood is the optic sheath. There is at least one report (25) in which 40% (10 out of 25) of patients with orbital meningiomas were under 20 years of age and 24% (6 out of 25 patients) were under 10 years of age. This age distribution has not been verified by others. Most intraorbital meningiomas are seen in middle-aged women rather than in children. Nonetheless, despite their rarity, intraorbital and optic canal meningiomas figure prominently in the differential diagnosis of an intraorbital mass in children.

TABLE 17-3. *Location of meningiomas in children*

	Crouse and Berg (11) (1972)	Merten et al. (35) (1974)	Cooper and Donn (9) (1974)	Sano et al. (47) (1991)	Kolluri et al. (26) (1987)	Ferrante et al. (18) (1989)
Intraventricular	0	8	1	5	1	36
Sphenoid	1	7	2	4	1	26
Parasagittal	0	7	1	9		
Convexity	2	7	2	7	12	141
Parasellar	0	3	1	2	1	
Posterior fossa	6	9	0	5	2	27
Intracerebral	1	7	0	4	Not reported	Not reported
Other	0	0	0	0	1	62
TOTAL	36	48	7	36	18	197

TABLE 17-4. *Presenting signs and symptoms of children with mengiomas*

	Crouse and Berg (11) (1972)	Merten et al. (35) (1974)	Copper and Dohn (9) (1974)	Sano et al. (47) (1981)	Kolluri et al. (1987)	Ferrante et al. (18) (1989)
Pressure	39%	52%	29%	46%	83%	57%
Visual defect		52%				
Cranial neuropathy		33%	29%	62%	16%	
Seizures	14%	31%		31%	11%	27%
Behavior	6%	10%		15%	5%	
Focal features	36%	23%	29%	23%	22%	25%

CLINICAL SIGNS AND SYMPTOMS

The most common presenting sign of meningioma in childhood is that of increased intracranial pressure followed by visual loss and/or visual field defects. Surprisingly, cranial neuropathies associated with lesions of either the sphenoid wing or the posterior fossa are the third most common sign. Seizures are seen in approximately 8 to 31% of the cases. Focal neurologic deficits are found in 23 to 36% of the patients. Behavior changes are the least common symptoms, occurring in 6 to 15% of cases (Table 17-4). Because of an expansile head and the large size of the mass at diagnosis, presentation is a bit different in infancy than in other age groups (Table 17-5).

Intraventricular meningiomas present with signs of intermittent obstruction of cerebrospinal fluid outflow tracts (3). Headaches, vomiting, visual impairment, and papilledema may be prominent. If the tumor becomes large enough, persistent obstructive hydrocephalus may develop. Ptosis, nystagmus, gait disturbances, seizures, akinetic episodes, narcolepsy, and polyuria have all been reported with intraventricular tumors. Headaches may be either frontal, parietal, or occipital. Intermittent loss of consciousness implies compromise of the reticular formation, whereas focal signs suggest involvement of projecting systems either ascending or descending from the cortex. Autonomic signs and cranial neuropathies imply involvement of hypothalamic or brain-stem structures.

Optic canal or orbital tumors occur with signs of afferent pupillary defects,

TABLE 17-5. *Characteristics of meningiomas in infancy (<1 yr)*

Male preponderance
Convexity location
Lack of dural attachment
Rapid growth, large size
Large head

central or central cecal scotomas, and a variety of visual field abnormalities. As the tumor fills the optic canal, optic nerve dysfunction associated with pain may be an early finding and thus helps to differentiate this lesion from the relatively painless optic glioma. Orbital meningiomas are more likely to be associated with x-ray changes on plain skull films, tomography, and angiography than tumors of the optic sheath. Funduscopic examination may reveal shunt vessels, atrophy, or edema of the optic disc (39,58).

Because meningiomas of the optic nerve sheath are thought to arise from the arachnoid cells of the dura, an enlarging tumor is prone to compress underlying functional tissue. Thus, early in the course of the disease there may be pain and visual loss. Ptosis occurs when the tumor breaks through the dural capsule and subsequently acts as a space-occupying mass. Restriction of eye movement results from contraction of the extraocular muscles, and is thought to be a response to the mechanical resistance and limitation of motion produced by a rigid optic nerve. The development of disc edema and shunt vessels, in large measure, reflects the pressure of an enlarging tumor produced by a rigid optic nerve (58).

DIAGNOSTIC STUDIES

As with all intracranial neoplasms, diagnosis of a meningioma begins with clinical evaluation followed by neuroimaging. Regardless of the patient's age, plain skull films provide inferential evidence of a mass. Some signs are more specific than others. Decalcification of the dorsum sella and remodeling of the sella turcica are consistent with increased intracranial pressure. Calcification of the falx with a subsequent lateralized shift may be seen in adults but is rarely found in childhood. Changes on plain skull films suggesting a meningioma are calcification, hyperostosis, bone destruction, and increased vascularity (21). Hyperostosis has been associated with invasion of the bone by tumor, although a cause-and-effect relationship between bone growth and meningioma has not been definitively established. Bone destruction may occur as a result of infiltration of the bone by tumor, or may be secondary to erosion of bone by a pressure effect. Bone destruction is more commonly seen in tumors arising from the cribriform plate or over the convexities. Psammomatous meningiomas, more than other forms of meningiomas, are apt to calcify.

Vascular changes seen on skull films may also suggest the presence of a meningioma. An increase in the size of the middle meningeal groove, enlargement of the foramen spinosum, and increase of the diploic channels suggest increased vascularity and may be associated with the presence of an underlying tumor. Branches of the middle meningeal artery penetrating the bone supplying a tumor may give rise to clusters of small, punctate radiolucencies, which can be identified on plain films.

Although plain skull films are highly informative, the advent of CT scans has made screening skull films relatively obsolete. The CT scan not only allows visualization of size and location of the tumor but also gives information concerning displacement of other tissue and allows assessment of the degree of calcification. When used with contrast, CT provides information relative to the vascularity and draining vessels of the tumor. Arteriograms may still be necessary to determine if the vascular supply is arising from either an internal or an external arterial source.

CT features of meningiomas are relatively typical and consist of well circumscribed or somewhat lobulated irregular high-density lesions that readily enhance with contrast. Infrequently, low-density or isodense CT lesions are identified. The density of the tumor in all probability relates to the presence of connective tissue, extracellular water, fat, or calcification within psammoma bodies (51). Hilal and Chang (22) correlated the initial density of the tumor seen on the CT scan and the extent of contrast uptake. These authors suggested that the relationship of uptake versus density is rectilinear and bears some relationship to pathologic specificity. The higher the initial density, the less likely there is to be contrast enhancement. Tumors with the greatest amount of contrast enhancement are those associated with the lowest density. Radiolucency relates to cerebral edema and in turn may relate to the alteration of the blood–brain barrier.

MRI may be superior to CT in defining the location and extent of meningiomas. The MRI characteristics of meningiomas are generally a decreased signal on T1-weighted images and increased signal on T2-weighted images relative to cerebral white matter. MRI characteristics tend to be heterogeneous secondary to tumor vascularity, cysts, and calcification. An interface may be found between the meningioma and the brain consisting of a cerebrovascular cleft, vascular rim, or dural margin. Calcification appears as coarse irregular foci of decreased intensity on all sequences. In those tumors that do not infiltrate the brain, there is a clear interface between the brain and the periphery of the tumor. In comparison with CT, MRI permits more complete delineation and anatomic definition of the tumor. Higher energy MRI scans are more readily able to differentiate an extraaxial from an intraaxial location of the tumor. MRI allows discrimination of the interface of the meningioma with normal brain. High field signals have been associated with three different types of interfaces. A signal void represents marginal blood vessels. The cerebrospinal space is recognized by high signal intensity on T2 and low signal on T1, and a dural margin is recognized by low signal intensity on T2 and T1 (37,53). Thus, refinements in imaging have helped to define the extent of margins of the tumor, the anatomic nature of the tumor, whether the tumor invades the brain, and the interface between tumor and normal brain. Even with this degree of sophistication, histologic correlations cannot be made (Fig. 17-1).

SERIES RELATED SPECIFICALLY TO CHILDREN

Most information concerning the course and natural history of meningiomas is found in the adult literature. Few series are specifically limited to children. Although meningiomas are seen in all age groups, there is a predilection for early adolescence (Table 17-1). The largest single series of meningiomas found in childhood is that reported by the University of California at San Francisco (35). These authors reported their experience in 48 cases of meningiomas occurring in childhood. Sixty-six percent were found to be supratentorial, 19% were found in the posterior fossa, and 17% were intraventricular. The authors did not include angioblastic and sarcomatous meningiomas in this series. Histologically, the tumors were classified into psammomatous, fibroblastic, and meningothelial types. Tumors were found in all age groups varying from 4 months to 20 years, with a slight preference for the hemidecade between 10 and 14 years of age. Six of the 48 children with meningiomas had multiple tumors. Symptoms depended on the location of the tumor. The most commonly involved cranial nerves were the facial and auditory nerves. Other symptomatology included visual complaints, seizures, ataxia, endocrine abnormalities, behavioral disturbances, proptosis, increased intracranial pressure, and motor and sensory loss. Seizures, when they occurred, were associated with supratentorial tumors and, in one case, with a tumor that had risen in the posterior fossa but had extended into the middle cranial fossa. Calcification on skull films was not found in children under 5 years of age. Of the 48 patients, 28 had surgical removal with a presumptive cure. Of the remaining 20, 15 had died.

Crouse and Berg (11) reviewed the records of children with meningiomas seen in a large teaching hospital between 1936 and 1969. Only 13 patients were identified. The most frequent presenting signs in this group were headaches, followed by nausea, vomiting, diplopia, gait disturbances, diminished visual acuity, and hemiparesis. As expected, there were no characteristic signs or symptoms. Patients with cranial neuropathies were found to have posterior fossa lesions, whereas those presenting with hemiparesis or papilledema were apt to have a supratentorial mass. If the mass was supratentorial, the EEG showed a slow-wave focus, and if the mass was below the tentorium, the EEG was likely to be normal. Total removal was accomplished in only 1 patient. Three out of 13 were still alive at the time of the report. Another was lost to follow-up, and in a third, diagnosis was made at the time of autopsy. Of the remaining 8, the average survival was 6.7 years. The length of survival correlated mostly with histologic type rather than location. Two patients with meningeal sarcoma survived less than 1 year, although several patients with sarcomatous changes survived several years. Because this was a small series, little information was obtained regarding natural history.

The series by Cooper and Dohn (9) from the Cleveland Clinic, and also that of Sano et al. (47) from Japan, suffer from insufficient case material. The Cleveland Clinic reported the results in seven patients. The ratio of boys to girls in this series was 5:2, whereas in other series it was generally 1. Two out of seven patients were free of symptoms, and the other three were alive with either residual neurologic deficit or seizures. Two had died. Of interest, in one patient, a meningioma developed at the site of previous radiation for a medulloblastoma. A falcine meningothelial meningioma was removed from the occipital area 12 years after diagnosis and radiation of a medulloblastoma (9). This association of radiation and development of meningiomas is well known (4,8,38) (see Chapter 23).

The report by Sano et al. (47) of 8 cases from Japan is no less anecdotal. They included another 10 cases and combined these with the original 8 for analysis. Four out of the 18 had seizures. Intraventricular location and sarcomatous changes were the predominant features of this group of patients. Prognosis appeared to be somewhat more optimistic than that of other series. Eight out of 12 cases were alive after 10 years, with the longest patient surviving 20 years without evidence of recurrence. Three out of 5 patients had a sarcomatous form of meningioma and survived for more than 10 years.

The most recent report on meningeal tumors in pediatrics is a series from the Hospital for Sick Children in Toronto. Davidson et al. (14) reported their experience over 18 years. There were 22 meningiomas in this series. Histologic types for the most part were either sclerosing, transitional, or meningothelial. The age range was 4 months to 16 years. Of the 22 patients, 1 died a year and another 4 years following diagnosis. A third patient experienced a recurrence after 4 years. Of the remaining 17 patients, all were alive with a follow-up of 4 months to 12 years. Results were unknown in 2 patients.

Perhaps the largest series in children to date is that of Ferrante et al. (18). They reviewed the data on 197 patients accumulated from the literature as well as their own series. The mean age of this group was 9.1 years; the male-to-female ratio was 1.3:1. The most frequent sites were the frontal lobe in 19.2%, the ventricular system in 16.6%, middle cranial fossa in 12.3%, and posterior cranial fossa in 10.2%. In their series of 19 patients, there was only 1 death; and follow-up time varied from 6 months to 22 years. Five out of 19 experienced recurrences over a period of 1 to 10 years.

Meningiomas occurring in the first year of life, although reported, are distinctly rare. Because of the expansibility of the head in infancy, congenital tumors are apt to present somewhat differently than those in the older age group. A high-pitched cry, focal seizures, or myoclonic seizures may be associated with cortical irritation. Vomiting of a projectile nature, intermittent opisthotonos, or rigidity reflect either increased intracranial pressure or involvement of midline structures. Mendiratta et al. (34) reported a case in which a child presented with myoclonic seizures and was found to have subdural cysts associated with a retro Sylvian meningioma (34). In Cuneo and Rand's book (12), there is a description of a 3-month-old boy who had vomiting and rigidity since birth. Surgery revealed a large calcified angioblastic meningioma. Others have reported a meningioma occurring in a 2-month-old boy who presented with an enlarged head circumference and papilledema. What initially was thought to be a subdural hematoma was found to be a large fibroblastic meningioma.

Sakai (46) makes the point that the characteristics of meningiomas occurring in infancy consist of predominance of location on the convexity, a peritumoral cyst larger than the tumor itself, no dural attachment or limited adhesions to the dura, and a rapid increase in head circumference. Seizures may present in up to 20 to 25% of the cases. Prognosis relates to degree of surgical removal. Total surgical removal has been associated with long survival and potential cure.

Overall, the clinical spectrum of meningiomas in childhood, as in adults, is quite broad. These tumors, when seen in the child, tend to be large and have a greater tendency than in the adult to occur in the posterior fossa or in the ventricular system. In children, meningiomas are more likely to be sarcomatous in nature. All these features account for the failure to remove the tumor surgically and the reported high rate of recurrence.

TREATMENT

Because total surgical removal is associated with a cure, aggressive surgery is the treatment of choice (36). Most posterior fossa meningiomas require an operative tour de force and are difficult to remove. Several authors, commenting on the rarity of cerebellar pontine angle tumors in childhood, have suggested that when tumors in this region are identified, they are invariably meningiomas or neuromas. Cranial nerve signs may be the major key to diagnosis.

Wara et al., (55) in reviewing 188 meningiomas in all locations, reported a 44% total surgical removal, none of which recurred. Of the remaining 104 patients, 58 had subtotal removal without radiation. The recurrence rate in this group was 74%. Of 16 patients who had radiation after surgery, 7 were alive 1 to 7 years after radiation; 6 died from disease, and 2 died of intercurrent infection; 1 remained alive with a persistent tumor. Twenty-seven patients had recurrent operations. Of these, 17 died 1 to 18 years after the second operation; 5 were alive without recurrence; and 5 were alive with recurrence 1 to 19 years after operation. Thirty-four patients were irradiated immediately after subtotal operation; 29% of these recurred, the majority within 5 years.

The Royal Marsden (20) experience with 186 patients was reported in 1989, and their results with radiotherapy for meningiomas was reviewed between 1963 and 1983. The 10-year actuarial survival was 67% for all cases; progression-free survival was 61%. Radiotherapy was reserved for treatment of residual or unresectable disease, recurrent tumors, and those thought to have a frankly malignant histology. Children under 20 years of age represented somewhere between 3 and 4% of the total. Prognosis was related to the success of surgery. Those who had subtotal or total resection had an actuarial survival of 77%, while the survival for inoperable patients treated with radiotherapy was 46%. This study strongly supported the role of radiotherapy for treatment of incompletely resected inoperable meningiomas regardless of histologic type.

As with other tumors, many factors influence radiation responsiveness to meningiomas. These include vascularity of the tumor, volume of brain irradiated, location of the tumor, growth rate of the tumor, and treatment technique. Least important in planning irradiation is the histology of the tumor (54). Friedman (19) suggested that certain regions of the brain tolerate high doses of radiation better than others. In his report, patients with sphenoid ridge, parasagittal, and posterior fossa meningiomas who received radiation doses greater than 8,000 cGy did relatively well. He infers that the frontal lobes, certain portions of the temporal lobes, and occipital lobes are less susceptible to radionecrosis than the motor areas of the brain or spinal cord and thus can tolerate larger doses of radiation. In addition, like others, Friedman suggests that the smaller the volume of brain irradiated, the larger can be the radiation dose. Unlike Friedman, we suspect that all parts of the brain are equally radiosensitive. Those portions of the central nervous system that do not have a clear-cut functional signature may incorrectly appear to be relatively immune to radiation. More detailed examination with attention to cognitive function, both long-term and short-term memory, and other particularly human traits such as judgment and affect may uncover significant abnormalities.

Radiation needs to be looked at circumspectly because, paradoxically, there have been a number of reports of meningiomas occurring years following radiation to the head for other types of neoplasms. Latency of this complication may be as long as 20 years and as short as 3 to 7 years. Radiation-induced meningiomas have been identified with low-dose (70 to 175 cGy) intermediate-dose (1,500 to 2,000 cGy), and high-dose radiation (3,600 to 6,600 cGy). Unlike that of meningiomas occurring in nonirradiated patients, the histologic pattern is characterized by increased cellularity, giant cells, and gross nuclear pleomorphism (4,5,28,52) (also see Chapter 23).

PROGNOSIS

The recurrence rate of meningiomas after total removal has variously been estimated from 5 to 21% (23,50). In a large series reported by Jellinger and Slowik (24), there was a 13% recurrence rate. Melamed et al. (33) have suggested that recurrence was more likely if the tumor was found either parasagittally or in the posterior fossa. Recurrence in the former was related to the proximity and invasion of the superior sagittal sinus and in the latter to the technical difficulties associated with surgery in the posterior fossa. Recurrence has been inversely related to the extent of tumor removal. Focal invasion of the dural sinus, although not considered a malignant feature, is associated with recurrent disease. Prognostic variables affecting recurrence of meningiomas have been assessed in a few series. The most often quoted is the series of Crompton and Gauteir-Smith (10). They examined 181 tumors, all of which were parasagittal and falcine in location. The majority of these tumors recurred within 5 years of the original operation. Focal necrosis, cerebral infiltration, and mitosis were most likely associated with recurrence, whereas central necrosis of the tumor was more apt to be an indication of tumor size rather than a reflection of possible recurrence. Histologic type, presence of psammoma bodies, foam cells, pleomorphism, vacuolated nuclei, nuclear inclusions, adiposity, and bone formation were of no predictive value. Mitoses, although correlating with recurrence, have been considered by most to reflect the rate of growth rather than malignant potential. Invasion of brain parenchyma is generally not seen and when found is considered to be a malignant feature. Changes in histology to that of a sarcomatous, anaplastic, or papillary pattern also suggest malignancy.

Remote metastasis by definition implies malignant behavior. Metastasis has been described in the lungs, liver, bone, kidney, and lymph nodes (6,46,50). Cerebrospinal fluid metastases generally reflect malignant behavior, although isolated meningioma deposits in cerebrospinal fluid found at autopsy, distant from the site of the original tumor, have been considered by some to represent benign passively transported seeding rather than malignant behavior (32).

SUMMARY

In conclusion, the meningioma is considered to be a benign tumor, although malignant behavior and remote metastasis are well known. Criteria used to estimate malignancy include tendency to recur, local invasiveness, percent of mitosis, atypical histology, and remote metastasis. Recurrence tends to be inversely related to the extent of the tumor removed. Local invasion of the dura, venous sinuses, and bones is well known and in and of itself does not imply malignancy. Changes of histology to a sarcomatous, anaplastic, or papillary pattern suggest malignancy. Invasion of the brain parenchyma is generally not seen, and when it occurs is also considered a sign of malignancy.

The meningioma of childhood presents a bit differently than in the adult. Meningiomas in childhood are more frequently apt to invade the brain, are not associated with the dural attachment, and tend to be cystic in nature.

Unlike the adult, there is no clearly demonstrated female preponderance and, in fact, in infancy the males may predominate. On presentation, childhood meningiomas may be larger and can be sarcomatous. Because total removal is difficult, recurrence is to be expected. Treatment is primarily surgical; and if the tumor is totally removed, like the craniopharyngioma and juvenile astrocytoma of the cerebellum, cure can be achieved. On the basis of experience obtained from adults, radiation should be considered for those tumors that surgery has failed to remove completely.

REFERENCES

1. Annegers JF, Laws ER, Kurland LT, Grabow JD. Head trauma and subsequent brain tumors. *Neurosurgery* 1979;4:203–206.
2. Auster LS. The role of trauma in oncogenesis: a juridicial consideration. *JAMA* 1961;175: 946–950.
3. Avman N, Dincer C. Meningiomas of the third ventricle. *Acta Neurochir* 1978;42:217–224.
4. Balasubramaniam C, Armstrong D, Cheek W, Laurent J. Postradiation meningioma in a child. *Pediatr Neurosci* 1988;14:319–323.
5. Beller AJ, Feinsod M, Sahar A. The possible relationship between small dose irradiation to the scalp and intracranial meningiomas. *Neurochirurgie* 1972;4:135–143.
6. Bellur SM, Chandra V, McDonald LW. Association of meningiomas with extraneural primary malignancy. *Neurology* 1979;29:1165–1168.
7. Bodian M, Lawson D. The intracranial neoplastic diseases of childhood: a description of their natural history based on a clinicopathological study of 129 cases. *Br J Surg* 1953;40: 368–392.
8. Bogdanowicz WM, Sachs E. The possible role of radiation in oncogenesis of meningioma. *Surg Neurol* 1974;2:379–383.
9. Cooper M, Dohn DF. Intracranial meningiomas in childhood. *Cleve Clin Q* 1974;41:197–204.
10. Crompton MR, Gautier-Smith PC. The prediction of recurrence in meningiomas. *J Neurol Neurosurg Psychiatr* 1970;33:80–87.
11. Crouse SK, Berg BO. Intracranial meningiomas in childhood and adolescence. *Neurology* 1972;22:135–141.
12. Cuneo HM, Rand CW. *Brain tumors of childhood*. Springfield IL: Charles C Thomas; 1952: 121.
13. Cushing H, Eisenhardt L. *Mengiomas: their classification, regional behavior, life history and surgical end results*. Springfield IL: Charles C Thomas; 1938:69–73.
14. Davidson GS, Hope JK. Meningeal tumors of childhood. *Cancer* 1989:63:1205–1210.
15. Dinakar I, Balaparameswara R. Cystic meningiomas in child. *Ind J Pediatr* 1971;38: 223–224.
16. Drake JM, Hendrick EB, Becker LE, Chuang SH, Hoffman HJ, Humphreys RP. Intracranial meningiomas in children. *Pediatr Neurosci* 1985–86;12:134–139.
17. Evard M, Passy V. Von Recklinghausen's disease with multiple meningiomas. *Laryngoscope* 1972;82:2222–2225.
18. Ferrante L, Acqui M, Artico M, Mastronardi L, Rocchi G, Fortuna A. Cerebral meningiomas in children. *Childs Nerv Syst* 1989;5:83–86.
19. Friedman M. Irradiation of meningioma: a prototype circumscribed tumor for planning high-dose irradiation of the brain. *Int J Radiat Oncol Biol Phys* 1977;2:949–958.
20. Glaholm J, Bloom HJG, Crow JH. The role of radiotherapy in the management of intracranial meningiomas: the Royal Marsden Hospital experience with 186 patients. *Int J Radiat Oncol Biol Phys* 1989;18:755–761.
21. Gold HA, Kieffer SM, Peterson HO. Intracranial meningiomas: a retrospective analysis of the diagnostic value of plain skull films. *Neurology* 1969;19:873–878.
22. Hilal SK, Chang CH. Specificity of computed tomography in the diagnosis of supratentorial

neoplasma: consideration of metastases and meningiomas. *Neuroradiology* 1978;16: 537–539.
23. Hoessly GF, Olivecrona H. Report of 280 cases of verified parasagittal meningiomas. *J Neurosurg* 1955;12:614–626.
24. Jellinger K, Slowik F. Histological subtypes and prognostic problems in meningiomas. *J Neurol* 1975;208:279–298.
25. Karp LA, Zimmerman LE, Borit A, Spencer W. Primary intraorbital meningiomas. *Arch Ophthalmol* 1974;91:24–28.
26. Kolluri VRS, Reddy DR, Reddy PK, Naidu MRC, Rao SBP, Sumathi C. Meningiomas in childhood. *Childs Nerv Syst* 1987;3:271–273.
27. Kolluri VRS, Reddy DR, Reddy PK, Naidu MRC, Devi S. CT findings in cystic meningiomas. *Acta Neurochir* 1987;87:31–33.
28. Koos ThW, Miller MH. Intracranial tumors of infants and children. St Louis: CV Mosby; 1972:118–123.
29. Kumar PP, Good RR, Skultety FM, Leibrock LG, Severson GS. Radiation-induced neoplasms of the brain. *Cancer* 1987;59:1274–1282.
30. Lee YY, Lin SR, Horner FA. Third ventricle meningioma mimicking a colloid cyst in a child. *AJR* 1979;132:669–671.
31. Lipper S, Dalzell JC, Watkins PJ. Ultrastructure of psammoma bodies of meningioma in tissue culture. *Arch Pathol Lab Med* 1979;103:670–675.
32. Ludwin SK, Conley FK. Malignant meningioma metastasizing through the cerebrospinal pathways. *J Neurol Neurosurg Psychiatr* 1975;38:136–142.
33. Melamed SH, Sahar A, Beller AJ. The recurrence of intracranial meningiomas. *Neurochirurgia (Stuttg)* 1979;22:47–51.
34. Mendiratta S, Rosenblum J, Strobos R. Congenital meningioma. *Neurology* 1967;17: 914–918.
35. Merten DF, Gooding CA, Newton TH, Malamud N. Meningiomas of childhood and adolescence. *J Pediatr* 1974;84:696–700.
36. Mircevski M, Mircevska D, Bojadziev I, Basevska R. Surgical treatment of intraventricular meningiomas in childhood. *Acta Neurochir* 1985;35:89–91.
37. Nakasu S, Nakasu Y, Matsumura K, Matsuda M, Handa J. Interface between the meningioma and the brain on magnetic resonance imaging. *Surg Neurol* 1990:33:105–116.
38. Norwood CW, Kelly DL, Davis CH. Irradiation induced mesodermal tumors of the central nervous system: report on two meningiomas following x-ray treatment for glioma. *Surg Neurol* 1974;2:161–164.
39. Olivecrona H. The parasagittal meningiomas. *J Neurosurg* 1947;4:327–341.
40. Quest DO. Meningiomas: an update. *Neurosurgery* 1978;3:219–225.
41. Reddy DR, Kolluri VRS, Rao KS, Reddy PK, Naidu MRC. Cystic meningiomas in children. *Childs Nerv Syst* 1986;2:317–319.
42. Rohringer M, Sutherland GR, Louw DF, Sima AAF. Incidence and clinicopathological features of meningioma. *J Neurosurg* 1989;71:665–672.
43. Rozario R, Adelman L, Prager RJ, Stein BM. Meningiomas of the pineal region and third ventricle. *Neurosurgery* 1979;5:489–495.
44. Rubinstein LJ. Tumors of the central nervous system. In: *Atlas of tumor pathology*. Washington, DC: Armed Forces Institute of Pathology; 1972:169–170.
45. Russell DS. Meningeal tumors: a review. *J Clin Pathol* 1950;3:191–211.
46. Sakaki S, Nakagawa K, Kimura H, Ohue S. Intracranial meningiomas in infancy. *Surg Neurol* 1987;28:51–57.
47. Sano K, Wakai S, Ochiai C, Takakura K. Characteristics of meningiomas in childhood. *Childs Brain* 1981;8:98–106.
48. Satyanarayana K, Chandy SM, Rao TS. Congenital meningioma with subdural hygroma and proencephaly (a case report). *Neurol India* 1975;23:57–58.
49. Shaffi CM, Lekias JS. Meningiomas: treated and untreated. *Med J Aust* 1975;1:589–594.
50. Simpson D. The recurrence of intracranial meningiomas after surgical treatment. *J Neurol Neurosurg Psychiatr* 1957;20:22–39.
51. Skullerud J, Loken AC. The prognosis in meningiomas. *Acta Neuropathol* 1974;29:337–344.
52. Soffer C, Gomori JM, Sirgal T, Shalt MN. Intracranial meningiomas after high-dose irradiation. *Cancer* 1989;63:1514–1519.

53. Spagnoli MV, Goldberg HI, Grossman RJ, et al. Intracranial meningiomas: high-field MR imaging. *Radiology* 1986;161:369–375.
54. Tans JT, deJongh IE. Computed tomography of supratentorial meningioma. *Clin Neurol Neurosurg* 1977;80:10–21.
55. Wara WM, Sheline GE, Newman H, Townsend JJ, Boldrey EB. Radiation therapy of meningiomas. *AJR* 1975;123:453–458.
56. Wasserkrug R, Peyser E, Lichtig C. Extracranial bone metastases from intracranial meningiomas. *Surg Neurol* 1979;12:480–484.
57. Whatmore WJ, Hitchcock ER. Meningioma following trauma. *Br J Surg* 1973;60:496–498.
58. Wilson WC, Gordon M, Lehman RAW. Meningiomas confined to the optic canal and foramina. *Surg Neurol* 1979;12:21–28.
59. Wright JE. Primary optic nerve meningiomas: a clinical presentation and management. *Trans Am Acad Ophthalmol Otol* 1977;83:617–625.

18

Choroid Plexus Tumors

Choroid plexus papillomas are rare, representing 0.4 to 0.6% of intracranial tumors in all age groups; however, they represent a larger proportion of tumors seen in children. The first case report describing a choroid plexus papilloma was by Guerard in 1833 (33). By 1937, only 72 additional cases of choroid plexus papillomas were reported in the world literature (51). Referral patterns may bias incidence figures. In the Connecticut Tumor Registry, which registers all patients in the state of Connecticut, choroid plexus papillomas were found to represent 1% of 467 tumors in children (14). Higher incidence figures have been reported by the London Hospital for Sick Children and the Boston Children's Hospital (21,33). Incidence figures from London revealed that 2.3% of 600 brain tumors in children less than 17 years of age were choroid plexus papillomas. The incidence of this tumor in a series of 408 children under 12 years of age reported from Boston was 3.9%. Approximately 70% of choroid plexus tumors occur in children less than 2 years of age, with a median age at onset of 9 months (1). Choroid plexus papillomas may be congenital and have been reported in premature infants (31).

Location varies with the patient's age. Fourth ventricular choroid plexus papillomas are more commonly found in adults, whereas the lateral ventricles are the usual site of tumors in children (32,41). Although early reports suggested a left lateral ventricular predominance, this is no longer believed to be the case (20). The third ventricle is an unusual site for choroid plexus papillomas, with only about 10% occurring in this location (18,49).

PATHOLOGY

Kernohan and Fletcher-Kernohan (27) considered choroid plexus papillomas under the rubric of ependymomas, which included epithelial, myxopapillary, and cellular ependymomas, and papillomas of the choroid plexus. Rubinstein (43) also considered choroid plexus papillomas as a variant of ependymomas; others (4) view them as distinct nosologic entities.

The tumors may vary greatly in size, described in one study (41) as ranging from the size of a walnut to that of an egg. The tissue is soft and vascular and often contains a thin transparent capsule (32,33). On the cut surface the neoplasm is gray-red or red in color and quite friable. The surface is finely

Brain Tumors in Children: Principles of Diagnosis and Treatment, 2/e, edited by M.E. Cohen and P.K. Duffner, Raven Press, Ltd., New York, 1994.

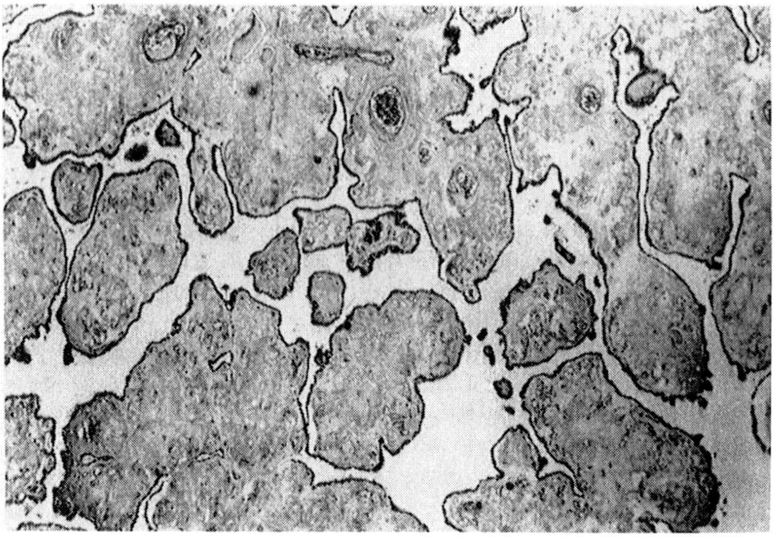

FIG. 18-1. Choroid plexus papilloma. Several papillary structures sectioned transversely resemble normal choroid plexus. The epithelium is generally arranged in a single layer around a core of vascular connective tissue. In this case, the fibrovascular stroma is more abundant than in normal choroid plexus (Gomori Trichrome).

granular or coarsely nodular. The tumors are usually attached to normal choroid plexus. Those that arise in the lateral ventricles tend to have their site of origin in the ventricular trigone.

The microscopic appearance of choroid plexus papillomas is that of normal choroid plexus (Fig. 18-1). A single layer of cuboidal or columnar cells covers highly vascularized connective tissue stroma. There are numerous branching papillary formations (16). Cytoplasm is pale and vacuolar with large nuclei, but mitoses are not present. Many have droplets of mucus (47). The cells are more columnar, crowded, and slightly more pleomorphic than normal choroid plexus (4).

Malignant choroid plexus papillomas (choroid plexus carcinomas), unlike the benign variety, are characterized by cellular pleomorphism, mitoses, multinucleated cells, necrosis, and hemorrhage and may invade surrounding brain (10). Lewis (29) and Russell and Rubinstein (44) established criteria for the diagnosis of the malignant choroid plexus papilloma: (a) invasion of adjacent neural tissue with infiltrating cells that assume a diffuse growth pattern; (b) loss of regular papillary structure in areas of invasion and malignant alterations of cells; and (c) transition of normal choroid plexus architecture to an undifferentiated pattern. Up to 20% of choroid plexus papillomas are malignant (48).

Cerebrospinal fluid seeding occurs with both benign and malignant papillomas. In those cases in which a benign choroid plexus papilloma seeds the leptomeninges, the histologic character of the metastases may remain benign. Conversely, malignant papillomas, which may disseminate widely throughout the CSF pathways, behave in a malignant fashion. There has been at least one case of a choroid plexus papilloma that has metastasized extracranially (52).

Immunohistochemical markers have been used to help differentiate choroid plexus papillomas from either choroid plexus carcinomas or metastatic carcinomas in older patients. The number of cases studied to date has been quite limited. Early on, it appeared that CEA strongly correlated with the presence of choroid plexus carcinomas (7,15). More recent data suggest that CEA is only rarely present in choroid plexus tumors but is often positive in metastatic carcinoma (38). Another marker, S100, is positive in most cases of choroid plexus tumors, but its absence does not necessarily negate the diagnosis (23). S100 reportedly correlates with choroid plexus tumors of low malignant potential and is rare in choroid plexus carcinomas. Another marker, reported by Herbert et al. (22) in 1990, was transthyretin (TTR), a transport protein for thyroxin and retinol. TTR distinguished choroid plexus tumors (both choroid plexus papillomas and choroid plexus carcinomas) from papillary ependymomas. The authors theorized that TTR was synthesized by choroid plexus epithelium and hence was an excellent marker for primary choroid plexus neoplasms. This marker allowed the investigator to distinguish choroid plexus tumors from both metastatic carcinomas and papillary ependymomas. As with S100, although TTR is often positive in choroid plexus tumors, its presence is not universal.

Paulus and Janisch (38) correlated histologic features with immunohistochemical tests in 67 patients with choroid plexus tumors. A poor prognosis, characterized by either progressive disease or death, correlated significantly with (a) less than 50% of the tumor cell staining heavily for S100, (b) presence of mitoses, (c) absence of TTR in tumor cells, (d) brain invasion by neoplastic cell nests, (e) absence of marked stromal edema, and (f) necrotic areas. Of interest, increased cellular density, nuclear pleomorphism, or blurred papillary structure did not correlate with prognosis. The three histologic features seen most often with recurrent rather than nonrecurrent choroid plexus papillomas were mitoses, less than 50% of tumor cells staining positive for S100, and absence of TTR. Analysis of immunohistochemical markers in more patients is necessary before the reliability of these markers for either diagnosis or prognosis is established.

DIAGNOSIS

Children with choroid plexus papillomas usually present with signs and symptoms of increased intracranial pressure. The most common presenting symptoms are vomiting, clumsiness, headaches, weakness, and seizures (3,21). There is generally a short duration of time from the onset of symptoms to diagnosis. In one series (33), most patients had an abrupt onset of symptoms before diagnosis ranging from 1 week to 2 months, with only two patients having a duration of symptoms of 1 year or greater. Physical examination reflects increased intracranial pressure and is characterized by macrocephaly, papilledema, sixth nerve palsy, and pyramidal tract signs. Choroid plexus tumors should be suspected when hydrocephalus in childhood has an acute onset and no apparent cause. In addition, the presence of papilledema is unusual in infantile hydrocephalus, whereas it is extremely common in children presenting with choroid plexus tumors.

Plain skull films, although rarely diagnostic, reflect signs of increased intracranial pressure and are characterized by suture diastasis and a large cranial vault. Since calcification of the choroid plexus is distinctly unusual in children less than 10 years of age, unilateral calcification in the region of the choroid plexus in the first decade of life is strongly suggestive of choroid plexus papilloma. Because many papillomas are pedunculated, the calcification may shift with movement of the head. Overall, calcification of choroid plexus papillomas occurs in approximately 4% of cases. The presence of a large mottled calcification, forming a cast of the ventricular pathways, is highly suggestive of a papilloma (42,48).

Cerebrospinal fluid examination may be of diagnostic importance. Most patients will have elevated CSF pressure, and the majority will have elevation of CSF protein. Because the choroid plexus papilloma is highly vascular, cerebrospinal fluid may show evidence of bleeding. Hence, the most important finding on CSF examination may be the presence of either xanthochromia or frank blood (49) (Fig. 18-2).

On CT, the choroid plexus papilloma is a well marginated, smooth or lobulated mass that is either isodense or slightly hyperdense prior to contrast

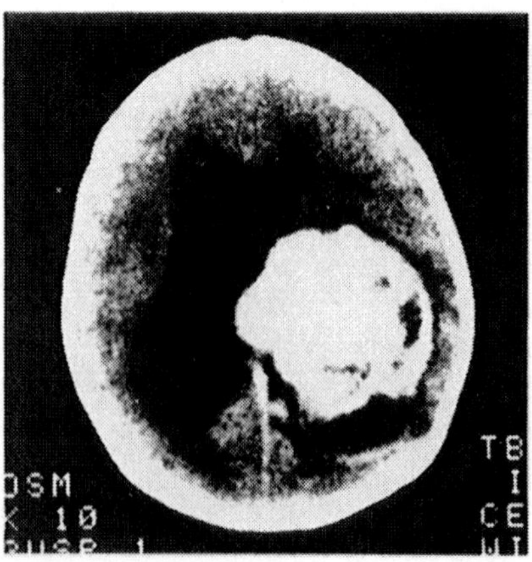

FIG. 18-2. Six-week-old baby presented with irritability, low-grade fever, and bulging anterior fontanelle. Lumbar puncture revealed xanthochromia, secondary to protein of 558 mg%. CT scan demonstrated large choroid plexus tumor, which markedly enhanced with contrast.

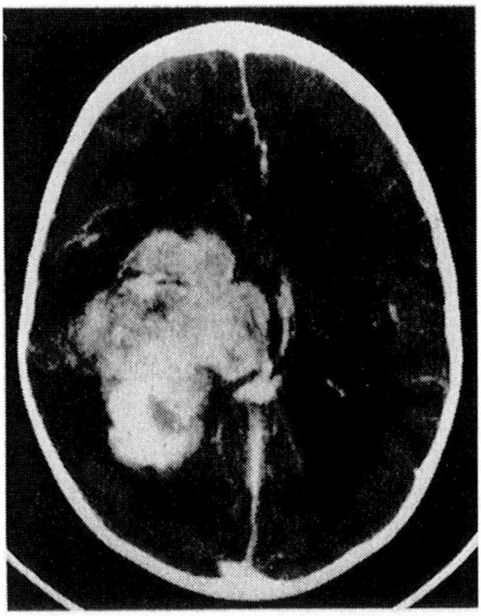

FIG. 18-3. Four-month-old with choroid plexus carcinoma. Note marked contrast enhancement, edema, and irregular margins.

enhancement (6). Calcification may be identified in the precontrast scan. In general, choroid plexus papillomas have punctate calcification, whereas choroid plexus carcinomas have larger and more globular calcification (25). Following administration of contrast, the tumor has marked homogeneous enhancement. Benign choroid plexus papillomas generally have smooth bor-

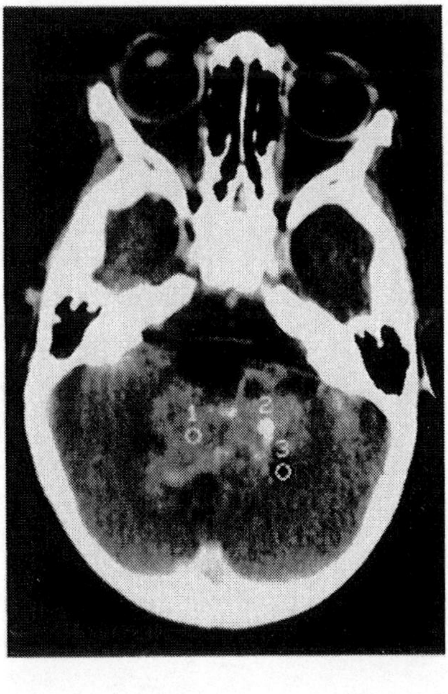

FIG. 18-4. Fourth ventricular choroid plexus carcinoma in 6-month-old baby. Most choroid plexus tumors in infants occur in the lateral ventricles.

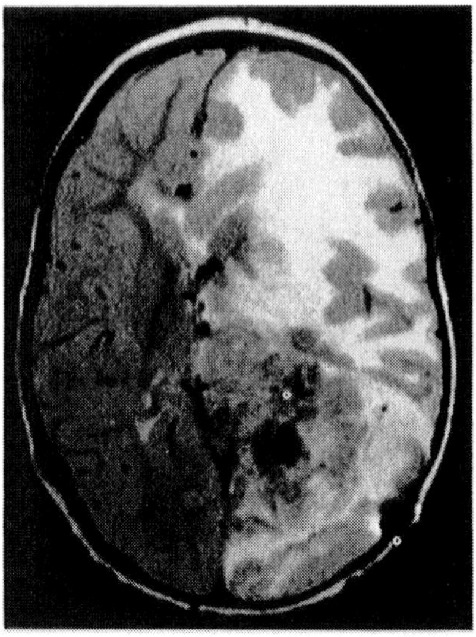

FIG. 18-5. MRI of a 3-year-old child with recurrent CPC, first diagnosed at 6 weeks of age. Mass of complex signal is predominantly located in the left occipital and posterior/superior parietal lobe. A large amount of edema is present.

ders with little or no extension into parenchyma, whereas irregular margins and extension of tumor into surrounding brain is more typical of the choroid plexus carcinoma (Figs. 18-3 and 18-4). Hydrocephalus and peritumoral edema are common (24).

On MRI, the choroid plexus papilloma is homogeneous on both short TR/TE and long TR/TE sequences (53). The choroid plexus carcinoma is less homogeneous because of central necrosis, hemorrhage, and cyst formation. A curvilinear signal void is often identified, characteristic of enlarged intratumoral vessels. Inhomogeneity on CT or MRI suggests carcinomatous change, as does invasion of the adjacent brain parenchyma (6) (Fig. 18-5).

Angiography is still used in the preoperative evaluation of children with choroid plexus papillomas because it is essential in defining the vascular supply of the tumor (39,43).

TREATMENT

The treatment of choroid plexus papillomas is total surgical excision. Although operative mortality has been high because of the tumor's hemorrhagic tendency, operative deaths have been decreasing in recent years. A surgical series from 1952 to 1968 (20) reported a 31% mortality, whereas in the same center, from 1969 to 1978, surgical mortality was 16%. It is anticipated that postoperative survival rates from the 1980s and 1990s will be even better.

Hydrocephalus is a well-known complication of choroid plexus papillomas. Whether the hydrocephalus develops as a result of hypersecretion of

CSF by the tumor or develops from a failure of resorption of CSF due to tumor bleeding has been debated for years. Ray and Peck (40) reported a 3-year-old child with hydrocephalus who initially had a ventriculoureteral shunt. The child urinated in such profusion that she became dehydrated. Subsequently, the ureteral shunt was replaced with a ventriculoperitoneal shunt, which led to massive ascites. This child was ultimately found to have bilateral choroid plexus papillomas. A variety of sophisticated studies employing ventricular perfusion techniques have documented increased secretion of CSF. Milhorat et al. (35) determined the rate of CSF formation in a 2-year-old child before and after removal of a lateral ventricular choroid plexus papilloma. The rate of CSF formation preoperatively was 1.05 ± SD 0.01 ml/min or 1,656 ml per day, compared with a postoperative CSF rate of formation of 0.2 ± SD 0.01 ml/min or 288 ml per day. Similarly, Eisenberg et al. (12) and Gudeman et al. (19) found the rate of CSF fluid formation 4 to 5 times higher in their patients compared with normal. Those who favor overproduction point to the elimination of hydrocephalus after the complete removal of tumor (19). However, according to some reports removal of the tumor has not corrected the hydrocephalus (45). Choroid plexus papillomas are known to be friable and bleed easily. At least some patients will develop a resorptive defect owing to this bleeding and hence will develop a communicating hydrocephalus. It is likely that both overproduction and decreased absorption of CSF act jointly to produce hydrocephalus. Although the use of preoperative shunting in choroid plexus papillomas has been debated, all neurosurgeons would recommend shunting postoperatively if the hydrocephalus does not abate with tumor removal.

In general, most neurosurgeons recommend radical en bloc removal of tumor. After occlusion of the main arterial feeders and division of the pedicle, the mass will generally shrink in size, permitting easier removal. The surgical approach to the fourth ventricle is generally a suboccipital craniectomy. The third ventricle is often approached through a frontal transcortical incision across the dilated ventricle of the nondominant hemisphere via the foramen of Monro. The transcallosal route to the third ventricle has been recommended by others. In particular, this approach avoids a cortical incision and the possibility of creating an epileptic focus (26). Finally, the papilloma of the lateral ventricle is usually approached via a posterior parietal central incision (33,39). The least possible manipulation of the tumor is necessary to prevent bleeding as well as to prevent cerebrospinal fluid seeding of malignant cells. Hemostasis must be complete after surgical closure to eliminate bleeding and prevent communicating hydrocephalus. An important complication of gross total resection, in particular, has been the development of subdural collections secondary to cortical mantel collapse. It is believed that these collections develop because of ventricular subdural fistulas (2).

Although operative mortality has been quite high, recurrence after total removal of the tumor is rare. Several studies have reported recurrence rates of 0 to 7% following gross total resection (7,13,20,33,46). In general, if the child with a choroid plexus papilloma survives a gross total resection, late recurrences are unusual and no further treatment is necessary.

Radiotherapy: Choroid Plexus Papillomas

Experience with radiation therapy in choroid plexus papillomas is limited, primarily because these tumors can be cured with surgery alone. Indeed postoperative radiation is not indicated in children who have had a gross total resection of a benign choroid plexus papilloma. In those cases of subtotally resected tumors, some studies have demonstrated a prolonged progression-free survival with postoperative radiation (13,34). These data are confounded by reports of children with subtotal resection who have survived for prolonged periods without adjuvant treatment. Some authors (5) have suggested that preoperative radiation be given to shrink the tumor. In at least one case reported by Hawkins (21), tumor removal was made easier by preoperative radiation. Unfortunately, it has also been reported that radiation may cause adhesions of the tumor to surrounding structures, sometimes making total removal impossible. In view of this and other well-known risks of cranial irradiation, many authors suggest radiation only if there is evidence of recurrence, or if the tumor is malignant.

Radiation: Choroid Plexus Carcinomas

Choroid plexus carcinomas must be viewed differently than benign choroid plexus papillomas. The likelihood of achieving a gross total resection is less with the malignant varieties because there is much more invasion of surrounding tissue. Whether postoperative radiation following gross total resection offers a survival advantage has not yet been clarified. In a combined series of 50 children with choroid plexus carcinomas, 17 had a gross total resection (Table 18-1). Of these, 10 were treated with surgery alone: 6 had no evidence of recurrent disease and 4 either progressed or died. Six children had gross total resection followed by radiation in varying dosages and volumes. Of these, 4 remain alive and well, 1 progressed, and 1 developed a second malignancy 18 years following diagnosis. There has been one report of a child treated with a gross total surgical resection and chemotherapy. That child remained progression-free for at least 5 months, but the long-term outcome was not specified. Although some authors suggest that gross total resection is the only treatment necessary for children with choroid plexus carcinomas, the literature suggests that there is a significant failure rate following surgical removal alone.

A much more dismal picture comes from a review of those children who have had less than gross total surgical resection. In the same literature review

TABLE 18-1. *Treatment of choroid plexus carcinomas*

Author	Location	Age	Surgery	RT	CT	PFS	Status
Pascual-Castroviejo (37)	RLV	21 m	"S"	—	—	—	Dead, 22 m
	RLV	2 m	"S"	—	—		Dead
	RLV	22 m	"S"	—	—		Dead, 24 m
Coffin (7)	LLV	3 yr	"S"	—	—	—	Alive, 9 m+
Packer (36)	LLV	15 m	GTR	—	+	5 m	
	4TH V	5 m	PR (>50%)	+		3 m	
	LLV	1 wk	GTR	—	—	9.5+ yr	
	RLV	15 m	GTR	—	—	18+ m	
	L THAL	33 m	ST/BX	+	+ (PD)	6 m	
	LLV	31 m	ST/BX	—	+	2 m	
	R THAL	26 m	ST/BX (×2)	—	—	2 m	
	LLV	7.5 yr	PR	+	—	52 m	
	RLV	7.7 yr	GTR	+	—	60+ m	
	LLV	9.5 yr	ST/BX	+	—	44+ m	
	LLV	19 m	GTR	—	—	46+ m	
Gianella-Borradori (17)		2 yr	PR	—	+	2 yr	2 yr+
		7 wk	GTR	—	+ (PD)		5 yr+
Matson (31)	RLV	2 yr	PR (invasive)	—	—		5 m
	LLV	4 m	PR (invasive)	—	—		Died, 2 wks
	LLV	9 m	GTR	+	—	3 yr	Alive
	LLV	20 m	PR × 2 (invasive)	—	—	—	Died 2nd "S"
Allen (1)	LLV	9 m	ST	—	+	9	46
	L & RLV	18 m	ST	—	+	16	57
	LLV	27 m	ST	—	+	10	11
Ho (23)	RLV	24 m	PR	—	—		Dead, 1 m
	CP	6 yr	PR	—	—		Dead, 3 m
Lewis (29)	LLV	20 m	PR	3-wk			3yr, dead
	CPA	13 m	?	course			4 m, dead
	LLV	4 yr	BX	+	—		Dead, 6 wks
Boyd (2)	4TH V	18 m	BX	—	+		Dead, 2 m
	LLV	5 m	PR	—	—		Dead, postop.
Humphreys (24)	LLV		Decompress	—	—		Dead, 3 m
	LLV		GTR	+	—		Dead, 3 m
	LLV		BX	+	—		Dead, 6 m
	4TH V		ST	—	—		Dead, 3 m
	RLV		GTR	+	—		26+
Ellenbogen (13)		Pt. 1	GTR	+	—		Alive + +
		Pt. 2	GTR	—	—		Alive + +
		Pt. 3	GTR	—	—		Alive + +
		Pt. 4	GTR	—	—		Alive + +
		Pt. 5	GTR	+	—		18 yr[c]
		Pt. 6[a]	GTR × 2	+ (PD)	+ (PD)		Alive
		Pt. 7[a]	GTR × 2	—	+ (PD)		Alive, 1 yr
		Pt. 8[a]	GTR × 2	—	+ (PD)		Dead, 6 wk
		Pt. 9[a]	BX – GTR	—	+		Alive, 3 yr
		Pt. 10	ST				Dead[b]
		Pt. 11	ST				Dead[b]
		Pt. 12	ST				Dead[b]
		Pt. 13	ST				Dead[b]
		Pt. 14	ST				Dead[b]

+ +, alive average 9.8 yr; RLV, right lateral ventricle; LLV, left lateral ventricle; 4TH V, fourth ventricle; THAL, thalamus; m, month; yr, year; GTR, gross total resection; PR, partial resection; ST, subtotal resection; BX, biopsy; PD, progressive disease.

[a] Progressed despite gross total resection; three salvaged with chemotherapy, repeat surgery, radiotherapy.

[b] Dead within 7 months.

[c] Died of second malignancy.

of 50 patients with choroid plexus carcinomas, 32 had either subtotal resection, partial resection, or biopsy. All 19 children treated with less than gross total resection alone either progressed or died; many died in the postoperative period. Seven children were treated with less than gross total resection followed by radiation. Of these, only 2 remain disease-free. Finally, 6 children were treated with less than gross total resection and chemotherapy; only 1 remains alive and well. Thus, although recent articles have suggested that the prognosis of choroid plexus carcinomas is not as poor as previously thought, this rosy outlook is not supported by the literature. Unquestionably those children with gross total surgical resection have the best prognosis, but even in this group, survivals are limited. Although most authors recommend postoperative radiation for older children with choroid plexus carcinomas, the literature does not demonstrate a convincing argument that radiation is effective.

Many choroid plexus carcinomas occur in extremely young children. As such, because of the known neurotoxicity associated with radiating the infant's brain, there has been an increasing interest in using chemotherapy as the first postsurgical approach (10). Durable responses to chemotherapy following recurrence have already been reported. The most commonly used agents have been vincristine, Cytoxan, cis-platinum, and VP-16 in varying combinations. Two of three children in one series treated with vincristine and cis-platinum at the time of recurrence were doing well at the time of publication (13). It should be noted, however, that two of these patients received gross total resections at the time of recurrence prior to beginning chemotherapy and one also received radiation. A child with a progressive choroid plexus carcinoma was treated successfully by Maria et al. (30) with a combination of cis-platinum, bleomycin, and vinblastine. There have now been several reports of young children with choroid plexus carcinomas treated with chemotherapy following initial surgery. Five infants treated on a Pediatric Oncology Group (11) protocol with Cytoxan, vincristine, cis-platinum, and VP-16 and delayed radiation were free of progression at 5+, 15+, and 29+ months. One child failed after 6 months and then was irradiated. She remained disease-free for 18 months. The fifth child had disease control for 21 months prior to progression and died 24 months later, after failing several salvage therapies. Progression-free survivals lasting from 9 to 16 months were also reported by Allen (1) in three subtotally resected children treated with a protocol similar to the POG study, i.e., cis-platinum, VP-16, Cytoxan, and vincristine, with overall survivals of 11, 46, and 57 months. Primary postoperative chemotherapy was also used by Packer (36) in two children. The first child received a combination of CCNU, vincristine, and intrathecal methotrexate and was progression-free for 5 months; the second failed on cyclophosphamide and vincristine after 2 months. Although chemotherapy regimens are in a state of flux and the number of patients so treated is limited, disease-free survivals following subtotal resection and chemotherapy have surpassed previous results of surgery with and without radiation. Whether chemotherapy will ultimately add to the disease-free survival of children with gross total resection awaits future studies.

PROGNOSIS

The 5-year survival of children with choroid plexus papillomas reported by Farwell et al. (14) from the Connecticut Tumor Registry was 67%. Of interest, the 1-year and 5-year survivals were identical. Thus, if the patient survives 1 year after surgery, the likelihood of cure is quite good. This is not the case with children with choroid plexus carcinomas. In these cases, the duration from symptoms to death has been reported to be 9 months (9).

Unfortunately, the quality of life of young children following aggressive surgery for choroid plexus papillomas is poor. Spallone et al. (46) noted that although their results in children over 5 years of age were consistently good, only 2 of 7 children operated under 5 years of age enjoyed a good quality of life. Complications included pyramidal tract weakness, mental retardation, and persisting hydrocephalus. In another study (37) of 14 children less than 2 years of age with choroid plexus neoplasms, only 1 child lived "normally." Of the remaining 13, 9 died, 3 were mentally retarded with hydrocephalus and subdural collections, and 1 had a borderline seizure disorder. Whether these complications are solely due to aggressive surgery or relate, in part, to the long-standing presence of tumor with coincident hydrocephalus is unclear. Adding cranial radiation to this already damaged group of young children will increase the incidence of neurotoxicity. Prospective studies coupled with neuropsychological testing are necessary to assess the various toxicities associated with different treatment regimens.

SUMMARY

Choroid plexus papillomas represent 0.4 to 0.6% of intracranial tumors in all age groups but represent 1 to 4% of brain tumors in children. The tumors are more commonly located in the lateral ventricles in children, with a predominance in the left lateral ventricle. In adults, choroid plexus papillomas are more often in the fourth ventricle. The tumors are usually benign, and their pathology is nearly identical to that of the normal choroid plexus. The tumors may occasionally be malignant with pleomorphism, mitoses, endothelial proliferation, and invasion of normal surrounding brain. Patients present with typical signs of increased intracranial pressure. In the past, the infant or young child who presented with signs of increased intracranial pressure of nonfocal nature may have spuriously been diagnosed as having congenital hydrocephalus rather than a choroid plexus papilloma. Today, the diagnosis may be readily made on CT scan or MRI as an intraventricular mass of high density that markedly enhances with contrast. Whether the associated hydrocephalus is due to overproduction of cerebrospinal fluid by the choroid plexus papilloma or the result of decreased absorption of cerebrospinal fluid is unclear; in all likelihood, it represents a combination of both processes.

The treatment of choroid plexus papillomas is surgery. Because of the tumor's known vascularity, operative mortality even today remains high. If total removal is accomplished, late recurrences are limited. Postoperative shunts have been advocated for those patients with persistent hydrocephalus following total removal of the tumor. Radiation is restricted to children with recurrent tumors.

The treatment of choroid plexus carcinomas is in a state of evolution. Gross total resection offers the best possibility of prolonged disease-free survival; but the invasiveness of the tumor, and its tendency to metastasize, limits the likelihood that this can be successfully accomplished in most patients. Moreover, even with gross total resection, the likelihood of cure is very limited. Survivals are sufficiently dismal with anything less than a gross total resection that either postoperative radiation or chemotherapy is recommended. In the very young child, postoperative chemotherapy is the most promising area of study.

REFERENCES

1. Allen J, Wisoff J, Helson L, et al. Choroid plexus carcinoma: responses to chemotherapy alone in newly diagnosed young children. *J Neurooncol* 1992;12:69–74.
2. Boyd MC, Steinbok P. Choroid plexus tumors: problems in diagnosis and management. *J Neurosurg* 1987;66:800–805.
3. Branch CE, Dyken PR. Choroid plexus papilloma and infantile spasms. *Ann Neurol* 1979; 5:302–304.
4. Burger PC, Vogel FS. *Surgical pathology of the nervous system and its coverings*. John Wiley & Sons; 1982:321–326.
5. Carrea R, Polak M. Preoperative radiotherapy in the management of posterior fossa choroid plexus papillomas. *Childs Brain* 1977;3:12–24.
6. Coates TL, Hinshaw DB, Peckman N, et al. Pediatric choroid plexus neoplasms: MR, CT, and pathologic correlation. *Radiology* 1989;173:81–88.
7. Coffin CM, Wick MR, Braun JT, Dehner LP. Choroid plexus neoplasms: clinicopathologic and immunohistochemical studies. *Am J Surg Pathol* 1986;10(6):394–404.
8. Davis LE, Cushing H. Papillomas of the choroid plexus. *Arch Neurol Psychiatr* 1925;13: 681–710.
9. Dohrmann GJ, Collias JC. Choroid plexus carcinoma: case report. *J Neurosurg* 1975;43: 225–232.
10. Duffner PK, Cohen ME. Treatment of brain tumors in babies and very young children. *Pediatr Neurosci* 1986;12:304–310.
11. Duffner PK, Cohen ME, Horowitz M, et al. The treatment of choroid plexus carcinoma in infancy with chemotherapy. *Ann of Neurol* 1989;26:460.
12. Eisenberg HM, McComb JG, Lorenzo AV. Cerebrospinal fluid reproduction and hydrocephalus associated with choroid plexus papilloma. *J Neurosurg* 1974;50:381–385.
13. Ellenbogen RG, Winston KR, Kupsky WJ. Tumors of the choroid plexus in children. *Neurosurgery* 1989;25(3):327–335.

14. Farwell JR, Dohrmann GJ, Flannery JT. Central nervous system tumors in children. *Cancer* 1977;40:3123–3132.
15. Felix I, Phudhichareonrat WC, Halliday WC, Becker LE. Choroid plexus tumors in children: immunohistochemical and scanning-electron-microscopic features. *Pediat Neurosci* 1987;13:263–269.
16. Ghatak NR, McWhorter JM. Ultrastructural evidence for CSF production by a choroid plexus papilloma. *J Neurosurg* 1976;45:409–415.
17. Gianella-Borradori A, Zeltzer PM, Bodey B, Nelson M, Britton H, Martin A. Choroid plexus tumors in childhood: response to chemotherapy and immunophenotypic profile using a panel of monoclonal antibodies. *Cancer* 1991;69:809–816.
18. Gradin WC, Taylon C, Fruin AH. Choroid plexus papilloma of the third ventricle: case report and review of the literature. *Neurosurgery* 1983;12(2):217–220.
19. Gudeman SK, Sullivan HG, Rosner MH, Becker RP. Surgical removal of bilateral papillomas of the choroid plexus of the lateral ventricles with resolution of hydrocephalus. *J Neurosurg* 1979;50:677–681.
20. Guidetti B, Spallone A. The surgical treatment of choroid plexus papillomas: the results of 27 years experience. *Neurosurg* Rev 1981;4:129–137.
21. Hawkins JC. Treatment of choroid plexus papillomas in children: a brief analysis of twenty years' experience. *Neurosurgery* 1980;6:380–384.
22. Herbert J, Cavallaro T, Dwork AJ. A marker for primary choroid plexus neoplasms. *Am J Pathol* 1990;136(6):1317–1324
23. Ho DM, Wong TT, Hung-Chuang L. Choroid plexus tumors in childhood: histopathologic study and clinicopathological correlation. *Childs Nerv Syst* 1991;7:437–441.
24. Humphreys RP, Nemoto S, Hendrick EB. Childhood choroid plexus tumors. *Concepts Pediatr Neurosurg Karger, Basel* 1987;7:1–18.
25. Johnson DL. Management of choroid plexus tumors in children. *Pediatr Neurosci* 1989; 15:195–206.
26. Jooma RD, Grant N. Third ventricle choroid plexus papillomas. *Childs Brain* 1983;10: 242–250.
27. Kernohan JW, Fletcher-Kernohan EM. Ependymomas, study of 109 cases. *Res Publ Assoc Res Nerv Ment Dis* 1937;16:182–209.
28. Laurence KM, Hoare RD, Till K. The diagnosis of the choroid plexus papilloma of the lateral ventricle. *Brain* 1961;84:628–641.
29. Lewis P. Carcinoma of the choroid plexus. *Brain* 1967;90:177–186.
30. Maria B, Graham M, Strauss L, Wharam M. Response of a recurrent choroid plexus tumor to combination chemotherapy. *J Neurooncol* 1985;3:259–262.
31. Matson DD. Hydrocephalus in a premature infant caused by papilloma of the choroid plexus. With report of surgical treatment. *J Neurosurg* 1953;10:416–420.
32. Matson DD. Intracranial tumors of the first two years of life. *West J Surg Obstet Gynecol* 1964;72:117–122.
33. Matson DD, Crofton FDL. Papilloma of the choroid plexus in childhood. *J Neurosurg* 1960; 17:1002–1027.
34. McGirr SJ, Ebersold MJ, Scheithauer BW, Quast LM, Shaw EG. Choroid plexus papillomas: long-term follow-up results in a surgically treated series. *J Neurosurg* 1988;69:843–849.
35. Milhorat TH, Davis DA, Hammock MK. Choroid plexus papilloma. II: Ultrastructure and ultracytochemical localization of Na-K-ATPase. *Childs Brain* 1976;2:290–303.
36. Packer RJ, Perilongo G, Johnson D, et al. Choroid plexus carcinoma of childhood. *Cancer* 1992;69:580–585.
37. Pascual-Castroviejo I, Villarejo F, Perez-Higueras A, Morales C, Pascual-Pascual SI. Childhood choroid plexus neoplasms. *Eur J Pediatr* 1983;140:51–56.
38. Paulus W, Janisch W. Clinicopathologic correlations in epithelial choroid plexus neoplasms: a study of 52 cases. *Am J Neuropathol* 1990;80:635–641.
39. Raimondi AJ, Gutierrez FA. Diagnosis and surgical treatment of choroid plexus papillomas. *Childs Brain* 1975;1:81–115.
40. Ray BS, Peck FC. Papilloma of the choroid plexus of the lateral ventricles causing hydrocephalus in an infant. *J Neurosurg* 1956;13:405–410.
41. Ringertz N, Reymond A. Ependymomas and choroid plexus papillomas. *J Neuropathol Exp Neurol* 1949;8:355–380.

42. Rovit RL, Schecter MM, Chodroff P. Choroid plexus papilloma: observations on radiographic diagnosis. *AJR* 1970;110:608–617.
43. Rubinstein LJ. *Tumors of the central nervous system.* Washington, DC: Armed Forces Institute of Pathology; 1972:85–104, 154–157, 259–262.
44. Russell DS, Rubinstein LJ. *Pathology of tumors of the nervous system.* London: Edward Arnold; 1989:163–166.
45. Simpson DA, Carter RT, Ducrou W. Intracranial tumors in infancy. *Dev Med Child Neurol* 1968;10:190–199.
46. Spallone A, Pastore FS, Giuffre R, Guidetti B. Choroid plexus papillomas in infancy and childhood. *Childs Nerv Syst* 1990;6:71–74.
47. Svien HJ, Mabon RF, Kernohan JW, Crain WMcK. Ependymoma of the brain: pathologic aspects. *Neurology* 1953;3:1–15.
48. Thompson JR, Harwood-Nash D, Fritz CR. The neuroradiology of childhood choroid plexus neoplasms. *AJR* 1973;118:116–133.
49. Tomasello F, Albanese V, Bernini FP, Picozzi P. Choroid plexus papilloma of the third ventricle. *Surg Neurol* 1981;16:69–71.
50. Turcotte JF, Copty M, Bedard F, Michaud J, Verret S. Lateral ventricle choroid plexus papilloma and communicating hydrocephalus. *Surg Neurol* 1980;13:143–146.
51. Turner OA, Simon MA. Malignant papillomas of choroid plexus: report of two cases with review of literature. *Am J Cancer* 1937;30:289–297.
52. Valladares JB, Perry RH, Kalbag RM. Malignant choroid plexus papilloma with extraneural metastasis. *J Neurosurg* 1980;52:251–255.
53. Vazquez E, Ball WS, Prenger EC, Castellote A, Crone KR. Magnetic resonance imaging of fourth ventricular choroid plexus neoplasms in childhood. *Pediatr Neurosurg* 1991–92; 17:48–52.

19

Miscellaneous: Primitive Neuroectodermal Tumors and Oligodendrogliomas

Primitive neuroectodermal tumors and oligodendrogliomas, although infrequent, are of sufficient interest to warrant inclusion in a book on pediatric brain tumors. Both tumors raise unanswered questions concerning management, prognosis, and biology. The primitive neuroectodermal tumor, and to a lesser extent the oligodendroglioma, represents a pathologic quagmire. There is much confusion regarding the pathologic criteria for separating primitive neuroectodermal tumors from other neuroectodermal malignancies of the central nervous system, such as cerebral neuroblastomas, medulloepitheliomas, medulloblastomas, ependymoblastomas, and pineoblastomas. Although features of oligodendrogliomas are relatively clear-cut, the mixed gliomatous elements frequently found in this tumor raise questions regarding natural history. Because the pathology relative to the degree of clinical malignancy is confusing for oligodendrogliomas, framing treatment protocols that will allow firm conclusions has been difficult. In the following sections, the problems associated with each of these tumors will be addressed separately.

PRIMITIVE NEUROECTODERMAL TUMORS

In 1973, Hart and Earle (23) described a group of tumors with common pathological and clinical features, which they termed primitive neuroectodermal tumors. The tumors were found in the cerebrum of children and young adults. They were clinically malignant and had a rapid course from diagnosis to death. It is this group of classical PNETs that will be addressed in this chapter.

There does not appear to be a sex preference in the cases reported to date. Most primitive neuroectodermal tumors occur in very young children. In Tomita's (71) study of 17 children, 15 were less than 5 years of age at diagnosis. In contrast, Grant (21) reported 10 patients with primitive neuroectodermal tumors, of whom 5 were from 20 to 66 years of age. From a compiled series of 47 recently reported cases, the average age at diagnosis was 12 years; and of these, 24 were 5 years or less at diagnosis (15,19,21,24,54,66).

Brain Tumors in Children: Principles of Diagnosis and Treatment, 2/e, edited by M.E. Cohen and P.K. Duffner, Raven Press, Ltd., New York, 1994.

Location

Primitive neuroectodermal tumors are primarily hemispheric in location, most typically involving the frontal, temporal, and/or parietal lobes. There have also been reports of primitive neuroectodermal tumors located in the spinal cord (12).

Pathology

Grossly, primitive neuroectodermal tumors are sharply delineated from surrounding brain tissue. Necrotic areas and cyst formations are commonly present. The tumors have been variably described as hemorrhagic, soft, lobulated, and occasionally encapsulated. Calcification may be identified. As the tumor may reach considerable size, increased intracranial pressure and mass effect are to be expected.

Microscopically, primitive neuroectodermal tumors consist of small, undifferentiated cells without observable cytoplasm and dark oval to irregular nuclei. Because of their marked cellularity, they appear grossly basophilic with hematoxylin and eosin stain (35). Numerous mitotic figures, areas of vascular endothelial hyperplasia, and necrosis are often present. Although the tumor is 90 to 95% undifferentiated, focal areas of differentiation may be recognized (Fig. 19-1). Differentiation may be along either neuronal or

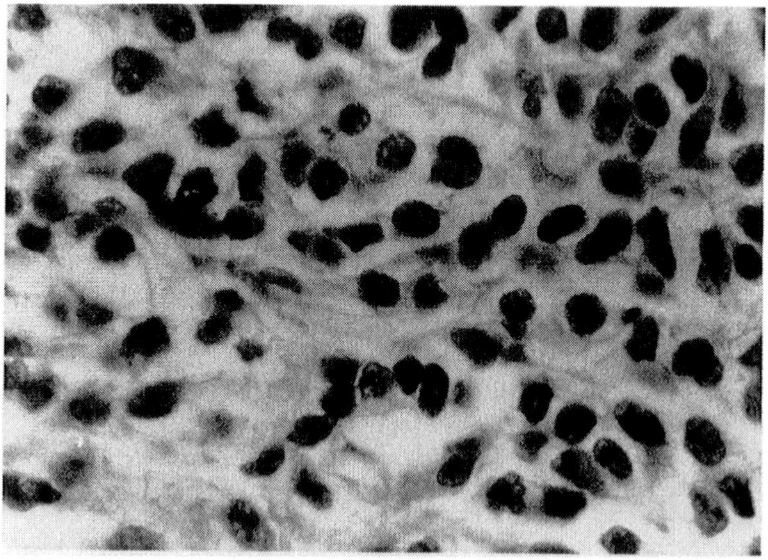

FIG. 19-1. Microscopic pathology of primitive neuroectodermal tumor characterized by small, undifferentiated cells with little cytoplasm.

glial cell lines. The neuronal differentiation is characterized by an increase in cell size and an increase in the amount of cytoplasm. As the tumor differentiates along neuronal lines, Homer-Wright rosettes with central fibrillary tangles and prominent nucleoli are recognized. Glial differentiation is characterized by an increase in cell size and formation of glial processes. Early glial differentiation is demonstrated by a spongioblastic appearance of the cells. At times ependymomatous features are recognized, characterized by the presence of perivascular pseudorosettes. Other areas of the tumor may reflect oligodendroglial differentiation. A prominent mesenchymal component has been frequently reported in series of patients with primitive neuroectodermal tumors.

On ultrastructural examination, the tumor cells have been noted to have similarities to the developing cortical plate of the fetus, suggesting that the predominant cell is a primitive undifferentiated neuroectodermal cell of the cerebrum. The cells are small with a high nuclear-to-cytoplasmic ratio and small processes. They do not have significant junctional complexes or cytoplasmic differentiation (6,44).

Cellular differentiation may at times be recognized only by electron microscopy. For instance, in one study reported by Markesbery and Challa (44), ultrastructural evaluation revealed characteristics suggestive of ependymal differentiation. However, because the tumor lacked ependymal rosettes or central canals, ependymal features would not have been recognized on light microscopy. In another study, the presence of Nissl substance and dense-core vesicles in the cytoplasm of several small cells suggested the capacity for neuronal differentiation. Such dense-core vesicles have been found in nerve terminals in the autonomic nervous system and the central nervous system, and in a variety of neuron-containing tumors and pheochromocytomas. Astrocytes are identified on ultrastructural evaluation by the presence of 80 to 90 A filaments in the cytoplasm and glial processes. As with light microscopy, ultrastructural features have supported the concept that this is a primitive multipotential cell of the cerebral hemispheres with the potential for divergent differentiation.

Immunohistochemistry is a recent adjunct in the evaluation of primitive neuroectodermal tumors. Immunohistochemistry allows differentiation of PNETs from cerebral lymphomas and undifferentiated secondary tumors. While cerebral lymphomas stain positively with antibodies to common leukocyte antigen, this staining has not been found in patients with primitive neuroectodermal tumors (21). GFAP may also be helpful in differentiating PNET from cerebral lymphomas because GFAP may be found in PNETs in the absence of obvious astrocytic differentiation. Unlike medulloblastomas, in which neuroblastic differentiation can be found in as many as 40% of cases, astrocytic differentiation is more common in cerebral PNETs (21). The theory that primitive neuroectodermal tumors, although beginning from a presumed pluripotential stem cell, may differentiate along different cell lines, is also supported by immunohistochemical studies. The finding of vimentin (suggesting cells of mesenchymal origin), GFAP (suggesting those of astrocytic origin), and cytokeratin proteins (CKP) (typically specific for epithelial cells) in PNETs suggests the differentiation possible in these tumors. It has been questioned whether the presence of CKP and vimentin are reliable indicators of tumor cell differentiation or whether they indicate abnormal protein synthesis of neoplastic cells. Grieshammer (22) has suggested that the presence of the cytokeratin proteins associated with vimentin is an indicator of an early developmental stage of the tumor cells.

Differentiation of primitive neuroectodermal tumors from a variety of other tumors with similar pathologic characteristics is often difficult. In particular, pathologically medulloblastoma and PNET have often been considered synonymous. Both are histologically malignant, with variable differentiation. Like the cerebellar medulloblastoma, PNETs may spread along the CSF axis and extraneurally. The pathologic differentiation of medulloblastomas from primitive neuroectodermal tumors, without knowledge of the site from which the tumor arose, is extremely difficult. However, GFAP staining, positive in over 90% of cases in one series of patients with PNETs, is not common in medulloblastomas and, when positive, staining is less extensive and less intense (19). Moreover, the incidence of either glial, neuronal, or mesenchymal differentiation is much higher in PNETs than in medulloblastomas, where reports of differentiation range from 20 to 25%. Furthermore, when medulloblastomas differentiate they tend toward neuronal elements, whereas PNETs are more often astrocytic. Large cysts and dense calcification are also more prominent in PNETs than in medulloblastomas. From a biologic point of view, the tumors are quite different as well. Medulloblastomas are radiosensitive, whereas PNETs are less so. Furthermore, survivals are far worse for children with PNETs than for those with medulloblastomas.

Horten and Rubinstein (27) believe that primitive neuroectodermal tumors are cerebral neuroblastomas. Cerebral neuroblastomas also occur in children, in similar locations, and have similar pathology to primitive neuroectodermal tumors. Their biologic behavior, however, is far less malignant than that of primitive neuroectodermal tumors, and they have a generally longer duration of survival. Furthermore, ultrastructural evaluation of primitive neuroectodermal tumors has shown limited evidence of neuroblastic or neuronal elements, although focal early neuroblastic differentiation has been found frequently by light microscopy. Thus, because these tumors are not purely neuroblastic, the concept that cerebral neuroblastomas and primitive neuroectodermal tumors are the same entity may not be tenable. Alternatively, cerebral neuroblastomas may represent one end of the spectrum of this highly undifferentiated tumor.

Separation of primitive neuroectodermal tumors from other primitive central nervous system malignancies is also difficult. Perhaps the major differentiating point identifying primitive neuroectodermal tumors is that although 90 to 95% of primitive neuroectodermal tumors are undifferentiated, they often show focal areas of glial and/or neuronal differentiation in addition to a prominent mesenchymal component. This should be contrasted with other neuroectodermal tumors, which are generally composed of one cell type. In addition, although primitive neuroectodermal tumors offer a wide pathologic spectrum, their clinical behavior is remarkably consistent. Unfortunately, this confusion in nosology has confounded analysis of therapeutics in the literature.

Signs And Symptoms

Clinical presentation is generally one of increased intracranial pressure and long-tract signs. Seizures are occasionally the presenting symptom. The striking clinical finding in our patients and those of others has been that, despite the huge mass of tumor bulk, the children were relatively asymptomatic. They went to school and functioned almost normally, without motor deficit, until death. Their major neurologic findings were inappropriate affect and papilledema reflecting increased intracranial pressure. Hemiparesis, when present, was mild. Seizures were readily controlled with anticonvulsant medication. These signs and symptoms are echoed in other reports in the literature. The most common presenting symptom in the literature has been headache followed by nausea, vomiting, and seizures. Motor abnormalities, including hemiparesis and paraparesis, as well as papilledema, have been common presenting physical abnormalities. Symptoms at presentation vary with age at diagnosis. Therefore, the very young child is more likely to present with an enlarged head circumference whereas the older patients more commonly have papilledema. Abnormalities of vision have also been reported in several studies.

In general, the duration of symptoms to diagnosis is short. Hart and Earle (23) reported an average duration of 4.8 months with a range of 0 to 3 years; Kosnik et al. (35) reported an average duration of symptoms before diagnosis of 3 weeks. In our own study (15), symptoms occurred over a period of 6 weeks to 6 months with an average of 3.5 months. Short duration of symptoms is more typical in the young child. For example, in a study by Pigott (54), the patients' age at diagnosis ranged from 11 months to 5 years, and duration of symptoms ranged from 1 week to a maximum of 12 weeks. Although there are occasional cases in the literature (21) with duration of symptoms prior to diagnosis exceeding 8 years, long duration before diagnosis is distinctly unusual. Indeed, in one case reported by Hart and Earle (23), symptoms preceded diagnosis by 3 years, a sufficiently unusual period of time for them to bring it specifically to the readers' attention.

Diagnosis

Primitive neuroectodermal tumors are characterized on CT scan as large supratentorial mass lesions (Fig. 19-2). Compression of adjacent brain and

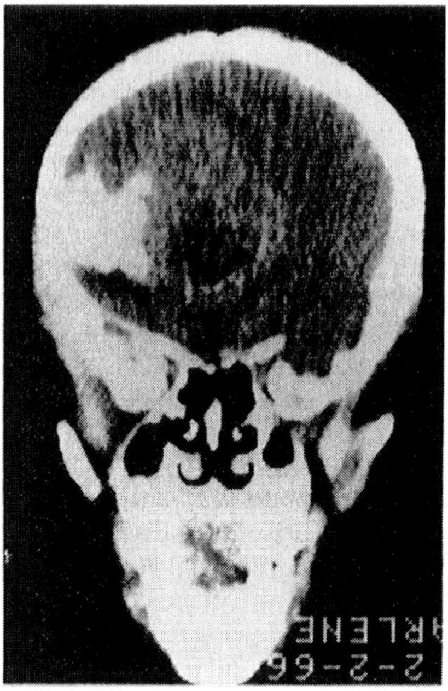

FIG. 19-2. CT scan in coronal projection of a 13-year-old patient with PNET. Note extensive calcification and ring-like enhancement of tumor.

lateral ventricles and a midline shift are typical. On the noncontrast-enhanced scan, the tumors are isodense to hyperdense with some foci of hypodensity. The areas of hypodensity are typically associated with tumor necrosis. Calcification is readily identified on CT and can be quite extensive. Cystic lesions are also recognized. The tumors enhance with contrast to varying degrees, ranging from modest to dense. Of note, the tumors are associated with little or no surrounding brain edema. Invasion of the meninges is seen at times (24).

Magnetic resonance imaging typically reveals a well defined mass without significant edema in adjacent brain. Although MRI provides a more accurate estimate of tumor size and anatomical definition than CT, calcification is not identified as well as on CT. Cystic areas are characterized by short T1 and long T2, suggesting hemorrhagic origin (Fig. 19-3). Angiography may also be useful prior to surgery because it identifies arterial and venous drainage as well as the vascular blush of the tumor nodules (18,54). Extensive neovascularity is sometimes seen (24). Since PNETs often seed the subarachnoid space, a metastatic workup, including an MRI of the spine as well as evaluation of CSF for cytology, should be performed.

Treatment

The initial approach to PNETs is surgical. Although gross total resection is often attempted, the extensive nature of the tumor as well as its vascularity

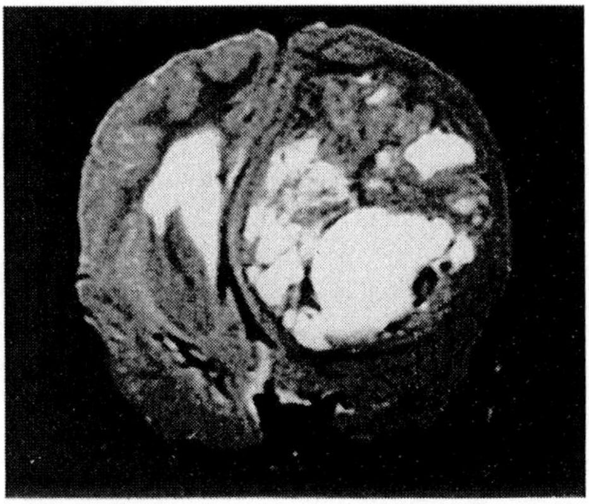

FIG. 19-3. MRI of infant with PNET. Note large mass, shift of midline structures, and lack of edema.

often limits success. Extrapolating from the medulloblastoma experience would suggest that maximum surgical removal would be beneficial. The actual number of patients with PNETs in the literature having achieved gross total resection is limited. Some authors have reported better survivals with this tumor type when gross total resection is achieved (66). Alternatively, Tomita (71) analyzed 10 of his own patients and 4 in the literature who had received gross total resection without resulting in surgical death. Four of the 14 survived 2 years or more, while 12 of 39 who had had subtotal resection or less survived 2 years. Statistical analysis did not reveal that degree of surgical resection correlated with survival.

Surgery alone is not curative and, except in infants, is typically followed by cranial irradiation with and without radiation to the neuraxis. There are no large studies of children with supratentorial PNETs by which to assess various treatment options. Since the tumors are well known to seed the cerebrospinal fluid axis, most authors recommend craniospinal radiation. Others provide only whole-brain radiation with a boost to the primary if a metastatic workup is negative. This approach is based on the assumption that the first site of failure (as in ependymomas) is the primary site. The risks of this approach were demonstrated in one study (19). Of 16 evaluable patients, 10 received only local radiation and an additional 5 received a maximum of 2500 cGy to the spine. Of these, 4 did not progress and 4 experienced recurrence only in the primary site. Of the remainder, recurrence occurred only in the subarachnoid space in 4 patients and simultaneously in the primary and subarachnoid space in 3. Although 1 child experienced failure in the subarachnoid space after having received adequate spinal radiation, i.e., 3450 cGy, this child had a positive myelogram at diagnosis. These data suggest that the high incidence of neuraxis failures should mandate craniospinal radiation (in standard doses) at the outset.

The role of chemotherapy has yet to be determined. We (15) previously reported three patients treated with surgery, radiation, and a chemotherapy protocol consisting of methotrexate, vincristine, 1,3 Bis (2-chlorethyl)-1-nitrosourea (BCNU), and dexamethasone. All children were committed to as complete a surgical removal as possible. The patients received whole-brain radiation in doses of 6,000 cGy. Chemotherapy included intermediate dose i.v. methotrexate 500 mg/m^2, intrathecal methotrexate 12 mg/m^2, weekly i.v. vincristine 2 mg/m^2, and dexamethasone 8 mg/m^2 by mouth. One child was neurologically stable for 11 months. When his CT scan showed evidence of tumor increasing in size and clinical examination revealed increasing proptosis, we added procarbazine 100 mg/m^2 by mouth. The proptosis responded readily, and the patient was stable for another 6 months before death. In a second case, the patient responded to initial surgery and radiotherapy for 14 months. At the time of recurrence she was treated with a repeat operation and the chemotherapy protocol outlined above. The patient remained symptom-free for 16 months, after which recurrent tumor was documented on neuroradiologic and clinical studies. At this point she was treated with 100 mg/m^2 procarbazine. She had prompt clinical and radiologic improvement for the next 6 months. The third case responded to initial surgery, radiation, and chemotherapy for a total of 13 months. At the time of diagnosis of recurrence, diffuse intracranial and extracranial involvement was found and no further therapy was attempted.

On the basis of these cases, we were encouraged that chemotherapy might be effective. However, Tomita (71) surveyed the literature on 24 patients with either primary or recurrent PNETs. He found no statistical difference in long-term survival between those treated with or without adjuvant chemotherapy. Despite this, since many PNETs occur in infancy, chemotherapy is the treatment modality of choice for these children. Results have been extremely poor. In recently published data, infants with primitive neuroectodermal tumors on the Pediatric Oncology Group protocol treated with postoperative Cytoxan, vincristine, cis-platinum, and VP16 fared significantly worse in both progression-free and overall survival compared with infants having tumors of different histologies.

"Eight-in-one" is another chemotherapeutic regimen that has been used in young children with PNETs. The regimen includes VCR, CCNU, procarbazine, hydroxyurea, cis-platinum, cytosine, arabinoside, methylprednisolone, and either cyclophosphamide or DTIC. In Figueroa's (18) study, three children were treated with eight-in-one. Two had stable disease for periods less than 1 year, and the third remained stable for 7 years. These encouraging results are contrasted with another study in which eight-in-one was used on three children either preoperatively or postoperatively. Of these, two failed between 3 and 4 months following onset of treatment, and a third is alive 16 months later. The use of eight-in-one at recurrence was ineffective in one child. The three long-term survivors in Gaffney's (19) study (7 to 11 years) had been treated with vincristine and CCNU. Thus, data are insufficient at this time to make firm recommendations regarding chemotherapy.

Overall, the outcome for children with PNETs is quite poor. We reviewed the literature up to 1991 and found 75 cases of children less than 18 years of age with PNETs, of whom one was lost to follow-up (4,8,15,18,19,21,24, 31,33,50,54,66,71,76) (Table 19-1). Of these, 55 are dead. Of the 19 survivors, only 12 have been followed beyond 2 years. Those patients with 90% or more undifferentiated tumors have a worse survival, with an 11% 2-year survival in one study (19). There have been reports of recurrence not only in the primary site and in the neuraxis but also extraneurally (50). One of our patients had metastases to the spinal cord as well as to the lungs; tracheal, bronchial, and pulmonary hilar lymph nodes; the pericardium; the diaphragm; and the liver. A child with a congenital cerebral PNET was reported by Yu et al. (76). The infant presented with a large head as well as cutaneous lesions in the neck and enlarged cervical lymph nodes. On biopsy, the cervical lymph nodes were almost totally replaced by metastatic tumor. In addition, cutaneous lesions in the posterior auricular region had similar findings as that found in the lymph nodes. Another child treated 3 years earlier for a PNET developed a retroperitoneal mass while his head CT remained normal (24).

In summary, primitive neuroectodermal tumors are highly malignant tumors found in the cerebral hemispheres of children and young adults. They are grossly cystic with sharp borders and hemorrhagic features. Microscopic examination reveals 90 to 95% undifferentiation with the capacity to differentiate along neural and glial lines. A prominent mesenchymal component may be seen. In general, primitive neuroectodermal tumors are associated with a short course from onset of symptoms to diagnosis and death with an estimated 5-year survival of only 20% (28). The tumors may spread along the cerebrospinal fluid axis as well as extraneurally. Aggressive treatment with surgery, radiation, and chemotherapy has been attempted, but results are still extremely poor. Because of their propensity to seed the cerebrospinal fluid, craniospinal radiation is recommended.

OLIGODENDROGLIOMAS

Oligodendrogliomas are relatively uncommon tumors, accounting for 4 to 7% of all primary intracranial gliomas. They are much more unusual in children, representing less than 1% of tumors seen in childhood. There were no reports of oligodendrogliomas in Matson's (45) pediatric series of 751 cases; and in the series by Farwell et al. (17) from the Connecticut Tumor Registry, oligodendrogliomas were found to be less than 1% of the 467 childhood brain tumors reported. Although the tumor is found in all age groups, it is rare in the young child and is more likely to be seen in the adolescent (5,70). There

TABLE 19-1. *Cerebral PNETs in children*

Author	Surgery	RT (cGy) Brain (tumor)	RT (cGy) SPCD	Chemotherapy	Outcome
Tomita (71)	GTR	5040	—	—	Dead, 10 mos
	PR	5040 (6120)	—	—	Dead, 6 mos
	GTR	4120 (5020)	—	—	Dead, 9 mos
	PR	5040	—	—	Dead, 10 mos
	PR	—	—	—	Dead, 4 days
	GTR	5040	—	—	Alive, 60 mos
	BX	5018	2583	BCNU + VCR + IT-MTX (post-RT) AZQ (recurrence)	Alive, 56 mos
	GTR	4482 (5020)	2500	8-in-1 (pre-RT) VCR + cyclo (recurrence) VP-16 + ifosfamide (recurrence)	Dead, 15 mos
	STR	5040	2500	8-in-1 (recurrence) VP-16 + ifosfamide (recurrence)	Dead, 13 mos
	GTR	4448	3450 (4448)	8-in-1 (post-RT)	Dead, 4 mos
	GTR	—	—	—	Alive, 18 mos
	GTR	—	—	CCNU + VCR + PCZ	Dead, 4.5 mos
	GTR	5040	2520	none	Dead, 6 mos
	STR	—	—	8-in-1	Alive, 16 mos
	GTR	2520 (5400)	2520	VP-16 + ifosfamide (recurrence)	Dead, 15 mos
	GTR	2520 (6000)	2520	—	Alive, 12 mos
	PR	—	—	CCNU (postop)	Dead, 2 mos
Figueroa (18)	STR	5040	2995	+ (8-in-1)	Alive, 5 yr
	PR	—	—	+ (8-in-1)	Alive, on chemo
	STR	—	—	+ (8-in-1)	Alive, on chemo
	+	—	—	—	Dead, postop
Pigott (54)	STR	—	—	—	Dead, 2 wks
	STR	+	—	+	Dead, 8 mos
	GTR	—	—	+	Dead, 3 mos
	STR	+	+	+	Dead, 6 mos
	STR	—	—	—	Dead, 15 mos
Grant (21)	STR	6000	—	—	Alive, 70 mos
	BX	—	—	—	Dead, postop
	GTR	4500	—	—	Dead, 3 mos
	STR	5280	—	+	Dead, 10 mos
	STR	—	—	—	Dead, 2 mos
Yu (76)	BX	—	—	+	Dead, 2 mos
Songpaibool (66)	BX	6000	3000	—	Dead, 7 mos
	GTR	—	—	—	Dead, postop
	GTR	5000	—	—	Alive, 32 mos
	PR	5000	2000	—	Dead, 6 mos
Gaffney (19)	PR	5000	+	—	Dead, 7 mos
	PR	5700	+	+	Alive, 7 yr
	?	5500	—	—	Dead, 8 mos
	PR	5500	+	+	Dead, 31 mos
	PR	5500	+	+	Dead, 10 mos
	BX	5000	—	—	Lost
	STR	5000	+	+	Alive, 11 yr
	STR	5000	—	—	Dead, 8 mos

TABLE 19-1. *(Continued)*

		RT (cGy)			
Author	Surgery	Brain (tumor)	SPCD	Chemotherapy	Outcome
Parker (50)	"S"	—	—	—	Dead, postop
	"S"	—	—	—	Dead, postop
	"S"	—	—	—	Alive, 3 yr
	"S"	+	—	—	Dead, 21 mos
	"S"	—	—	—	Dead, postop
	"S"	—	—	—	Dead, 1 day
	"S"	+	—	—	Dead, 18 mos
Knapp (33)	STR	3500 (5100)	2800	VCR, cyclo, trifluorodeoxithymidine	Dead, 7 mos
	PR	3000 (5000)	—	VCR, BCNU, VCR, cyclo, TFD (rec)	Dead, 10 mos
Baum (4)	PR	+	+	—	Dead, 20 mos
	GTR	+	+	HD, MTX	2nd malignancy
	PR	+	+	VCR, CCNU, PCZ	Dead, 9 mos
	STR	+	+	—	Dead, 7 mos
	STR	+	+	—	Dead, 3 mos
	STR	early			Alive
Hinshaw (24)	PR	4928 (5504)	—	—	Alive, 2 yr
	GTR	5200	—	Cyclo, VCR, adri, actino	Dead, 4 yr
	STR	Begun	—	—	Dead, 1 mo
	PR	3500	—	—	Alive, 3 yr
Duffner (15)	PR	5000 (6000)	—	MTX, VCR, BCNU, dex	Dead, 18 mos
	STR	6000	—	MTX, VCR, BCNU, dex	Dead, 39 mos
	STR	5000	—	MTX, VCR, BCNU, dex	Dead, 16 mos
Jenkin (31)	STR	5250	—	—	Dead
	STR	5100	—	—	Alive, 4 yr
	STR	5000	—	—	Dead
	GTR	5200	—	—	Alive, 4 yr
	STR	5250	—	CCNU, VCR	Dead
Bruno (8)	"S"	—	—	—	Dead, 1 day
	"S"	—	—	—	Dead, 3 days
	"S"	3780	—	—	Alive, 12 mos
	—	—	—	—	Dead, 4 days

Adapted (in part) from Tomita T, McLone DG, Yasue M. Cerebral primitive neuroectodermal tumors in childhood. *J Neurooncol* 1988;6:233–243.

S, surgery; GTR, gross total resection; PR, partial resection; MTX, methotrexate; VCR, vincristine; DEX, dexamethasone; cyclo, cyclophosphamide; actino, actinomycin; HD, high dose; PCZ, procarbazine; 8-in-1, VCR, CCNU, PCZ, hydroxyurea, cis-platinum, cytosine arabinoside, methylprednisolone, and either cyclo or DTIC.

is a male/female distribution of approximately 2:1 (13). Although there is no hereditary predisposition, an association among siblings has been reported (51). Most oligodendrogliomas occur in the cerebral hemispheres with a frontal lobe predominance. However, rare cases of intraventricular as well as posterior fossa oligodendrogliomas have been identified (14,49). Occasionally, this tumor has been reported in the spinal cord.

Pathology

Oligodendrogliomas, as with many other neoplasms of the central nervous system, were originally described by Bailey and Bucy (2). Pure forms of the tumor are usually not encountered. Rather, the oligodendroglioma is found to represent the predominant cell type in a mixed glioma. During surgery a festoon-like pattern has been recognized (34). As a result, the neoplastic tissue appears flattened and pale when compared to surrounding brain. Occasionally, mucoid and cystic degeneration are recognized. Koos and Miller (34) indicate that blue-red lumps may be encountered, projecting to the surface like mushrooms. In general, oligodendrogliomas are firm and gray-red in nature. The tumor may be friable, calcified, or necrotic. Although foci of calcification may not be identified roentgenographically, microcalcification is invariably seen on histologic sections (58).

The tumor has a characteristic honeycomb appearance consisting of a monotonous collection of uniform cells with spheroid appearance and clear cytoplasm (Fig. 19-4). In addition to pale perinuclear halos, the cytoplasm may contain basophilic material that stains for mucin. Compact areas of tumor may lack the honeycomb appearance. Mitotic figures are variable and may be easily identified from field to field. According to Gilles et al. (20), the finding of oligodendrogliocytes in mixed glioma, regardless of the predominant histologic cell, suggests a benign prognosis. Rubinstein (58) has emphasized the presence of connective tissue, which may separate oligodendrogliocytes into clusters and clumps. Recognition of perivascular collars, pseudorosettes, and gemistocytic astrocytes may add to the diagnostic confusion. Palisading of tumor cells similar to that seen in astrocytomas is not unusual.

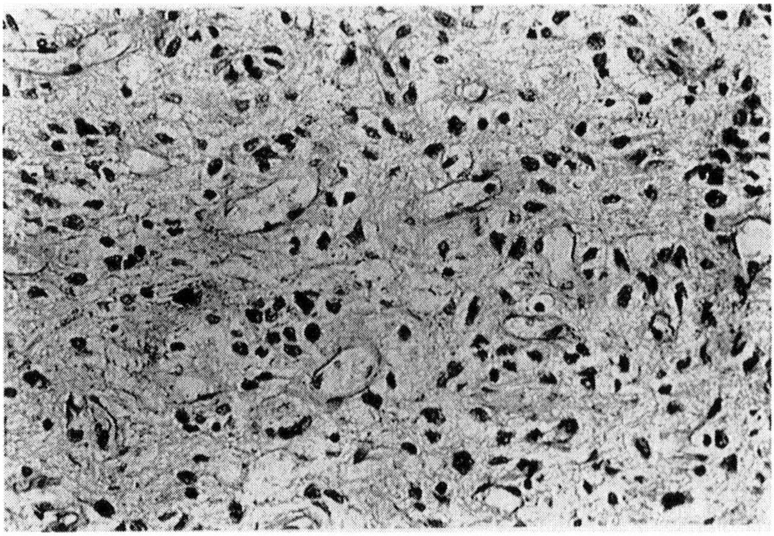

FIG. 19-4. Microscopic section of oligodendroglioma showing honeycomb appearance, which consists of uniform cells with perinuclear halos.

Attempts have been made to identify histologic features that predict transition of the tumor from a benign to a malignant pattern of behavior (3). Unlike the transition of astrocytoma to glioblastoma multiforme, there are no specific features of the oligodendrogliocyte that enable the pathologist to identify characteristics suggesting malignant transformation. Although Kernohan (16) initially suggested a classification of oligodendroblastoma for the more malignant-appearing tumors, later publications refuted this nosology. The pathologic features that characterize malignancy in other gliomas have not shown a similar correspondence between pathology and clinical behavior in patients with oligodendrogliomas (16). Despite these qualifications, Barnard (3) has suggested several histologic features that correlate with malignant behavior. In citing the clinical course of five cases, he suggests two ways in which malignant changes may occur. In the first instance malignancy is related to the degree of cellular differentiation; and in the second instance, although oligodendrogliomatous features may remain constant, concomitant neoplastic proliferation of astroglial cells may be found. The neoplastic cells are theorized to arise by proliferation of astroblasts attached to blood vessels or from the surrounding fibrous glia. This transition from benign to malignant behavior may not occur for many years, thus accounting for the protracted courses seen in many patients. The malignant behavior of the tumor may subsequently accelerate, resulting in a rapidly progressive terminal course.

Oligodendrogliomas have been graded according to a variety of classifications. The system most commonly used is Smith's (64) from the Armed Forces Institute of Pathology. Five histologic features are the basis for grading a tumor from A to D. Features include endothelial proliferation, necrosis, high nuclear-to-cytoplasmic ratio, high cell density, and pleomorphism. In grade A tumors all five features are either absent or low. In grade B tumors, either pleomorphism is present and/or the cell density and nuclear-to-cytoplasmic ratio is high. Grade C tumors are characterized by pleomorphism, high nuclear-to-cytoplasmic ratio, high cell density, and endothelial proliferation. Grade D tumors are those in which all five features are both present and high. On the basis of this classification, median survivals for grade A tumors were 94 months, grade B tumors 51 months, grade C tumors 45 months, and grade D tumors 17 months. Pleomorphism was the only factor significantly correlated with survival by itself (64). Others have also developed grading systems. Burger (10) evaluated histologic variables in patients with oligodendroglioma and compared them with postoperative survival. The most important prognostic factors in a univariate analysis were mitoses, necrosis, nuclear cytologic atypia, vascular hypertrophy, and vascular proliferation. The only independently significant variable was necrosis. When Burger analyzed cases according to the Smith classification, he found that most tumors in his study lacked a marked degree of pleomorphism. Thus, although pleomorphism was associated with shorter survivals, a statistically significant association could not be determined.

In yet another histologic classification, Mork et al. (46) correlated histologic features with survival in patients from Norway with oligodendrogliomas. Histologic features of prognostic significance were microcysts, necrosis, and cell density. Of interest, endothelial proliferation, calcification, nuclear atypia, perivascular lymphocytic infiltration, and leptomeningeal invasion were not prognostic. Overall, those patients whose tumors had low cell density, microcystic changes, and no necrosis survived longer. A poor but not significantly worse prognosis was also found in patients who had subpial tumor cell infiltration. Unlike in Smith's grading system, endothelial proliferation was not prognostic, and unlike in Burger's classification, mitoses were not associated with a worse prognosis.

Kros et al. (36) compared Kernohan's grading system of four grades based on cell density, neuropil, cell appearance, pleomorphism, hyperchromasia, vascular and endothelial proliferation, mitotic rate, necrosis, cysts, and calcium with the Smith classification. The relationship between grade of tumor and survival was determined in 72 patients. The authors found that the longest survivals were in Smith's grade A and Kernohan's grade 1 categories, while patients in Smith's grade D and Kernohan's grade 4 categories were associated with a shorter survival. The intermediate grades of B and C and 2 and 3 did not differ significantly from each other. On the basis of this study, Kros et al. suggested that reducing the grading system from four grades to three would provide a more concise classification for oligodendrogliomas.

The same authors analyzed the prognostic relevance of DNA flow cytometry in oligodendrogliomas. Although approximately a third of the tumors were diploid, tetraploid, or aneuploid, there was no correlation with survival. Gemistocytes were identified as associated with a poor prognosis. Kros' analysis supported the validity of Smith's grading system as well as Burger's (10) premise that mitoses impacted adversely on prognosis. Since the number of mitoses was of prognostic significance, Kros (38) recommended that this factor should be incorporated into Smith's grading system (38).

Clinical Signs and Symptoms

Because most oligodendrogliomas occur in the cerebral hemispheres, symptomatology and clinical signs relate in large measure to the area of the brain involved. Seizures are by far the most common presenting symptom in most series of patients with oligodendrogliomas (1,13,73). The incidence of patients with oligodendrogliomas presenting with seizures approaches 50 to 70% (1). Many children with oligodendrogliomas are diagnosed as part of a seizure evaluation. Over one-third of patients in one study (13) had no neurologic deficit and had presented for evaluation only because of seizure disorders. Pelc et al. (53) reported an interesting, albeit unusual, case of an infant 5 months of age with right-sided seizures. Over the next 9.5 years the patient was evaluated on many occasions for generalized and focal motor seizures. At age 10, the findings of optic atrophy, left temporal bone protrusion, and intracranial calcification led to surgical identification of a large oligodendroglioma. In adult series, patients with seizures have a longer duration of survival than those without. This may relate to the fact that the patients are in better condition at the time of presentation and also have had a slower clinical course than patients who present with signs and symptoms of increased intracranial pressure. Other prominent symptoms include nausea, vomiting, headaches, lethargy, and dementia.

Usual clinical features are those of increased intracranial pressure (papilledema) and focal motor signs. Ataxia was present in 39% of patients in Ludwig's (42) series. The ataxia was believed to be secondary to frontal lobe dysfunction rather than cerebellar disease. In addition, in the same series hemorrhage was identified in 22% of patients. The hemorrhage was, at times, associated with coma or stroke. When cerebrovascular accident occurred in the presence of an intracranial glioma, oligodendrogliomas were the most likely underlying tumor. Finally, meningismus was found in 13% of patients, reflecting leptomeningeal spread. Of interest, none of these symptoms correlated with tumor grade. In another study (69) the presence of dementia was associated with a shorter postoperative survival than the presence of other symptoms.

Neuroimaging

Before CT, radiologic diagnosis of an oligodendroglioma was often based on the finding of a calcified intracerebral mass in a patient with a longstanding history of seizures. The presence of a mass lesion was further confirmed by either air encephalography, angiography, or both. The advent of CT and MRI has allowed preoperative characterization of the lesion. The masses are typically sharply demarcated without much surrounding edema (40). Tumor calcification is common but not invariable. The morphology of the calcification is either nodular, shell-like, or ring-like (73). Hemorrhage and cysts are also found frequently. Contrast enhancement, although present in about 50% of cases, is usually mild or poorly defined.

Oligodendrogliomas may commonly be confused with either nonneoplastic cysts or old infarcts since the lesions are typically hypodense or isodense on CT scan. This is particularly true in those patients in whom the tumors do not enhance with contrast (Fig. 19-5). Two points are useful in differentiating old infarcts from oligodendrogliomas. Because oligodendrogliomas are typically located in the frontal lobe, erosion of the inner table is common. Erosion of the inner table of the skull may not be identified on skull films but is readily identified on CT scan. Bony erosion suggests a chronic expanding process rather than an infarct. In addition, whereas nonneoplastic cysts tend

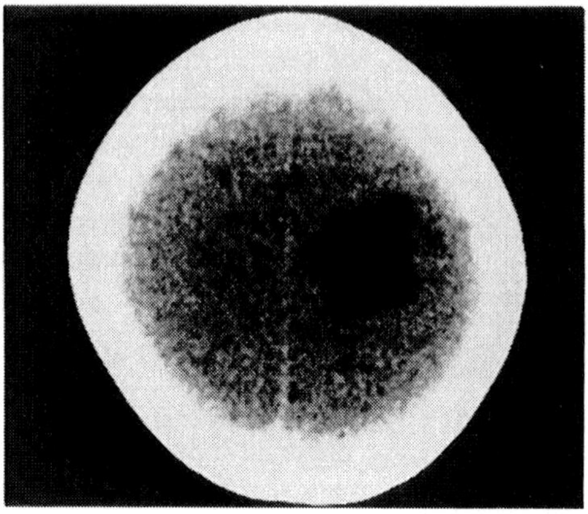

FIG. 19-5. Axial CT showing nonenhancing low-density mass in midportion of left parietal lobe. Patient had presented with focal seizures. Initial CT diagnosis was infarct.

to have smooth borders, oligodendrogliomas have irregular margins, suggesting that the lesion is neoplastic rather than cystic. The absence of enhancement, as in astrocytomas, is not diagnostic and does not exclude neoplasm (72). Although the presence of enhancement and cystic components is said to be strongly suggestive of malignancy, this concept is not universally supported (73).

There are rare cases of intraventricular oligodendrogliomas (14). These are unusual lesions representing only 1.3 to 10% of all oligodendrogliomas. The tumors are typically located in the anterior portion of the lateral ventricles. They have different CT characteristics than typical cerebral oligodendrogliomas in that they are usually hyperintense with small cystic hypodense lesions in the bulk of the matrix. As in most oligodendrogliomas, there is clumped calcification. Hydrocephalus is a constant feature of these lesions.

MRI has also been a useful adjunct not only in diagnosing patients with oligodendrogliomas but also in planning radiation therapy (63). The typical MR features are hypointensity on T1 and hyperintensity on T2. MR allows better differentiation of margins than CT and hence allows more accurate radiation planning.

Extraneural Metastases

Extraneural metastases have been reported with oligodendrogliomas (29,48,67). Among a series of 240 primary CNS gliomas that metastasized extraneurally, oligodendrogliomas represented the seventh most frequent neoplasm (2.7%) (52). The duration following diagnosis to metastases ranged from 18 to 86 months. MacDonald et al. (43) reported 7 of their own patients with oligodendrogliomas and 15 in the literature whose tumors had metastasized to lymph nodes, bone, scalp, muscle, and pleura. Whereas some studies have suggested that extraneural metastases occur in patients with longer than anticipated survivals (allowing the metastatic implants to become clinically significant), in their series patients with extraneural metastases did not have longer survivals than those without. Two patterns of spread were identified. Pattern 1 was defined as spread to the scalp and regional lymph nodes followed by subsequent distant metastases. This pattern was found in patients who had had multiple craniotomies. In pattern 2, distant metastases occurred in the absence of local scalp or regional lymph node involvement. Patients with pattern 2 typically had received early aggressive therapy with radiation and chemotherapy. MacDonald et al. and others have queried whether aggressive treatment changes tumor biology, allowing the recurring tumor to become more aggressive and more widely disseminated. Of importance, systemic metastases responded to both focal radiotherapy and chemotherapy.

Spread within the central nervous system is also frequently present (68). Jellinger (30) reported that of 65 oligodendrogliomas in his series, 29% had invaded meninges. Thus, although extraneural metastases from anaplastic oligodendrogliomas are still relatively unusual, spread within the central nervous system is quite common. A neuraxis evaluation should be done before one embarks on radiation and/or chemotherapy.

Treatment

Surgery

Radical tumor resection should be the goal of the neurosurgeon. A gross total resection has been associated with the best progression-free survivals, with the average postoperative survival greater than 7 years (26). However, many studies that emphasize the improved survival for patients with gross total resection do not emphasize the fact that those tumors that can be gross totally resected are typically of lower histologic grade and often occur in patients less than 20 years of age. Both young age and low histologic grade are good prognostic factors regardless of degree of surgical resection (60).

The role of radiation in the treatment of oligodendrogliomas is still in dispute. Most of the literature from the late 1980s and early 1990s recommends that radiation be given to patients with subtotal resections. Unfortunately, virtually all the studies published to date have been retrospective. Thus, these studies must be viewed with some skepticism. Shaw et al. (60) reported 81 patients with pure oligodendrogliomas. There was no advantage identified in adding radiation to patients with gross total resection. In contrast, those patients who had had subtotal resection had significantly better survivals if they were irradiated with greater than 5,000 cGy. Lindegaard (41) retrospectively reviewed 170 patients with oligodendrogliomas from 1953 to 1977. In this study, postoperative radiation was also found to improve survival significantly in subtotally resected patients ($P = 0.0089$). However, the influence on survival was only temporary. Although the 5-year survival without radiation was 27% compared to 36% with radiation, by 8 years there was no significant difference in survival between the two groups. In contrast, Wallner et al. (74) reported a retrospective study of 42 patients with intracranial oligodendrogliomas. Postoperative radiation, greater than 45 Gy, provided a significant survival advantage. The 10-year survival of 14 patients treated with more than 45 Gy following surgery was 56% versus 18% in 11 patients treated with surgery alone.

Others (55) have questioned the role of radiation even in subtotally resected patients with oligodendrogliomas. Bullard (9) reported a retrospective study of 71 patients with oligodendrogliomas. There was no significant difference in survival between those patients treated with surgery and those treated with surgery plus radiation. Similarly, Reedy (55) reported 57 cases from the Cleveland Clinic and found no advantage to postoperative radiation. However, the limits of retrospective reviews extending over 30 years are well known and preclude definitive conclusions.

The presence or absence of radiation is not the only prognostic factor to have been identified. Factors associated with improved survival include young age (i.e., less than 20 years), frontal or parietal location, calcification, lack of enhancement on CT scan, and low grade of tumor (60). Tumor grade has been a consistently strong prognostic factor (7). As noted earlier in this chapter, grading systems of Smith, Burger, Mork, and Kernohan have attempted to prognosticate on the basis of histologic criteria. The presence or absence of seizures, temporal lobe location, tumor size, and partial versus whole-brain radiation were not associated with changes in survival in one study, but focal neurologic deficit at diagnosis was associated with a poor prognosis (75).

The vast majority of the oligodendroglioma literature is based on adult patients. Although many series have younger patients within their groups, the numbers are extremely limited. Since the incidence of oligodendrogliomas in childhood is probably less than 1%, it is unrealistic to expect a prospective study to be undertaken. One of the only reviews of children with oligodendrogliomas was published in 1978 by Dohrman et al. (13) based on the Connecticut Tumor Registry. Only 12 children were diagnosed as having oligodendrogliomas over a 41-year period. On the basis of this very limited sample, no statistically significant advantage to postoperative radiation was found. Survivals of children with oligodendrogliomas were 70% at 5 years and 58% at 10 years. Hirsch et al. (25) reported a retrospective study of 42 children with astrocytic and oligodendrocytic tumors of the cerebral hemispheres in children. Surgery was recommended as the primary treatment modality, as recurrences were extremely limited in those patients who had survived gross total resection, with a resulting 95% progression-free survival at 5 years. Radiation was limited to those patients with recurrence. Admittedly, this was a mixed group of astrocytic tumors, but the results are impressive and suggest a better prognosis than in adults.

Rarely, oligodendrogliomas may occur in the cerebellum. Four children with malignant oligodendrogliomas of the cerebellum were reported by Packer (49). Three patients received local radiation, and all tumors recurred outside the radiation field. Of importance, the disease at the primary tumor site was unchanged. Because of the high incidence of leptomeningeal disease, the authors suggested that a metastatic workup routinely be performed (as has been previously recommended) and that craniospinal radiation be strongly considered.

In summary, the value of radiation has not been conclusively demonstrated. Although recent adult literature recommends postoperative radiation with subtotally resected tumors, risk factors must be taken into consideration. Since patients with high-grade oligodendrogliomas are at increased risk for early recurrence, radiation therapy should be considered in these patients. Alternatively, others have suggested that a child with a low-grade oligodendroglioma should be followed after surgery and given radiation only at time of progression (61,62). Because recurrence of oligodendrogliomas is variable and may not be manifest for long periods of time, continuous assessment may be the most prudent approach (65).

Chemotherapy appears to be effective for malignant oligodendrogliomas. This approach has been advanced by Cairncross et al. (11). A combination of procarbazine, CCNU, and vincristine (PCV) was associated with both clinical and neuroradiologic responses. Eight patients with malignant oligodendrogliomas were treated with chemotherapy at recurrence. Six of them were treated with PCV, one with BCNU, and one with AZQ. All patients had partial responses, with the exception of one patient who achieved a complete response. Responses were durable; at least half lasted longer than a year at the time of report. Similarly, good results were reported by Kyritsis et al. (39) using a PCV regimen in recurrent anaplastic oligodendrogliomas. Of interest, those patients treated at initial diagnosis with adjuvant chemotherapy actually fared worse than those treated with conventional radiotherapy.

Because large series of children with oligodendrogliomas are limited, statistical information regarding survival is, at best, presumptive. In the Connecticut series, the mean duration of survival was 103.5 months (13). Long-term survivals in the isolated patient are scattered throughout the literature (56,57). In Dohrmann's (13) study of 11 children with intracerebral gliomas, the 1-year survival was 80%, 5-year survival 70%, and 10-year survival of 58%. The lack of information regarding pathologic grade in Dohrmann's study makes this study difficult to interpret. Oligodendrogliomas are part of a Pediatric Oncology Group/Children's Cancer Group Study in which children with low-grade hemispheric tumors are treated with either total resection and follow-up or, if partially resected, either observation or local radiation. It is hoped that this study will establish whether or not radiation is necessary in this patient population and provide a better understanding of prognosis.

Summary

Oligodendrogliomas are rare tumors seen in childhood. Pathologically, although the histology is characteristic, features suggestive of a mixed glioma are usually identified. The findings of oligodendrogliocytes in a mixed glioma suggest a benign prognosis. Oligodendrogliomas may be associated with a protracted course. However, seeding of cerebrospinal fluid and extraneural metastasis are well known, as is aggressive behavior. In general, the tumor presents without signs of increased pressure or changes on neurologic examination. Focal motor seizures are the predominant symptomatology. A CT scan may show a low-density lesion intermixed with calcium with little or no shift of midline structures. As the tumor grows slowly and, other than seizures, is generally unassociated with clinical deficit, treatment initially consists of maximal surgical resection. Upon evidence of dissemination, recurrence, or high pathologic grade, radiation or combined modality therapy should be considered. The need for routine postoperative radiation following subtotal resection has not been clarified in the pediatric population.

REFERENCES

1. Backus RE, Millichap JG. The seizure as a manifestation of intracranial tumor in childhood. *Pediatrics* 1962;29:978–984.
2. Bailey P, Bucy PC. Oligodendrogliomas of the brain. *J Pathol Bacteriol* 1929;32:735–751.
3. Barnard RO. The development of malignancy in oligodendrogliomas. *J Pathol Bacteriol* 1968;96:113–123.
4. Baum ES, Morgan ER, DalCanto MC, West PM. Review of experience with primitive neuroectodermal tumors of childhood. In: Humphrey GB, Dehner LP, Grindey GB, Acton RT, eds. *Pediatric oncology 1*. The Hague:Martin Nijhoff; 1981:239–242.
5. Berkheiser SW. Oligodendrogliomas in the young age group. *J Neurosurg* 1956:13:170–175.
6. Boesel CP, Suhan JP, Bradel EJ. Ultrastructure of primitive neuroectodermal neoplasms of the central nervous system, with special note in regard to children: 20 years experience: 1939–1958. *Cancer* 1978;42:194–201.
7. Bruner JM. Oligodendroglioma: diagnosis and prognosis. *Semin Diagn Pathol* 1987;4: 251–261.
8. Bruno LA, Rorke LB, Norris DG. Primitive neuroectodermal tumors of infancy and childhood. In: Humphrey GB, Dehner LP, Grindey GB, Acton RT, eds. *Pediatric oncology 1* The Hague:Martin Nijhoff; 1981:265–267.
9. Bullard DE, Rawlings CE, Phillips B, et al. Oligodendroglioma: an analysis of the value of radiation therapy. *Cancer* 1987;60:2179–2188.
10. Burger PC, Rawlings CE, Cox EB, et al. Clinicopathologic correlations in the oligodendroglioma. *Cancer* 1987;59:1345–1352.
11. Cairncross JG, Macdonald DR. Successful chemotherapy for recurrent malignant oligodendroglioma. *Ann Neurol* 1988;23:360–364.
12. Dehner LP. Primitive neuroectodermal tumors of the central nervous system in childhood: Retrospective and overview. In: Humphrey GB, Dehner LP, Grindey GB, Acton RT, eds. *Pediatric oncology 1*. The Hague:Martinus Nijhoff; 1981:277–288.

13. Dohrmann GJ, Farwell JR, Flannery JT. Oligodendrogliomas in children. *Surg Neurol* 1978; 10:21–25.
14. Dolinskas CM, Simeone FA. CT characteristics of intraventricular oligodendrogliomas. *AJNR* 1987;8:1077–1082.
15. Duffner PK, Cohen ME, Heffner RR, Freeman AI. Primitive neuroectodermal tumors of childhood: an approach to therapy. *J Neurosurg* 1981;55:376–381.
16. Earnest F III, Kernohan JW, Craig W McK. Oligodendrogliomas: a review of 200 cases. *A M A Arch Neurol Psychiatr* 1950;63:964–976.
17. Farwell JR, Dohrmann GJ, Flannery JT. Central nervous system tumors in children. *Cancer* 1977;40:3123–3132.
18. Figueroa RE, Gammal TE, Brooks BS, et al. MR findings on primitive neuroectodermal tumors. *J Comput Assist Tomogr* 1989;13(5):773–778.
19. Gaffney CC, Sloane JP, Bradley NJ, Bloom HJG. Primitive neuroectodermal tumours of the cerebrum. *J Neurooncol* 1985:3:23–33.
20. Gilles FH, Winston J, Fulchiero A. Leviton A. Histologic features and observation variation in cerebellar gliomas in children. *J Neurosurg* 1976;45:409–415.
21. Grant JW, Steart PV, Gallagher PJ. Primitive neuroectodermal tumors of the cerebrum: a histological and immunohistochemical study of 10 cases. *Clin Neuropathol* 1988;7:228–233.
22. Grieshammer T, Zimmer C, Vogeley KT. Immunohistochemistry of primitive neuroectodermal tumors in infants with special emphasis on cytokeratin expression. *Acta Neuropathol* 1991;82:494–501.
23. Hart MN, Earle KM. Primitive neuroectodermal tumors of the brain in children. *Cancer* 1973;43:890–897.
24. Hinshaw DB Jr, Ashwal S, Thompson JR, Hasso AN. Neuroradiology of primitive neuroectodermal tumors. *Neuroradiology* 1983;25:87–92.
25. Hirsch JF, Sainte Rose C, Pierre-Kahn A, Pfister A, Hoppe-Hirsch E. Benign astrocytic and oligodendrocytic tumors of the cerebral hemispheres in children. *J Neurosurg* 1989; 70:568–572.
26. Horrax G, Wu WQ. Postoperative survival of patients with intracranial oligodendroglioma with special reference to radical tumor removal: a study of 26 patients. *J Neurosurg* 1951; 8:473–479.
27. Horten BC, Rubinstein LJ. Primary cerebral neuroblastoma: a clinicopathological study of 35 cases. *Brain* 1976;99:735–756.
28. Humphrey GB, Dehner LP, Kaplan RJ, Waters KD, Jenkin RDT, Wara WM. Overview on the management of primitive neuroectodermal tumors. In: Humphrey GB, Dehner LP, Grindey GB, Acton RT, eds. *Pediatric oncology 1*. The Hague:Martinus Nijhoff, 1981: 289–294.
29. James TGI, Pagel W. Oligodendroglioma with extracranial metastases. *Br J Surg* 1961;39: 56–65.
30. Jellinger J, Minauf M, Salzer-Kuntschik M. Oligodendroglioma with extraneural metastases. *Neurosurg Psychiatr* 1969;32:249–253.
31. Jenkin D. Primitive neuroectodermal tumour. In: Humphrey GB, Dehner LP, Grindey GB, Acton RT, eds. *Pediatric oncology 1*. The Hague:Martinus Nijhoff; 1981:243–246.
32. Kernohan JW, Maybon RF, Svien JG, et al. Symposium on new and simplified concepts of gliomas: a simplified classification of gliomas. *Proc Staff Meet Mayo Clin* 24 1949;24: 71–75.
33. Knapp J, Francini D, VanEys J, Cangir A. Primitive neuroectodermal tumors of brain in childhood: literature review and the M.D. Anderson experience. In: Humphrey GB, Dehner LP, Grindey GB, Acton RT, eds. *Pediatric oncology 1*. The Hague:Martinus Nijhoff; 1981: 215–224.
34. Koos WTh, Miller MG. *Intracranial tumors of infants and children*. St. Louis: CV Mosby; 1971.
35. Kosnik EJ, Boesel CP, Bay J, Sayers MP. Primitive neuroectodermal tumors of the central nervous system in children. *J Neurosurg* 1978;48:741–746.
36. Kros JM, Troost D, van Eden CG, Van Der Wert AJM, Uylings HBM. Oligodendroglioma: a comparison of two grading systems. *Cancer* 1988;61:2251–2259.
37. Kros JM, van Eden CG, Stefanko SZ, Waayer-Van Batenburg M, van der Kwast ThH. Prognostic implications of glial fibrillary acidic protein containing cell types in oligodendrogliomas. *Cancer* 1990;66:1204–1212.

38. Kros JM, van Eden CG, Vissers CJ, et al. Prognostic relevance of DNA flow cytometry in oligodendroglioma. *Cancer* 1992;69:1791–1798.
39. Kyritsis AP, Yung WK, Bruner J, Gleason MJ, Levin VA. The treatment of anaplastic oligodendrogliomas and mixed gliomas. *Neurosurgery* 1993;32:365–371.
40. Lee YY, Van Tassel P. Intracranial oligodendrogliomas: imaging findings in 35 untreated cases: *AJR* 1989;152:361–369.
41. Lindegaard KF, Mork SJ, Eide GE, et al. Statistical analysis of clinicopathological features, radiotherapy, and survival in 170 cases of oligodendroglioma. *J Neurosurg* 1987;67:224–230.
42. Ludwig CL, Smith MT, Godfrey AD, Armbrustmacher VW. A clinicopathological study of 323 patients with oligodendrogliomas. *Ann Neurol* 1986;19:15–21.
43. Macdonald DR, O'Brien RA, Gilbert JJ, Cairncross JG. Metastatic anaplastic oligodendroglioma. *Neurology* 1989;39:1593–1596.
44. Markesbery WR, Challa VR. Electron microscopic findings in primitive neuroectodermal tumors of the cerebrum. *Cancer* 1979;44:141–147.
45. Matson DD. *Neurosurgery of infancy and childhood.* Illinois:Charles C Thomas; 1969.
46. Mork SJ, Halvorsen TB, Lindegaard KF, Eide GE. Oligodendroglioma: histologic evaluation and prognosis. *J Neuropathol Exp Neurol* 1986;45(1):65–78.
47. Mork SJ, Lindegaard KF, Halvorsen RB, et al. Oligodendroglioma: incidence and biological behavior in a defined population. *J Neurosurg* 1985;63:881–889.
48. Ordonez NG, Ayala NG, Leavens ME. Extracranial metastases of oligodendroglioma: report of a case and review of the literature. *Neurosurgery* 1981;8:391–395.
49. Packer RJ, Sutton LN, Rorke LB, et al. Oligodendroglioma of the posterior fossa in childhood. *Cancer* 1985;56:195–199.
50. Parker JC, Mortara RH, McCloskey JJ. Biological behavior of the primitive neuroectodermal tumors: significant supratentorial childhood gliomas. *Surg Neurol* 1975;52:245–247.
51. Parkinson D, Hall CW. Oligodendrogliomas: simultaneous appearance in frontal lobes of siblings. *J Neurosurg* 1962;19:424–426.
52. Pasquier B, Pasquier D, Golet AN, Panh MH, Couderc P. Extraneural metastases of astrocytomas and glioblastoma: clinicopathological study of two cases and review of the literature. *Cancer* 1980;45:112–125.
53. Pelc S, Brihaye J, Perier O, Heimann R, Baleriaux D. Temporal lobe oligodendroglioma developing from infancy into adulthood. *Ann Neurol* 1977;2:537–540.
54. Pigott TJD, Punt JAG, Lowe JS, et al. The clinical, radiological and histopathological features of cerebral primitive neuroectodermal tumours. *Br J Neurosurg* 1990;4:287–298.
55. Reedy DP, Bay JW, Hahn JF. Role of radiation therapy in the treatment of cerebral oligodendroglioma: an analysis of 57 cases and a literature review. *Neurosurgery* 1983;5:499–503.
56. Roberts M, German W. A long term study of patients with oligodendrogliomas: Follow-up of 50 cases, including Dr. Harvey Cushing's series. *J Neurosurg* 1966;24:697–700.
57. Roberts M, German WJ. Oligodendroglioma: a 40-year survival—case report. *J Neurosurg* 1969;31:355–357.
58. Rubinstein LJ. *Tumors of the central nervous system.* Washinton, DC: Armed Forces Institute of Pathology; 1972:85–104, 259–262.
59. Russell DS, Rubinstein LJ. *Pathology of tumours of the nervous system.* Baltimore:William & Wilkins; 1989.
60. Shaw EG, Scheithauer BW, O'Fallon JR, Tazelaar HD, Davis DH. Oligodendrogliomas: the Mayo Clinic experience. *J Neurosurg* 1992;76:428–434.
61. Sheline GE. Radiation therapy of primary tumors. *Semin Oncol* 1975;2:29–42.
62. Sheline GE, Boldrey E, Karlsberg P, Phillips TL. Therapeutic considerations in tumors affecting the central nervous system: oligodendrogliomas. *Radiology* 1964;82:84–89.
63. Shuman WP, Griffin BR, Haynor DR, Jones DC. The utility of MR in planning the radiation therapy of oligodendroglioma. *AJNR* 1987;8:93–98.
64. Smith MT, Ludwig CL, Godfrey AD, Armbrustmacher VW. Grading of oligodendrogliomas. *Cancer* 1983;52:2107–2114.
65. Solitare GB, Robinson F, Lamarche JB. Oligodendroglioma: recurrence following an exceptionally long post-operative symptom-free period. *Can Med Assoc J* 1967;97:862–865.
66. Songpaibool P, Shuangshoti S, Phonprasert C, et al. Intracranial primitive neuroectodermal tumors: experience of 7 cases with particular reference to survival. *J Med Assoc Thai* 1991; 74(3):165–171

67. Spataro J, Sacks O. Oligodendroglioma with remote metastases: case report. *J Neurosurg* 1961;18:683–687.
68. Strang RR, Nordenstam H. Intracerebral oligodendroglioma with metastatic involvement of the cauda equina. *J Neurosurg* 1961;18:683–687.
69. Sun ZM, Genka S, Shitara N, Akanuma A, Takakura K. Factors possibly influencing the prognosis of oligodendroglioma. *Neurosurgery* 1988;22:886–891.
70. Svoboda DJ. Oligodendroglioma in a six-week old infant. *J Neuropathol Exp Neurol* 1959; 18:569–574.
71. Tomita T, McLone DG, Yasue M. Cerebral primitive neuroectodermal tumors in childhood. *J Neurooncol* 1988;6:233–243.
72. Varma RR, Crumrine PK, Berman I, et al. Childhood oligodendrogliomas presenting with seizures and low-density lesions on computed tomography. *Neurology* 1983;33:806–808.
73. Vonofakos D, Marcu H, Hacker H. Oligodendrogliomas: CT patterns with emphasis on features indicating malignancy. *J Comput Assist Tomogr* 1979;3(6):783–786.
74. Wallner KE, Gonzales M, Sheline GR. Treatment of oligodendrogliomas with or without postoperative irradiation. *J Neurosurg* 1988;68:684–688.
75. Wilkinson IMS, Anderson JR, Holmes AE. Oligodendroglioma: an analysis of 42 cases. *J Neurol Neurosurg Psychiatr* 1987;50:304–312.
76. Yu IT, Ho DM, Wong TT, Liu HC. Congenital cerebral primitive neuroectodermal tumor with astrocytic differentiation and extracranial metastases. *Childs Nerv Syst* 1990;6: 179–182.

20

Brain Tumors in Infants and Very Young Children

Brain tumors in infants and very young children have unique properties that distinguish them from brain tumors occurring in the older child. Although the literature specifically addressing these problems is limited, the percentage of all childhood brain tumors occurring in children less than 2 years of age may approach 10%. We (17) reviewed data on 887 children, aged 0 to 14 years, with brain tumors from the Surveillance, Epidemiology, End Results (SEER) registries from 1973 through 1980. Of 887 brain tumors, 112, or approximately 12.6%, were found in children less than 2 years of age (Fig. 20-1). Koos and Miller (33) reviewed children with brain tumors aged 0 to 16 years from the Neurological Clinic at the University of Vienna Hospital and found 59 of 700 (8%) to be 2 years of age or younger at the time of diagnosis. Others have reported higher numbers of young children in their series. Fessard (24) evaluated children who had received surgery for brain tumors in several Parisian hospitals and found that 15% were less than 2 years of age. Studies by Tomita and McLone (60) as well as that of Albright (1) have reported that 15 to 16% of children treated with brain tumors at their institutions were less than 2 years of age at diagnosis.

Of those tumors occurring in children less than 2 years old, a substantial number are found in infants and neonates. In the SEER registries of Atlanta, Seattle, and Connecticut 534 brain tumors were identified in children aged 0 to 18 years from 1968 to 1979; of these, 27, or 5%, were less than 6 months of age at diagnosis. Others have reported similar incidence figures. For example, 12 of 228 children with brain tumors (5.3%) were less than 1 year of age in a series reported from Japan (59). The number of intracranial tumors diagnosed in children less than 1 year of age was somewhat higher (8 to 11%) in two additional series (4,48). Jellinger and Sunder-Plassman (30) reported 56 of 730 children with brain tumors in the Neurosurgical Department of Vienna whom they considered to have "congenital" tumors (8%). Of these, 12 were "definitely connatal" (i.e., the tumor was present or produced symptoms at birth or within the first 2 weeks of life); 20 were "probably connatal" (i.e., present or recognized within the first year of life); and 25 were "possible" (i.e., diagnosed after 1 year of age, but symptoms were traced to less than 1 year of age). With these criteria in mind, Jellinger and Sunder-Plassman, in the same article, reviewed the world's literature and found 132 cases

---

Brain Tumors in Children: Principles of Diagnosis and Treatment, 2/e, edited by M.E. Cohen and P.K. Duffner, Raven Press, Ltd., New York, 1994.

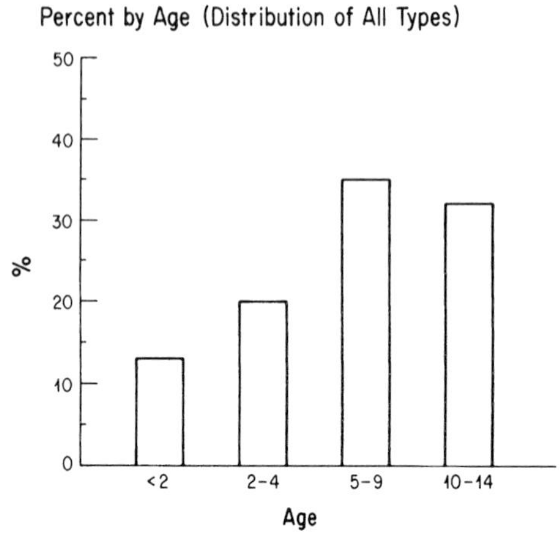

FIG. 20-1. Distribution by age of brain tumors in children 0 to 14 years from the SEER registries (1973 to 1980) (17).

of "connatal brain tumors" with 34 "definite," 40 "probable," and 58 "possible."

CLINICAL PRESENTATION

By the time of diagnosis most tumors in infants are quite large. This may reflect the aggressive biology of many infant tumors as well as the fact that these tumors are often diagnosed quite late in their course. Delay in diagnosis occurs, in part, because infants are able to expand their skulls to accommodate increased intracranial pressure, hence masking for some time the typical signs and symptoms associated with a mass lesion (Fig. 20-2). The most common presenting signs of infants with brain tumors are enlarged heads and bulging fontanelles (6,37). Forty-five percent of infants in a study by Farwell et al. (22) had increased head circumferences, and 27% had bulging anterior fontanelles. Increased intracranial pressure, when present, is commonly due to the development of hydrocephalus secondary to obstruction of the ventricular system by a mass (5,45). Alternatively, a supratentorial hemispheric mass, because of sheer bulk, may present with increased intracranial pressure without evidence of hydrocephalus. Asai (6), in a review of intracranial neoplasms in the first year of life, found that the average diameter of the tumors was 4.6 cm, with the largest being 16 cm in diameter (Fig. 20-3). The head circumference in some of these neonates may be so large that maternal dystocia develops and babies may have to be delivered by cesarean section (55). Before the advent of the CT scan, congenital brain tumors were often misdiagnosed as congenital hydrocephalus, subdural effusions, or hematomas.

Vomiting is the most common presenting symptom of infants with brain

A

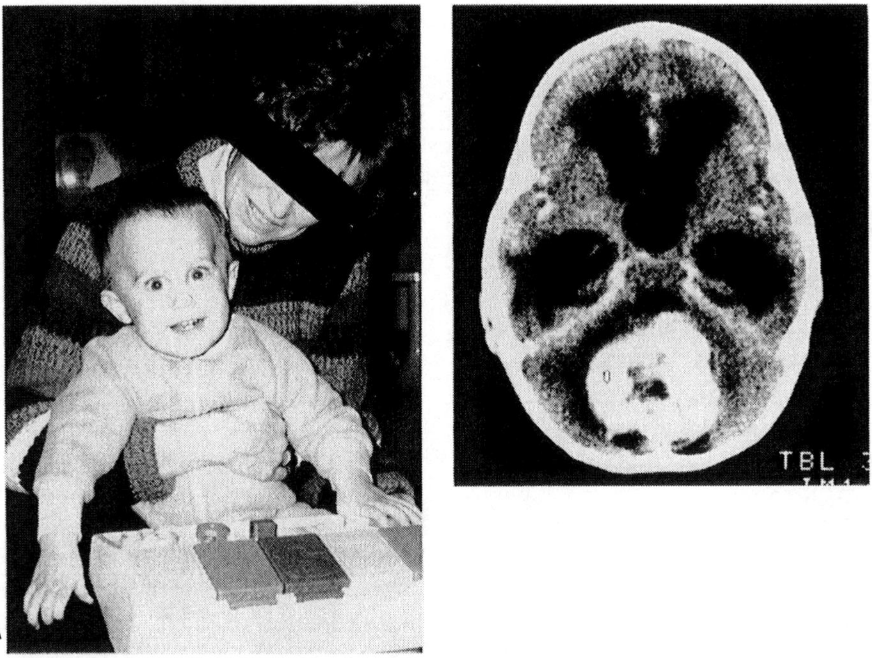

B

FIG. 20-2. A. Fourteen-month-old child with rapidly increasing head circumference. Mother had noted changing hat sizes. He was otherwise bright, alert, and asymptomatic. **B,** CT scan of child in A demonstrating large enhancing posterior fossa mass and hydrocephalus. Diagnosis, medulloblastoma.

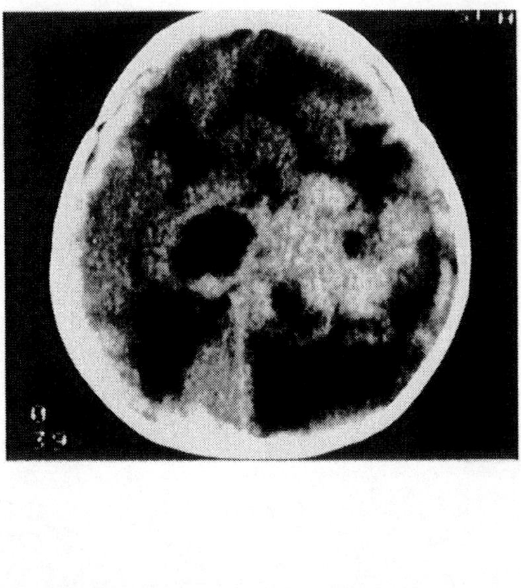

FIG. 20-3. Two-month-old with glioblastoma multiforme. CT reveals enormous enhancing tumor.

tumors (5). Even when symptoms are divided according to age, i.e., neonates, infants, and toddlers, vomiting represents one of the most frequently reported symptoms in all age groups (1). Vomiting may be either due to increased intracranial pressure or the result of tumor on the floor of the fourth ventricle. Since, in these cases, signs of increased intracranial pressure may be absent, some babies with brain tumors have been initially misdiagnosed as having gastrointestinal disease.

Infants with supratentorial mass lesions may present with focal neurologic signs, typically hemiparesis. As opposed to older children, in whom the finding of hemiparesis suggests acquired structural disease, those presenting with hemiparesis in the first 2 years of life more commonly have a static encephalopathy. Clinical differentiation between children with mass lesions and those with hemiparetic cerebral palsy may be difficult (49) (Fig. 20-4). A potentially important historical point is the presence of early hand preference. In general, children with hemiparetic cerebral palsy have strong hand dominance from early infancy, in contrast to the patient with a supratentorial tumor, who may be described as ambidextrous prior to the development of hemiparesis. This observation should raise the suspicion that there is progressive intracranial pathology rather than a static encephalopathy of infancy. In those cases of congenital brain tumors, however, hemiparesis may be present from birth, making the diagnosis extremely difficult.

Convulsions may be another symptom of supratentorial brain tumors in young children (22). Although partial seizures with elementary symptomatology with or without secondary generalization are most common, infantile

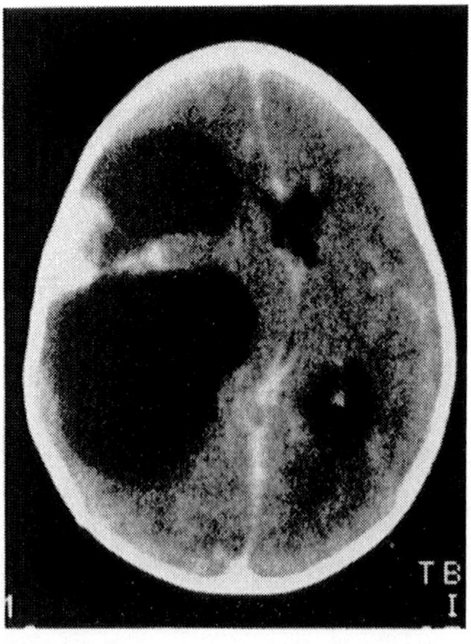

FIG. 20-4. CT of a 15-month-old who presented for evaluation of left hemiparesis. The child had been ambidextrous for the first 6 months of life prior to developing a strong right-handed predominance. Diagnosis, low-grade astrocytoma.

spasms occasionally have been associated with an underlying brain tumor (24). There has been at least one report of two infants with brain tumors and infantile spasms who attained good seizure control on ACTH and normalization of the EEG prior to diagnosis and treatment of their brain tumors (51).

Infants with midline tumors may present with failure to thrive, endocrinopathies, and visual symptoms. A characteristic presentation of the child with a hypothalamic tumor is the diencephalic syndrome. Originally described by Russell (52) in 1951, the syndrome is characterized by severe failure to thrive despite good appetite and food intake (52). These babies are typically alert and happy despite severe emaciation. Those children with midline tumors involving the optic nerves and chiasm may present with decreased visual acuity and nystagmus. Because detailed examinations of visual acuity are difficult in this young age group, diagnosis is often delayed. Moreover, an incorrect diagnosis of congenital nystagmus has been made in many of these children. Although congenital nystagmus may be associated with optic atrophy, chiasmatic gliomas should be excluded by CT scan or MRI (see Chapter 15).

As in older children, tumors of the posterior fossa are characterized by signs and symptoms of increased intracranial pressure as well as ataxia. Although ataxia in the toddler is difficult to diagnose, a change in gait is always suspicious. Meningismus and opisthotonos, when identified, may signify irritation of the cervical roots due to tonsillar herniation.

In summary, although the presence of a large head circumference, split sutures, and bulging fontanelle strongly suggests the presence of increased intracranial pressure, other symptoms with which these babies present, such as vomiting, failure to thrive, and early hand preference, are often attributed to either a non-CNS etiology or developmental abnormality. Thus, diagnosis may be delayed until the tumor is quite large. Alternatively, some infants with brain tumors present initially with catastrophic neurologic deterioration as a result of hemorrhage into the tumor. Bleeding may occur spontaneously or following a minor head injury. In these cases, children with previously unsuspected tumors may present in an obtunded state.

DIAGNOSTIC STUDIES

Suture separation and thinning of the vault are characteristically found in skull films of infants with increased intracranial pressure. Asymmetric expansion of the cranial vault may further localize the mass lesion (24). At times, the mass may actually erode through the inner table of the skull (Fig. 20-5). The presence of calcification on x ray must be differentiated from that associated with congenital infection (7,54).

EEGs are generally nonspecific and nondiagnostic. They commonly reflect diffuse changes of increased intracranial pressure. Localized asymmetry and

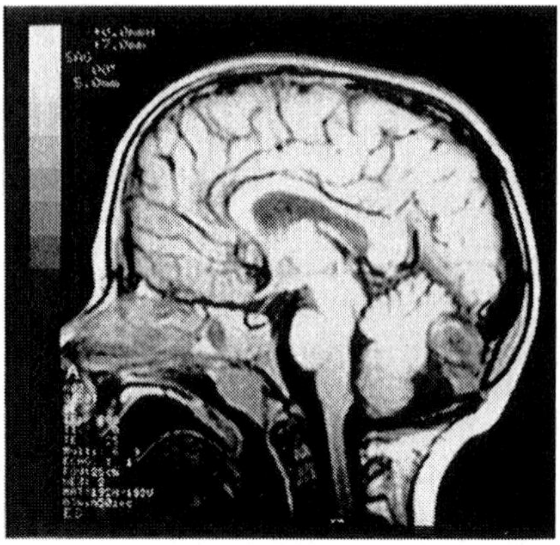

FIG. 20-5. Eighteen-month-old child who cried when his mother brushed his hair. He had point tenderness of the lower occipital region. Skull film revealed a lesion directly at the site of pain. MRI demonstrated a dermoid, which had eroded through the skull.

focal delta may be observed with supratentorial tumors. EEG abnormalities associated with posterior fossa tumors are generally diffuse or found predominantly in the occipital region. Occasionally, a pattern of hypsarrhythmia accompanying infantile spasms may be identified (24).

CT and, more recently, MRI have replaced other modalities in the diagnosis of brain tumors in infancy. The most striking neuroradiologic difference between infant tumors and those of older children is their extremely large size. In one study (8) of neonatal brain tumors, tumor occupied more than one-third of the intracranial volume in 75% of patients. Moreover, hydrocephalus is often massive (4,8,46) (Fig. 20-6). CT readily identifies tumor calcification, which, although typically found in teratomas, may also be noted in primitive neuroectodermal tumors and ependymomas. Both MRI and CT scan features vary according to tumor type. As noted earlier in this book, MRI provides better anatomical definition than CT. However, at present, the significantly longer study time (2 minutes versus 30 to 45 minutes) limits

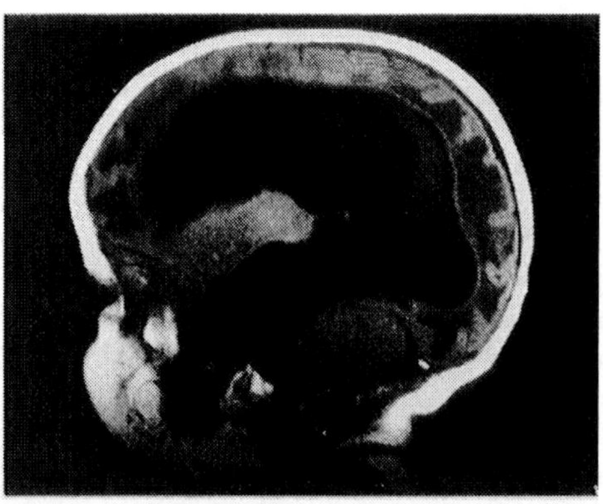

FIG. 20-6. Massive hydrocephalus in an infant with a fourth ventricular anaplastic ependymoma.

this modality because of the necessity for prolonged sedation in the very young child.

Tumors in infants not only are extremely large at diagnosis but also are often widely disseminated throughout the subarachnoid space. In one study (2), 9 of 11 children less than 5 years of age had disseminated medulloblastoma at diagnosis, compared with 0 of 8 who presented at 11 years of age or older. This high incidence of neuraxis dissemination at diagnosis has been confirmed in the Pediatric Oncology Group infant brain tumor study, particularly in patients with medulloblastoma and embryonal tumors (18).

CSF examination, often performed in these babies to exclude meningitis, can be misleading. In one study (24), 14 babies with supratentorial tumors had lumbar punctures; 10 had evidence of increased CSF protein and 4 had pleocytosis of 5 to 15 cells. Seventeen patients with posterior fossa tumors in the same study also received lumbar punctures. Six patients with fourth ventricular ependymomas had pleocytosis (24 to 575 cells) and three cases of "malignant tumors" of the posterior fossa had pleocytosis and increased protein. The presence of blood in the CSF may reflect either subarachnoid or intraventricular hemorrhage or may be the result of a hemorrhage into a necrotic tumor. Thus, the presence of red cells, white cells, and/or elevated protein does not exclude the possibility of an intracranial tumor (7,50) and must be differentiated from meningitis, intraventricular or subarachnoid hemorrhage, and extracerebral fluid collections.

Because of neuraxis dissemination, CT myelograms or MRI examinations of the spine are mandatory in the evaluation of infants with brain tumors. The possibility of herniation should temper the decision to obtain a myelogram in those patients who have not had total surgical resections and continue to have increased intracranial pressure. Despite this caveat, assessment of neuraxis dissemination, when possible, will not only affect choice of treatment but also allow more realistic prognostication.

TUMOR TYPES AND LOCATION

Although brain tumors in children less than 2 years of age are more common in the posterior fossa than in the supratentorial regions, these differences are not as striking as in the older child. Fessard (24) reported a predominance of 57% versus 43% of posterior fossa tumors over supratentorial tumors in children less than 2 years, whereas in older children 60 to 70% of brain tumors were located in the posterior fossa. Children in the first 6 months of life have a higher proportion of supratentorial than infratentorial tumors compared with children between 7 and 12 months of age (24). The younger the child, the more likely is the tumor to be supratentorial. Seventy-one percent of children with brain tumors in the first year of life in a series (6) from Toronto were supratentorial in location. Jellinger and Sunder-Plass-

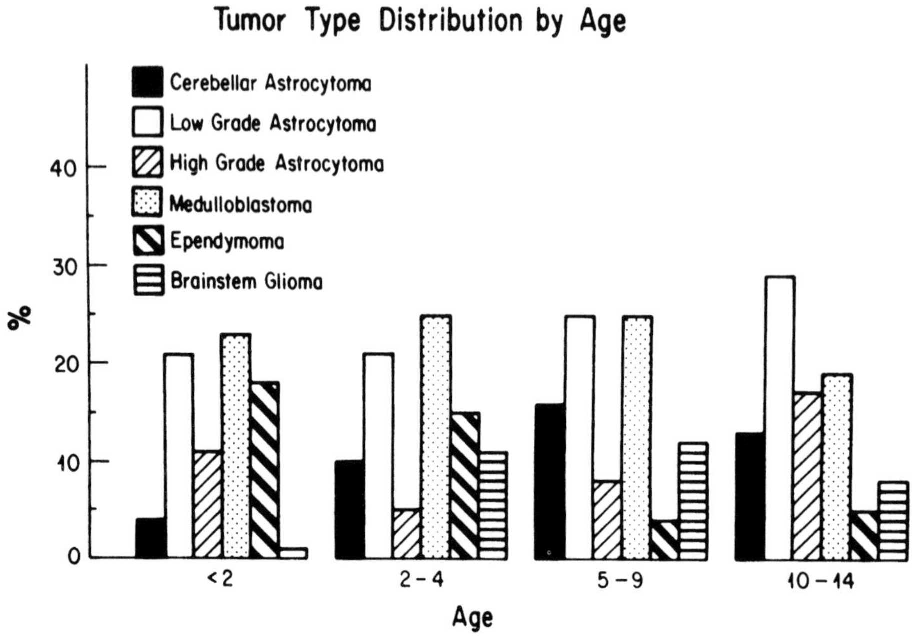

FIG. 20-7. Tumor type distribution by age: SEER registries 1973 to 1980 (17).

man (30) likewise reported that approximately 70% of brain tumors diagnosed at birth or in the first week of life were supratentorial in location. Similarly, in a series (8) of 45 congenital brain tumors diagnosed within the first 60 days of age, two-thirds were supratentorial in location.

Of 887 tumors identified in the SEER registry (17) from 1973 through 1980, 112 were found in children less than 2 years of age (Fig. 20-7). The most common tumor in children less than 2 years old was medulloblastoma, representing 23% of the total; low-grade astrocytomas represented 21%; ependymomas were the third most common tumor, followed by high-grade astrocytomas including glioblastoma multiforme. Brain stem gliomas and cerebellar astrocytomas were rare before 2 years of age.

In both the SEER registries and Matson's (38) series, medulloblastomas were found in 23% of children less than 2 years old with brain tumors. Medulloblastomas were the most common malignant brain tumor identified in the Pediatric Oncology Group infant brain tumor study (18) of children less than 3 years of age, representing 31% of the 198 children. In a series (23) of even younger children with brain tumors, i.e., less than 18 months of age, reported by Farwell et al., 30% had medulloblastomas. Medulloblastomas are also relatively common in neonates. The concept (if true) that medulloblastomas are congenital tumors that develop from embryonic rests in the posterior medullary velum or the fetal external granular layer of the cerebellum helps explain the high incidence in infancy. Of 27 children between birth and 6 months of age diagnosed as having brain tumors from the SEER registries of Atlanta, Seattle, and Connecticut, 6 had medulloblastomas. In another study, 2 of 12 patients with brain tumors diagnosed at birth or within 1 week of life had medulloblastomas (17%). Four additional children with medulloblastomas diagnosed at birth or in the neonatal period were culled from 74 cases in the literature (30).

Astrocytomas represent a high proportion of brain tumors in young children. In the SEER registry data, low-grade supratentorial astrocytomas represented 21% of brain tumors in children less than 2 years and were the second most frequently identified histologic grouping. High-grade astrocytomas, i.e., anaplastic astrocytomas and glioblastomas, represented 11% of tumors in the SEER registry data in young children and 12% of the tumors in the infant malignant brain tumor study of the Pediatric Oncology Group. In contrast, brain stem gliomas and cerebellar astrocytomas are rare, representing 2 to 5% of the whole (17).

Ependymomas were the third most common brain tumor in children less than 2 years old in the SEER registry series. Indeed, the highest incidence of ependymomas in the SEER registries (0 to 14 years) occurred in this very young age group, whereas ependymomas represented only 4% of tumors in children ages 5 to 9 (17). Others have also found that as a group ependymomas occur more commonly in the very young, representing 20% of tumors in children 0 to 2 years, whereas they represent only 8% of tumors in older children (23,24,33,36,54). Twenty-three percent of malignant brain tumors in children less than 3 years of age in the Pediatric Oncology Group infant brain tumor protocol were ependymomas (18).

Primitive neuroectodermal tumors or embryonal tumors predominantly occur in the very young child. As a group, embryonal tumors represented the third most common malignant brain tumor in the Pediatric Oncology Group infant brain tumor study (18). Since this is still a relatively poorly understood designation, the incidence of this grouping is unknown. If pineoblastomas, ependymoblastomas, cerebral neuroblastomas, and medulloepitheliomas are included under the rubric of PNET, the number of infants with this diagnosis increases proportionately (Fig. 20-8).

Congenital intracranial teratomas are more common in Japan than in the United States or Europe. Although teratomas were distinctly unusual in the SEER series, in a Japanese series (58,59) of 103 neonatal intracranial tumors, 53 (51%) were teratomas. Many of these were found in stillborn fetuses. Teratomas have been found in the pineal region, suprasellar region, cerebellar vermis, and lateral ventricles (62). As with medulloblastomas, the concept that teratomas arise from embryonic germ layers suggests that these tumors are derived from fetal rest cells. This may account in part for the frequency of these tumors in infancy.

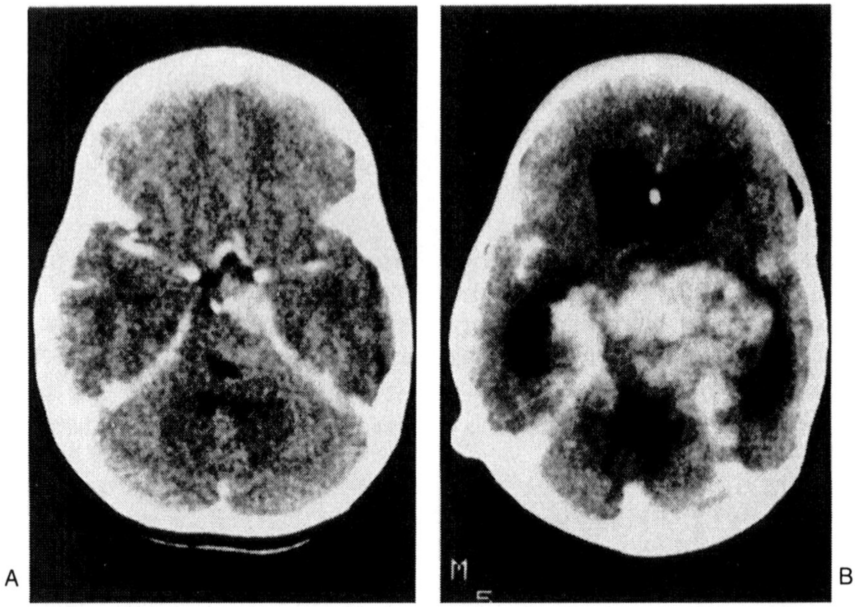

FIG. 20-8. A, Eighteen-month-old who presented for evaluation of new onset of limp. Exam revealed mild hemiparesis. Biopsy = PNET. **B,** Six weeks later, despite chemotherapy, tumor had widely disseminated.

The choroid plexus papilloma, although not common in the SEER registry data, was reported in 10% of Matson's series (38). He operated on 21 tumors located in the lateral ventricle. Nineteen of the 21 patients were less than 3 years of age, reflecting the observation that most choroid plexus tumors occur in children less than 2 years of age with a median age at diagnosis of 9 months (3). Choroid plexus papillomas are most common in the lateral ventricles in infancy, whereas in older age groups they are more often present in the fourth ventricle. Choroid plexus carcinomas are most common in the very young child, in whom they may represent 20 to 30% of choroid plexus tumors overall (Chapter 18).

TREATMENT AND PROGNOSIS

The overall survivals of 112 children less than 2 years of age from the SEER registry (17) (1973 to 1980) were significantly worse than those of other age groups, having a 36% 5-year survival compared with a 57% survival in children 10 to 14 years ($P < 0.001$) (Fig. 20-9). Other series have confirmed this poor outcome. Nearly one-third of Fessard's (24) infants died within 1 month after surgery, and only 16 of 66 survived more than 2 years. Farwell

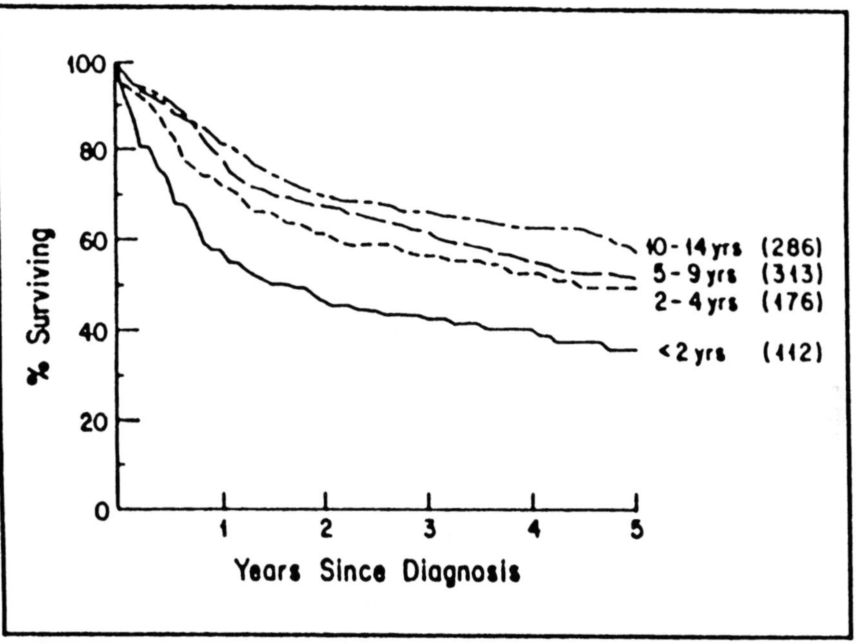

FIG. 20-9. Survival according to age at diagnosis: SEER registry 1973 to 1980 (17).

et al. (23) reviewed survivals in 54 children less than 18 months of age with brain tumors. Of the 54, 20 died within 1 month after diagnosis, and 31 died within 6 months. Overall, she found a 23% probability of a 5-year survival.

Prognosis varies with tumor type and location. Children with cerebral hemisphere tumors had a 39% 1-year and a 28% 5-year survival rate in her study, whereas there were no 5-year survivals in children with brain stem tumors. The longest survivals were found in children with dermoids, teratomas, and choroid plexus papillomas. Tomita (60) found that in children less than 2 years of age with medulloblastomas, ependymomas, and primitive neuroectodermal tumors the 1-year survival was 20.7%.

Very young children with medulloblastomas have significantly worse survivals than older children. Children less than 4 years of age treated on a CCG study (21) in which postoperative radiation was delivered with and without CCNU, vincristine, and prednisone had 5-year survivals of 35%. These survivals should be compared with reports (21,48) of 40 to 60% in older children with medulloblastomas. In most studies, failures tended to occur early, typically in the first year following diagnosis.

Young children with ependymomas also do poorly compared to older patients. A median survival of 8.5 months and a 32% 12-month and 12% 5-year survival were reported in a registry population (17). Poor results were also found by Nazar (41) in a single-institution study of children with infratentorial ependymomas. Children less than 2 years of age had a 5-year survival of 20%, significantly worse than that of older children with ependymomas.

Reasons for the poor prognosis of infants and very young children with brain tumors relate in part to the risk of surgery and the reluctance to treat very young children with potentially neurotoxic therapy. Until recently, many parents chose to withhold therapy entirely rather than commit their child to aggressive therapy since the likelihood of efficacy was limited while the likelihood of neurotoxicity was high. These concerns have led in the past 10 years to increased attention to this population of children and the subsequent development of innovative treatment approaches.

In 1964, Matson (38) wrote that the risks of operating on children in the first 2 years of life should be no greater than those of operating on older children or adults. This optimistic view was not supported by subsequent reports of surgical mortality in this age group. The operative mortality in Pittsburgh in children less than 2 years of age over a 30-year period was 20% (1). Other series (31) have reported surgical mortality as high as 33%. In the past decade, operative mortality has decreased. The operative mortality in Pittsburgh, for example, from 1979 to 1984 dropped to just 1 operative death in 24 children (1). Similarly, Tomita (60) reported an operative mortality in "recent years" of 5.6% among 36 patients diagnosed by computed tomography. The high operative mortality and postoperative morbidity associated with surgery in very young children relates in part to their relatively small blood volume, i.e., 75 ml/kg. If blood loss occurs too rapidly during surgery, the patients are prone to develop hypotension leading to cardiac arrhythmias and cardiovascular collapse. In addition, infants are at risk for hypothermia, which may further complicate their operative course. Although with advances in anesthesia and surgical techniques operative mortality has decreased, morbidity remains quite high. Since the tumors are often very vascular, intraoperative hemorrhage and stroke may occur.

Surgical techniques used in infants differ from those used in older children. Since infants are prone to hypotension, some surgeons recommend that posterior fossa tumors be removed with the infant in the prone or lateral position rather than the sitting position (which is typically favored in the older child). Infants are at additional risk because the large tumor often displaces the major cerebral vessels. Attention to the aberrant location of cerebral vessels is necessary to prevent inadvertent damage to vasculature. In addition, since the degree of hydrocephalus is often enormous, the surgeon must be careful not to allow rapid decompression of the ventricular system with resultant collapse of the ventricles and subsequent tearing of cortical veins. This sequence of events may lead to hematomas in either the intraoperative or postoperative period (1).

With decreasing operative mortality, surgery has become increasingly aggressive. In children with low-grade astrocytomas and other low-grade tumors, maximal cytoreduction may eliminate the need for either chemotherapy or radiation until such time as the tumor recurs. Although the data are limited on high-grade tumors such as medulloblastomas and ependymomas, early data from the Pediatric Oncology Group infant study (18) suggest that gross total resection is associated with significantly better survivals than incomplete resection. Surgical cure can be achieved in children with choroid plexus papillomas. Prognosis also appears to be significantly improved in children with choroid plexus carcinomas if gross total resection is achieved (Chapter 18). Despite maximal surgical resection, recurrence is to be expected in medulloblastomas, ependymomas, glioblastomas, and embryonal tumors unless postoperative adjuvant therapy is delivered.

A major area of concern in the treatment of brain tumors in young children is the risks associated with cranial irradiation (13–16,35). Before 3 years of age, decreases in the dose of radiation to the whole brain of 10 to 20% have been recommended. This reduction in radiation is likely inadequate for tumor control, and may be a major reason that infants do significantly worse than older children with the same tumors. Unfortunately, even with reduced dose radiation, neurotoxicity is to be expected (39,56) (Chapter 23). Spinal irradiation is also fraught with potential long-term consequences. Neuhauser et al. (42) related the effects of increasing doses of radiation to the spine with the age of the patient. Overall, growth disturbances produced by radiation were directly related to dosage and inversely related to age (Fig. 20-10).

These concerns have resulted in interest in delaying or eliminating radiation in this young population by way of postoperative chemotherapy (13). In one of the early studies (61), MOPP (nitrogen mustard, vincristine, prednisone, and procarbazine) was given as primary therapy for infants less than 4 years of age with brain tumors. Seven had astrocytomas (three grade 1, three grade 2, 1 grade 3), 6 had medulloblastomas, 2 had mixed gliomas, 1 had an ependymoma, and 1 had a primitive neuroectodermal tumor. Fifteen of 17 responded, and of these 6 remained in continuous complete remission with a median duration of follow-up of 28.9 months. Horwitz et al. (29) treated 12 infants less than 27 months of age with postoperative chemotherapy and delayed radiation. One group received MOPP therapy, and the second received a combination of Cytoxan, vincristine, cis-platinum, and procarbazine. The latter group were part of a Pediatric Oncology Group pilot. The original goal of the study was to continue chemotherapy until the child was at least 2 years of age. After 1985 the protocol was changed such that children less than 2 years of age were treated for 24 months and those between the ages of 2 and 3 were treated for 12 months. Radiation was then administered. Objective responses were identified in 6 of 8 children who had residual tumor postoperatively. In addition, 8 children remained disease-free for a minimum of 7 months with a median time of 28 months from date of diagnosis.

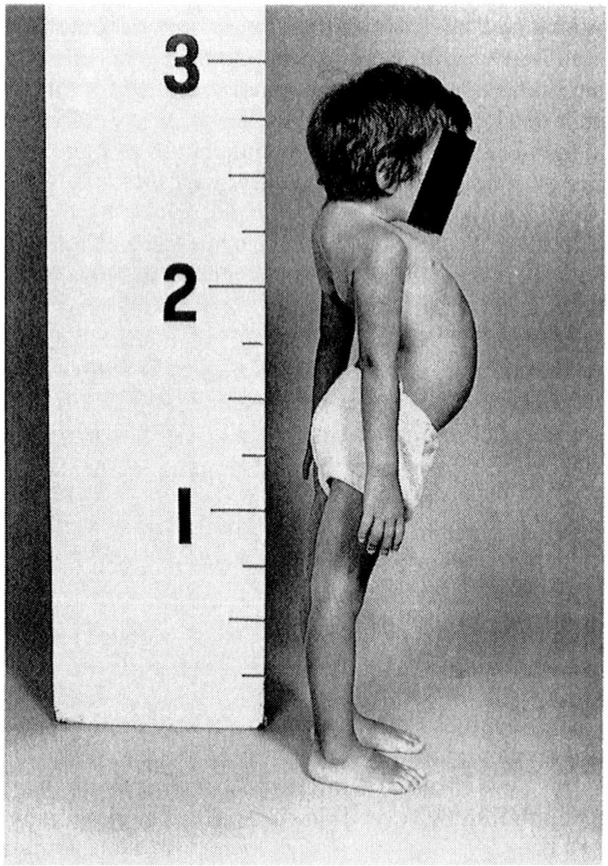

FIG. 20-10. Four-year-old child radiated at 6 months of age for rapidly progressive cervical cord astrocytoma. Note severe spinal deformity.

The largest study of prolonged postoperative chemotherapy and delayed radiation in infants with brain tumors has come from the Pediatric Oncology Group (18). One hundred ninety-eight infants less than 3 years of age with malignant brain tumors were treated with a combination of Cytoxan, vincristine, cis-platinum, and VP16. Thirty-nine percent of patients with measurable postoperative disease had complete or partial responses (>50% reduction in tumor size) following two cycles of Cytoxan, vincristine. Response rates were highest for medulloblastoma (48%), malignant glioma (60%), and ependymoma (48%). Brain stem gliomas and PNETs showed little or no response. Overall, the 1-year progression-free survival was 47% in children 0 to 23 months old and 42% for children 24 to 36 months old. Most failures occurred within the first year, with few late failures. The progression-free and overall survivals of children with ependymomas, medulloblastomas, and high-grade gliomas compared favorably with historical controls using standard postoperative radiation. Moreover, preliminary results suggest that cognitive abilities did not decline during chemotherapy.

Another study of postoperative chemotherapy with delayed radiation in infants less than 3 years of age with medulloblastoma was presented at the SIOP meetings in Hanover, Germany in 1992 (34). Twenty-three infants were treated with either a combination of procarbazine, ifosphamide, VP16, high-dose methotrexate, cis-platinum, and cytosine arabinoside or a protocol consisting of procarbazine, high-dose methotrexate, and vincristine. Radiation was delayed until age 3 years. Partial or complete responses were observed in 50% of cases. The overall event-free survival at 4 years was 56% and 80% in those patients with gross total resection. There was a high rate of dissemination at relapse with 7 of 9 having evidence of CSF metastases. A French study (32) used vincristine, carboplatinum, and procarbazine in children less than 3 years of age with malignant brain tumors. Ten children were entered on study, and 4 remained in complete remission from 12 to 15 months duration. An additional 2 had stable residual disease. Finally, Geyer et al. (26) reported at ASCO preliminary results of the Children's Cancer Study Group trial for infants with malignant brain tumors. In this trial 78 infants less than 18 months of age with medulloblastoma, primitive neuroectodermal tumor, or malignant ependymoma, and 37 infants less than 24 months of age with malignant astrocytoma were treated with "eight-in-1." The 1- and 2-year progression-free survival was 33% and 25% for the group of children with medulloblastoma, primitive neuroectodermal tumor, or malignant ependymoma. Eighty-seven percent of the children with progressive disease had died. Of the infants with malignant astrocytoma, the 1- and 2-year progression-free survival was 44% and 35%.

In the first edition of this book concerns were raised about how well infants would tolerate aggressive chemotherapy (25). These fears have not been realized. With the advent of hematopoietic protectors, e.g., granulocyte stimulating factor, leukopenia has been greatly reduced. These studies have demonstrated that infants can tolerate aggressive chemotherapy as well as older children. Moreover, in several trials, survivals have been at least as good as those achieved with standard radiation. Whether the long-term toxicity of these chemotherapy regimens will be less than with cranial irradiation awaits follow-up studies.

Long-Term Effects

The long-term effects of cranial irradiation on infants with brain tumors include adverse effects on intellect and endocrine function and the development of leukoencephalopathy. Farwell et al. (23) found that 8 of 18 infants who survived their brain tumors (1935 to 1974) were retarded or handicapped. Four were institutionalized, 2 were in schools for retarded children, and 2 were quadriplegic or hemiplegic. Only 3 children were normal. Fessard (24) also found poor results in children treated in this age group. Only 5 of 66 children were normal. The remainder had blindness, epilepsy, hydrocephalus, "backwardness," and "neurologic symptoms."

Spunberg et al. (56) analyzed the effects of cranial irradiation on 14 children less than 2 years with brain tumors. Radiation doses ranged from 2,400 to 5,000 cGy over 3 to 9.5 weeks. Five children had epilepsy, 3 were deaf, 3 had decreased visual acuity, 4 had hemiplegia or quadriplegia, 10 had cerebellar dysfunction, and 4 had cranial nerve deficits. Only 4 were felt to be neurologically intact. A composite of Quality of Survival Scale revealed one patient to be grade I, i.e., no evidence of physical, neurologic, or endocrine abnormality, average to superior intelligence, high educational achievement, and full employment potential. Five were considered grade II, i.e., "minimal" physical or neurologic disability, clinical evidence of mild endocrine dysfunction, borderline IQ, elementary educational achievement, and limited employment potential. Two were grade III, suggesting moderate disability, requiring special education and potential for employment only under supervision. Six were grade IV or V, suggesting severe or total disability.

A retrospective study of 20 long-term survivors diagnosed as having brain tumors under the age of 3 and followed for more than 5 years was reported by Suc et al. (57). Eighty-five percent of those infants developed impaired cognitive function. In addition, 65% had a neurologic handicap. In another study (28) of children with medulloblastomas, 54% of 11 children treated before 3 years of age had IQs less than 80.

These and other studies (19,44) have consistently found that when children are irradiated at a young age, they are prone to develop significantly more intellectual problems than older children. However, most of these studies are retrospective in nature. Mulhern et al. (40) prospectively evaluated a group of infants with brain tumors treated with preirradiation chemotherapy. None of eight patients scored in the normal range of mental development at the time of their initial assessment. During chemotherapy, two improved, five were stable, and only one showed a decline. After radiation no child improved, one remained stable, and the remaining children all showed significant declines. These results are important as they suggest that the baseline IQ of many of these infants may be abnormal. Thus, treatment with chemotherapy and delayed or no radiation may prevent decline over baseline, but the children may still be subnormal. The large size of these tumors at diagnosis as well as the extensive damage following attempts at gross total resection makes this hardly surprising. Although prospective intellectual assessments were performed in the Pediatric Oncology Group infant brain tumor study, the results are not yet available.

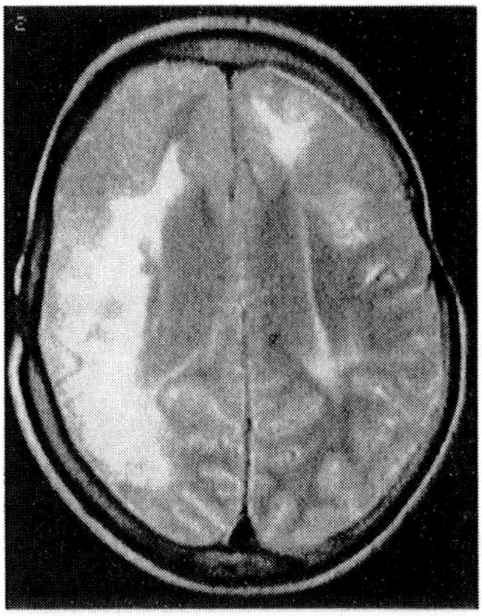

FIG. 20-11. Ten-year-old child treated with cranial irradiation at 2 years of age. MRI reveals both leukoencephalopathy and infarct, the latter secondary to moyamoya disease.

The most severe effects of radiation on endocrine function in the very young child are adverse effects on growth. Although all prepubertal children are susceptible to growth failure from radiation damage to the hypothalamic pituitary axis, infants are at further risk because of radiation damage to the spine (Chapter 23). Infants who receive radiation to the spine before 1 year of age have a potential loss of ultimate adult height of 10 cm, compared with older children who will lose approximately 5 cm (53). There is no information at this time regarding the influence of young age on susceptibility to radiation-induced hypothyroidism or gonadal dysfunction. It is known, however, that when chemotherapy is added to radiation the likelihood of hypothyroidism and ovarian dysfunction rises dramatically (9,43). Since young infants are increasingly treated with prolonged chemotherapy, these complications will likely be identified in the future.

Leukoencephalopathy has also been reported more commonly in children radiated before 3 years of age (10,11). Intracranial calcification has been reported in radiated young children even in the absence of chemotherapy. The dose of radiation associated with leukoencephalopathy has ranged from 3,500 to 5,000 cGy. In addition, radiation vasculopathy, characterized by occlusive arteriovascular disease and the development of moyamoya, is more common in the very young (Fig. 20-11).

SUMMARY

Ten percent of childhood brain tumors occur in children less than 2 years of age. In the first 6 months of life the tumors are more commonly supratentorial than infratentorial, while in the second 6 months of life the numbers of supratentorial and infratentorial tumors are approximately equal. After 1 year of age, the tumors follow the usual childhood pattern of posterior fossa predominance. In general, although the types of tumor are similar to those found in older age groups, the relative incidence of the tumor types is different. Ependymomas represent as many as 20% of tumors in this age group, whereas their incidence in older children is approximately 10%. Alternatively, brain stem gliomas and cerebellar astrocytomas are common in older age groups and relatively unusual in infancy. Medulloblastomas represent

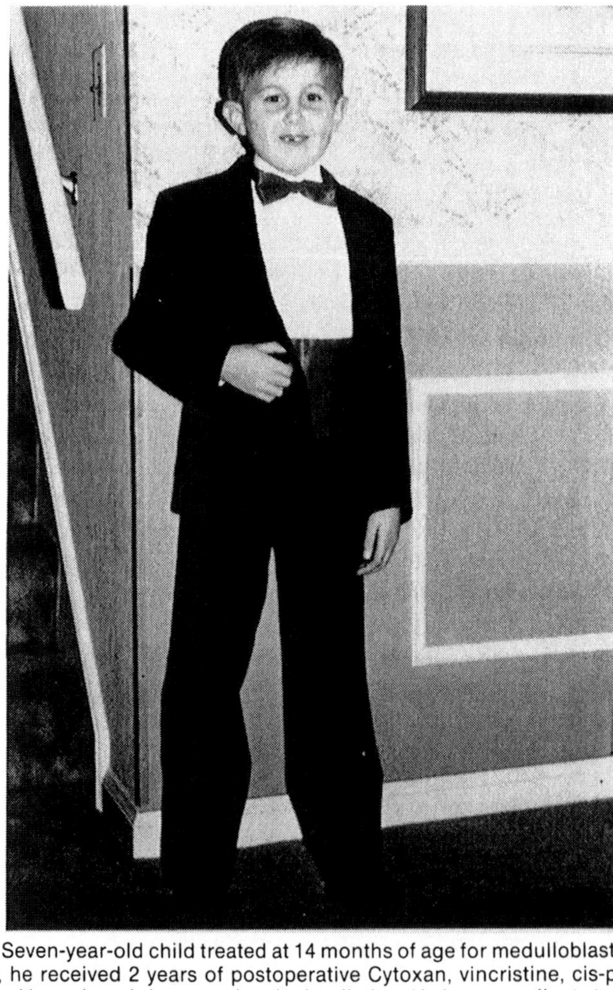

FIG. 20-12. Seven-year-old child treated at 14 months of age for medulloblastoma. Following surgery, he received 2 years of postoperative Cytoxan, vincristine, cis-platinum, and VP16 followed by reduced-dose craniospinal radiation. He is an excellent student and free of disease. He is the same child shown in Fig. 20-2A.

approximately 20 to 30% of tumors in this age group, which is comparable to the incidence found in older children.

Treatment represents a major problem. Infants and very young children have worse survivals than older children with the identical tumor types and yet suffer the brunt of radiation-induced neurotoxicity. To address these concerns, current studies are delaying or even eliminating radiation in infants with malignant brain tumors by using prolonged postoperative chemotherapy. Early data suggest that results are as good as or better than those achieved with standard radiation. Current infant brain tumor studies withhold radiation entirely in those children without evidence of disease following completion of chemotherapy. Whether the long-term side effects of these chemotherapy regimens will be less than those associated with radiation awaits follow-up of infants treated in this manner (Fig. 20-12).

REFERENCES

1. Albright AL. Brain tumors in neonates, infants, and toddlers. *Contemp Neurosurg* 1985; 7(22):1-6.
2. Allen JC, Epstein F. Medulloblastoma and other primary malignant neuroectodermal tumors of the CNS. *J Neurosurg* 1982;57:446.
3. Allen J, Wisoff J, Helson L, Pearce J, Arenson E. Choroid plexus carcinoma: responses to chemotherapy alone in newly diagnosed young children. *J Neurooncol* 1992;12:69–74.
4. Ambrosino MM, Hernanz-Schulman M, Genieser NB, Wisoff J, Epstein F. Brain tumors in infants less than a year of age. *Pediatr Radiol* 1988;19:6–8.
5. Arnstein LH, Boldrey E, Naffziger HC. Case reports and survey of brain tumors during the neonatal period. *J Neurosurg* 1951;8:315–319.
6. Asai A, Hoffman HJ, Hendrick EB, Humphreys RP, Becker LE. Primary intracranial neoplasms in the first year of life. *Childs Nerv Syst* 1989;5:230–233.
7. Azar-Kia B, Krishnan UR, Schechter MM. Neonatal craniopharyngioma. *J Neurosurg* 1975;42:91–93.
8. Buetow PC, Smirniotopoulos JG, Done S. Congenital brain tumors: a review of 45 cases. *AJR* 1990;155:587–593.
9. Clayton PE, Shalet SM, Price DA. Gonadal function after chemotherapy and irradiation for childhood malignancies. *Horm Res* 1988;30:104–110.
10. Cohen ME, Duffner PK. Long-term consequences of CNS treatment for childhood cancer. I: Pathologic consequences and potential for oncogenesis. *Pediatr Neurol* 1991;7:157–163.
11. Davis PC, Hoffman JC, Pearl GS, Braun IF. CT evaluation of effects of cranial radiation therapy in children. *AJR* 1986;147:587–592.
12. Deutsch M. Radiotherapy for primary brain tumors in very young children. *Cancer* 1982; 50:2785–2789.
13. Duffner PK, Cohen ME. Changes in the approach to central nervous system tumors in childhood. *Pediatr Neurol* 1992;39(4):859–877.
14. Duffner PK, Cohen ME. Long-term consequences of CNS treatment for childhood cancer. II: Clinical consequences. *Pediatr Neurol* 1991;7:237–242.
15. Duffner PK, Cohen ME. The long-term effects of central nervous system therapy on children with brain tumors. *Neurol Clin* 1991;9(2):479–495.
16. Duffner PK, Cohen ME. Treatment of brain tumors in babies and very young children. *Pediatr Neurosci* 1986;12:304–310.
17. Duffner PK, Cohen ME, Myers MH, Heise HW. Survival of children with brain tumors: SEER Program, 1973–1980. *Neurology* 1986;36:597–601.
18. Duffner PK, Horowitz M, Krischer J, et al. Postoperative chemotherapy and delayed radiotherapy in children less than 3 years of age with malignant brain tumors. *NEJM* 1993;328: 1725–1731.

19. Ellenberg L, McComb JG, Siegel SE, Stowe S. Factors affecting intellectual outcome in pediatric brain tumor patients. *Neurosurgery* 1987;21:638–644.
20. Ellenbogen RG, Winston KR, Kupsky WJ. Tumors of the choroid plexus in children. *Neurosurgery* 1989;25:327–335.
21. Evans AE, Jenkin DT, Sposto R, et al. The treatment of medulloblastoma: results of a prospective randomized trial of radiation therapy with and without CCNU, vincristine and prednisone. *J Neurosurg* 1990;72;572–582.
22. Farwell JR, Dohrmann GJ, Flannery JT. Central nervous system tumors in children. *Cancer* 1977;40:3123–3132.
23. Farwell JR, Dohrmann GJ, Flannery JT. Intracranial neoplasms in infants. *Arch Neurol* 1978;35:533–537.
24. Fessard C. Cerebral tumors in infancy. *Am J Dis Child* 1968;115:302–308.
25. Gale GB, D'Angio GJ, Uri A, Chatten J, Koop CE. Cancer in neonates: the experience at the Children's Hospital of Philadelphia. *Pediatrics* 1982;70:409–413.
26. Geyer J, Zeltzer P, Finlay J, et al. Chemotherapy for infants with malignant brain tumors: report of the Children's Cancer Study Group trials. *ASCO* 1992;1005.
27. Geyer R, Levy M, Berger MS, Milstein J, Griffin B, Bleyer WA. Infants with medulloblastoma: a single institution review of survival. *Neurosurgery* 1991;29:707-711.
28. Hope-Hirsch E, Renier D, LaBouch-Tubiana A, Sainte-Rose C, Pierre-Kahn A, Hirsch JF. Medulloblastoma in childhood: progressive intellectual deterioration. *Childs Nerv Syst* 1990;6:60–65.
29. Horowitz ME, Mulhern RK, Kun LE, et al. Brain tumors in the very young child. *Cancer* 1988;61:428–434.
30. Jellinger K, Sunder-Plassman M. Connatal intracranial tumors. *Neuropaediatrie* 1973;4: 46–63.
31. Jooma R, Hayward RD, Grant DN. Intracranial neoplasms during the first year of life: analysis of one hundred consecutive cases. *Neurosurgery* 1984;14:31–41.
32. Kalifa C, Flamant F, Hartmann O, Vassal G, Lemerle J. Postsurgical chemotherapy without radiation therapy in patients less than three years with malignant brain tumors. *Pediatr Neurosci* 1988;14:163.
33. Koos WT, Miller MH. *Intracranial tumors of infants and children*. Stuttgart:Thieme; 1971: 14-22.
34. Kuhl J, Gnekow A, Havers W, et al. Primary chemotherapy after surgery and delayed irradiation in children under three years of age with medulloblastoma: pilot trial of the German Pediatric Brain Tumor Study Group. *Med Pediatr Oncol* 1992;20:387.
35. Littman P, D'Angio GJ. Radiation therapy in the neonate. *Am J Pediatr Hematol Oncol* 1981;3:279–285.
36. Lorentzen M, Hagerstrand I. Congenital ependymoblastoma. *Acta Neuropathol* 1980;49: 71–74.
37. Mapstone TB, Warf BC. Intracranial tumor in infants: characteristics, management, and outcome of a contemporary series. *Neurosurgery* 1991;28(3):343–348.
38. Matson DD. Intracranial tumors of the first two years of life. *West J Surg Obstet Gynecol* 1964;72:117–122.
39. Meadows AT, Massari DJ, Fergusson J, Gordon J, Littman P, Moss K. Declines in I.Q. scores and cognitive dysfunctions in children with acute lymphocytic leukaemia treated with cranial irradiation. *Lancet* 1981;2:1015–1018.
40. Mulhern RK, Horowitz ME, Kovnar EH, Langston J, Sanford RA, Kun LE. Neurodevelopmental status of infants and young children treated for brain tumors with preirradiation chemotherapy. *J Clin Oncol* 1989;7(11):1660–1666.
41. Nazar GB, Hoffman HJ, Becker LE, Jenkin D, Humphreys RP, Hendrick B. Infratentorial ependymomas in childhood: prognostic factors and treatment. *J Neurosurg* 1990;72: 408–417.
42. Neuhauser EBD, Wittenborg MH, Berman CZ, Cohen J. Irradiation effects of roentgentherapy on the growing spine. *Radiology* 1952;59:637–650.
43. Oberfield SE, Allen JC, Pollack J, New MI, Levine LS. Long-term endocrine sequelae after treatment of medulloblastoma: prospective study of growth and thyroid function. *J Pediatr* 1986;108:219–223.
44. Packer RJ, Sutton LN, Atkins TE, et al. A prospective study of cognitive function in

children receiving whole-brain radiotherapy and chemotherapy: 2-year results. *J Neurosurg* 1989;70:707–713.
45. Papadakis N, Millan J, Grady DF, Segerberg LH. Medulloblastoma of the neonatal period and early infancy. *J Neurosurg* 1971;34:88–91.
46. Radkowski MA, Naidich TP, Tomita T, Byrd SE, McLone DG. Neonatal brain tumors: CT and MR findings. *J Comput Assist Tomogr* 1988;12(1):10–20.
47. Raimondi AJ, Tomita T. Brain tumors during the first year of life. *Childs Brain* 1983;10: 193–207.
48. Raimondi AJ, Tomita T. Medulloblastoma in childhood. *Acta Neurochir* 1979;50:127-138.
49. Raskind R, Beigel F. Brain tumors in early infancy: probably congenital in origin. *J Pediatr* 1964;65:727–732.
50. Rothman SM, Nelson JS, DeVivo DC, Coxe WS. Congenital astrocytoma presenting with intracerebral hematoma. *J Neurosurg* 1979;51:237–239.
51. Ruggieri V, Caraballo R, Fejerman N. Intracranial tumors and West Syndrome. *Pediatr Neurol* 1989;5:327–329.
52. Russell A. A diencephalic syndrome of emaciation in infancy and childhood. *Arch Dis Child* 1951;26:274.
53. Shalet SM, Gibson B, Swindell R, Pearson D. Effect of spinal irradiation on growth. *Arch Dis Child* 1987;62:461–464.
54. Simpson DA, Carter RF, Ducrou W. Intracranial tumours in infancy. *Dev Med Child Neurol* 1968;10:190–199.
55. Solitare GB, Krigman MR. Congenital intracranial neoplasm: a case report and review of the literature. *J Neuropathol Exp Neurol* 1964;23:280–292.
56. Spunberg JJ, Chang CH, Goldman M, Auricchio E, Bell JJ. Quality of long-term survival following irradiation for intracranial tumors in children under the age of two. *Int J Radiat Oncol Biol Phys* 1981;7:727–736.
57. Suc E, Kalifa C, Brauner R, Habrand JL, et al. Brain tumours under the age of three: the price of survival. *Acta Neurochir (Wien)* 1990;106:93–98.
58. Takaku A, Kodama N, Ohara H, Hori S. Brain tumors in newborn babies. *Childs Brain* 1978;4:365–375.
59. Takaku A, Mita R, Suzuki J. Intracranial teratoma in early infancy. *J Neurosurg* 1973;38: 265–268.
60. Tomita T, McLone DG. Brain tumors during the first twenty-four months of life. *Neurosurgery* 1985;17(6):913–919.
61. van Eys J, Cangir A, Coody D, Smith B. MOPP regimen as primary chemotherapy for brain tumors in infants. *J Neurooncol* 1985;3:237–243.
62. Whittle IR, Simpson DA. Surgical treatment of neonatal intracranial teratoma. *Surg Neurol* 1981;15:268–273.

21

Extraneural Metastasis in Childhood Brain Tumors

Although extraneural metastases are known to occur with primary tumors of the CNS, they are considered a rarity. In 1969 Smith et al. (35) reviewed 8,000 primary neuroectodermal CNS tumors from the Armed Forces Institute of Pathology. Thirty-five patients had extraneural metastases, an incidence of 0.4%. Similarly low incidence figures were reported by the Department of Pathology at Grenoble (29). In this study of 750 patients with primary brain tumors, only 4 tumors were associated with extraneural metastases, an incidence of 0.5%. A more recent study (5) of pediatric brain tumors from Toronto, Canada, reported 21 of 917 cases (2.3%) as having extraneural metastases. In another study (10), 6 out of 36 children with brain tumors treated at the Roswell Park Cancer Institute with surgery, radiation, and chemotherapy had documented evidence of extraneural metastases. Fifteen of these 36 patients had autopsies, which included examination of the head and body, and extraneural involvement was found in 5. An additional child, who did not have an autopsy, had extraneural involvement diagnosed during life. The incidence of extraneural metastases in our autopsy series was 33% with an overall incidence of 16%.

Overall, glial tumors account for approximately 30 to 40% of primary brain tumors associated with extraneural metastases (13,29). As expected, of all gliomas, glioblastomas are the most prone to metastasize (23).

Glasauer and Yuan (13) analyzed 88 published reports of children and adults with brain tumors who had developed extracranial metastases. To this series, they added one of their own. Of 89 patients, 66 were adults and 23 were children. Of the adults with extracranial metastases, 47% had either meningiomas or meningosarcomas. The majority of the remainder had gliomas. Of the children with brain tumors in this series, tumor types included 8 medulloblastomas, 5 ependymomas, 2 gliomas, 2 meningosarcomas, 2 pinealomas, and 1 choroid plexus papilloma. Thirty-three cases of extraneural metastases from non-germinomatous intracranial germ-cell tumors have also been reported.

In childhood, the most common brain tumor associated with the development of systemic metastases is the medulloblastoma. Although this association has been known since the 1930s, there have been increasing reports of

Brain Tumors in Children: Principles of Diagnosis and Treatment, 2/e, edited by M.E. Cohen and P.K. Duffner, Raven Press, Ltd., New York, 1994.

this complication in recent years. Chatty and Earle (6) reported extraneural metastases in 4 out of 201 patients with medulloblastomas, an incidence of 2%. Campbell (5) reported a higher incidence, i.e., 10% of 152 children with medulloblastoma had extracranial metastates. Kleinman et al. (20) reviewed 13 series of children with medulloblastomas. Of a total of 686 patients, 33 (5%) were found to have extraneural metastases. In smaller series, the incidence of extraneural metastases with medulloblastomas has been even higher. Paterson (30) reported systemic metastases in 7 of 35 patients with medulloblastoma (20%). Hoffman et al. (17) reported an incidence of 14.6%; Das and Dalby (7) reported 13.6%; and Schnitzler et al. (33) reported 14%. Thus, the incidence of documented extraneural metastases in children with medulloblastomas appears to be far higher than was previously believed.

AGE

An age-related predilection for extraneural metastases does not appear to exist (13). Children with meningeal tumors and extraneural metastases ranged in age in one study from 7 days to 12 years, and children with cerebral tumors and extraneural metastases ranged in age from 8 weeks to 16 years. In a study (6) analyzing extraneural metastases in children with medulloblastomas, there was no significant difference between children with and without metastases either in age or sex. The usual male-to-female ratio held true.

SITE OF METASTASES

The site of metastasis varies with the primary tumor. Medulloblastomas most commonly spread to bone, bone marrow, and lymph nodes (22). The pelvis is the most common bony site for metastatic spread from medulloblastomas, followed by involvement of the femur and vertebral column (20,22). In long bones, the metaphyses are the most common site of metastatic involvement (21). Lymphatic metastases most frequently involve the cervical chain (20). Although medulloblastomas may spread to the lung, pleura, liver, and breast, these sites are far less common (31).

Glioblastomas most commonly spread to the lung and lymph nodes, with less frequent involvement of bone, pleura, and liver. Metastases from ependymomas most commonly involve the lung and lymph nodes, and less commonly bone, pleura, and liver (23) (Fig. 21-1) (see Chapter 11). Meningiomas spread to the lung and pleura, and less commonly to the lymph nodes, liver, and bone (13,40). Pituitary carcinomas most often invade the liver (13). Metastatic implants in lymph nodes, bone, and, less commonly, scalp have been reported with anaplastic oligodendrogliomas (24).

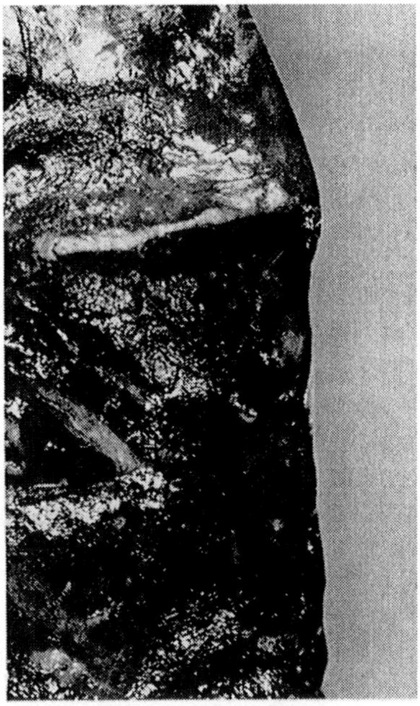

FIG. 21-1. Lung metastasis from supratentorial malignant ependymoma.

DIAGNOSIS

Weiss (42) described four criteria necessary for the diagnosis of extraneural metastases from a primary CNS tumor:

1. The proven presence of a single histologically characteristic tumor of the CNS
2. A clinical history compatible with the premise that this tumor accounted for the initial symptoms
3. An autopsy to exclude the presence of another primary tumor
4. Identical morphology of the primary lesion and the metastases with allowance for variation in anaplasia

Many authors have adhered to the Weiss criteria in their reports of children and adults with extraneural metastases. However, because more patients are diagnosed as having extraneural metastases during life, these criteria need to be expanded. The true incidence of extraneural metastases may become established in the future as collaborative brain tumor studies include sequential bone scans and skeletal surveys as part of treatment protocols.

The most common presenting symptom of bony metastases is pain. Differentiation from root compression is sometimes difficult. Consequently, myelography is often performed before obtaining plain x-ray studies and bone scans. A differentiating clinical point favoring bony metastases is the absence of increased pain on Valsalva maneuvers. These maneuvers, by increasing cerebrospinal fluid pressure, would intensify root pain caused by secondary deposits within the spinal subarachnoid space. In addition, skeletal metastases, unlike root pain, are at times accompanied by severe localized tender swelling in the area of the bone involved. Signs of generalized disease including loss of weight, appetite, and energy are commonly seen in patients with skeletal metastases, although this symptom complex is not pathognomonic of this complication (21).

Technetium bone scans are usually but not always abnormal in the presence of bony metastases (Fig. 21-2). Ho et al. (16), for example, described a patient with a medulloblastoma who had diffuse osteoblastic bony lesions identified on plain films in the presence of a normal bone scan. Plain x-ray studies may reveal either osteolytic or osteosclerotic abnormalities. Often there is a mixture of both bone destruction and sclerosis (14,17) (Fig. 21-3). The bone lesions on x-ray studies are similar to those seen with neuroblastomas, leukemia, Hodgkin's disease, and Wilms' tumor (21). Calcium, phosphorus, and acid phosphatase may be normal in the face of diffuse osteoblastic lesions, but alkaline phosphatase can be elevated (16).

The bone marrow is a common site for the spread of medulloblastomas. The resulting leukoerythroblastic anemia, along with tumor infiltration, may be diagnosed by bone marrow aspiration (2,21). Unfortunately, anemia in

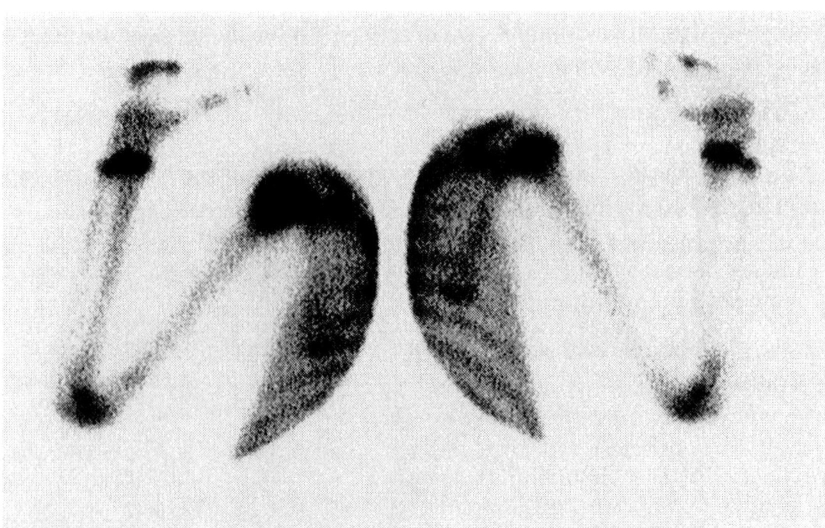

FIG. 21-2. Technetium pyrophosphate bone scan reveals an increased uptake in the proximal metaphysis of the left humerus. The patient had a medulloblastoma diagnosed 6 months previously.

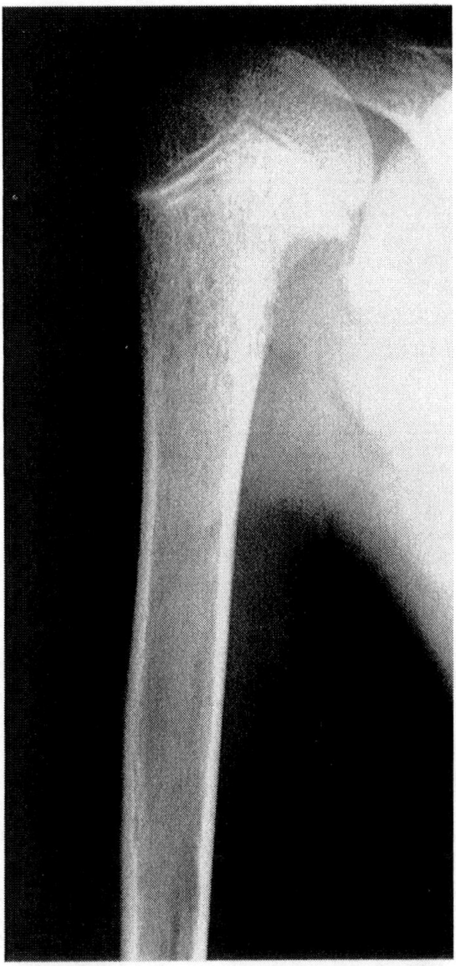

FIG. 21-3. The patient presented with hip pain but no complaints of pain in the arm, 6 months after the diagnosis of a medulloblastoma. The x-ray study reveals mottled areas of decreased density in the metaphysis of the left humerus with subperiosteal resorption of the bone.

children with brain tumors may be falsely attributed to the bone marrow depression caused by spinal irradiation and/or chemotherapeutic agents, rather than to bone marrow replacement by tumor cells. Thus, any unexplained anemia in a child with a brain tumor should raise the suspicion of bone marrow metastasis.

Lymph nodes are another common metastatic site for medulloblastomas, and when suspected a biopsy should be done. Involvement of the lung and pleura may be diagnosed on the basis of chest films, again followed by biopsy for definitive diagnosis. Liver involvement may be suggested by hepatomegaly or pain in the right upper quadrant (Fig. 21-4). Diffuse nonspecific abdominal pain may reflect seeding of the peritoneum.

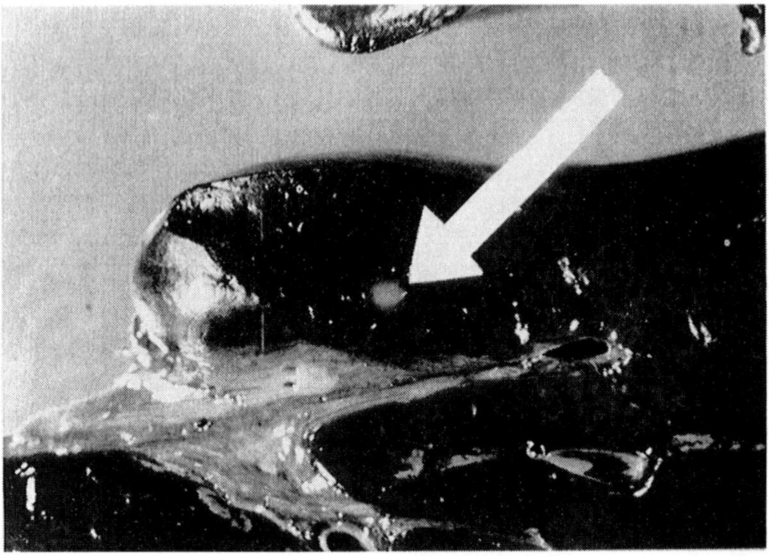

FIG. 21-4. Extraneural metastases of a primitive neuroectodermal tumor to the liver.

INVOLVEMENT OF THE CNS

Although systemic metastases are usually accompanied by recurrence of tumor in the CNS, this is by no means always the case. Out of 88 patients in one series (20), 6 had evidence of systemic metastases an average of 5 months before the diagnosis of a recurrent tumor within the CNS. There has been at least one isolated report (25) of a case of metastasis discovered before diagnosis of the primary brain tumor. It is of interest that at the time of autopsy, 87% of patients with extraneural metastases in one series (20) had recurrent tumor in the posterior fossa. However, there were 2 patients in whom there was no tumor identified in the CNS, despite the presence of extraneural metastases.

The interval after diagnosis of the primary tumor and before the development of extraneural metastases is variable. The average duration before the development of extraneural metastases is approximately 2 years. However, metastases have been reported as early as 5 months after diagnosis (7). In another series reported by Paterson (30), extraneural metastases associated with medulloblastomas appeared as early as 4 months after surgery . We recently had a patient with a medulloblastoma [not included in our published series (10)] who developed extraneural metastases 6 months after diagnosis. Metastases were in the pelvis, humerus, and mandible. It is of interest that this patient did not have evidence of CNS disease at the time that bony metastases were diagnosed.

FACTORS INFLUENCING METASTASES

It is well recognized that brain tumor cells are capable of extracranial growth, as has been demonstrated by the successful transplantation of experimental murine glioma into pleural and peritoneal cavities (44). Despite this, until recently the number of reports of brain tumors with extracranial spread has been quite limited. The rarity of extracranial spread of brain tumors has been explained by several theories, including the early occlusion of venous channels by tumor compression, the absence of cerebral lymphatics, the possible immune responses to tumor cells by other organs, and the short lifespan of patients with primary brain tumors (36).

The overwhelming majority of patients who develop extraneural metastases have had surgery for their primary brain tumor. Therefore, several authors (23) implicate surgery as at least one mechanism by which tumor cells bypass the blood–brain barrier. It is theorized that craniotomy may induce a negative pressure in cerebral veins, creating a suction effect on tumor cells (29). This will then provide the tumor cell entree to the systemic circulation. Indeed, it has been demonstrated that the venous blood of patients with brain tumors examined during and after surgery often contains tumor cells (35). Another theory suggests that blood vessels in the glial scars that develop after surgery are more patent and less easily compressible than those in the original tumor bed. Consequently, they may be more easily infiltrated by tumor cells (14). Entree to the systemic circulation may also be accomplished by invasion of the dura's vascular structures at the operative site (9,43). Finally, surgery may allow the tumor to migrate into bone and scalp flaps, thus providing access to the lymphatic as well as the vascular circulation (11).

There have, however, been isolated cases in which spontaneous metastases have occurred before surgery. Rubinstein (32) reported a patient with an anaplastic astrocytoma, with metastases to bone marrow and abdominal lymph nodes, prior to any surgical intervention. Glasauer and Yuan (13), and Pasquier et al. (29) found another seven cases of gliomas in the literature with extraneural metastases prior to craniotomy. It is of interest that there are no differences in the metastatic sites of implants in operated and nonoperated patients (13,29). Thus, although surgery may allow primary brain tumor cells access to extracranial regions, other potential routes must also be available.

Another factor favoring metastases has been ventriculoperitoneal and ventriculoatrial shunting (3). Kleinman et al. (20) reviewed 103 patients with medulloblastomas and extraneural metastases. Of these, 23 had undergone shunt procedures. He found that metastases occurred earlier in those patients with shunts than in those children without shunts. Patients with shunts developed metastases an average of 1.3 years after the diagnosis, whereas patients without shunts developed metastases an average of 2 years after the diagnosis. Seven patients with pineal germinomas and ventriculoperitoneal shunts have been reported (27) with peritoneal metastases. Latency between initial diagnosis and metastases ranged from 5 months to 3 years.

Precraniotomy shunts have been employed in the surgical approach to posterior fossa tumors in order to decrease the morbidity of surgery in those patients with elevated intracranial pressure. Hoffman et al. (17) reported 6 out of 41 patients with medulloblastomas who had received precraniotomy ventriculoperitoneal shunts and subsequently developed systemic metastases. Two of these patients had local recurrences. The remaining 4 had no recurrences in the CNS either clinically or at the time of autopsy. The patients presented with abdominal complaints and were found to have medulloblastoma cells seeding the peritoneum. Ultimately, the tumor invaded the bone marrow and bone. One patient also developed pulmonary metastases. Because precraniotomy ventriculoperitoneal shunts presumably provide access for malignant cells to enter the abdominal cavity, the authors proposed the use of a millipore filter to eliminate this route of entree. Unfortunately, the millipore filter has not been as successful as previously thought, largely because of the occurrence of shunt obstruction by tumor cells. Thus, at the present time, routine preoperative shunting is not advisable in patients with medulloblastomas.

Whereas surgery and shunts allow brain tumor cells access to areas outside the CNS, prolonging the life of patients with brain tumors by aggressive multimodality therapy may allow transplanted cells time to become clinically evident. This theory has been proposed by Alvord (1) and others (10). The basis of this theory rests on the concept of exponential tumor growth, which suggests that as tumor cells double in number, there should be a predictable increase in tumor mass over a given period of time (18). The survival of patients with brain tumors relates in part to mass of the tumor, which can be predicted if the doubling time of the tumor cell line is known (36). After 20 doublings, the average cancer cell produces a volume of 1 mm^3, which is presumably the smallest size at which a macroscopic diagnosis of cancer can be made (34). After 30 doublings, the single tumor cell reaches a diameter of 1 cm, the earliest that the lesion can be detected radiographically. The average glioma will not be diagnosed until it reaches a diameter of approximately 2.5 cm, or four generations after it has reached a diameter of 1 cm. A glioblastoma is thought to be fatal approximately eight doublings after the tumor has reached 1 cm in diameter. Thus, the clinically detectable life span of the glioma may be only four or five generations (1). This relatively short survival may be explained in part by the rigid structure of the skull, which is unable to compensate for an enlarging mass and allows early compromise of vital structures. Conversely, patients with malignancies in the abdominal cavity may accommodate an enlarging tumor for eight or nine generations from diagnosis until death from visceral carcinomatosis (1). Hence, if a CNS tumor metastasizes at surgery, it would take up to 30 generations before the metastases reached 2 cm^3, a size that could be easily diagnosed at the time of autopsy. This would be long after most patients had already died of their primary tumors. In our series, several patients were long-term survivors by the time they developed extraneural metastases. One child with a malignant ependymoma survived 45 months, and a patient with an unclassified malignant glioma survived 7 years. A third child with a primitive neuroectodermal tumor survived only 16 months, but this is a relatively long survival—the usual life span of patients with these tumors is reported to be 7 to 8 months (10). Hitchcock et al. (15) reported a patient with glioblastoma multiforme with multiple metastases diagnosed during life who survived a total of 20 years. The aggressive therapy and consequent prolongation of life in these patients presumably allowed the necessary doubling times for extracranial metastases to become clinically evident. One doubling time of the tumor is altered in vivo by many factors, including necrosis, exfoliation, and cell death (38). Nevertheless, the Alvord hypothesis is intriguing because it suggests that if patients with brain tumors survive longer, extracranial metastases may reach a sufficient size to be readily diagnosed on pathologic and clinical examination. Ironically, prolonging the survivals of patients with brain tumors may also increase the incidence of extraneural metastases.

The influence of radiation and chemotherapy on the development of extraneural metastases is not yet known. Chemotherapeutic agents, by destroying proliferating cells, may enhance the nutritional environment of the remaining tumor cells. This would indirectly allow nonproliferating cells to enter the cell cycle (38). Theoretically, then, suboptimal chemotherapy may have the potential to promote tumor growth. Chemotherapy may also alter immune systems and allow the spread and growth of tumor cells in extracranial locations. Although radiation has a known oncogenic effect, it is not known whether it may also influence the development of extraneural metastases. The treatment of brain tumors with chemotherapy is still relatively new, and it is unclear if this type of treatment will influence the development of extraneural metastases. As the phenomenon of extraneural metastases in childhood brain tumors becomes better appreciated, the influence of chemotherapy and radiotherapy on the development of these lesions will become clarified.

Finally, the increasing number of reported cases of extraneural metastases may reflect in part the medical community's enhanced awareness of this problem. Previously, failure to recognize extracranial metastasis clinically may have contributed to a low reporting yield. As discussed, bone pain may not be present with skeletal metastases and even if present is often attributed to neural involvement. Evaluation of such patients with plain radiographs and bone scans, in addition to myelography, may increase the number of extraneural metastases found. Likewise, awareness that anemia may be the result of bone marrow replacement, rather than as a result of iatrogenic causes, may increase the reports of this complication. A meticulous autopsy examination is also necessary. In one study, extensive autopsies were performed on patients who had died from melanomas. Close pathologic examination of the bone increased the incidence of skeletal metastases in that series from a historical incidence of 7 to 50% (Mindel, personal communication, 1981). Occult metastatic lesions of bone and soft tissue in children with brain tumors may be asymptomatic and thus may not be diagnosed during life. Therefore, extensive and detailed autopsies will be necessary to establish the true incidence of these lesions. Greater awareness by both clinicians and pathologists of the possibility of extraneural metastases with brain tumors may increase the detection of this phenomenon.

TREATMENT

The diagnosis of extraneural metastases is of more than academic interest, because these lesions may respond to treatment. Moreover, the rising incidence of extraneural metastases raises the question of whether systemic chemotherapy should be administered to patients with brain tumors at initial diagnosis. Nathanson and Kovaks (26) in 1978 reviewed several reports of patients who had had metastatic medulloblastomas treated with chemotherapy (Table 21-1). Chemotherapy regimens differed and included varying combinations of vincristine, actinomycin D, nitrogen mustard, cyclophosphamide, 1,3 Bis(2-chlorethyl)-1-nitrosourea (BCNU),1-(2-chlorethyl)3-cyclohexyl-1-nitrosourea (CCNU), and adriamycin. Responses were achieved in 12 of 22 courses of chemotherapy delivered to 19 patients with a mean duration response of 5.2 months. The range of response was from 2 to 12 months. Responses to treatment were obtained in 9 of 15 patients with bone metastases, 2 of 5 children with lymph node involvement, 2 of 3 patients with skin and soft tissue metastases, and 0 of 2 patients with metastatic involvement of the lungs. Nathanson and Kovacs employed a regimen of vincristine, actinomycin D, cyclophosphamide, and adriamycin on the assumption that because medulloblastomas and neuroblastomas have common origins in embryologic neural crest tissue, they might respond to similar chemotherapeutic agents. Indeed, they found that extraneural metastases did respond to this regimen, whereas CNS tumors did not. Consequently, they suggested that if neural involvement was also present, the patient should be treated additionally with nitrosoureas. It should be noted that when these patients received treatment, there was radiologic as well as clinical improvement. For example, Lassman (21) treated patients with bony metastases with vincristine alone or in combination with cyclophosphamide. X-ray studies of bone after treatment revealed gradual reossification of the osteolytic lesion and disappearance of the periosteal new bone. Osteoblastic areas became more homogenous and smooth and lost their irregularity. The quality of survival in these patients was good until the final recurrence. We have treated two children with bony metastases with cyclophosphamide, vincristine, and

TABLE 21-1. *Chemotherapeutic experience with extraneural metastatic medulloblastomas*

Author	Patients	Drug	Response
Drachman et al. (9)	1	Vincristine	PR, 3 months
Gyepes and D'Angio (14)	3	Actinomycin D	NR, 1 patient Unknown, 2 patients
Lassman (21)	2	Vincristine	Response, 26 months Response, 10 months
	2	Vincristine and cyclophosphamide	Response, 14 months NR, 1 patient
Debnam and Staple (8)	2	Vincristine and cyclophosphamide	Stable disease, 12 months NR, 1 patient
Kessler et al. (19)	1	Vincristine and CCNU	PR, 2 months
Ward (35)	1	Vincristine and cyclophosamide	Response, 8 months
Brutschin and Culver (4)	3	Vincristine	NR, 1 patient Unknown, 2 patients
Parkinson et al. (28)	1	Vincristine and cyclophosphamide	NR, 1 patient
Stolzenberg et al. (37)	1	Cyclophosphamide	PR, 2 months
Nathanson and Kovacs (26)	2	Vincristine, cyclophosphamide and actinomycin D	PR, 11 months PR, 4 months PR, 4 months
Duffner and Cohen (10)	2	Vincristine, cyclophosphamide and adriamycin	Response, 10 months Response, 2 years
Duffner and Cohen	1	Vincristine, BCNU, procarbazine	Response, 10 months

Adapted from Nathanson L, Kovacs SG. Chemotherapeutic response in metastatic medulloblastoma: Repeat of two cases and a review of the literature. *Med Pediatr Oncol* 1978; 4:105–110.

adriamycin with resolution of symptoms for 10 months and 2 years, respectively. A third child has been treated with BCNU, vincristine, and procarbazine, with resolution of pain and improvement on plain x-ray studies. Seven adult patients with metastatic anaplastic oligodendrogliomas were treated with either focal radiation or nitrosourea-based chemotherapy. The systemic metastases responded to therapy for 6 to 18 months. However, five of seven died 14 to 24 months following diagnosis of extraneural metastases (24). VP16, cis-platin, vinblastine, and bleomycin were used effectively in a case of extraneural metastasis to lung in a child with a pineal region nongerminomatous germ cell tumor. Control lasted over 46 months (41). Another child with a germinoma and bone metastases responded for over 30 months to a similar chemotherapy regimen, i.e., vinblastine, bleomycin, doxorubicin, and cis-platin (12). Obviously, because the number of treatment reports is quite limited, a consistent therapeutic program has yet to be established (Table 21-1).

SUMMARY

Extraneural metastases may occur with brain tumors of both children and adults. The most common childhood brain tumor to spread beyond the CNS axis is the medulloblastoma. However, ependymomas, glioblastomas, meningiomas, astrocytomas, pinealomas, and choroid plexus tumors have been reported to develop extraneural metastases as well. There is no age- or sex-related predilection for this phenomenon. The site of metastasis varies with the primary tumor. In general, medulloblastomas spread to bone, bone marrow, and lymph nodes, whereas gliomas and meningiomas commonly involve lung and pleura. The average interval from diagnosis of the primary tumor to metastatic spread is 2 years. Systemic metastases are not always associated with recurrent tumors in the CNS. Factors influencing the development of extraneural metastases include prior surgery, ventriculoperitoneal or ventriculoatrial shunts, and, possibly, the use of cranial irradiation and systemic chemotherapy. The increasing reports of patients with extracranial metastases may be related in part to the prolongation of lifespans of patients with brain tumors, which allows extracranial tumor cells the necessary doubling times to become either clinically significant or easily identifiable on autopsy. In addition, awareness of this complication by clinicians and pathologists may be leading to more realistic incidence figures. The diagnosis of extraneural metastases is of clinical importance, because some may respond to local radiation and systemic chemotherapy. Several centers have reported extraneural metastases in 10 to 15% of children with medulloblastomas. If these reports are confirmed, primary adjuvant chemotherapy may be necessary to prevent the development of extraneural metastases.

REFERENCES

1. Alvord EC. Why do gliomas not metastasize? *Arch Neurol* 1976;33:73–75.
2. Bach M, Simpson WJ, Platts ME. Metastatic cerebellar sarcoma (desmoplastic medulloblastoma) with diffuse osteosclerosis and leukoerythroblastic anemia. *AJR* 1968;18:649–653.
3. Brust JCM, Moiel RH, Rosenberg RN. Glial tumor metastases through a ventriculo-pleural shunt. *Arch Neurol* 1968;18:649–653.
4. Brutschin P, Culver GJ. Medulloblastoma: extracranial metastases from medulloblastomas. *Radiology* 1973;107:359–363.
5. Campbell AN, Chan HSL, Becker LE, Daneman A, Park TS, Hoffman HJ. Extracranial metastases in childhood primary intracranial tumors. *Cancer* 1984;53:974–981.
6. Chatty E, Earle K. Medulloblastoma: a report of 201 cases with emphasis on the relationship of histologic variant to survival. *Cancer* 1971;28:977–983.
7. Das E, Dalby JE. Distant metastases from medulloblastoma. *Acta Radiol Ther* 1977;16: 117–123.
8. Debnam JW, Staple TW. Osseous metastases from cerebellar medulloblastoma. *Radiology* 1973;107:363–365.
9. Drachman DA, Winter TS, Karon M. Medulloblastoma with extracranial metastases. *Arch Neurol* 1963;9:86–98.
10. Duffner PK, Cohen ME. Extraneural metastases in childhood brain tumors. *Ann Neurol* 1981;10:261–265.

11. Eade OE, Urich H. Metastasizing gliomas in young subjects. *J Pathol* 1971;103:245–256.
12. Gay JC, Janco RL, Lukens JN. Systemic metastases in primary intracranial germinoma. *Cancer* 1985;55:2688–2690.
13. Glasauer FE, Yuan RHP. Intracranial tumors with extracranial metastases. *J Neurosurg* 1963;20:474–493.
14. Gyepes MT, D'Angio GJ. Extracranial metastases from central nervous system tumors in children and adolescents. *Radiology* 1966;87:55–63.
15. Hitchcock MH, Hollinshead AC, Chretien P, Rizzoli HV. Soluble membrane antigens of brain tumors. *Cancer* 1977;40:660–666.
16. Ho EP, Lieber A, DeLand FH, Maruyama Y. Generalized osteoblastic bony metastases from medulloblastoma. *Oncology* 1976;33:253–256.
17. Hoffman HJ, Hendrick EB, Humphreys RP. Metastasis via ventriculoperitoneal shunt in patients with medulloblastoma. *J Neurosurg* 1976;44:562–566.
18. Hoshino T, Wilson CB. Review of basic concepts of cell kinetics as applied to brain tumors. *J Neurosurg* 1975;42:123–131.
19. Kessler LA, Dugan P, Concannon JP. Systemic metastases of medulloblastoma promoted by shunting. *Surg Neurol* 1975;3:147–152.
20. Kleinman GM, Hochberg FH, Richardson EP. Systemic metastases from medulloblastoma: report of two cases and review of the literature. *Cancer* 1981;48:2296–2309.
21. Lassman LP. Diagnosis and management of skeletal metastases from cerebellar medulloblastoma. *Childs Brain* 1976;2:38–45.
22. Lewis MB, Nunes LB, Powell DE, Shnider BI. Extraaxial spread of medulloblastoma. *Cancer* 1973;31:1287–1297.
23. Liwnicz B, Rubinstein LJ. The pathways of extraneural spread in metastasizing gliomas: a report of three cases and critical review of the literature. *Hum Pathol* 1979;10:453–467.
24. MacDonald DR, O'Brien RA, Gilbert JJ, Cairncross JG. Metastatic anaplastic oligodendroglioma. *Neurology* 1989;39:1593–1596.
25. McComb JG, Davis RL, Isaacs H, Landing BH. Medulloblastoma presenting as neck tumors in two infants. *Ann Neurol* 1980;7:113–117.
26. Nathanson L, Kovacs SG. Chemotherapeutic response in metastatic medulloblastoma: repeat of two cases and a review of the literature. *Med Pediatr Oncol* 1978;4:105–110.
27. Pallini R, Bozzini V, Scerrati M, Zuppi C, Zappacosta B, Rossi GF. Bone metastasis associated with shunt-related peritoneal deposits from a pineal germinoma. *Acta Neurochir* 1991; 109:78–83.
28. Parkinson D, Ross RT, Shields C. Metastatic medulloblastoma. *Can J Neurol Sci* 1974;1: 253–254.
29. Pasquier B, Pasquier D, Golet AN, Panh MH, Coudere P. Extraneural metastases of astrocytomas and glioblastoma: clinicopathological study of two cases and review of the literature. *Cancer* 1980;45:112–125.
30. Paterson E. Distant metastases from medulloblastoma of the cerebellum. *Brain* 1961;84: 301–308.
31. Raimondi AJ, Tomita T. Medulloblastoma in childhood. *Acta Neurochir* 1979;50:127–138.
32. Rubinstein LJ. Development of extracranial metastases from a malignant astrocytoma in the absence of previous craniotomy: case report. *J Neurosurg* 1967;26:542–547.
33. Schnitzler ER, Richards MJS, Chun RWM. Cerebellar medulloblastoma: an analysis of four cases of extraneural metastases. *Am J Dis Child* 1978;132:1004–1008.
34. Schwartz M. A biomathematical approach to clinical tumor growth. *Cancer* 1961;14: 1272–1294.
35. Smith DR, Hardman JM, Earle KM. Metastasizing neuroectodermal tumors of the central nervous system. *J Neurosurg* 1969;31:50–58.
36. Steel GG. Cytokinetics of neoplasia. In: Holland JF, Frei E III, eds. *Cancer medicine*. Philadelphia:Lea & Febiger; 1973:125–140.
37. Stolzenberg J, Fischer JJ, Kligerman MM. Extraneural metastasis in medulloblastoma 10 years after treatment. *AJR* 1970;108:71–74.
38. Valeriote F, Vietti TJ. Cellular kinetics and conceptual basis of chemotherapy. In: Sutow WW, Vietti TJ, Fernbach DJ, eds. *Clinical pediatric oncology*. St Louis:CV Mosby; 1977: 182–196.
39. Ward HWC. CCNU in treatment of recurrent medulloblastoma. *Br Med J* 1974;1:642.

40. Wasserkrug R, Peyser E, Lichtig C. Extracranial bone metastases from intracranial meningiomas. *Surg Neurol* 1979;12:480–484.
41. Watterson J, Priest JR. Control of extraneural metastasis of a primary intracranial nongerminomatous germ cell tumor. *J Neurosurg* 1989;71:601–604.
42. Weiss L. A metastasizing ependymoma of the cauda equina. *Cancer* 1955;8:161–171.
43. Winkelman NW, Cassel C, Schlesinger B. Intracranial tumors with extracranial metastases. *J Neuropathol Exp Neurol* 1952;11:149–168.
44. Zimmerman HM. The natural history of intracranial neoplasms with special reference to the gliomas. *Am J Surg* 1957:93:913–924.

22

Long-Term Pathologic Effects of Cancer Treatment on the Nervous System

Michael E. Cohen, Daniel J. Lacey, and Patricia K. Duffner

The clinical consequences of treatment of cancer of the nervous system have been well documented and are reviewed in Chapter 23. The structural substrate of these abnormalities has been less well detailed. Despite these misgivings, there is a growing literature dealing with imaging and pathologic changes following both radiation and chemotherapy to the nervous system (44,45,49,94,95). Where possible, this chapter will review structural changes and correlate them with known clinical syndromes.

Structural damage to the CNS resulting from therapeutic irradiation of the head and neck has been known since the 1930s (44). Most of the early literature consists of scattered reports of patients, mostly adults, given large doses of radiation and treated for skull cancer, pituitary disorders (acromegaly), and brain tumors. Reports of the potential hazards of therapeutic CNS irradiation in children were initially derived from the treatment and prophylaxis of CNS leukemia and, surprisingly, were not reported in detail until the 1970s. Since then, many papers have described the long-term effects of radiation on the CNS in children with leukemia (75). Radiation damage to the spinal cord (myelopathy) after treatment for spinal malignancy was initially reported in 1941, and although hundreds of cases have been subsequently published, few have included children (15,20).

Therapeutic strategies aimed at the prevention of CNS leukemia received a great deal of attention in the 1960s because of its extremely grave prognosis. Craniospinal irradiation, combined with systemic and lumbar subarachnoid administration of chemotherapeutic agents, was shown to be an effective regimen in preventing CNS relapse. What had been a virtually uniformly fatal disease has become "curable" in up to 50% of patients. However, it became apparent in the early and middle 1970s that the prolonged survival of children was not free of complications. Neurologic, psychologic, and endocrinologic symptoms developed which could not be explained by either infections from immune suppression or meningeal leukemia. Neuropathologic reports describing previously unrecognized lesions in treated leukemic

Brain Tumors in Children: Principles of Diagnosis and Treatment, 2/e, edited by M.E. Cohen and P.K. Duffner, Raven Press, Ltd., New York, 1994.

children followed shortly thereafter. A series of papers (40,70,71,79) from 1974 to 1978 described the two major pathologic features seen in some brains of treated leukemic patients, namely, destruction of white matter (leukoencephalopathy) and damage to smaller and medium-sized blood vessels (microangiopathy).

Information is limited regarding long-term pathologic complications of treatment of the solid tumors of the CNS in children. In part, this reflects the relative rarity of pediatric brain tumors, the poor survival rates, and the declining frequency of postmortem examinations. As in leukemia, the use of a variety of therapeutic regimens for the histologic myriad of CNS tumors has resulted in significantly improved survivals. Pari passu with increased survival has been an increased awareness of the potential consequences of therapy itself.

Limitations in predicting the long-term iatrogenic CNS effects in children include the fact that although considerable pathologic data are available from adult patients, this information cannot be extrapolated to the child. It is well known that the immature nervous system has different tolerances to radiation and drugs than the adult nervous system. Therefore, identical therapeutic regimens given to children and adults with different types and loci of tumors could theoretically result in different pathologic (and clinical) consequences. Another limitation has been the inability to adequately define the pathologic potential of the therapeutic agents in current use, since multiagent chemotherapy regimens, in addition to radiation therapy, remain the rule in childhood cancer, specifically in the treatment and prophylaxis of CNS neoplasia. Finally, remote effects of cancer on the nervous system may need to be considered when clinical and pathologic findings develop long after completion of therapy. Although a host of syndromes have been described in adults, the only well accepted "remote" CNS effect of cancer in children is the opsoclonus–polymyoclonus syndrome associated with neuroblastoma.

The ability to detect deleterious effects of cancer treatment on the CNS is continually being improved through the development of sophisticated neuroinvestigative techniques. CT and MRI permit verification of clinical leukoencephalopathy as well as presymptomatic detection (67). Sensory evoked responses, to a minimal extent, are helpful in detecting neurotoxicity of chemotherapeutic agents (47). In the future, magnetic resonance angiography, magnetic resonance spectroscopy, and positive emission tomography will be useful in assessing untoward treatment effects.

HEMISPHERIC PATHOLOGY

Although cortical gray matter symptoms of seizures and dementia are commonly described in patients as adverse effects of therapy, pathologic involvement of cortical neurons has been only infrequently reported. Most series have emphasized white matter and vascular changes, and have not paid attention to neuronal morphology or cortical architecture (91). In those few studies (5,31,72) that include neuronal descriptions, few if any significant changes have been seen. Hendin et al. (40) described frontoparietal laminar cortical necrosis in a leukemic patient treated with radiation, methotrexate, and other drugs. These authors also described prominent Alzheimer type II cortical neuronal change presumably secondary to hepatic dysfunction. In an autopsy series of 22 treated leukemics, Crosley (23) found a high percentage of atrophic brains, the majority of which were only mildly to moderately affected. Microscopically, irregular neuronal loss and gliosis were present in all cortical layers.

Absence of prominent neuronal cytopathology is difficult to reconcile with clinical symptoms of gray matter involvement. One possibility is that cognitive effects are secondary to an altered neurochemical transmission between cellular elements not reflected in neuronal structural integrity. Another possible reason for this discrepancy is that structural alterations of neurons may not be revealed by standard neurohistologic methods or cytoarchitecture. For instance, Golgi stains have been useful in Down's syndrome to demonstrate alterations in the structure and number of neurons. This methodology has been applied in other dementing illnesses (i.e., phenylketonuria) to identify change not observed by standard neurohistologic procedures (74).

LEUKOENCEPHALOPATHY

Multifocal destructive lesions of white matter have been described in patients treated with radiation, methotrexate, other chemotherapeutic agents, and combination therapies (5,10,18,23,54). The clinical implications of leukoencephalopathy were not appreciated until 1975 when two pathologic series (56,62) of children with acute lymphocytic leukemia were published. Most, but not all, patients developed neurologic symptoms and signs weeks to months after completion of treatment (25). The clinical features were drooling, dysphagia, dementia, hemiparesis, ataxia, and labored speech. Focal or generalized seizures were also common but difficult to explain on the basis of white (rather than gray) matter damage. Progression of symptoms was usually subacute and at times relentless, leading to death or a persistent vegetative state. Conversely, there have been other patients who have partially or completely recovered (8).

The areas of white matter most frequently involved are the deep cerebral hemisphere (centrum semiovale) and periventricular regions. Involvement is usually multifocal and asymmetric (48). Microscopically, loss of oligodendroglia and myelin are evident in affected lesions, with axonal swelling and fragmentation (25). Discrete areas of coagulative necrosis extend and meld by confluence (84). Astrocytosis and phagocytosis occur late. Dystrophic calcification often develops, as well as compensatory dilatation of the ventricles and subarachnoid space (31,56). Fibrinoid necrosis of blood vessels has been reported in some series but not in others, even though radiation therapy was similarly employed (52). A histologic inflammatory response within and around these lesions is not usually present.

The pathogenesis of this complication has been, like cancer treatment itself, multimodal. Leukoencephalopathy is seen in patients receiving radiation therapy for primary CNS tumors in doses, for the most part, greater than 5,000 cGy and in fractions exceeding 200 cGy a day (15,53,54). Leukoencephalopathy is much less frequent with total radiation doses below 5,500 cGy and fractions per dose of 150 to 180 cGy per day. However, clinical, neuroradiologic, or pathologic evidence of leukoencephalopathy has been found in leukemic children who received more than 1,800 cGy to the head (8). Demyelination has also been reported in patients given methotrexate by any of the following routes of administration: intraventricular, intrathecal, or intravenous (5,11,62,72,85). Methotrexate is one of the most common chemotherapeutic agents used in leukemic treatment, and the one most often implicated as having the greatest potential of producing leukoencephalopathy. Cytosine arabinoside and 1,3 Bis(2-chlorethyl)-1-nitrosourea (BCNU) have also been identified as causing leukoencephalopathy (3,14). Methotrexate's contribution to the development of leukoencephalopathy appears to depend on total dosage, route of administration, timing, and CSF flow dynamics (86). Bleyer and Griffin (8) emphasized that methotrexate given during or following radiation treatment is of greater concern than that given prior to radiation. Since combined radiation and chemotherapy has been the standard protocol for leukemic patients, the relative contributions of these modalities have been questioned.

Disruption of the CSF and blood–brain barriers is thought to be instrumental in causing leukoencephalopathy. Capillary damage and blood–brain barrier (BBB) alterations are well-known sequelae of radiation, especially in already compromised brains (18). First, subsequent intravenous methotrexate administration has been shown to result in increased brain levels of methotrexate, which more easily diffuses through a "leaky" blood–brain barrier (28). Second, the ependymal cell tight junction–CSF barrier may be altered by radiation and drugs. Egress of intrathecally or intraventricularly administered drugs from ventricular CSF into brain parenchyma will result in the highest concentrations in deep white matter (70). Altered spinal fluid clearance also results in prolongation of exposure to potentially toxic drugs in the CSF. Finally, barrier disruption at the cellular level (neuronal, glial, ependymal), induced by one mode of therapy, may enhance the toxic effects of another administered at a later time (31). Both radiation and methotrexate have been reported to sensitize tissue exposed to the damaging effects of subsequently administered agents (8,69,78). Leukoencephalopathy has also been associated with loss of oligodendroglia and myelin, axonal swelling, and fragmentation. Changes of reactive astrocytosis, dystrophic calcification, and coagulative necrosis may become confluent, leading to a leukoencephalopathic picture (34). Secondary effects of capillary damage result in alterations of the blood–brain barrier. Disruption of blood–brain barrier and CSF–brain barrier may lead to periventricular damage and damage to the Virchow-Robin spaces.

Leukoencephalopathy and CT

With the emergence of computed tomography in the early 1970s, clinical pathologic correlations began to emerge. Hypodense areas in the white matter, cerebral atrophy, areas of necrosis, increase in sulci width, and enlargement of ventricles have been associated with seizures, long tract signs, and dementia (5,19). These findings are thought to reflect demyelination with focal or diffuse areas of white matter necrosis, glial damage, calcification, and microangiopathy (15). Although a relationship between CT features and total dose of radiation dose per fraction, volume of radiation, overall treatment time, and patient age have been indirectly inferred, precise correlations are not known. On CT, white matter changes are characterized by decreased attenuation in injured areas. The hypodensities may have scalloped lateral margins with sparing of cerebral cortex and subcortical arcuate fibers. Ventricular dilatation and increased width of the cerebral sulci reflect cerebral atrophy. Intracranial calcifications, recognized primarily in the white matter and basal ganglia, represent long-standing microangiopathy (56). These findings can be observed years following treatment (75).

CT leukoencephalopathy was initially recognized in 1978 in children with leukemia (51,52). These children were treated with radiation and methotrexate as part of the treatment of sanctuary sites for leukemia. Of those studied, 53% had CT scans characterized by increased size of the cerebral sulci, hypodense areas, and areas of calcification especially in the basal ganglia. Ochs et al. (63) subsequently described CT scans in children with acute lymphocytic leukemia whose CNS prophylaxis did not include radiation. In contrast to the earlier reports, only 18% of these patients had abnormalities on CT scan and all were of a mild degree (63). On further examination of the original material reported by Peylan-Ramu (67), there were a few patients who had not received cranial radiation. Only 9% of this group had CT abnormalities. The conclusion from these studies has been that patients with CNS leukemia treated only with methotrexate are less likely to develop CT leukoencephalopathy than those treated with both radiation and chemotherapy. It is noteworthy, however, that high-dose intravenous methotrexate is also capable of producing CT leukoencephalopathy even without concomitant radiation. The tendency to develop leukoencephalopathy increases in those patients who have central nervous system disease at the time of treatment.

In our own review (28) of patients with CNS leukemia who received methotrexate but who did not receive cranial radiation, 80% had CT scans compatible with leukoencephalopathy. Furthermore, all our patients with CNS leukemia who were radiated developed leukoencephalopathy. The etiology for this may, in part, be related to altered cerebrospinal fluid clearance of methotrexate. Others (28) had obtained methotrexate levels from Ommaya reservoirs in leukemic children with and without CNS disease. Methotrexate concentrations in patients with CNS leukemia were significantly higher at 24 and 48 hours when compared to a control group. These findings raised the possibility that delayed intraventricular clearance of drugs may occur in patients with meningeal disease. Because of this, CT abnormalities in children with CNS leukemia were compared with CSF methotrexate clearance. Not surprisingly, those patients with more severe CT leukoencephalopathy had significantly higher CSF methotrexate levels at 24 and 48 hours following administration. This observation suggests that delayed clearance of methotrexate from the ventricles permits transependymal flow of drug across the ventricular walls, resulting in periventricular damage. Leukoencephalopathy is more likely in those children with leukemia who have CNS disease and who have been treated with both radiation and methotrexate (11). In contrast, children without meningeal disease who have not received radiation are less likely to develop this complication. Thus, the relative risk of developing CT leukoencephalopathy in leukemic children can be assessed as follows: least—children without CNS involvement who received only chemotherapy prophylaxis; moderate—children without CNS leukemia who received both radiation and chemotherapy; and greatest—children with CNS leukemia who were treated with either radiation or chemotherapy. Whereas the total dose of radiation to the CNS given to children with leukemia is 1,800 to 2,500 cGy, the dose of radiation given to children with CNS neoplasms is significantly higher, i.e., 5,500 to 6,500 cGy to the tumor bed. As expected, the increased dose is associated with an increased frequency and severity of leukoencephalopathy.

Leukoencephalopathy and MRI

Because of its multiple paradigms of imaging and the ability to recognize alterations in water content, MRI provides a detailed assessment of the nervous system (64). Zimmerman et al. (96) have graded white matter changes on MR from 4 to 0. Grade 4, the worst, consists of diffuse white matter abnormalities manifested by irregular increased T2 signals extending from the ventricle to the cortical medullary junction. Grade 3 (Fig. 22-1) consists of a periventricular halo or band of hyperintensity of variable thickness forming smooth lateral margins around the ventricle. Grade 2 consists of a pencil-thin continuous line of hyperintensity around the ventricles. Grade 1 consists

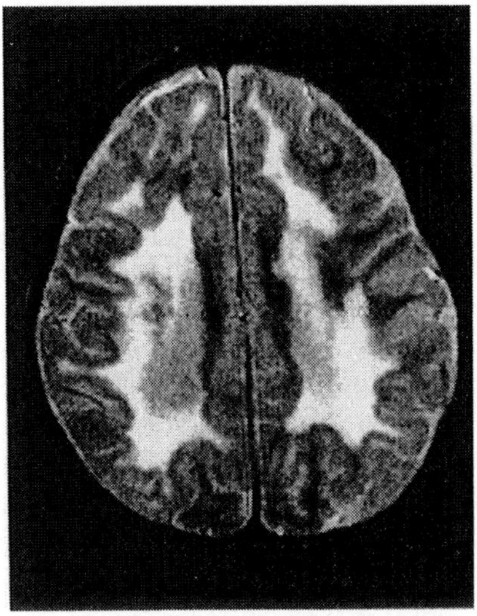

FIG. 22-1. Grade 3 leukoencephalopathy as identified by MRI and defined in the article by Zimmerman (96).

of a discontinuous area of periventricular hyperintensity. Grade 0 consists of no evidence of periventricular hyperintensity.

Constine et al. (21) have correlated white matter changes with dose, patient age, volume of radiation, and the time after radiation. Also considered was the relationship between clinical signs and white matter changes. These authors suggested that patients who receive more than 7,000 cGy in 180 cGy per fraction were more apt to have periventricular hyperintensity than those who had received less than 6,000 cGy. Of interest is the observation that periventricular hyperintensities were more of a problem in adults than in children, contradicting both the clinical experience and observation based on CT imaging. Fifty percent of patients with whole-brain radiation were reported to have grade 3 to 4 changes, compared with only 14% of those in whom radiation was confined to local regions. Again, although no specific correlations have been made, this paper inferred that the combination of large-volume radiation and a longer interval to the time of scanning is associated with an increased frequency of white matter changes. Frank dementia appeared to be associated with more severe involvement, although direct relationships between clinical abnormalities and MRI grade could not be established because many patients with the lower MRI grades also had cognitive difficulties.

The sensitivity and lack of specificity provided by MRI imaging can, at times, be quite confusing. Changes seen in patients with leukoencephalopathy have been reported in normal individuals, although the frequency varies in different series and the meaning of these changes has not been established (35). Grades 1 and 2 changes have been recognized in elderly patients with either trauma or tumor. The more severe changes have been limited to those who have had radiation for neoplasms. The most frequently demonstrated periventricular hyperintensities have been in areas adjacent to the frontal occipital horns and the centrum semiovale. Scalloped configuration is thought to occur as a result of damage to arcuate fibers that interconnect the cerebral gyri (24). This may be associated with cognitive changes.

There has been some speculation that younger children are less apt to have severe changes on MRI than are adults, reflecting the putative limited ability of the elderly to repair damage to white matter. Alternatively, white matter changes in adults can result from microvascular changes associated with the normal aging process (10). This finding is not expected in the young.

Despite the above qualifications, the white matter changes seen as a consequence of radiation therapy can be observed in different degrees on both MRI and CT examinations. The correlation of the degree and intensity of these changes with clinical symptoms continues to be limited. With the development of MRI spectroscopy and PET scanning, specific clinical pathologic correlations should be forthcoming. To date, MRI spectroscopy has been used primarily to differentiate shifts of aerobic to anaerobic metabolism and, by inference, to distinguish radiation necrosis from tumor recurrence.

POSITRON MISSION TOMOGRAPHY

Increasingly, positron emission tomography is providing another dimension in the evaluation of adverse effects of therapy. PET scanning, because of its ability to monitor regional metabolism, provides the potential of defining cerebral diaschisis, that is, abnormalities of function remote from disease site as well as changes at the site of treatment (66). Alterations in local metabolism and in those distant from the lesion will permit correlation between structural changes and function. PET scanning has also been used to distinguish radiation necrosis from tumor. In those patients who develop signs of a mass lesion with edema months to years after surgery and radiotherapy, decreased glucose metabolism, as measured by PET, may suggest radiation necrosis rather than recurrent tumor. Unfortunately, reports that glucose metabolism in low-grade astrocytomas may be lower than in contralateral brain, in contrast to the increased metabolism seen in glioblastoma multiforme, has made the distinction of low-grade astrocytomas from radiation necrosis difficult or even impossible (26).

RADIATION NECROSIS

Radiation necrosis has been reported in patients who receive high-dose radiation, usually greater than 6,000 cGy. Radiation necrosis, in all likelihood, is an intensification of the pathologic processes observed with leukoencephalopathy and consists of vascular damage with infarction, astrogliosis, patchy demyelination, and frank necrosis (79). Necrosis is found in the areas of vascular damage and results from infarction secondary to reduction of blood flow to these areas. Encephalopathy occurs without necrosis from ischemia in terminal or border-zone blood areas. This may explain, to some extent, the periventricular lesions described in leukoencephalopathy because these regions are supplied by periventricular arterial border-zone vessels (16).

Radiation necrosis, like recurrent tumor, is associated with edema and mass effect. Radiation necrosis is found in isodense curves representing 89% of the maximum radiation dose (13). On neuroimaging, heterogeneity of contrast-enhanced zones intermixed with low-density areas, an irregular contour, and localization in the areas of greatest radiation should suggest radiation necrosis rather than tumor. Neuroimaging features of recurrent tumor tend to be homogeneity of the image and growth at the margins rather than at the center of the original tumor. Radiation necrosis and tumor can both be associated with mass effect requiring surgical debulking. The former does not require additional therapy; the latter may lead to adjuvant treatment (27,59,80).

Descriptions of pathologic radiation necroses in animals have been reported in several papers. These consist of astrocytic or glial reactions with perivascular collections of mononuclear cells. Following these changes tissue breaks down, resulting in demyelination, proliferative astrogliosis, and necrosis. Vascular changes include capillary occlusion, hemorrhagic exudates, endothelial proliferation, and fibrinoid necrosis. Vasogenic edema may develop either at the site of the lesion or remote from the areas of radiation damage. Necrosis, vacuolation, and petechial hemorrhage occurs months to years after exposure to radiation (37).

VASCULOPATHIES

Vasculopathies may arise as a result of occlusion of large vessels at the base of the brain with resultant ischemia in the area supplied by the vessel. This may allow for the subsequent development of a moyamoya pattern (Fig. 22-2). There have also been isolated reports of occlusive arterial disease (65) following the injection of chemotherapeutic agents such as L-asparaginase (73).

Although large-vessel diseases can be readily identified by angiography, the microangiopathy observed in leukoencephalopathy and other forms of radiation necrosis can be observed only histopathologically. Mineralizing microangiopathy was reported in several papers by Price and Birdwell (70–72) in the late 1970s. They described mineralizing microangiopathy in 17% of 168 autopsied leukemic patients treated with whole-brain radiation

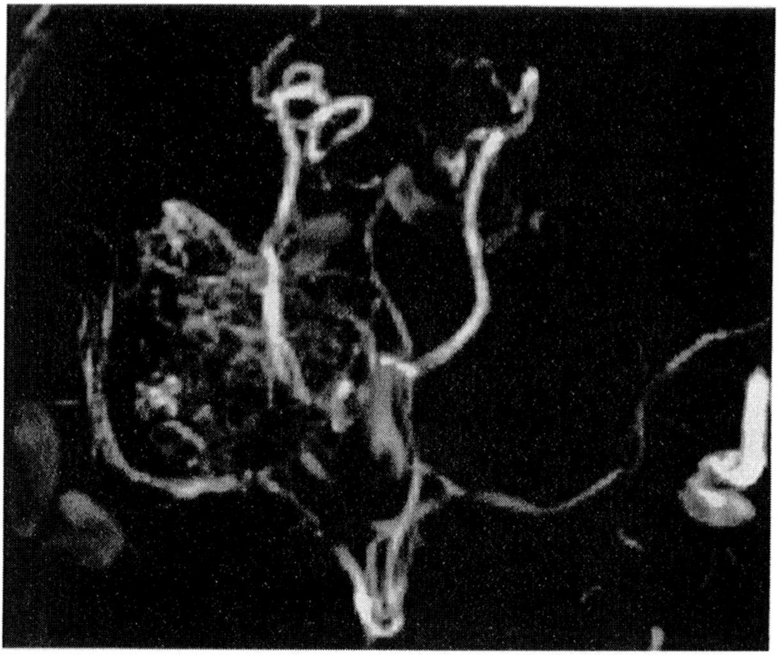

FIG. 22-2. Moyamoya in a 12-year-old boy irradiated for a thalamic glioma. Note the "puff of smoke" pattern in the basal ganglia on the right side.

and intrathecal methotrexate. Small blood vessels were affected, and luminal occlusion was often present. Microangiopathy is associated with deposition of calcium, mucopolysaccarides, and necrotic material found in and around small vessels. Areas in the brain most commonly affected are the basal ganglia, primarily the putamen (31). Cerebellar and cortical vessels are less involved (25,39). These pathologic changes have correlated most directly with neuroimaging findings of leukoencephalopathy.

BRAIN STEM AND SPINAL-CORD PATHOLOGY

Demyelination of the pons has been reported in both adults and children. Clinical findings consist of long tract signs, ataxia, cranial neuropathies, and pseudobulbar paresis. Although demyelination has been described in the cerebellum, midbrain, and medulla, the pons is the site most extensively damaged (13,17,23,48). Myelinolysis is characterized by neuronal atrophy, intense gliosis with sparing of the axons, and limited involvement of blood vessels (38). Two major forms of pontine damage have been recognized. The first consists of multifocal bilateral lesions in the basis pontis (12). Myelin loss, axonal swelling, and fragmentation are evident. Blood vessels are spared, and inflammation is absent. Multifocal pontine lesions have also been reported in adults and animals after intrathecal injection of the antibiotic gentamicin, suggesting that this form of pathology is not specific for cancer or its treatment. The second form, central pontine myelinolysis (CPM), typically spares axons. Myelination tends to be more diffuse. Central pontine myelinolysis was first described by Adams (1) in 1959 in malnourished adult alcoholics. Since then, it has been reported in fewer than 50 children (92). In addition to cancer therapy, other etiologic factors have been implicated in the pathogenesis of CPM. These include chronic debilitation and malnutrition, electrolyte and other metabolic derangements, and hepatic damage.

In addition to CPM, demyelination and frank necrosis, either diffusely scattered or localized to the dorsolateral pons and medulla, have been described. The latter has been identified after radiation therapy and is thought to reflect secondary effects of vascular damage (14,15). Periventricular necrosis and gliosis at the bulbar level have been reported in children with ventricular obstruction or altered CSF flow who have received intraventricular methotrexate. At the medullary level, neuronal atrophy with intense gliosis was reported by Hendin et al. (40) in leukemic children.

Cerebellar effects have been infrequently reported in pathologic series and clinical populations. Crosley and associates (23) described six patients with leukemia in whom cerebellar pathology was prominent. Neuronal loss with gliosis and demyelination were the most frequent lesions. In two, these were limited to the deep cerebellar nuclei. Of note is the report of a clinically reversible cerebellar syndrome after administration of the pyrimidine antagonist 5-fluorouracil (94,95).

The spinal cord has been even less frequently implicated in iatrogenic effects of treatment than the brain stem. Spinal cord pathology may be spuriously low in that most large pathologic series do not include examination of the spinal cord. Most children with late-onset myelopathy have received spinal radiation, but some have also received chemotherapy (6,20,83). The risk of developing delayed radiation myelopathy, for the most part, is dependent on dose and fraction per dose. Numerous attempts have been made to correlate the risk of radiation myelopathy with specific dose levels. The first dose equivalency was the NSD, or nominal standard dose, devised by Ellis (29), which compared the biologic effects of treatment of skin and connective tissue. Using this formula, Wara (93) has estimated the risk of delayed radiation myelopathy to be 1% at 1,015 rets and 50% at 1,480 rets. Sheline (86) introduced the neuroret in an effort to act to assess the risk of neurotissue injury. A neuroret was defined as $TD \times N^{-0.44} \times T^{-0.06}$, where *TD* is the total dose in rads (cGy), *N* is the number of doses per fraction and T is the total of treatment duration in days. These units, although of some interest, have not been universally adopted. Rather, the general assumption has been that a spinal cord dose of more than 4,500 cGy, or doses per fraction of 180 cGy, enhances the risk of radiation myelopathy. Myelopathy increases substantially with higher doses per fraction and higher total dose, shorter total treatment duration, and the extent of spinal cord irradiated. These are merely generalizations; there is significant variation in sensitivity from individual to individual.

Onset of spinal cord symptoms typically occurs weeks to months after radiation. These symptoms have been described as acute, subacute, remitting, or progressive. Obliteration of the spinal subarachnoid space has been observed with marked degrees of leptomeningeal reactions and spinal cord swelling (20) (Fig. 22-3). Vascular changes vary from minimal to extreme. Most severe cases show necrosis of the cord, chromolytic changes, axonal swelling, fragmentation, and loss of oligodendroglia. Nerve roots, ganglion, and peripheral nerves are usually intact. Transudation from blood vessels into the surrounding tissue may be associated with significant edema. Occlusion of blood vessels produces ischemia, necrosis, and tissue destruction (33,55).

Four syndromes have been described with radiation myelopathy (89). The first is a myelopathy consisting of mild sensory signs. This is usually transient and self-limited over a period of months. The second is manifested by signs of lower motor neuron disease with selective injury to the anterior horn cells. This syndrome is rare and, for the most part, has been reported in adults. The third form of radiation myelopathy presents as an acute paraplegia or quadriplegia secondary to infarction of the spinal cord and is associated with

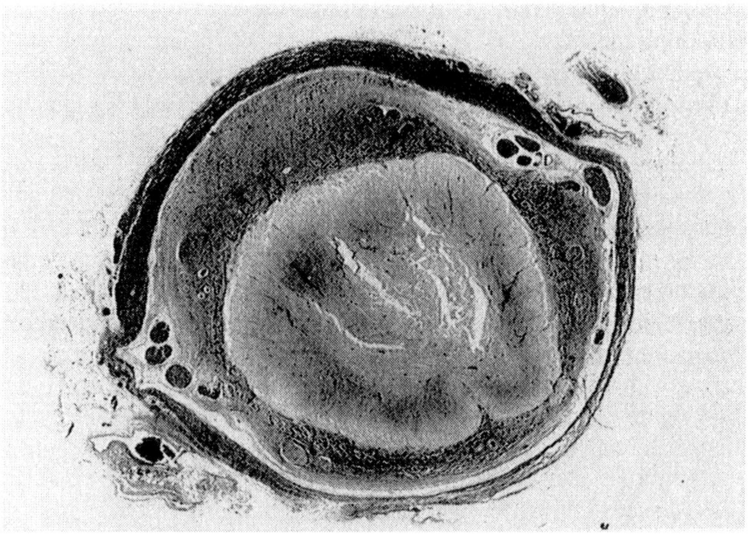

FIG. 22-3. Cervical cord section of a child with a medulloblastoma treated with neuraxis radiation and chemotherapy. Intensely fibrotic meninges compress the cord. There is cavitation of gray and white matter, especially on the right. Note the demyelination of dorsal and lateral fascicles. Trichrome stain (20).

radiation-induced damage to blood vessels. This syndrome is paroxysmal in nature and reaches its zenith in several hours, after which stabilization occurs. The fourth syndrome consists of a progressive myelopathy beginning years to months following radiation. Sensory signs are the earliest symptoms, consisting of burning, paresthesias, and inability to perceive pain and temperature. A multisystem disease of the cord evolves, manifested by motor weakness, sensory impairment, and bowel and bladder dysfunction. This has been seen with the use of combined radiation and intrathecal therapy, and substantiates the perception that multimodality treatment may be additive or synergistic in its iatrogenic effects (33,41,51,58,74,81).

PERIPHERAL NERVOUS SYSTEM

Unlike the brain and spinal cord, cranial and peripheral nerves tend to be resistant to radiation effects (7,43,77,87). No series of long-term radiation-induced peripheral neuropathies have been reported in children (22). On the other hand, the association of chemotherapy with neuropathies is well recognized. For instance, vincristine, which acts by binding to tubulin, prevents microtubular formation and thus affects axonal plasmic flow. As a result, neuropathy is universal and usually dose-limiting (76,82). Onset begins with loss of deep tendon reflexes, and the effects may progress to symmetric sensory loss, weakness, and muscle atrophy. Constipation, secondary to an autonomic neuropathy, is well described and consists of ileus, urinary retention, impotence, and, less commonly, orthostatic hypotension. Cranial neuropathies described with vincristine have involved the ocular motor nerves, abducens, and the facial nerves (88). Muscle pain involving the jaws and legs is commonly reported. Fatal myelopathies and encephalopathy have been described following the inappropriate intrathecal administration of vincristine (17,42,61).

As with vincristine, cis-platinum neurotoxicity is common and dose-limiting. Cis-platinum effects the hair cells of the organ of Corti and is characterized by high-frequency neurosensory hearing loss. Peripheral neuropathies consist of a large-fiber sensory polyneuropathy with paresthesias, vibratory and proprioceptive loss with relative sparing of pain and temperature. Neuropathies have also been reported with VP16 (60,77,83). Vincristine and VP16 may act in a synergistic way. Radiation sensitizers such as misonidazole have also been reported to cause a dose-limited symmetrical polyneuropathy (57).

There are at least four patients with Hodgkin's disease who developed a typical Guillain-Barré polyneuropathy weeks to 9 months after VCR treatment. One patient, a child, had also received irradiation and other drugs (46). In one, a sural nerve biopsy was normal; the sural nerve of another patient showed pronounced loss of axons and myelin (46,50). Another child with Hodgkin's disease who received no radiation or chemotherapy also developed progressive weakness of the limbs over a 2-year period. Pathologic examination revealed severe spinal cord anterior horn cell loss, diffuse demyelination, and peripheral nerve myelin loss with axonal preservation. Because the first symptoms in the four patients developed much later than the usual VCR neurotoxicity, and because the last patient never received vincristine, the polyneuropathies were judged not to be VCR-induced. Rather, they were considered to represent one of the "remote" effects of cancer on the nervous system. Most of these patients were immune-suppressed. In view of what is known about potential long-term and delayed neuropathological effects of chemotherapy at other levels of the neuraxis, absolving vincristine from a causative role may be premature.

SUMMARY

All anatomic levels of the nervous system can be adversely affected by the treatment in use. Demyelination has been the most consistently described neuropathologic sequela. The second most common pathologic feature has been mineralizing microangiopathy with occlusion of small blood vessels. Dystrophic calcification, when identified, is most commonly found in the basal ganglia.

Most of the pathologic results described have been associated with radiation rather than chemotherapy and, in general, have been dose-related. As a result, in young children and infants, radiation dose is now universally decreased by 10 to 20% of that used in adults. Although not well documented, a 1980 report (36) suggested that CNS damage may be reversible. In this report, following 5,000 cGy for a third ventricular tumor, a 21-year-old man developed clinical and CT evidence of leukoencephalopathy. Six months following completion of therapy, clinical symptoms disappeared and CT reverted to normal. Isolated reports such as this suggest that serial assessments during treatment can lead to interventions to limit complications. The identification of delayed CNS effects of treatment should temper early enthusiasm for new treatments until sufficient time has elapsed for potential long-term complications to become apparent.

REFERENCES

1. Adams RD, Victor M, Mancall EL. Central pontine myelinalysis: a hitherto undescribed disease occurring in alcoholic and malnourished patients. *Arch Neurol Psychiatr* 1959;81: 154–172.
2. Albert DM, Wong VG, Henderson ES. Ocular complications of vincristine therapy. *Arch Ophthalmol* 1967;78:709–713.
3. Allen JC. The effects of cancer therapy on the nervous system. *J Pediatr* 1978;93:903–909.
4. Allen JC, Deck MDF, Howieson J, Brown M. CT scans of long-term survivors of various childhood malignancies. *Med Pediatr Oncol* 1981;9:109–117.

5. Allen JC, Rosen G, Mehta BM, Horten B. Leukoencephalopathy following high-dose IV methotrexate chemotherapy with leucovorin rescue. *Cancer Treat Rep* 1980;64:1261–1273.
6. Ballweg GP, Donnenfeld H, Chusid J. Subacute radiation myeopathy in a 12-year-old boy. *Childs Brain* 1976;2:195–201.
7. Berger PS, Bataini JP. Radiation-induced cranial nerve palsy. *Cancer* 1977;40:152–155.
8. Bleyer WA, Griffin TW. White matter necrosis, mineralizing, microangiopathy, and intellectual abilities in survivors of childhood leukemia: associations with central nervous system irradiation and methotrexate therapy. In: Gilbert HA, Kagan AR, eds. *Radiation damage to the nervous system*. New York: Raven Press; 1980:155–174.
9. Bode U, Oliff A, Bercu BB, DiChiro G, Glaubiger DL, Poplack DG. Absence of CT brain scan and endocrine abnormalities with less intensive CNS prophylaxis. *Am J Pediatr Hematol Oncol* 1980;2:21–24.
10. Brant-Zawadzki M, Fein F, Van Dyke C, Kiernan R, Davenport I, deGrout J. Magnetic resonance imaging of the aging brain: patchy white matter lesions and dementia. *AJNR* 1985;6:675–682.
11. Bresnan MJ, Gilles FH, Lorenzo AV, Watters GV, Barlow CF. Leukoencephalopathy following combined irradiation and intraventricular methotrexate therapy of brain tumors in childhood. *Trans Am Neurol Assoc* 1972;97:204–206.
12. Breuer AC, Blank NK, Schoene WC. Multifocal pontine lesions in cancer patients treated with chemotherapy and CNS radiotherapy. *Cancer* 1978;41:2112–2120.
13. Brismar J, Roberson GH, Davis KR. Radiation necrosis of the brain: neuroradiological considerations with computerized tomography. *Neuroradiology* 1976;12:109–113.
14. Burger PC, Kamenar E, Schold SC, Fay JW, Phillips GL, Herzig GP. Encephalomyelopathy following high-dose BCNU therapy. *Cancer* 1981;48:1318–1327.
15. Burger PC, Mahaley MS, Dudka L, Vogel FS. The morphologic effects of radiation administered therapeutically for intracranial gliomas: a postmortem study of 25 cases. *Cancer* 1979; 44:1256–1272.
16. Cantini R, Giorgetti W, Valleriani AM, Murchianti M, Amodero C. Radiation-induced cerebral lesions in childhood. *Childs Nerv Syst* 1989;5:135–139.
17. Casey EG, Jellife AM, LeQuesnem, et al. Vincristine neuropathy: clinical and physiologic observations. *Brain* 1973;96:69.
18. Caveness WF. Experimental observations: delayed necrosis in normal monkey brain. In: Gilbert HA, Kagan AR, eds. *Radiation damage to the nervous system*. New York: Raven Press; 1980:1–37.
19. Cohen ME, Duffner PK. Long-term consequences of CNS treatment for childhood cancer. I: Pathologic consequences and potential for oncogenesis. *Pediatr Neurol* 1991;7:157–163.
20. Cohen ME, Duffner PK, Terplan KL. Myelopathy with severe structural derangement associated with combined modality therpy. *Cancer* 1983;52:1590–1596.
21. Constine LS, Konski A, Ekholm S, McDonald S, Rubin P. Adverse effects of brain irradiation correlated with MR and CT imaging. *Int J Radiat Oncol Biol Phys* 1988;15:319–330.
22. Coplan J, Grimes CT, Richman RA, Post EM. Sensorineural hearing loss in children following radiation therapy. *Pediatr Res* 1982;6:333A.
23. Crosley CJ, Rorke LB, Evans A, Nigro M. Central nervous system lesions in childhood leukemia. *Neurology* 1978;28:678–685.
24. Curnes JT, Laster DW, Ball MR, Dixon MM, Witcofski RL. MRI of radiation injury to the brain. *AJR* 1986;147:119–124.
25. DeReuck J, Eecken Vander H. The anatomy of the late radiation encephalopathy. *Eur Neurol* 1975;13:481–494.
26. DiChiro G, Oldfield E, Wright DC, et al. Cerebral necrosis after radiotherapy and/or intraarterial chemotherapy for brain tumors: PET and neuropathologic studies. *AJR* 1988;150: 189.
27. Dooms GC, Hecht S, Brant-Zawadzki M, Berthiaume Y, Norman D, Newton TH. Brain radiation lesions: MR imaging. *Radiology* 1986;158:149–155.
28. Duffner PK, Cohen ME, Berger P, Brecher M, Bakshi S. Abnormalities of CT scans and altered methotrexate clearance in children with central nervous system leukemia. *Ann Neurol* 1981;10:286–287.
29. Ellis F. Dose time and fractionation: a clinical hypothesis. *Clin Radiol* 1969;20:1–7.
30. Eyster EF, Wilson CB. Radiation myelopathy. *J Neurosurg* 1970;32:404–420.

31. Flament-Durand J, Ketelbant-Balasse P, Maurus R, Regnier R, Spehl M. Intracerebral calcifications appearing during the course of acute lymphocytic leukemia treated with methotrexate and x-rays. *Cancer* 1975;35:319–325.
32. Foley KM, Woodruff JM, Posner JB. Radiation-induced malignant schwannomas. *Neurology* 1975;25:354.
33. Gagliano RG, Costanzi JJ. Paraplegia following intrathecal methotrexate: report of a case and review of the literature. *Cancer* 1976;37:1663–1668.
34. Gangji D, Reaman GH, Cohen SR, Bleyer WA, Poplack DG. Leukoencephalopathy and elevated levels of myelin basic protein in the cerebrospinal fluid of patients with acute lymphoblastic leukemia. *N Engl J Med* 1980;303:19–21.
35. Gerard G, Weisberg L. MRI periventricular lesions in adults. *Neurology* 1986;36:998–1001.
36. Godwin-Austen RB, Howell DA, Worthington B. Observations on radiation myelopathy. *Brain* 1975;98:557–568.
37. Groothuis DR, Vick NA. Radionecrosis of the central nervous system: the perspective of the clinical neurologist and neuropathologist. In: Gilbert HA, Kagan AR, eds. *Radiation damage to the nervous system.* New York:Raven Press; 1980:93–106.
38. Harris JR, Levene MB. Visual complications following irradiation for pituitary adenomas and craniopharyngiomas. *Radiology* 1976;120:167–171.
39. Harwood-Nash DCF, Reilly BJ. Calcification of the basal ganglia following radiation therapy. *AJR* 1970;108:392–395.
40. Hendin B, DeVivo DC, Torack R, Lell M, Ragab AH, Vietti TJ. Parenchymatous degeneration of the central nervous system in childhood leukemia. *Cancer* 1974;33:468–482.
41. Howell DA. Radiation myelopathy. *Dev Med Child Neurol* 1979;21:653–662.
42. Kaufman IA, Kung FH, Koenig HM, Giammona ST. Overdosage with vincristine. *J Pediatr* 1976;89:671–674.
43. Kinsella T, Weichselbaum RR, Sheline GE. Radiation injury of cranial and peripheral nerves. In: Gilbert HA, Kagan AR, eds. *Radiation damage to the nervous system.* New York:Raven Press; 1980:145–153.
44. Kramer S. The hazards of therapeutic irradiation of the central nervous system. *Clin Neurosurg* 1968;15:301–318.
45. Kramer S, Lee KF. Complications of radiation therapy: the central nervous system. *Semin Roentgenol* 1974;9:75–83.
46. Kurczynski TW, Choudhury AA, Horwitz SJ, Roessmann U, Gross S. Remote effect of malignancy on the nervous system in children. *Dev Med Child Neurol* 1980;22:205–222.
47. Lavenstein B, Chugani H, Woo S, Sinks L. Effectiveness of the brain stem auditory evoked response to monitor clinical course and response to chemotherapy in children with brain stem tumors. *Neurology* 1982;32:A219.
48. Lee Y, Nauert C, Glass JR. Treatment-related white matter changes in cancer patients. *Cancer* 1986;57:1473–1482.
49. Levitt LJ, Dawson DM, Rosenthal DS, Moloney WC. CNS involvement in the non-Hodgkin's lymphomas. *Cancer* 1980;45:545–552.
50. Lisak, RP, Mitchell M, Zweiman B, Orrechio E, Asbury AK. Guillain-Barré syndrome and Hodgkin's disease: three cases with immunological studies. *Ann Neurol* 1977;1:72–78.
51. Littman P, Rosenstock JG, Bailey C. Radiation myelitis following craniospinal irradiation with concurrent actinomycin-D therapy. *Med Pediatr Oncol* 1978;5:145–151.
52. Liu HM, Mauer HS, Vongsvivut S, Conway JJ. Methotrexate encephalopathy: a neuropathologic study. *Hum Pathol* 1978;9:635–648.
53. Marks JE, Baglan RJ, Prassad SC, Blank WR. Cerebral radionecrosis: incidence and risk in relation to dose, time, fractionation and volume. *Int J Radiat Oncol Biol Phys* 1981;7: 243–252.
54. Martins AN, Johnston JS, Henry JM, Stoffel TJ, DiChiro G. Delayed radiation necrosis of the brain. *J Neurosurg* 1977;47:336–345.
55. Mastaglia FL, McDonald WI, Watson JV, Yogendran K. Effects of x-radiation on the spinal cord: an experimental study of the morphological changes in central nerve fibres. *Brain* 1976;99:101–122.
56. McIntosh S, Fischer DB, Rothman SG, Rosenfield N, Lobel JS, O'Brien RT. Intracranial calcifications in childhood leukemia: an association with systemic chemotherapy. *J Pediatr* 1977;91:909–913.

57. Melgaard B, Hansen HS, Kamieniecka Z, et al. Misonidazole neuropathology: a clinical electrophysiological and histologic study. *Ann Neurol* 1982;12:10–17.
58. Mena H, Garcia JH, Velandia F. Central and peripheral myelinopathy associated with systemic neoplasia and chemotherapy. *Cancer* 1981;48:1724–1737.
59. Mikhael MA. Radiation necrosis of the brain: correlation between patterns on computerized tomography and dose of radiation. *J Comput Assist Tomogr* 1979;3:241–249.
60. Mollman JE. Cisplatin neurotoxicity. *N Eng J Med* 1990;322:126.
61. Moress GR, D'Agostino AN, Jarcho LW. Neuropathy in lymphoblastic leukemia treated with vincristine. *Arch Neurol* 1967;16:377–384.
62. Norrell H, Wilson CB, Slagel DE, Clark DB. Leukoencephalopathy following the administration of methotrexate into the cerebrospinal fluid in the treatment of primary brain tumors. *Cancer* 1974;33:923–932.
63. Ochs JJ, Berger P, Brecher ML, Sinks LF, Kinkel W, Freeman AI. Computed tomography brain scans in children with acute lymphocytic leukemia receiving methotrexate alone as central nervous system prophylaxis. *Cancer* 1980;45:2274–2278.
64. Packer RJ, Zimmerman RA, Bilaniuk LT. Magnetic resonance imaging in the evaluation of treatment: related central nervous system damage. *Cancer* 1986:58:635–640.
65. Painter MJ, Chutorian AM, Hilal SK. Cerebrovasculopathy following irradiation in childhood. *Neurology* 1975;25:189–194.
66. Patronas NJ, Di Chiro, Brooks RA, et al. Work in progress: (^{18}F) fluorodeoxyglucose and positron emission tomography in the evaluation of radiation necrosis of the brain. *Radiology* 1982;144:885–889.
67. Peylan-Ramu N, Poplack DG, Blei CL, Herdt JR, Vermess M, DiChiro G. Computer assisted tomography in methotrexate encephalopathy. *J Comput Assist Tomogr* 1977;1: 216–221.
68. Peylan-Ramu N, Poplack DG, Pizzo PA, Adornato BT, DiChiro G. Abnormal CT scans of the brain in asymptomatic children with acute lymphocytic leukemia after prophylactic treatment of the central nervous system with radiation and intrathecal chemotherapy. *N Engl J Med* 1978;298:815–818.
69. Phillips TL, Fu KK. Quantification of combined radiation therapy and chemotherapy effects on critical normal tissues. *Cancer* 1976;37:1186–1200.
70. Price RA. Histopathology of CNS leukemia and complications of therapy. *Am J Pediatr Hematol Oncol* 1979;1:21–29.
71. Price RA, Birdwell DA. The central nervous system in childhood leukemia. III: Mineralizing microangiopathy and dystrophic calcification. *Cancer* 1978;42:717–728.
72. Price RA, Jamieson PA. The central nervous system in childhood leukemia. II: Subacute leukoencephalopathy. *Cancer* 1975;35:306–318.
73. Priest JR, Ramsay NC, Latchaw RE, et al. Thrombotic and hemorrhagic strokes complicating early therapy for childhood acute lymphoblastic leukemia. *Cancer* 1980;46:1548–1554.
74. Reagan TJ, Thomas JE, Colby MY Jr. Chronic progressive radiation myelopathy: its clinical aspects and differential diagnosis. *JAMA* 1968;203:128–132.
75. Riccardi R, Brouwers P, DiChero G. Abnormal computed tomography brain scans in children with acute lymphoblastic leukemia: serial long-term follow-up. *J Clin Oncol* 1985;3: 12–19.
76. Rosenthal S, Kaufman S. Vincristine neurotoxicity. *Ann Int Med* 1974;80:733–737.
77. Rozencweig M, Von Hoff DD, Slavik M, Muggia FM. Cis-diammine-dichloroplatinum (II): a new anticancer drug. *Ann Intern Med* 1977;86:803–812.
78. Rubinstein LJ, Herman MM, Long TF, Wilbur JR. Disseminated necrotizing leukoencephalopathy: a complication of treated central nervous system leukemia and lymphoma. *Cancer* 1975;35:291–305.
79. Safadari GH, Fuentes JM, Dubois JB, Alirezai M, Castan P, Viahovitch B. Radiation necrosis of the brain: time of onset and incidence related to total dose and fractionation of radiation. *Neuroradiology* 1985;27:44–47.
80. Safdari H, Boluix B, Gros C. Multifocal brain radionecrosis masquerading as tumour dissemination. *Surg Neurol* 1984;21:35–41.
81. Saiki JH, Thompson S, Smith F, Atkinson R. Paraplegia following intrathecal chemotherapy. *Cancer* 1972;29:370–374.
82. Sandler SG, Tobin W, Henderson ES. Vincristine-induced neuropathy: a clinical study of fifty leukemia patients. *Neurology* 1969;19:367–374.

83. Shaefer SD, Post JD, Close LG, et al. Ototoxicity of low and moderate dose cisplatin. *Cancer* 1985;56:1934.
84. Shapiro WR, Allen JC, Horten BC. Chronic methotrexate toxicity to the central nervous system. *Clin Bull* 1980;10:49–52.
85. Shapiro WR, Chernik NL, Posner JB. Necrotizing encephalopathy following intraventricular instillation of methotrexate. *Arch Neurol* 1973;28:96–102.
86. Sheline GE. Therapeutic irradiation and brain injury. *Int J Radiat* 1980;6:1215.
87. Shukovsky LJ, Fletcher GH. Retinal and optic nerve complications in a high dose irradiation technique of ethmoid sinus and nasal cavity. *Radiology* 1972;104:629–634.
88. Shurin SB, Rekate HL, Annable W. Optic atrophy induced by vincristine. *Pediatrics* 1982; 70:288–291.
89. Sundaresan N, Gutierrez FA, Larsen MB. Radiation myelopathy in children. *Ann Neurol* 1978;4:47–50.
90. Tiller-Borcich JK, Fike JR, Phillips TL, Davis RL. Pathology of delayed radiation brain damage: an experimental canine model. *Radiat Res* 1987;110:161–172.
91. Tsuruda JS, Kortman KE, Bradley WG. Radiation effects on cerebral white matter: MR evaluations. *AJNR* 1987;8:431–437.
92. Valsamis MP, Peress NS, Wright LD. Central pontine myelinolysis in childhood. *Arch Neurol* 1971;25:307–312.
93. Wara WM, Philip TL, Sheline GE, et al. Radiation tolerance of the spinal cord. *Cancer* 1975;35:1558.
94. Weiss HD, Walker MD, Wiernik PH. Neurotoxicity of commonly used antineoplastic agents. Part I. *New Engl J Med* 1974;291:75–80.
95. Weiss HD, Walker MD, Wiernik PH. Neurotoxicity of commonly used antineoplastic agents. Part II. *New Engl J Med* 1974;291:127–133.
96. Zimmerman RD, Fleming CA, Lee BCP, Saint-Louis LA, Deuk MDF. Periventricular hyperintensity as seen by magnetic resonance: prevalence and significance. *AJNR* 1986;7: 13–20.

23

Long-Term Clinical Effects

Cranial irradiation (CRT) and chemotherapy may produce significant long-term adverse effects on children treated for brain tumors. These effects of therapy, which include intellectual deterioration, endocrinopathies, and oncogenesis, have important implications: some are amenable to treatment, and others may be prevented by careful monitoring of drug and radiation administration (29).

The early delayed effects of radiotherapy have been best described after radiation of the spinal cord. The symptoms appear a few weeks to several months after spinal radiation and consist of Lhermitte syndrome, i.e., tingling and paresthesias induced by neck flexion (54). The syndrome is self-limited and usually abates after 2 to 36 weeks. This early delayed effect of radiation is thought to result from transient demyelination of the posterior columns (108).

The most common early delayed effect involving the cerebrum is the somnolence syndrome. The condition was first brought to the attention of the medical community in 1929, when Druckmann described a syndrome present in 3% of 1,100 children treated for ringworm of the scalp by radiation with 150-kV x rays (108). Somnolence associated with anorexia, apathy, and headaches occurred 6 to 8 weeks after radiation. The symptoms persisted 4 to 14 days and resolved completely and spontaneously with no mental or physical sequelae up to 4 years later. It is of interest that Druckmann could prevent the syndrome by reducing the x-ray energy to 70 kV, thus limiting the cerebral dose. In 1973, Freeman et al. (41) reported the presence of somnolence syndrome in children with acute lymphoblastic leukemia (ALL) (41). Thirty-nine percent of 28 leukemic children developed pronounced symptoms of somnolence, anorexia, and lethargy 6 weeks after the completion of cranial radiation, and a further 39% developed the features in a milder form. In all cases the symptoms were transient, no focal neurologic abnormalities were detected, and all children made a spontaneous and complete recovery. More recent studies (62) of children with ALL have reported somnolence syndrome in 58% to 63% of patients. A reduction in radiation from 2,400 to 1,800 cGy has not altered the incidence of somnolence syndrome (62). Another approach to reduce the intensity of this condition has been the administration of daily steroids. Mandell and others (71) found that if the daily prednisone

Brain Tumors in Children: Principles of Diagnosis and Treatment, 2/e, edited by M.E. Cohen and P.K. Duffner, Raven Press, Ltd., New York, 1994.

dose was greater than 15 mg/m^2, the incidence of somnolence syndrome was reduced to only 13%.

A severe form of the early delayed effects of radiation was reported by Lampert and Davis (57) in 1964. They described a rapidly progressive clinical picture of ataxia, focal motor signs, cranial neuropathies, nystagmus, and death which developed over 2 days, 13 weeks after the termination of radiotherapy. Necropsy revealed punched-out plaques of demyelination within the field of radiation with pronounced microglial and astrocytic proliferation. The vessels showed no degenerative changes but revealed lymphocytes and plasma cells in the perivascular spaces. The plaques resembled the lesions of acute multiple sclerosis.

Radiation necrosis is perhaps one of the most serious of the late delayed effects of radiation. It occurs from months to years following radiation therapy, with a peak incidence at 1 to 3 years. The clinical picture is one of insidious and progressive deterioration, characterized by focal neurologic signs, dementia, seizures, and often death. The incidence of radiation necrosis is likely to increase with the use of brachytherapy (123).

The pathology of radiation necrosis is necrosis of white matter with severe vasculopathy involving both large and small vessels. Protein-rich fluid in perivascular spaces and adjacent parenchyma suggests disturbances of the permeability of the vessel walls (27,61,72,73). Radiation necrosis often mimics a mass lesion; therefore, differentiation from tumor recurrence is sometimes difficult (16,28,72,73,82). Both tumor and radiation necrosis may be characterized by elevation in spinal-fluid protein, increased uptake on brain scan, focal EEG with delta activity, and an avascular mass on angiography. CT cannot reliably distinguish the two entities. On CT examination, both radiation necrosis and tumor present as mass lesions with decreased attenuation coefficients and variable enhancement. MR imaging has also not been helpful in differentiating the two entities, even with administration of gadolinium, since breakdown of the blood–brain barrier occurs in both radiation necrosis and tumor. Potentially differentiating points suggestive of radiation necrosis are irregular contours of the lesion, localization within the isodose curves representing 80 to 90% of the maximum dose of radiation, and the finding of contrast-enhanced zones intermixed with low-density areas. None of these findings is pathognomonic. It has been suggested that PET may help distinguish radiation necrosis from recurrent tumor, but at present only case reports are available for study (89). Differentiating the two entities is important for clinical care. Although both necrosis and tumor may require surgical debulking, radiation necrosis requires no further therapy, whereas recurrent tumor will likely require adjuvant treatment.

Beyond these acute and subacute effects of radiotherapy, the long-term toxicities of CNS therapy include adverse effects on intelligence and endocrine function as well as the development of second malignancies. Until recently, survivals of children with brain tumors were sufficiently limited so that concern over these long-term effects of therapy was unnecessary. As children with certain types of brain tumors now have a better prognosis, these long-term and possibly remediable late effects have important implications.

INTELLECTUAL FUNCTION

The long-term effects of radiation and chemotherapy on intellectual function have been studied most extensively in children with leukemia. This emphasis on children with leukemia, rather than on children with brain tumors, reflects in part their better overall prognosis as well as the larger numbers of children with leukemia available for study. Although early studies produced contradictory results, recent literature confirms significantly lower IQs and poorer learning ability in children who have received cranial irradiation as opposed to chemotherapy alone for CNS prophylaxis. Soni et al. (111) and Verzosa et al. (119) reported two groups of children with leukemia treated at St. Jude's Hospital with cranial irradiation and chemotherapy. In neither study was there believed to be prohibitive toxicity affecting neuropsychologic competence. These results differed from those obtained at other centers, where children who had been irradiated for leukemia were commonly found to have learning problems (60,69,76). In a later study, Goff et al. (44) reevaluated the children from the St. Jude's study. Neuropsychologic abnormalities, including distractibility and memory deficits, were identified and were most prominent in children treated before 8 years of age. Academic achievement, as measured by the Wide Range Achievement Test, was also worse in the younger long-term survivors. The majority of abnormalities on the Wechsler Intelligence Scale for Children (WISC) involved arithmetic and digit span. On the basis of Goff's data, the earlier results of Soni and Verzosa appeared to be unrealistically optimistic. In another study, Moss et al. (78) compared children who had been radiated for leukemia with sibling controls and found a significantly lower IQ in the treated subjects ($p < 0.001$). In comparison, children with leukemia who had not received CNS prophylaxis had no difference in IQ from their siblings.

The largest retrospective study of children with acute lymphocytic leukemia involved 104 children from the Roswell Park Cancer Institute, Rhode Island Hospital, West Virginia University Medical Center, and Mount Sinai Hospital (97). This study evaluated the neurotoxic effects of three different regimens of CNS prophylaxis from the Cancer and Leukemia Group B (CALGB) cooperative group: intrathecal methotrexate alone, intrathecal methotrexate plus cranial irradiation, and intrathecal methotrexate and intermediate-dose intravenous methotrexate (IDM). Statistically significantly lower IQs were found in those children who had received cranial irradiation. Radiated patients also did significantly worse on achievement tests and on tests of neuropsychologic function. Although differences were statistically significant, IQ scores of the radiated children were generally within the normal range. In a similar study, Copeland (23) evaluated long-term survivors of leukemia and lymphoma who had been treated with chemotherapy and radiation, but he extended the follow-up interval to between 7 and 8 years. As in the CALGB study, radiated children did significantly worse on IQ and achievement tests. Nonlanguage skills, especially visual motor functioning, and fine motor and spatial processing, were particularly effected.

Prospective evaluations have been done in a more limited number of patients. Meadows et al. (75,76) reported 31 children with ALL who had been treated with cranial irradiation and intrathecal methotrexate. IQ scores declined progressively over time, and the number of children with learning disabilities increased. Alterations in IQ were not evident until 3 or more years after diagnosis.

Several risk factors have been identified in the leukemic population. One of the most important is young age (35,76). Younger children with ALL, i.e., those less than 4 years old, have had the most severe intellectual abnormalities following CNS prophylaxis. Eiser and Lansdown (36) compared 9 children treated before 5 years of age and 6 children treated after 5 years of age with CRT and chemotherapy for ALL. Older children had no difference in IQ compared with controls, whereas the younger treated population had lower IQs with specific deficits in quantitative memory and motor skill performance. Another important risk factor is either the presence of CNS leukemia at diagnosis or at least one CNS relapse. Children who have had meningeal disease typically have below-normal full scale, verbal, and performance IQ scores and, in at least one study (80), 20% were in the profoundly retarded range. These children are at particular risk because they are likely to have an increased number of radiation courses, a higher incidence of epilepsy and are most prone to develop leukoencephalopathy: all of which are potent risk factors.

In summary, results of IQ scores, achievement tests, and tests of neuropsychologic function are significantly worse in those children with leukemia who have received cranial irradiation (66). These abnormalities are relatively subtle in those older children who have not had CNS leukemia. Unfortunately, children who have had at least one isolated CNS relapse, increased number of courses of radiation, seizures, CT leukoencephalopathy, and who are young at the time of CNS radiation may be significantly impaired.

The adverse effects of cranial irradiation on children with brain tumors are much more profound than on children with leukemia (Table 23-1). Bamford et al. (5), in 1976, reported on brain tumors in 30 children, 21 of which were posterior fossa in location. Patients were treated with radiotherapy but no chemotherapy. Forty-three percent were in the average to superior range in school, and 43% were educationally subnormal or severely retarded. Although none had formal psychometric testing, 20% were profoundly dis-

TABLE 23-1. *IQs of children treated for brain tumors*

Author	Surgery	RT	CT	IQ <70	IQ >90
Raimondi and Tomita* (91) *T* = 15	+	+	—	46%	20%
Hirsch et al.* (47) *T* = 21	+	+	+	31%	11%
Spunberg et al.* (112) *T* = 13	+	+	—	54%	23%
Duffner et al.* (32) *T* = 10	+	+	+	40%	20%
Danoff et al.* (25) *T* = 36	+	+	—	17%	56%
Jannoun** (49) *T* = 62	+	+	—	14.5%	59.7%
Packer**+ (86) *T* = 18	+	+	+	Mean IQ = 91	
Duffner**+ (31) *T* = 16	+	+	+/−	0%	50%

*, retrospective; **, prospective; +, 2 years following RT; RT, cranial radiation; CT, chemotherapy.

abled. Raimondi and Tomita (91) reported 18 children with medulloblastoma treated with surgery and radiotherapy. Intelligence testing was performed on 15 of 18 children. Only 3 children (20%) had IQs over 80, whereas 7 (46%) had IQs of 70 or less. Children with medulloblastomas treated with surgery, radiation, and chemotherapy including MTX, VCR, and CCNU were evaluated in another study (47). IQs ranged from 70 to 90 in 58% of the children and were below 70 in 31%; 82% had defective spatial orientation, dysphasia, and dysgraphia. We (32) studied 10 children with posterior fossa tumors treated with surgery, radiation, and chemotherapy at Roswell Park Cancer Institute. Children with supratentorial tumors were specifically excluded from this study in order to eliminate the possible influence of the tumor on intellectual functioning. The patients received intellectual evaluations at least 1 year after diagnosis and treatment. Six children had medulloblastomas, 1 child had an intraventricular ependymoma, 2 children had brain stem gliomas, and 1 child had a recurrent cerebellar astrocytoma. Four children had had intelligence testing in school before treatment of their tumors. In each case, results following treatment revealed deterioration of full scale IQ by at least 25 points. Six children did not have prior testing. Of these, 2 had IQs less than 20. Overall, 50% of the patients had IQs of less than 80 and 20% had IQs of over 100. Furthermore, 4 children with normal intelligence (IQ > 80) had learning problems requiring special classes. Of the 10 children evaluated, all had evidence of either dementia, learning disabilities, or intellectual retardation. Overall, the retrospective studies revealed that 30 to 50% of radiated children had IQs less than 70, whereas only 10 to 20% had IQs above 90 (15,25,32).

Prospective evaluations of children with brain tumors are limited. In general, results have not been as poor as were found in the retrospective studies. We (31) studied 16 children with brain tumors with a follow-up from 2 to 5 years. IQ scores significantly declined over time, but most remained in the normal range. More common than frank retardation was the presence of learning disabilities (present in 15 of 16 children). Eleven required special educational help. Packer (86) similarly prospectively evaluated children who had been irradiated for brain tumors. By 2 years following treatment, a statistically significant decline in full scale and verbal IQ was identified. As in our study, the majority of children had significant learning problems requiring special classes.

Various risk factors are associated with more severe intellectual deterioration. Hydrocephalus and increased intracranial pressure were at one time considered important risk factors. In an effort to assess the impact of hydrocephalus on intellectual function, children with cerebellar astrocytomas and medulloblastomas were compared (47). This analysis attempted to eliminate the role of increased intracranial pressure as the etiology for the patients' low IQs, as both groups had a history of obstructive hydrocephalus. There was a striking difference in the two populations: 62% of patients with cerebellar astrocytomas had IQs over 90 compared with 11% of patients with medulloblastomas. Since children with medulloblastomas had received postoperative radiation and chemotherapy whereas children with cerebellar astrocytomas had been treated with surgery alone, this study strongly implicated the postoperative treatment with radiation with or without chemotherapy as the cause of the children's intellectual difficulties.

Although hydrocephalus is no longer believed to play a significant role, several factors have been confirmed to increase the risk of intellectual deterioration in children with brain tumors. As in children with leukemia, one of the major risk factors for intellectual decline is young age at the time of treatment. Ellenberg (37), comparing children above and below 7 years of age at time of radiation, specifically evaluated age as a risk factor. Significantly lower IQs were identified in those children radiated before the age of 7. Younger children, i.e., less than 2 to 3 years of age, have developed the most profound intellectual disturbances following cranial irradiation (112).

The relationship between young age at the time of cranial irradiation and intellectual subnormalcy may be more complicated than at first glance. Mulhern (81) has shown that many infants and young children with brain tumors have abnormal development *before* treatment is begun. Less than 25% of children in his series had developmental quotients in the normal range prior to administration of either chemotherapy or radiation. This likely relates to the extremely large tumor size found in this population and the extensive surgery that is required for effective treatment. Nonetheless, in children with leukemia and brain tumors the young child bears the brunt of radiation-induced neurotoxicity.

Another risk factor for intellectual deterioration is location of tumor. Tumors that are supratentorial in location are more likely to be associated with low intellect than those that are located in the posterior fossa (37,56). Others have suggested that a midline location is similarly associated with poor prognosis. In Ellenberg's (37) study, patients whose tumors were supratentorial had significantly lower baseline IQs than the other groups. Thus, although all three groups (supratentorial, posterior fossa, and midline) had a loss of IQ following radiation, children with supratentorial tumors (since they were already at a lower baseline IQ) declined into the retarded range.

Other risk factors are the volume and dose of radiation. Although a safe dose of cranial radiation has not been identified, extrapolation from the leukemic population suggests that 1,800 to 2,400 cGy is associated with less intellectual deterioration than doses above that range. As might be anticipated, the child treated with whole-brain radiation has significantly more intellectual decline than the child who receives either local or no radiation (37,56).

Chemotherapy is also a risk factor. The concomitant use of intrathecal methotrexate and radiation is more likely to cause intellectual decline than radiation alone. Thus, when intrathecal methotrexate was added to the treatment of children with medulloblastomas, the 2-year posttreatment IQ scores were 74.6 in the methotrexate treated children compared to 91 and 92 in two other studies in which methotrexate was not given (49,86,94).

In summary, the adverse effects on intellect may range from mild to severe. Even in those cases in which the child has an IQ in the "normal range," intellectual deterioration from a previously higher level may be emotionally devastating to both child and family. The child who recognizes the loss of intellectual abilities is particularly tragic. Other children may maintain their previous IQ scores but do poorly in school because of learning disabilities. The severely demented child falls at the extreme of this spectrum. In all of these cases, educational and psychological support services must be provided to maximize the child's abilities. Too often, children with cancer are treated as "special" by school authorities and, as such, receive falsely elevated grades in the face of less stringent academic requirements. Because these children may now today be cured, this "kindness" may be counterproductive. Education should be realistic and when indicated, remedial.

ENDOCRINE FUNCTION

Detailed studies of children and adults have revealed a wide range of endocrine dysfunction following cranial irradiation (101). The most common of the endocrine complications of radiation is growth failure. Many investigators have studied children with leukemia and brain tumors to determine the various roles that growth hormone deficiency, poor nutrition, hypothyroidism, and abnormal vertebral growth play in this condition. The largest studies in children have involved patients with leukemia who received cranial irradiation for CNS prophylaxis. Sunderman and Pearson (114), in 1969, reviewed the growth patterns of 21 children with leukemia who had not received cranial irradiation and found normal linear growth patterns. Later, Fisher and Aur (40) and Swift et al. (115) studied children with ALL who had been treated with cranial irradiation. A total of 18 children in these two series had hypothalamic–pituitary axis testing and evaluation of linear growth. All were found to be within normal limits.

Most recent studies, however, have found at least biochemical growth hormone deficiency in radiated children with leukemia. Dacou-Voutetakis et al. (24) evaluated the acute effects of cranial irradiation on growth hormone release. They studied the patients before radiation and within 1 to 3 days after a 3-week 2,400-cGy course of cranial irradiation. Levels of growth hormone after irradiation were lower at both hourly intervals and peak than at pretesting. Thus, an immediate suppressive effect on the hypothalamic–pituitary axis by cranial irradiation was suggested.

The total dose of radiation appears to influence hypothalamic–pituitary function. Dickinson et al. (26) found that patients who had received 2,400 cGy had normal growth hormone response to arginine but not insulin stimulation, whereas patients who received more than 2,400 cGy had abnormal growth hormone responses to both. Insulin-induced hypoglycemia theoretically produces its effects on growth hormone release by acting on receptors in the hypothalamus. The mechanism of growth hormone release via arginine stimulation is not well established, but some suggest a direct effect on the pituitary gland. Because the pituitary is known to be relatively radioresistant, the radiation effects on growth hormone appear to be related to primary hypothalamic damage. Presumably, the lower doses of irradiation in the study by Dickinson et al. were sufficient to produce hypothalamic dysfunction, whereas the higher doses may have destroyed the pituicytes involved in growth hormone secretion. This study demonstrates the need for both arginine and insulin stimulation in the evaluation of patients with potential growth hormone deficiency.

The size and number of fractions, as well as the total dose of radiation, will also influence late effects. Shalet et al. (103) found that growth hormone deficiency was significantly more likely in those children who received 2,400 cGy of cranial irradiation over 2.5 weeks in 10 fractions, compared to those who received 2,400 cGy in 20 fractions over 4 weeks ($p < 0.002$). In both this study and that of Dickinson et al., patients who did not receive cranial irradiation had normal results on tests of growth hormone release.

A multi-institutional study (120) involving Roswell Park Cancer Institute in Buffalo, Mount Sinai Hospital in New York, West Virginia Hospital in Morgantown, and Rhode Island Hospital in Providence, evaluated endocrine function in 106 children with ALL treated with CNS prophylaxis consisting of intermediate dose methotrexate (IDM) and intrathecal (IT) methotrexate, radiation and IT methotrexate, and IT methotrexate. Abnormal growth hormone release on arginine and insulin stimulation was found significantly more often in patients treated with cranial irradiation, although a few children who received IDM and IT methotrexate were growth hormone deficient as well. At the time of the initial report, patients maintained their linear growth despite biochemical growth hormone deficiency. Brecher (14) recently reevaluated 59 of these patients who had remained in continuous complete remission. In contrast to the early results, male children who had been irradiated were found to have a mean height of 167.7 cm and those treated with chemotherapy alone, 179.1 cm. Similarly, girls who had been irradiated had a mean height of 154 cm and those treated with chemotherapy alone, 162.2 cm. The reasons for the disparity between these results and the earlier ones are unclear but may reflect the fact that many of the children at the time of the initial report had not yet undergone their pubertal growth spurt. Similar results were reported by Kirk (51). Seventy-seven children with acute lymphoblastic leukemia treated with chemotherapy and 2,400 cGy to the brain were evaluated 3 to 9 years following diagnosis. Sixty-five percent were growth hormone deficient. During treatment, growth was noted to slow and cross percentiles. Four years following diagnosis, heights had fallen by more than one standard deviation in 32% of patients. By 6 years following diagnosis, 71% had a fall in height of more than one standard deviation. Thus, children who have been irradiated for leukemia, if followed for sufficient time, may be found to have diminished adult stature.

It is becoming increasingly accepted that children with leukemia who receive cranial irradiation and chemotherapy have both a high incidence of growth hormone deficiency and abnormal adult stature. Abnormalities are more severe in those patients who receive higher total doses of radiation or those with higher doses per fraction. Abnormalities in growth have not yet been reported in patients treated with chemotherapy alone for CNS prophylaxis.

Whereas the dose of cranial irradiation for CNS prophylaxis in leukemia is 1,800 to 2,400 cGy, the dose of cranial irradiation for brain tumors may be 5,000 to 6,000 cGy. Thus, children with intracranial tumors, even those in whom the tumors are remote from the hypothalamic–pituitary axis, are at significant risk for endocrine dysfunction. The possible adverse effects of the brain tumor itself and the influence of increased intracranial pressure on endocrine function must be distinguished from effects of treatment. A limited number of prospective studies have been completed to date. Shalet et al. (100) prospectively studied children with brain tumors treated with surgery, radiation, and chemotherapy. All were normal before radiation. However, by 12 months after radiation, 6 of 14 children were growth hormone deficient, and by 24 months 7 of 14 were abnormal. The latency following radiation before damage becomes manifest has not yet been determined. In an attempt to answer this question, the same group evaluated growth hormone in children with brain tumors within 3 months after surgery (102). The majority of children had received approximately 2 weeks of radiotherapy. Although no growth hormone levels were distinctly abnormal, they were significantly lower than those of controls. By 1 to 2 years after treatment, 11 of 16 had abnormal growth hormone responses to insulin stimulation, and 10 of 11 were also abnormal with bovril. Thus, abnormalities in growth hormone release appear to become more severe over time.

We (34) prospectively evaluated 11 children with brain tumors whose tumors were remote from the hypothalamic pituitary axis. Provocative growth hormone testing was performed at baseline and at 3, 6, and 12 months following completion of radiation. All children had normal growth hormone values at diagnosis. By 3 months following radiation, 2 had evidence of growth hormone deficiency; by 6 months 9 of 11 were growth hormone deficient; and by 12 months 7 of 8 remaining children were growth hormone deficient. In our previous retrospective study (30), growth hormone deficiency was identified as late as 8 years following treatment. Thus, growth hormone deficiency occurs soon after cranial irradiation and the incidence appears to increase over time. In addition, more so than with leukemic children, children radiated for brain tumors typically develop growth failure (2). Approximately 80% of children radiated for brain tumors will have either decreased growth velocity or heights less than the tenth percentile (Table 23-2 and Fig. 23-1).

Patients are at risk for the development of growth hormone deficiency even if they receive radiation only to the posterior fossa. The radiation port to this region extends anteriorly to the posterior clinoids; thus although it excludes the pituitary gland, it includes within its confines the ventromedian nucleus of the posterior hypothalamus (the putative site of growth hormone releasing hormone) (Figs. 23-2 and 23-3). The etiology of growth hormone

TABLE 23-2. *Growth hormone deficiency in children with brain tumors*

Author	CRT	CT	Growth hormone deficiency		Decrease in growth velocity or height <10%	
Raimondi and Tomita (91)	+	—	Not tested		13/16	81%
Hirsch et al. (47)	+	+	19/29	66%	17/29	59%
Shalet et al. (100)	+	+	6/9	67%	5/9	56%
Broadbent et al. (15)	+	—	1/8	13%	3/8	38%
Danoff et al. (25)	+	—	6/6	100%	6/6	75%
Duffner et al. (30)	+	+	10/12	84%	10/10	100%
Pasqualini et al. (88)	+	+	9/13	69%	11/13	85%
Albertsson-Wikland et al. (2)	+	+	16/16	100%		56%
Shalet et al. (100)						
Pre RT	—	—	None			
Post RT	+	+	7/14	50%	12/13	92%
Bamford et al. (5)	+	—	Not tested			56%

CRT = Cranial radiation; CT = Chemotherapy.

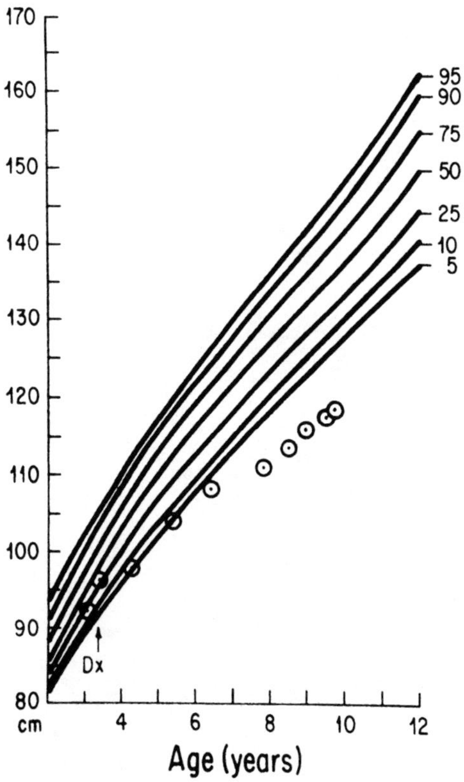

FIG. 23-1. Growth curve of a child radiated for medulloblastoma at age 2 years. Child was subsequently treated with growth hormone. Although growth improved, his adult height is only 151 cm.

deficiency may therefore lie with suppression of growth hormone releasing hormone in the hypothalamus rather than pituitary release of growth hormone. This postulate was supported by Lustig (67) when growth hormone deficient children previously radiated for brain tumors were given synthetic growth hormone releasing hormone. Following this treatment, growth hormone levels rose. This confirms the theory that the deficiency in part lies in the hypothalamic GHRH secreting neurons, owing to either failure of synthesis or delivery of GHRH to the pituitary. This point is important when treatment protocols are modified in an effort to reduce neurotoxicity because as long as the dose of radiation to the posterior fossa remains high, growth hormone deficiency on a hypothalamic basis can be anticipated.

Not all growth failure in children treated for brain tumors is caused by growth hormone deficiency. An important risk factor is spinal radiation (Fig. 23-4). Neuhauser (83) demonstrated that the effects of radiation on spinal growth were related to dose and age. The younger the child at the time of spinal irradiation, the more severe the adverse effects on vertebral body growth. Thus, the child who receives spinal radiation at 10 years may antici-

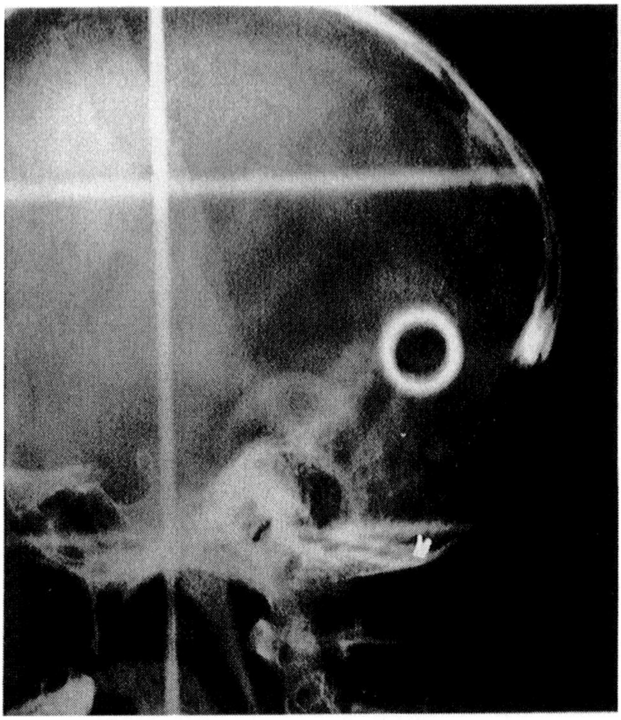

FIG. 23-2. Radiation port to the posterior fossa in a child with a medulloblastoma. Note that the anterior limit of the port is the posterior clinoid.

pate a 5.5-cm loss in adult height, whereas the child who is radiated at 1 year may anticipate a 9-cm loss (106). Brauner et al. (13) compared the heights of children treated with cranial versus craniospinal radiation. At the 2-year follow-up, children treated with craniospinal radiation had a significantly lower mean height than children treated with cranial radiation alone, even though the growth hormone response to arginine and insulin was the same in both groups. In this study, after the first 6-month period, poor spinal growth accounted for most of the subsequent growth retardation.

Another factor responsible for growth failure is precocious puberty. The actual incidence of precocious or early puberty in children treated for brain tumors is unknown, but the problem has been increasingly recognized (13). The impact of precocious puberty on eventual adult height is particularly important because growth ceases when there is fusion of the epiphyses. Thus, although there is an early growth spurt, most patients ultimately have short stature as adults.

The influence of chemotherapy on growth of children with brain tumors is as yet undetermined, although it is anticipated that growth may be abnormal

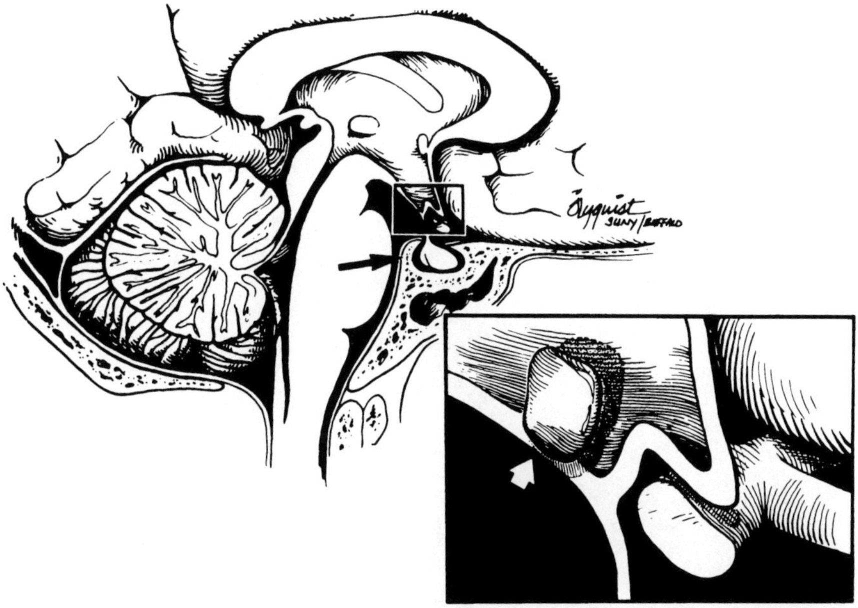

FIG. 23-3. Artist's rendition of the ventromedian nucleus in the hypothalamus *(white arrow)* and its relationship to the posterior clinoid *(black arrow)*. This nucleus is within the confines of the radiation port to the posterior fossa.

during chemotherapy due to poor nutrition. The actual impact of chemotherapy on adult stature is conjectural. In at least one study (104) children treated with chemotherapy in addition to craniospinal radiation were compared with those treated with craniospinal radiation alone. Those children who had received adjuvant chemotherapy had significantly lower standing heights than those not treated with chemotherapy.

Growth hormone deficiency can be treated with exogenous growth hormone. Unfortunately, most studies (21) have not shown results equivalent to those achieved in children with idiopathic growth hormone deficiency. At present dosages, exogenous growth hormone will improve leg growth but will not impact on spinal growth. Thus, those children whose vertebral bodies have been damaged by spinal radiation will tend to become increasingly disproportionate on growth hormone therapy. In addition, the advent of precocious puberty will limit the amount of time in which growth hormone can be effectively given before epiphyseal fusion occurs, resulting in an inadequate response. Another potential reason for the limited response to growth hormone treatment is that many endocrinologists wait at least 2 years following diagnosis before treatment is instituted, in order to be certain that there is no evidence of recurrent disease. Kanev (50) has suggested that growth

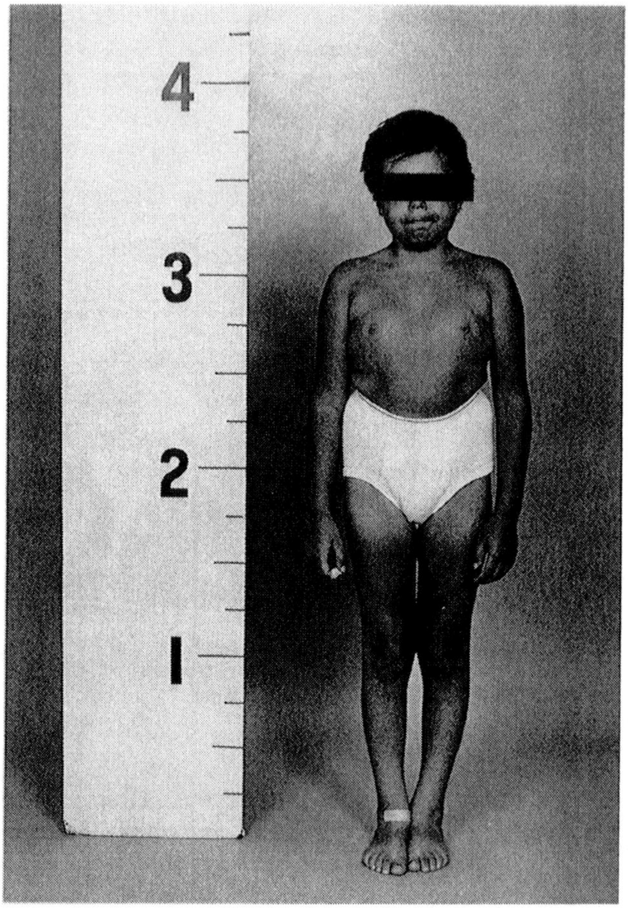

FIG. 23-4. Ten-year-old boy treated at age 2 years for a medulloblastoma with surgery, craniospinal radiation, and chemotherapy. Note skeletal disproportion with short trunk compared to length of arms and legs.

hormone should be given at the time of growth deceleration, regardless how long has elapsed since diagnosis, in order to maximize growth response.

Concerns about the use of exogenous growth hormone have primarily related to the theoretical consideration that growth hormone is oncogenic, capable of producing either early relapse or second malignancies. The literature offers surprisingly little about this very important problem. The Japanese (121) reported five children treated with synthetic growth hormone who developed acute lymphoblastic leukemia. However, among brain tumor patients, administration of growth hormone does not appear to be associated with early tumor recurrence. Most of the work in this area has come from

Shalet's group (19,105) in Manchester. They reported 14 children treated with exogenous growth hormone who developed tumor relapse and compared them with patients with the same types of tumor who relapsed but who were not treated with growth hormone. Growth hormone therapy did not significantly increase the relapse rate of children with medulloblastoma, glioma, or leukemia.

In summary, growth hormone deficiency is the most common endocrinopathy to develop following cranial irradiation. Although growth hormone replacement therapy will improve longitudinal growth, it has not been as effective as in children with idiopathic growth hormone deficiency. The advent of precocious puberty and the impact of radiation on the developing spine partly explain these poor results. At least one group (58) has suggested that when higher doses of growth hormone are administered, catch-up growth may occur. Earlier treatment with growth hormone and pharmacologically delaying puberty are other possible ways of improving the ultimate height of these children (113).

Thyroid dysfunction is the second most common endocrinopathy in children radiated for brain tumors. Hypothyroidism may be primary (due to radiation of the cervical spine) or secondary (due to damage of the hypothalamic–pituitary axis). Approximately 20% of children treated with craniospinal radiation may develop primary hypothyroidism. Recent data (63) have suggested that the addition of chemotherapy further increases the risk of hypothyroidism in patients treated with craniospinal radiation up to 69%. Compensated hypothyroidism is a risk factor for the development of thyroid tumors. Therefore, the child who has a normal T4 in the face of an elevated TSH should be placed on thyroxine even if the child is clinically euthyroid (63,64,84).

In addition to patients with primary hypothyroidism, those patients who have had radiation to the hypothalamic–pituitary axis as part of whole-brain radiation may develop secondary or tertiary hypothyroidism. Diagnosis of hypothyroidism is important because it may also adversely impact on both longitudinal growth and learning.

Gonadal dysfunction has only recently been reported in children with brain tumors. This likely reflects the fact that growth hormone deficiency and hypothyroidism usually occur within 2 or 3 years following treatment, whereas gonadal deficiency may not be manifest until the child reaches puberty or adulthood. Radiation to the spine has been associated with ovarian dysfunction. In one study (64), 35% of girls treated with spinal radiation developed ovarian dysfunction. Although the testes are relatively spared during spinal radiation, they are more susceptible to the toxic effects of chemotherapy. Cyclophosphamide, in particular, has an adverse effect on the testicular germinal epithelium. There is a high incidence of oligospermia or azoospermia in these patients, even though they may undergo normal pubertal maturation. Although the Leydig cells may also be affected by cyclophosphamide, androgen replacement has been only rarely necessary. In girls, the combination of chemotherapy and spinal radiation will exacerbate the likelihood of ovarian dysfunction; in one study 60% of girls were so affected. Both BCNU and CCNU have been associated with gonadal dysfunction (88). It is likely that as more chemotherapy is used and the patients are followed longer, a much higher incidence of gonadal dysfunction will be identified.

Thus, endocrinopathies are a common complication of treatment for children with brain tumors. The major risk factors appear to be young age at time of radiation, volume and dose of radiation, and adjuvant chemotherapy. Young children are most susceptible to the adverse affects of spinal radiation, resulting in short stature. It has not yet been determined whether they are also at greater risk for hypothalamic pituitary dysfunction.

The volume of radiation is an important risk factor for a variety of endocrine abnormalities. Children who receive spinal radiation have abnormal longitudinal growth and are also at risk for primary hypothyroidism. In addition, girls who receive spinal radiation are at risk for scatter to the ovaries, leading to gonadal dysfunction. Although restricting radiation to the posterior fossa will decrease the incidence of hypothyroidism, improve spinal growth, and reduce gonadal dysfunction in girls, growth hormone deficiency (on a hypothalamic basis) can still be anticipated.

The dose of radiation influences the time of onset of growth hormone deficiency. Clayton and Shalet (18) evaluated 82 children who were survivors of childhood malignant disease previously treated with 27 to 47.5 Gy to the hypothalamic–pituitary axis. Whereas growth hormone deficiency eventually developed throughout the dose range, the speed of onset was related to dose. Thus, children treated with doses greater than 30 Gy developed growth hormone deficiency earlier and experienced earlier growth deceleration.

Finally, the addition of chemotherapy to radiation is more likely than radiation alone to result in the development of hypothyroidism. One study (104) has also suggested that longitudinal height is more affected in those patients who have received a combination of chemotherapy and radiation rather than radiation alone. Certainly, chemotherapy is the major cause of gonadal dysfunction in boys treated for brain tumors, and adding chemotherapy to radiation may increase gonadal dysfunction in girls as well.

Thus, several risk factors need to be addressed. Future studies will attempt to reduce volume and dose of radiation, eliminate radiation entirely in very young children, and closely monitor the effects of chemotherapy on endocrine function. Endocrinopathies, which develop as a consequence of treatment, are potentially reversible. Administration of exogenous growth hormone will allow the child to improve longitudinal growth despite growth hormone deficiency, but only if the physician recognizes and treats the deficiency before the child reaches puberty and the epiphyses fuse. Unsuspected hypothyroidism may contribute to lethargy, poor linear growth, and learning difficulties. In a child with a brain tumor, these symptoms may often be attributed to either increased intracranial pressure or direct tumor effects. Evaluation of T4 and TSH function will allow early treatment of this problem. Low cortisol levels may be associated with potentially catastrophic complications, particularly if the child has to undergo a surgical procedure. The quality of life of these children will be greatly improved if appropriate hormonal replacement therapy is administered.

ONCOGENESIS

The oncogenic potential of radiation becomes of increasing significance as more patients survive their primary tumors. The likelihood that survivors of childhood cancer will develop a second malignancy is 10 times higher than that of age-matched controls (85). The reasons for the increased incidence are likely multifactorial and include, among others, environmental factors, genetic predisposition, susceptibility of the host, and previous central nervous system therapy. The Late Effects Study Group (75) identified 292 second malignancies since 1972 in 12 different pediatric oncology institutions from the United States, Canada, and Europe. Sixty-eight percent of these second malignancies developed in tissue previously exposed to radiation. Despite these caveats, there is clear-cut experimental evidence that radiation is oncogenic. Radiation therapy has been shown to cause brain tumors in animal studies. Both Haymaker (46) and Krupp (55) confirmed that radiation could produce brain tumors in a monkey population. The dose of radiation required to produce second malignancies is unknown; low, moderate, and high doses of radiation have all been associated with oncogenesis.

The clearest clinical evidence of the oncogenicity of radiation in humans has been in those patients who received low-dose radiation for benign conditions. Irradiation of the thymus for "status thymicolymphaticus" was common medical practice in the United States until the 1950s. In 1949, Scharnagel and Pack (99) reported a 5-year-old boy who had developed basal cell epitheliomas in the radiation port through which he had received thymic radiation soon after birth. This report was later followed by isolated reports of cancer of the thyroid developing in children previously irradiated for thymic hyperplasia (8). A statistically significant increase in thyroid carcinoma has since been found in children who had been radiated for thymic hyperplasia compared with their nonradiated siblings (39). Similarly, 1,644 patients who had received radiation of the head, neck, and chest in infancy were compared with 3,771 of their siblings. The incidence of cancer of the thyroid in radiated patients was 100 times the expected incidence (98).

Another benign condition treated with therapeutic radiation was tinea capitis. Radiation therapy was employed in the United States and Europe for tinea capitis until the discovery of griseofulvin in 1958 (9). In 1966, Albert et al. (1) reported a follow-up of 1,900 children who had been irradiated for tinea capitis compared with 1,801 children not treated with radiation. Nine cases of cancer developed in the radiated patients compared with only one case of cancer in the nonradiated patients. To date, the largest single follow-up study of patients treated for tinea capitis has come from Israel (77). Between 1949 and 1960, 17,000 children who immigrated to Israel were radiated for tinea capitis. The amount of radiation delivered to the brain was approximately 140 cGy. A significantly increased risk of malignant and benign neoplasms of the head and neck developed in the radiated group as compared to controls. The most striking increase was seen in tumors of the brain (especially meningiomas) as well as tumors of the parotid and thyroid. The long-term follow-up of the Israeli experience was reported by Ron et al. (96) in 1988. The 30-year relative risk for the development of tumors of the head and neck was 8.4. There was a direct relationship between dose and risk, with dosages of 250 cGy having a risk of 20 compared with a relative risk of 3.4 with doses less than 129 cGy. After 30 years, the most common of the second malignancies was meningiomas.

Moderate-dose radiation has also been associated with second malignancies. The bulk of the cases have been children treated for leukemia and lymphoma with 1,800 to 2,400 cGy CRT for CNS prophylaxis (Fig. 23-5). As of 1990, 26 cases of radiation-induced CNS tumors were reported (17) in children treated for acute lymphoblastic leukemia. Of these, 16 were glioblastomas, 8 astrocytomas, 1 primitive neuroectodermal tumor, and 1 ependymoma. The latency between radiation and second malignancy ranged from 4 to 11 years with an average of 7.5 years. The average total dose of radiation was 2,389 cGy. However, since most patients with leukemia are treated with both chemotherapy and radiation, a direct causal relationship cannot be confirmed (7,87).

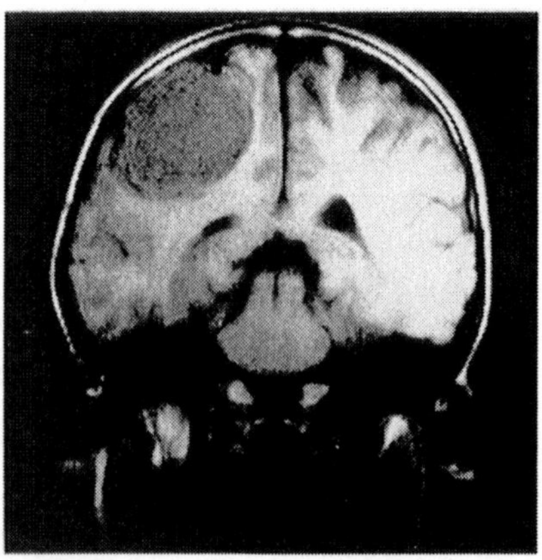

FIG. 23-5. Patient treated at age 2 years for ALL who presented with headaches at 16 years. Diagnosis of a meningioma was made, and tumor was removed successfully. Two years later the patient died of glioblastoma multiforme.

Of interest, whereas most of the brain tumors that developed following low-dose radiation for tinea capitis were meningiomas, most of the second malignancies in patients with acute lymphoblastic leukemia have been in the astrocytoma series. Radiation cannot be implicated in all cases. Malone (70) reported a child who developed an astrocytoma of the cervical cord outside the radiation port to the brain. Similarly, two patients previously reported by Regelson (93) and Tefft (117) were found at autopsy to have an astrocytoma of the cerebellum and of the pituitary gland. Neither patient had received cranial irradiation.

High-dose radiation for primary brain tumors has also been associated with increasing reports of second malignancies (Table 23-3). The definition of a second primary brain tumor is that the tumor must occur in the previous radiation port; it should develop after a sufficient latency period; the tumor must be of a different histology than the primary tumor; and the patient does not have one of the neurocutaneous syndromes such as neurofibromatosis or tuberous sclerosis (52). The duration from radiation to diagnosis of second tumor ranges from 2 to 47 years with a mean of 20 years. The most common secondary tumors are meningiomas and gliomas. Meningiomas tend to develop in those patients who had been irradiated in childhood. Radiation-

TABLE 23-3. *Second primary brain tumors in children*

Author	Age at diagnosis	Primary tumor	Radiation dose	Interval	Second tumor
Bogdanowicz and Sachs (11)	15 yr	Pit adenoma	6,114 cGy	16 yr	Meningioma
	3 yr	Medullo	6,000 cGy + 1,200 cGy	25 yr	Meningioma
Tanaka et al. (116)	17 yr	Oligo	6,600 cGy	23 yr	Meningioma
Bachman and Ostrow (4)	13 mo	Ependymoma	3,960 cGy	5 yr	Glioblastoma
Pearl et al. (90)	5 yr	Medullo	3,000 WB cGy 4,000 PF cGy	13 yr	Glioblastoma
Cohen et al. (22)	4 yr	Medullo	3,000 WB cGy 4,500 PF cGy	14 yr	Astrocytoma, frontal
Sogg et al. (110)	9 yr	Cranio	6,000 cGy	5 yr	Malig. Astro
Kleriga et al. (53)	10 mo	Medullo	5,000 cGy	11 yr	Malig. Astro
Maat-Schieman et al. (68)	5 yr	Cranio	6,000 cGy	14 yr	AA
Kitanaka (52)	13 yr	Germinoma	5,400 cGy	7 yr	AA
	7 yr	Cranio	6,000 cGy	16 yr	AA
Zampieri et al. (124)	11 yr	Sarcoma	5,600 cGy	7 yr	AA
Liwnicz et al. (65)	11 yr	Cranio	5,900 cGy	25 yr	Glioblastoma multiforme
	2 yr	Ependymoma	3,500 cGy	14 yr	Glioblastoma multiforme

Pit. adenoma, pituitary adenoma; medullo, medulloblastoma; oligo, oligodendroglioma; cranio, craniopharyngioma; AA, anaplastic astrocytoma.

ıeningiomas are often more aggressive than meningiomas arising (109). Those that have a more benign course tend to occur later se that are more aggressive, i.e., 20 years versus 6 years following on. The more aggressive tumors tend to arise in younger patients who been treated with lower doses of radiation than those who develop the ore benign variety.

Whereas astrocytomas were previously considered to be an unusual second primary, they have been increasingly reported over the past decade. Sixteen such cases were reported between 1984 and 1986, whereas previously only 40 were reported in the world literature (52). Cavin (17) identified 24 patients who developed intraaxial tumors following treatment for primary CNS neoplasia. Of the second tumors, 87% were glioblastomas. Radiation dosages have ranged from 4,000 to 6,000 cGy, and the latency from treatment to second tumor has varied from 1 to 26 years with a peak between 5 and 8 years. There is also a later peak between 21 and 28 years. As with meningiomas, the secondarily induced astrocytomas tend to be extremely aggressive. Their poor prognosis may relate as much to the biologic nature of the tumor as to the lack of aggressive treatment. Shapiro (107) has recommended that surgery, followed by modalities such as chemotherapy, brachytherapy, and repeat radiation, be considered in some of these patients. The risks of radiation necrosis, however, must be kept in mind if repeat radiation is to be delivered after a relatively short hiatus.

Extracranial second malignancies have also been reported in those children receiving radiation to the cervical spine. Thyroid neoplasia, in particular papillary carcinoma, has been reported in those individuals 10 to 20 years following radiation (3,39,92,95).

Another area of concern is the oncogenic potential of chemotherapy, which has been increasingly used in the treatment of patients with brain tumors. Although most cases of second malignancies have been confounded by coincident treatment with radiation, in a few reports (42), children and adults treated with chemotherapy alone for brain tumors later developed acute leukemia. At least two infants treated with MOPP therapy for primary brain tumors developed acute myelogenous leukemia (6). A third child, treated on the Pediatric Oncology Group study (33) with both chemotherapy (vincristine, Cytoxan, cis-platinum, VP16) and radiation subsequently died of acute myelogenous leukemia. This case is less clear than the MOPP cases because radiation was given subsequent to chemotherapy. Many of the new chemotherapy regimens for infants and older children employ drugs that are highly oncogenic. Thus, VP16, procarbazine, cyclophosphamide, and nitrogen mustard may further increase the incidence of second malignancies in this patient population (118,122).

Although radiation oncogenesis is a real phenomenon, many questions remain. The dose of radiation necessary to produce second malignancies is not well defined. It has been suggested (45) that low doses of radiation are more likely to be oncogenic than high doses. In one study (48), 6,000 women treated with low-dose radiation for benign gynecologic complaints were compared with women treated for malignant disease. Women who received low doses of radiation had a significantly higher incidence of leukemia than women treated for malignancies with high-dose radiation. In contrast, postirradiation sarcomas do not develop unless the dose of cranial irradiation is at least 3,000 cGy. Thus, the absolute dose of radiation required for the development of second malignancies is unknown. Similarly, the mechanism of radiation oncogenesis is not well defined. Cohen (22) has speculated that transformed cells present in areas of radiation necrosis, consisting of bizarre multinucleated glial cells within areas of intense astrogliosis, may represent the transition between necrosis and tumor. Clearly, the therapeutic efficacy of cranial irradiation for brain tumors outweighs its oncogenic potential. However, there is no indication for the use of radiation for cosmetic purposes or for benign lesions of the head or neck.

CONCLUSIONS

Since the first edition of this book, interest in the late effects of radiation and chemotherapy on children with brain tumors has increased remarkably. Whereas in the late 1970s and early 1980s it was sufficient to document these changes, it is now the focus of the cancer cooperative groups first to identify risk factors and then to alter treatment. As has been discussed in this chapter, one of the major risk factors for both radiation-induced dementia and growth failure is young age at the time of radiation. Thus, current cooperative group studies are treating infants and very young children who have brain tumors with prolonged postoperative (1 to 2 years) chemotherapy in an attempt either to delay radiation until the infant brain is better able to tolerate its effects or to eliminate cranial irradiation entirely. When the amount of radiation to the young child's nervous system is limited, less intellectual deterioration can be anticipated. Furthermore, delaying radiation to the spine until the child is older should lead to improved longitudinal growth.

Another risk factor being addressed in group studies is large volume of radiation. One treatment approach to reduce the volume of radiation is the elimination of neuraxis radiation in children with certain tumor types. For example, although children with posterior fossa ependymomas have been traditionally treated with craniospinal radiation, current studies are testing whether posterior fossa radiation alone will produce the same progression-free survivals achieved previously with neuraxis radiation. If spinal radiation is eliminated, one can anticipate better longitudinal growth, a decreased incidence of primary hypothyroidism, and a lower incidence of gonadal failure in females. Unfortunately, since the posterior fossa will still receive the full

5. Bamford FN, Morris-Jones P, Pearson D, Ribeiro GG, Shalet SM, Beardwell CG. Residual disabilities in children treated for intracranial space-occupying lesions. *Cancer* 1976;37: 1149–1151.
6. Baram TZ, Van Eys J, Pack B. Optimal surgery and MOPP chemotherapy in infants with primitive neuroectodermal tumors of the posterior fossa. *Ann Neurol* 1986;20:423.
7. Barasch ES, Altieri D, Decker RE, Ahmed S, Lin V. Primitive neuroectodermal tumor presenting as a delayed sequela to cranial irradiation and intrathecal methotrexate. *Pediatr Neurol* 1988;4:375–378.
8. Becker FO, Economou SG, Southwick HW, Eisenstein R. Adult thyroid cancer after head and neck irradiation in infancy and childhood. *Ann Intern Med* 1975;83:347–351.
9. Beller AJ, Feinsod M, Sahar A. The possible relationship between small dose irradiation to the scalp and intracranial meningiomas. *Neurochirurgia* 1972;4:125–143.
10. Blacklay A, Growwman A, Ross RJM, et al. Cranial irradiation for cerebral and nasopharyngeal tumors in children: evidence for the production of a hypothalamic defect in growth hormone release. *J Endocrinol* 1986;108:25–29.
11. Bogdanowicz WM, Sachs E. The possible role of radiation in oncogenesis of meningioma. *Surg Neurol* 1974;2:379–383.
12. Brauner R, Czernichow P, Rappaport P. Precocious puberty after hypothalamic and pituitary irradiation in young children. *N Engl J Med* 1984;311:920.
13. Brauner R, Rappaport R, Prevot C, et al. A prospective study of the development of growth hormone deficiency in children given cranial irradiation, and its relation to statural growth. *J Clin Endocrinol Metab* 1989;68:346–351.
14. Brecher ML, Voorhees MM, Ritchey AK, Harris MB, Forman E. Adult heights achieved by long-term survivors of childhood acute lymphocytic leukemia (ALL) prophylaxis. Proc Soc Pediatr Res 1992; 812:138 (abst).
15. Broadbent VA, Barnes ND, Wheeler TK. Medulloblastoma in childhood: long-term results of treatment. *Cancer* 1981;1:3–29.
16. Cantini R, Giorgetti W, Valleriani AM, Burchianti M, Amodeo C. Radiation-induced cerebral lesions in childhood. *Childs Nerv Syst* 1989;5:135–139.
17. Cavin LW, Dalrymple GV, McGuire EL, Maners AW, Broadwater JR. CNS tumor induction by radiotherapy: a report of four new cases and estimate of dose required. *Radiat Oncol Biol Phys* 1989;18:399–406.
18. Clayton PE, Shalet SM. Dose dependency of time of onset of radiation-induced growth hormone deficiency. *J Pediatr* 1991;118:226–228.
19. Clayton PE, Shalet SM, Gattamaneni HR, Price DA. Does growth hormone cause relapse of brain tumors? *Lancet* 1987;1:711–713.
20. Clayton PE, Shalet SM, Price DA. Gonadal function after chemotherapy and irradiation for childhood malignancies. *Horm Res* 1988;30:104–110.
21. Clayton PE, Shalet SM, Price DA. Growth response to growth hormone therapy following cranial irradiation. *Eur J Pediatr* 1988;147:593–596.
22. Cohen MS, Kushner MJ, Dell S. Frontal lobe astrocytoma following radiotherapy for medulloblastoma. *Neurology* 1981;31:616–619.
23. Copeland DR, Fletcher JM, Pfefferbaum-Levine B, Jaffe N, Ried H, Maor M. Neuropsychological sequelae of childhood cancer in long-term survivors. *Pediatrics* 1985:75: 745–753.
24. Dacou-Voutetakis C, Xypolyta A, Haidas A, Constantinidis M, Papavasiliou C, Zannos-Mariolea L. Irradiation of the head: immediate effect on growth hormone secretion in children. *J Clin Endocrinol Metab* 1977;44:791–794.
25. Danoff BF, Cowchock FS, Marquette C, Mulgrew L, Kramer S. Assessment of the long-term effects of primary radiation therapy for brain tumors in children. *Cancer* 1982;49: 1580–1586.
26. Dickinson WP, Berry DH, Dickinson L, et al. Differential effects of cranial radiation on growth hormone response in arginine and insulin infusion. *J Pediatr* 1978;92:754–757.
27. DiLorenzo N, Nolletti A, Palma L. Late cerebral radionecrosis. *Surg Neurol* 1978;10: 281–290.
28. Dooms GC, Hecht S, Brant-Zawadski M, Berthiaume Y, Norman D, Newton TH. Brain radiation lesions: MR imaging. *Radiology* 1986;158:149–155.
29. Duffner PK, Cohen ME. Long-term consequences of CNS treatment for childhood cancer. II: Clinical consequences. *Pediatr Neurol* 1991;7:237–242.

30. Duffner PK, Cohen ME, Anderson SW, et al. Long-term effects of treatment on endocrine function in children with brain tumors. *Ann Neurol* 1983;14:528–532.
31. Duffner PK, Cohen ME, Parker MS. Prospective intellectual testing in children with brain tumors. *Ann Neurol* 1988;23:575–579.
32. Duffner PK, Cohen ME, Thomas PRM. Late effects of treatment on the intelligence of children with posterior fossa tumors. *Cancer* 1983;51:233–237.
33. Duffner PK, Horowitz M, Kirscher J, et al. Postoperative chemotherapy and delayed RT in infants with brain tumors: a Pediatric Oncology Group study. *Ann Neurol* 1991;30:484.
34. Duffner PK, Voorhees MD, MacGillivray MH, et al. Long-term effects of cranial irradiation on endocrine function in children with brain tumors: a prospective study. *Cancer* 1985;56:2189.
35. Eiser C. Intellectual abilities among survivors of childhood leukemia as a function of CNS irradiation. *Arch Dis Child* 1978;53:391–395.
36. Eiser C, Lansdown R. Retrospective study of intellectual development in children treated for acute lymphoblastic leukemia. *Arch Dis Child* 1977;52:525–529.
37. Ellenberg L, McComb JG, Siegel SE, Stowe S. Factors affecting intellectual outcome in pediatric brain tumor patients. *Neurosurgery* 1987;21:638–644.
38. Farwell J, Flannery JT. Second primaries in children with central nervous system tumors. *J Neurooncol* 1984;2:371–375.
39. Favus MH, Schneider AB, Stachura ME, et al. Thyroid cancer occurring as a late consequence of head-and-neck irradiation. *N Engl J Med* 1976;294:1019–1025.
40. Fisher JN, Aur RJA. Endocrine assessment in children with lymphocytic leukemia. *Cancer* 1982;49:145–151.
41. Freeman JE, Johnston PGB, Voke JM. Somnolence after prophylactic cranial irradiation in children with acute lymphoblastic leukemia. *Br Med J* 1973;4:523–525.
42. Genot JY, Krulik M, Poisson M, et al. Two cases of leukemia following treatment of malignant glioma. *Cancer* 1983;52:222–226.
43. Glauser TA, Packer RJ. Cognitive deficits in long-term survivors of childhood brain tumors. *Childs Nerv Syst* 1991:7:2–12.
44. Goff JR, Anderson HR, Cooper PF. Distractibility and memory deficits in long-term survivors of acute lymphoblastic leukemia. *Dev Behav Pediatr* 1980;1:158–163.
45. Haselow RE, Nesbit M, Dehner LP, Khan FM, McHugh R, Levitt SH. Second neoplasms following megavoltage radiation in a pediatric population. *Cancer* 1978;42:1185–1191.
46. Haymaker W, Rubinstein LJ, Miguel J. Brain tumors in irradiated monkeys. *Acta Neuropathol* 1972;20:267–277.
47. Hirsch JF, Reiner D, Czernichow P, Beneveniste L, Pierre-Kahn A. Medulloblastoma in childhood: survival and functional results. *Acta Neurochir* 1978;48:1–15.
48. Hutchinson GB. Leukemia in patients with cancer of the cervix treated with radiation. *J Natl Cancer Inst* 1968;40:951–982.
49. Jannoun L, Bloom HJG. Long-term psychological effects in children treated for intracranial tumors. *Int J Radiat Oncol Biol Phys* 1989;18:747–753.
50. Kanev PM, Lefebvre JF, Mauseth RS, Berger MS. Growth hormone deficiency following radiation therapy of primary brain tumors in children. *J Neurosurg* 1991;74:743–748.
51. Kirk JA, Raghupathy P, Stevens MM. Growth failure and growth hormone deficiency after treatment for acute lymphoblastic leukemia. *Lancet* 1987;1:190–193.
52. Kitanaka C, Shitara N, Nakagomi T, Nakamura H. Postradiation astrocytoma. *J Neurosurg* 1989;70:469–474.
53. Kleriga E, Sher JG, Nallainathan SK, Stein SC, Sacher M. Development of cerebellar malignant astrocytoma at site of a medulloblastoma treated 11 years earlier. *J Neurosurg* 1978;49:445–449.
54. Kramer S, Lee KF. Complications of radiation therapy: the central nervous system. *Semin Roentgenol* 1974;9:75–83.
55. Krupp JH. Nine-year mortality experience in proton-exposed Macaca Mulatta. *Radiat Res* 1976;67:244–251.
56. Kun LE, Mulhern RK, Crisco JJ. Quality of life in children treated for brain tumors. *J Neurosurg* 1983;58:1–6.
57. Lampert PW, Davis RL. Delayed effects of radiation on the human central nervous system: "early" and "late" delayed reactions. *Neurology* 1964:14:912–917.

58. Lannering B, Albertsson-Wikland K. Improved growth response to GH treatment in irradiated children. *Acta Pediatr Scand* 1989;78:562–567.
59. Lansdown R, Eiser C. Retrospective study of intellectual development in children treated for acute lymphoblastic leukemia. *Arch Dis Child* 1977;52:525–529.
60. Larkins RG, Martin FIR. Hypopituitarism after extracranial irradiation: evidence for hypothalamic origin. *Br Med J* 1973;1:152–153.
61. Lindgren M. Tolerance of brain tissue and sensitivity of brain tumors to irradiation. *Acta Radiol* 1958;170:1–73.
62. Littman R, Rosenstock J, Gale G, et al. The somnolence syndrome in leukemic children following reduced daily dose fractions of cranial radiation. *Int J Radiat Oncol Biol Phys* 1984;10:1851–1853.
63. Livesey EA, Brook CGD. Thyroid dysfunction after radiotherapy and chemotherapy of brain tumors. *Arch Dis Child* 1989;64:593–595.
64. Livesey EA, Hindmarsh PC, Brook CGD, et al. Endocrine disorders following treatment of childhood brain tumors. *Br J Cancer* 1990;61:622–625.
65. Liwnicz BH, Berger TS, Liwnicz RG, et al. Radiation associated gliomas: a report of four cases and analysis of postradiation tumors of the central nervous system. *Neurosurgery* 1985;17:436–445.
66. Longeway J, Mulhern R, Crisco J, et al. Treatment of meningeal relapse in childhood acute lymphoblastic leukemia. II: A prospective study of intellectual loss specific to CNS relapse and therapy. *Am J Pediatr Hematol Oncol* 1990;12:45–50.
67. Lustig RH, Schriock EA, Kaplan SL, Grumbach MM. Effect of growth hormone-releasing factor on growth hormone release in children with radiation-induced growth hormone deficiency. *Pediatrics* 1985;76:274–280.
68. Maat-Schieman MLC, Bots GTAM, Thomeer RTWM. Malignant astrocytoma following radiotherapy for craniopharyngioma. *Br J Radiol* 1985;58:480–482.
69. McIntosh S, Klatskin EH, O'Brien RT. Chronic neurologic disturbance in childhood leukemia. *Cancer* 1976;37:853–857.
70. Malone M, Lumley H, Erdohazi M. Astrocytoma as a second malignancy in patients with acute lymphoblastic leukemia. *Cancer* 1986;57:1979–1985.
71. Mandell LR, Walker RW, Steinherz P, Fuks Z. Reduced incidence of the somnolence syndrome in leukemic children with steroid coverage during prophylactic cranial radiation therapy. *Cancer* 1989;63:1975–1978.
72. Marks JE, Baglan RJ, Prassad SC, Blank WF. Cerebral radionecrosis: incidence and risk in relation to dose, time, fractionation and volume. *Int J Radiat Oncol Biol Phys* 1981:7: 243–252.
73. Martins AN, Johnston JS, Henry JM, Stoffel TJ, DiChiro G. Delayed radiation necrosis of the brain. *J Neurosurg* 1977;47:336–345.
74. Meadows AT, Gordon J, Massari DJ, Littman P, Fergusson J, Moss K. Declines in IQ scores and cognitive dysfunctions in children with acute lymphocytic leukaemia treated with cranial irradiation. *Lancet* 1981;2:1015–1018.
75. Meadows ST, Baum E, Fossati-Bellani F, et al. Second malignant neoplasms in children: an update from the late effects study group. *J Clin Oncol* 1985;3:532–538.
76. Meadows AT, Evans AE. Effects of chemotherapy on the central nervous system: a study of parenteral MTX in long-term survivors of leukemia and lymphoma in childhood. *Cancer* 1976;37:1079–1085.
77. Modan G, Mart H, Baidatz D, Steinitz R, Levin SG. Radiation-induced head and neck tumors. *Lancet* 1974;23:277–279.
78. Moss HA, Nannis ED, Poplack DG. The effects of prophylactic treatment of the central nervous system on the intellectual functioning of children with acute lymphocytic leukemia. *Am J Med* 1981;71:47–52.
79. Mulhern RK, Crisco JJ, Kun LE. Neuropsychological sequelae of childhood brain tumors: a review. *J Clin Child Psychol* 1983;12:66–73.
80. Mulhern RK, Ochs J, Fairclough D, Wasserman AL, Davis KS, Williams JM. Intellectual and academic achievement status after CNS relapse: a retrospective analysis of 40 children treated for acute lymphoblastic leukemia. *J Clin Oncol* 1987;5:933–940.
81. Mulhern RK, Horowitz ME, Kovnar EH, Langston J, Sanford RA, Kun LE. Neurodevelopmental status of infants and young children treated for brain tumors with preirradiation chemotherapy. *J Clin Oncol* 1989;7:1660–1666.

82. Nelson DR, Yuh WTC, Wen BC, Ryals RJ, Cornell SH. Cerebral necrosis simulating an intraparenchymal tumor. *AJNR* 1990;11:211–212.
83. Neuhauser EBD, Wittenborg MH, Berman CZ, Cohen J. Irradiation effects of roentgen therapy on the growing spine. *Radiology* 1952;59:637–650.
84. Oberfield SE, Allen JC, Pollack J, New MI, Levine LS. Long-term endocrine sequelae after treatment of medulloblastoma: prospective study of growth and thyroid function. *J Pediatr* 1986;108:219–223.
85. Olsen JH. Risk of second cancer after cancer in childhood. *Cancer* 1986;57:2250–2254.
86. Packer RJ, Sutton LN, Atkins TE, et al. A prospective study of cognitive function in children receiving whole-brain radiotherapy and chemotherapy: 2-year results. *J Neurosurg* 1989;70:707–713.
87. Palma L, Vagnozzi R, Annino L, Ciaperta P, Maleci A, Cantore G. Post-radiation glioma in a child. *Childs Nerv Syst* 1988;4:296–301.
88. Pasqualini T, Diez B, Domene H, et al. Long-term endocrine sequelae after surgery, radiotherapy, and chemotherapy in children with medulloblastoma. *Cancer* 1987;59: 801–806.
89. Patronas NJ, DiChiro, Brooks RA, et al. Work in progress: (^{18}F) fluorodeoxyglucose and positron emission tomography in the evaluation of radiation necrosis of the brain. *Radiology* 1982;144:885–889.
90. Pearl GS, Mirra SS, Miles ML. Glioblastoma multiforme occurring 13 years after treatment of a medulloblastoma. *Neurosurgery* 1980;6:546–551.
91. Raimondi AJ, Tomita T. Advantages of "total" resection of medulloblastoma and disadvantages of full head post-operative radiation therapy. *Childs Brain* 1979;5:550–551.
92. Raventos A, Duszynski DO. Thyroid cancer following irradiation for medulloblastoma. *AJR* 1963;89:175–181.
93. Regelson W, Bross IDJ, Hananian J, Nigogosyan G. Incidence of second primary tumors in children with cancer and leukemia. *Cancer* 1965;18:58–72.
94. Riva D, Pantaleoni C, Milani N, Belani FF. Impairment of neuropsychological functions in children with medulloblastomas and astrocytomas in the posterior fossa. *Childs Nerv Syst* 1989;5:107–110.
95. Roggli VL, Estrada R, Fechner RE. Thyroid neoplasia following irradiation for medulloblastoma. *Cancer* 1979;43:2232–2238.
96. Ron E, Modan B, Boice JD, et al. Tumors of the brain and nervous system after radiotherapy in childhood. *NEJM* 1988;319:1033–1039.
97. Rowland JH, Glidewell OJ, Sibley RF, Holland JC. Effects of different forms of central nervous system prophylaxis on neuropsychologic function in childhood leukemia. *J Clin Oncol* 1984;2:1327–1335.
98. Saenger EL, Silverman FN, Sterling TD, Turner ME. Neoplasia following therapeutic irradiation for benign conditions in childhood. *Radiology* 1960;74:889–903.
99. Scharnagel IM, Pack GT. Multiple basal cell epitheliomas in a 5 year old child. *Am J Dis Child* 1949:77:647–651.
100. Shalet SM, Beardwell CG, Aarons BM, Pearson D, Morris-Jones PH. Growth impairment in children treated for brain tumors. *Arch Dis Child* 1978;42:491–494.
101. Shalet SM, Beardwell CG, MacFarlane IA, Morris-Jones PH, Pearson D. Endocrine morbidity in adults treated with cerebral irradiation for brain tumors during childhood. *Acta Endocrinol* 1977;84:673–680.
102. Shalet SM, Beardwell CG, Morris-Jones PH, Pearson D. Pituitary function after treatment of intracranial tumors in children. *Lancet* 1975:July 19:104–107.
103. Shalet SM, Beardwell CG, Pearson D, Morris-Jones PH. The effect of varying doses of cerebral irradiation on growth hormone production in childhood. *Clin Endocrinol* 1976;5: 287–290.
104. Shalet SM, Clayton PE, Price DA. Growth and pituitary function in children treated for brain tumors or acute lymphoblastic leukemia. *Horm Res* 1988;30:53–61.
105. Shalet SM, Clayton PE, Price DA. Growth impairment following treatment for childhood brain tumors. *Acta Pediatr Scan* 1988;343:137–145.
106. Shalet SM, Gibson B, Swindell R, Pearson D. Effect of spinal irradiation on growth. *Arch Dis Child* 1987;62:461–464.
107. Shapiro S, Mealey J Jr, Sartorius C. Radiation-induced intracranial malignant gliomas. *J Neurosurg* 1989;71:77–82.

108. Sheline GE. Radiation therapy of primary tumors. *Semin Oncol* 1975;2:29–42.
109. Soffer D, Gomori M, Siegal T, Shalit MN. Intracranial meningiomas after high-dose irradiation. *Cancer* 1989;63:1514–1519.
110. Sogg RL, Donaldson SS, Yorke CH. Malignant astrocytoma following radiotherapy of a craniopharyngioma. *J Neurosurg* 1978;48:622–627.
111. Soni SS, Marten GW, Pitner SE, Duenas DA, Powazek M. Effects of central nervous system irradiation on neuropsychologic functioning of children with acute lymphocytic leukemia. *N Engl J Med* 1975;293:113–118.
112. Spunberg JJ, Chang CH, Goldman M, Auricchio E, Bell JJ. Quality of long-term survival following irradiation for intracranial tumors in children under the age of two. *Int J Radiat Oncol Biol Phys* 1981;7:727–736.
113. Sulmont V, Brauner R, Fontoura M, Rappaport R. Response to growth hormone treatment and final height after cranial or craniospinal irradiation. *Acta Pediatr Scand* 1990;79: 542–549.
114. Sunderman CR, Pearson H. Growth effects of long-term antileukemic therapy. *J Pediatr* 1969;75:1058–1062.
115. Swift PGF, Kearney PJ, Dalton RG, Bullimore JA, Mott MG, Savage DCL. Growth and hormonal status of children treated for acute lymphoblastic leukemia. *Arch Dis Child* 1978; 53:890–894.
116. Tanaka J, Garcia JH, Netsky MG, Williams JP. Late appearance of meningioma at the site of partially removed oligodendroglioma: case report. *J Neurosurg* 1975;43:80–85.
117. Tefft M, Vawter GF, Mitus H. Second primary neoplasms in children. *AJR* 1968;103: 800–822.
118. Valagussa P, Santoro A, Fossati-Bellani F, Banfi A, Bonnadonna G. Second acute leukemia and other malignancies following treatment for Hodgkin's disease. *J Clin Oncol* 1986; 4:830–837.
119. Verzosa MS, Aur RJA, Simone JC, Hustu HG, Pinkel DP. Five years after central nervous system irradiation of children with leukemia. *Int J Radiat Oncol Biol Phys* 1976;1:209–215.
120. Voorhees ML, Brecher ML, Glicksman AS, et al. Hypothalamic-pituitary function of children with acute lymphoblastic leukemia after three forms of central nervous system prophylaxis. *Cancer* 1986;57:1287–1291.
121. Watanabe S, Tsunematsu Y, Fujimoto J, et al. Leukaemia in patients treated with growth hormone. *Lancet* 1988;1:159.
122. Whitlock JA, Greer JP, Lukens JN. Epidodophyllotoxin-related leukemia: identification of a new subset of secondary leukemia. *Cancer* 1991;68:600–604.
123. Wowra B, Schmitt HP, Sturm V. Incidence of late radiation necrosis with transient mass effect after interstitial low dose rate radiotherapy for cerebral gliomas. *Acta Neurochir* 1989;99:104–108.
124. Zampieri P, Zorat PL, Mingrino S, Soattin GB. Radiation-associated cerebral gliomas. *J Neurosurg Sci* 1989;33:271–279.

Subject Index